The Eponymous Atlas

Medical Innovations Through History

ORTHOPAEDICS

CUSTOMED

SERIES EDITORS

DR. RAVINDER SINGH CHANNEY
Ph.D., D.Sc. (Med. Journalism)

RIPUDAMAN SINGH CHANNEY
B. Pharm., M.B.A. (Pharma Marketing)

The Eponymous Atlas

Medical Innovations Through History

ORTHOPAEDICS

First Edition 2025.

For the use only of a Registered Medical Practionar or a Hospital, or a Laboratory.

Printed and Published by

CUSTOMED

D-71, Hauz Khas, New Delhi-110 016, India.

customedgroup.com

info@ customedgroup.com

ISBN: 9798284894422

DISCLAIMER

The authors, publisher, and printer of "The Eponymous Atlas: Medical Innovations Through History | ORTHOPAEDICS" have made every effort to ensure that the information presented in this book is accurate, up-to-date, and in line with current medical and legal standards at the time of publication. However, the field of pain management and medico-legal issues is constantly evolving, and new developments may occur that are not reflected in this book.

This book is intended for educational and informational purposes only. It is not a substitute for professional medical advice, diagnosis, or treatment. The techniques and approaches discussed in this book should only be performed by licensed healthcare professionals in accordance with local, regional, and national laws, guidelines, and best practices. It is the responsibility of each reader to ensure compliance with all applicable legal, ethical, and professional standards within their jurisdiction before applying any of the techniques described herein.

Neither the authors, publisher, nor printer can be held liable for any direct, indirect, incidental, or consequential damages, including but not limited to injury, malpractice claims, legal actions, or any other legal disputes arising from the use or misuse of the information contained in this book. Readers are strongly advised to consult with appropriate legal and medical professionals for personalized guidance related to their specific circumstances.

By using this book, readers acknowledge and agree that the authors, publisher, and printer assume no responsibility or liability for any outcomes associated with the use of the material presented.

This disclaimer is applicable internationally and covers all legal jurisdictions.

Dedication

To the visionary minds...
whose names became the language of orthopaedics,

To the surgeons, anatomists, and clinicians...
who saw beyond the fracture and into function,

To the mentors...
who taught not just techniques but the principles behind them,

To the students and residents...
who study every eponym not as a name, but as a key to understanding,

To the patients...
whose resilience brings meaning to every cast, correction, and reconstruction,

We dedicate The Eponymous Atlas: Orthopaedics.

May it stand as a tribute to the legacy of orthopaedic excellence
and a guide for all who seek to walk in its path.

Dr. Ravinder Singh Channey

Ripudaman Singh Channey

Preface

Orthopaedics, as both a science and a craft, has evolved through centuries of observation, innovation, and clinical refinement. Much of this progress is etched into the language we use daily—names that represent not just conditions or techniques, but legacies. The Eponymous Atlas: Orthopaedics is a comprehensive and structured compilation of these legacies, drawn from across disciplines and generations, offering a unique fusion of anatomical precision and historical depth.

Each entry in this atlas - from Abbott's Method to Zanca View - stands as a testament to the contributions of the pioneers whose names continue to define our understanding of fractures, deformities, surgical techniques, diagnostic views, and syndromes. These eponyms, far from being mere references, carry with them the clinical wisdom, diagnostic acumen, and procedural breakthroughs that have shaped orthopaedic education and practice.

This volume is not merely an alphabetical catalogue, but a contextual journey through the foundational pillars of musculoskeletal medicine. For each eponym, we have aimed to provide more than just definition - we offer historical insight, clinical relevance, diagnostic clarity, and, where appropriate, the continued role of these terms in modern-day orthopaedics.

From Bankart's Operation to Monteggia Fracture, Codman's Sign to Volkmann's Contracture, these names continue to echo through operating theatres, academic discussions, and exam halls. They are essential tools for orthopaedic surgeons, students, and healthcare professionals who seek not only to understand the condition but the heritage behind its naming.

The Eponymous Atlas: Orthopaedics is designed to be a reference, a teaching aid, and a historical lens through which readers can explore the depth and evolution of orthopaedic knowledge. Whether you are a medical student, orthopaedic trainee, educator, or seasoned practitioner, we hope this atlas will serve as a valuable companion - bridging clinical practice with the rich narrative of those who came before.

With admiration for the past and commitment to the future,

Dr. Ravinder Singh Channey

Ripudaman Singh Channey

Series Editors

Contents

Abbott's Method

Overview

Abbott's method is a historical technique for the gradual correction of scoliosis, primarily through the use of plaster jackets combined with lateral pulling and counterpulling forces. This method aimed to achieve spinal alignment and stabilization by applying continuous mechanical pressure to the spine, followed by immobilization in a corrected position.

Historical Background

- *Edville Gerhardt Abbott* (1871–1945), an orthopedic surgeon, developed this method in the early 20th century to address scoliosis, a condition characterized by abnormal lateral curvature of the spine.
- At a time when surgical options were limited and often risky, Abbott's method provided a non-invasive alternative for scoliosis management.
- The technique gained prominence during the first half of the 20th century, laying the groundwork for modern scoliosis treatment approaches.

Purpose

- **Primary Goal:** To correct the lateral curvature of the spine in scoliosis patients and prevent progression of deformity.
- **Secondary Objectives:** To improve posture and symmetry.
- To reduce associated pain and discomfort caused by spinal misalignment.

Procedure Overview

- **Initial Evaluation:** Assessment of the degree of spinal curvature through physical examination and imaging techniques, such as X-rays.
- **Application of Forces:** Wide bandages and pads are used to exert lateral pulling and counterpulling forces on the spinal column. These forces aim to over-correct the curvature.
- **Plaster Jacket:** Once the desired degree of spinal correction is achieved, a plaster jacket is applied.
- **The jacket provides:** Pressure to maintain spinal alignment.
- Counterpressure to prevent regression.
- Fixation to immobilize the spine in the corrected position.
- **Gradual Adjustments:** The process may involve periodic adjustments and replacement of jackets to accommodate changes in spinal alignment.

Results and Interpretation

- **Positive Outcomes:** Significant reduction in spinal curvature in patients with mild to moderate scoliosis.
- Improved posture and reduced risk of progression in younger patients during growth phases.
- **Limitations:**
- Variable success in severe or rigid scoliosis cases.
- Reliance on patient compliance for prolonged immobilization.

Physiological Basis

- **Mechanical Correction:** The lateral pulling forces create biomechanical pressure to realign vertebrae, counteracting the abnormal curvature.
- **Bone Remodeling:** Prolonged pressure on the spine facilitates gradual reshaping of the vertebrae and adjacent structures, particularly in younger patients with more flexible spines.
- **Stabilization:** Immobilization with plaster jackets helps maintain corrected alignment, promoting long-term adaptation of musculoskeletal structures.

Clinical Applications

- **Scoliosis Treatment:** Particularly effective in cases of adolescent idiopathic scoliosis where the spine retains some flexibility.
- **Spinal Deformities:** Used in conditions involving lateral curvature and associated asymmetries.
- **Prevention of Progression:** Aimed at halting further curvature progression in growing individuals.

Limitations and Technical Considerations

- **Patient Discomfort:** The use of plaster jackets can cause physical discomfort, skin irritation, and limitations in mobility.
- **Non-Applicability in Severe Cases:** Patients with rigid, severe, or neuromuscular scoliosis may not benefit significantly from this approach.
- **Time-Intensive:** Gradual correction requires multiple stages and patient compliance over an extended period.
- **Replacement by Modern Techniques:** With the advent of advanced bracing systems and surgical methods, Abbott's method has largely been replaced.

Modern Relevance

- While *Abbott's method* is no longer commonly used, it holds historical importance as a foundational approach in non-surgical scoliosis management.
- Its principles of *gradual mechanical correction* and immobilization inform modern techniques such as custom spinal braces (e.g., Boston Brace).

Associated Conditions

- **Adolescent Idiopathic Scoliosis:** Primary condition targeted by Abbott's method.
- **Congenital and Neuromuscular Scoliosis:** Limited applicability in these cases due to rigidity and associated comorbidities.
- **Kyphoscoliosis:** Occasionally adapted for cases involving combined lateral and posterior spinal deformities.

Clinical Importance

- **Historical Significance:** Introduced a systematic and non-invasive means of correcting spinal deformities in an era when surgical options were limited.
- **Advancement of Scoliosis Treatment:** Served as a stepping stone for modern bracing techniques and surgical interventions.
- **Pediatric Orthopedics:** Provided a non-surgical option for managing

scoliosis in growing children, reducing the risk of severe deformities in adulthood.

Bibliography

E. G. ABBOTT SCOLIOSIS: First Paper. The Physiological Postures of the Spine and Their Relations to Scoliosis." The Journal of Bone and Joint Surgery Am. 1917;s2-15:26-50.

Adams-Oliver Syndrome

Overview

Adams-Oliver syndrome (AOS) is a rare congenital condition characterized by defects of the scalp and skull (aplasia cutis congenita) and limb anomalies, often presenting as terminal transverse defects. This genetic disorder may also involve vascular abnormalities, with a significant portion of cases exhibiting autosomal dominant inheritance. AOS has considerable variability in its presentation, making early diagnosis and intervention essential.

Historical Background

- *Forrest H. Adams* and *C. P. Oliver* first described the syndrome in 1945, highlighting its distinct combination of congenital scalp defects and limb anomalies.
- Early reports of the condition focused on its genetic implications, establishing autosomal dominant inheritance patterns with variable expressivity and incomplete penetrance.
- Over time, additional associated features, such as vascular malformations and congenital heart defects, were identified, expanding the clinical spectrum of AOS.

Purpose

- **Clinical Recognition:** To identify characteristic features early, including scalp and limb abnormalities, to facilitate timely interventions.
- **Genetic Counseling:** To provide families with an understanding of the

autosomal dominant inheritance pattern and associated risks.

- **Multisystem Evaluation:** To detect and manage extracutaneous manifestations, such as cardiac or vascular anomalies.

Procedure Overview

- **Diagnosis:** Primarily clinical, based on characteristic findings of aplasia cutis congenita and limb anomalies.
- Imaging and genetic testing confirm the diagnosis and rule out other syndromes with overlapping features.
- **Management:** Wound care for scalp defects to prevent infection and promote healing.
- Orthopedic interventions for limb anomalies, including prosthetics or surgical reconstruction.
- Monitoring and treatment for associated vascular or cardiac complications.
- **Genetic Testing:** Identification of mutations in genes such as ARHGAP31, DOCK6, or EOGT, which are linked to AOS, providing confirmatory evidence and aiding family planning.

Results and Interpretation

- **Positive Findings:** Scalp and skull defects are readily identifiable at birth, often accompanied by limb malformations.
- Genetic testing confirms the presence of causative mutations in autosomal dominant cases.
- **Prognosis:** Dependent on severity; isolated scalp and limb defects have a good prognosis, while vascular or cardiac anomalies may result in more complex outcomes.

Physiological Basis

- **Developmental Disruption:** AOS results from disturbances in mesodermal development, affecting skin, bones, and vascular structures.
- **Skin and Skull Defects:** Aplasia cutis congenita arises due to incomplete formation of the epidermis and underlying tissues.
- **Limb Anomalies:** Terminal transverse limb defects stem from impaired vascular supply or mesenchymal growth during embryogenesis.

Clinical Applications

- **Early Identification:** Prenatal imaging may reveal limb defects or scalp anomalies, enabling early planning for delivery and postnatal care.
- **Surgical and Orthopedic Care:** Scalp reconstruction and limb prosthetics improve functional and cosmetic outcomes.
- **Vascular Management:** Monitoring for vascular complications, including arteriovenous malformations, is essential in comprehensive care.

Limitations and Technical Considerations

- **Variability in Presentation:** High variability can delay diagnosis, particularly in cases without classic findings.
- **Genetic Testing Access:** Limited availability in resource-constrained settings may hinder confirmation of the

diagnosis.

- **Complex Multisystem Involvement:** Requires a multidisciplinary approach, complicating management in patients with severe vascular or cardiac anomalies.

Modern Relevance

- **Advances in** *genetic testing* have improved diagnostic accuracy and expanded understanding of the molecular basis of AOS.
- *Prenatal screening techniques*, including high-resolution ultrasounds and fetal MRI, enable earlier recognition and intervention planning.
- Increased awareness of the syndrome among healthcare providers ensures more timely and effective management of affected individuals.

Associated Conditions

- **Aplasia Cutis Congenita:** The hallmark feature of AOS, involving congenital absence of skin and potentially underlying bone.
- **Limb Anomalies:** Including brachydactyly, syndactyly, or more severe terminal transverse defects.
- **Vascular Malformations:** Arteriovenous malformations and persistent pulmonary hypertension are reported in some cases.
- **Congenital Heart Defects:** Structural anomalies such as septal defects may occur in association.

Clinical Importance

- **Holistic Management:** Requires coordinated care involving dermatologists, orthopedists, cardiologists, and geneticists to address the wide-ranging manifestations.
- **Genetic Counseling:** Critical for families with autosomal dominant inheritance, helping guide family planning and early interventions in future pregnancies.
- **Improved Quality of Life:** Early recognition and intervention minimize complications, enabling affected individuals to lead functional lives.

References

F. H. Adams, C. P. Oliver: Hereditary deformities in man due to arrested development. Journal of Heredity, Washington, 1945, 36: 3-8.

Browning JC. Aplasia cutis congenita: approach to evaluation and management. Dermatol Ther. 2013;26:439–44.

Achilles' heel (Soft spot)

Overview

The term Achilles' heel is a metaphorical and anatomical reference derived from Greek mythology, symbolizing a person's or structure's point of greatest vulnerability. In medical terminology, the Achilles tendon and its associated conditions, such as achillobursitis (inflammation of the bursa near the tendon) and achillodynia (pain in the Achilles tendon), are named after the legendary Greek hero Achilles. His tale highlights both strength and vulnerability, with his heel representing a singular weakness despite overall might.

Historical Background

- The legend of *Achilles*, one of the greatest heroes of the Trojan War (12th century BC), originates in *Greek mythology* and is most famously recounted in Homer's *Iliad*.
- According to myth, Achilles' mother, Thetis, dipped him in the *river Styx* to make him invincible. However, the heel by which she held him remained untouched by the water, leaving it vulnerable.
- The concept of an "Achilles' heel" evolved as a metaphor for a critical weakness in an otherwise powerful entity.
- In medical terminology, anatomical structures and conditions related to the Achilles tendon draw from this myth, underscoring its cultural and scientific significance.

Purpose

- **Symbolism:** To signify a point of vulnerability, either metaphorical or literal, in otherwise robust systems or individuals.
- **Medical Significance:** To name and describe specific anatomical and pathological conditions associated with the Achilles tendon, the strongest yet prone-to-injury tendon in the human body.

Procedure Overview

(Medical Context)

- **Achillobursitis:** Inflammation of the bursa near the Achilles tendon is managed with rest, anti-inflammatory medications, and physical therapy.
- **Achillodynia:** Chronic pain in the Achilles tendon often requires a combination of therapies, such as stretching, strengthening exercises, and, in severe cases, surgical intervention.
- **Achillorraphy and Achillotomy:** Surgical procedures performed to repair or address injuries to the Achilles tendon.

Results and Interpretation

- **Medical Outcomes:** Properly managed Achilles tendon conditions result in restored mobility and pain reduction.
- Untreated or poorly managed issues can lead to chronic pain, reduced function, or tendon rupture.
- **Cultural Impact:** The metaphorical use of "Achilles' heel" has transcended mythology, becoming a universal term for vulnerability, extending its relevance beyond anatomy.

Physiological Basis

- **The Achilles tendon is the largest and strongest tendon in the body, connecting the calf muscles to the heel bone (calcaneus) and facilitating activities such as walking, running, and jumping.**
- **Despite its strength, its position and repetitive use make it susceptible to:** Overuse injuries, such as tendinitis.
- Ruptures, particularly during sudden or intense physical activity.
- The *bursa* near the tendon can become inflamed due to friction or overuse, leading to conditions like achillobursitis.

Clinical Applications

- **Orthopedic Treatment:** Management of Achilles tendon injuries through physical therapy, orthotics, and surgical interventions when necessary.
- **Sports Medicine:** Prevention and rehabilitation strategies for athletes prone to Achilles tendon injuries.
- **Podiatry:** Addressing biomechanical issues contributing to tendon stress and associated pain.

Limitations and Technical Considerations

- **Medical Context:** Treatments such as surgery or injections can have risks, including infection, incomplete recovery, or complications like scar tissue formation.
- **Mythological Context:** The tale of Achilles is allegorical, and its scientific relevance lies in its symbolic representation of strength and vulnerability.
- **Cultural MisInterpretation:** The metaphor may sometimes oversimplify complex vulnerabilities in medical or structural contexts.

Modern Relevance

- **Anatomical Significance:** The Achilles tendon remains a critical focus in orthopedic and sports medicine due to its functional importance and high injury susceptibility.
- **Metaphorical Use:** "Achilles' heel" continues to symbolize weakness in various fields, from literature to strategic planning.
- **Eponymous Medical Terms:** Conditions like achillobursitis, achillodynia, and surgical procedures such as achillorraphy are frequently encountered in medical practice.

Associated Conditions

- **Achillobursitis:** Inflammation of the bursa near the Achilles tendon.
- **Achillodynia:** Chronic pain in the Achilles tendon, often due to overuse or degenerative changes.
- **Tendon Rupture:** A complete tear of the tendon, typically requiring surgical intervention.
- **Tendinitis:** Inflammation of the Achilles tendon, usually due to overuse or biomechanical strain.

Clinical Importance

- **Functional Mobility:** The Achilles tendon plays a critical role in lower limb mobility; its injury can significantly impair movement and quality of life.

- **Cultural and Educational Significance:** The enduring story of Achilles and its associated terminology highlight the intersection of mythology, language, and medical science.

- **Vulnerability in Strength:** The metaphorical and anatomical "Achilles' heel" underscores the need to address weaknesses proactively, both in physical health and broader contexts.

References

Avery HC. 1998. Achilles' Third Father. Hermes 126(4):389-397.

Achilles' tendon

Overview

The Achilles tendon, the strongest and most well-known tendon in the human body, connects the calf muscles (gastrocnemius and soleus) to the heel bone (calcaneus). It is located at the posterior border of the Kager triangle. This tendon was historically named after the Greek hero Achilles, whose mythological vulnerability was his heel. First termed the "cord of Achilles" by Philip Verheyen in 1693, it has also been referred to as the "calcaneal tendon" in modern anatomical terminology. However, recent trends in medical nomenclature have reintroduced the eponym "Achilles tendon."

Historical Background

- The *Achilles tendon* has been recognized since antiquity, with early references describing its significance in movement and vulnerability.

- The Flemish anatomist *Philip Verheyen* was the first to name the tendon after Achilles in his anatomical text *Corporis Humani Anatomia* in 1693.

- Before Verheyen's eponym, it was known as the "tendo magnus" or "great tendon," a term attributed to *Hippocrates*.

- The tendon's association with Achilles reflects the mythical hero's heel as a symbol of strength coupled with vulnerability, a theme that has persisted across both mythological and scientific contexts.

Purpose

- **Functional Significance:** The Achilles tendon is essential for transmitting the force of the calf muscles to the foot, enabling activities such as walking, running, and jumping.
- **Symbolic Importance:** The tendon's name underscores its duality as both a powerhouse of strength and a site prone to injury, echoing the mythology of Achilles.

Procedure Overview

(Medical Context)

- **Assessment of Tendon Function:** Clinical evaluation of the Achilles tendon involves tests for flexibility, strength, and signs of injury (e.g., swelling, tenderness).
- **Intervention:** Injuries like tendonitis or ruptures may require conservative management (rest, physiotherapy, orthotics) or surgical repair in severe cases.
- **Rehabilitation:** Post-treatment care focuses on gradual strengthening and restoration of mobility to prevent re-injury.

Results and Interpretation

- **Anatomical Features:** The tendon is robust yet prone to overuse injuries due to its high load-bearing role in lower-limb movement.
- **Clinical Observations:** Injuries, such as Achilles tendinitis and tendon ruptures, are common, particularly among athletes and older individuals engaging in sudden physical activities.
- **Prognosis:** With proper treatment and rehabilitation, most patients recover fully; however, chronic issues like tendinosis may lead to lasting discomfort or reduced function.

Physiological Basis

- **Structure and Function:** Composed of collagen fibers, the Achilles tendon is designed to withstand significant tension, facilitating propulsion during gait and high-impact activities.
- **Biomechanical Role:** The tendon acts as a critical lever for the foot, amplifying the force generated by the calf muscles to lift the body off the ground.
- **Vulnerability:** Despite its strength, the tendon's limited vascular supply makes it susceptible to overuse injuries, degeneration, and ruptures.

Clinical Applications

- **Orthopedic Treatment:** Managing conditions like Achilles tendinitis, tendinosis, and ruptures through physical therapy, orthotics, or surgery.
- **Sports Medicine:** Developing prevention strategies for athletes, focusing on stretching, strengthening, and appropriate footwear.
- **Rehabilitation:** Post-injury or post-surgery protocols to restore full functionality and prevent recurrence.

Limitations and Technical Considerations

- **Prone to Injury:** The Achilles tendon is frequently affected by repetitive stress, poor biomechanics, and sudden increases in physical activity.
- **Challenges in Recovery:** Injuries, particularly ruptures, often require

long rehabilitation periods, and older individuals may experience slower recovery due to reduced tendon elasticity.

- **Terminological Debate:** The transition between eponyms and descriptive anatomical terms has caused some confusion, though "Achilles tendon" remains widely used.

Modern Relevance

- **Advances in** *biomechanical research* and *imaging techniques* have improved understanding of Achilles tendon function and injury mechanisms.
- *Sports medicine and orthopedics* continue to emphasize the importance of the tendon in both professional athletes and active individuals.
- The re-adoption of the term "Achilles tendon" reflects a broader trend toward preserving historical eponyms in medical terminology.

Associated Conditions

- **Achilles Tendinitis:** Inflammation of the tendon due to overuse or repetitive strain.
- **Tendinosis:** Chronic degeneration of tendon fibers, often caused by untreated or recurring tendinitis.
- **Tendon Rupture:** A complete tear of the tendon, usually resulting from acute trauma or excessive stress.
- **Bursitis:** Inflammation of the bursa near the tendon, often accompanying other conditions.

Clinical Importance

- **Functional Mobility:** The Achilles tendon is critical for basic and advanced motor functions, from walking to sprinting.
- **Injury Prevention and Recovery:** Understanding the tendon's biomechanics and vulnerabilities allows for better prevention and treatment of injuries.
- **Cultural and Scientific Legacy:** The enduring name "Achilles tendon" highlights the intersection of mythology and medicine, emphasizing the importance of historical and cultural context in anatomical nomenclature.

References

Kirkup J. Mythology and history. In: Helal B, Wilson D, eds. The Foot. New York: Churchill Livingstone, 1988: 1–8.

Albert's disease

Overview

Albert's disease, also known as Achilles tendon bursitis, Achilles tendinitis, or retrocalcaneal bursitis, is a painful condition characterized by inflammation of the bursae located between the os calcis (heel bone) and the Achilles tendon. This condition results in pain, swelling, and difficulty in walking, particularly during activities involving ankle movement. Named after Eduard Albert, who first described it in 1893, the disease is now synonymous with retrocalcaneal bursitis and is commonly managed using both conservative and endoscopic treatments.

Historical Background

- In *1893*, *Eduard Albert*, an Austrian surgeon, published an article on *achillodynia*, a term he coined to describe pain localized to the Achilles tendon. His work detailed a patient with intense pain and swelling at the tendon insertion.
- The disease was later expanded upon by *Alfred Schanz*, contributing to its alternative eponym, *Schanz's syndrome*.
- Historically, Albert's disease was managed using conservative measures, but advancements in imaging and surgical techniques have revolutionized its treatment.

Purpose

- **Symptom Relief:** To alleviate pain and inflammation at the Achilles tendon and surrounding structures.
- **Restoration of Mobility:** To improve walking and standing ability by addressing the underlying inflammatory process.
- **Prevention:** To avoid chronic complications, such as tendon degeneration or rupture, through timely intervention.

Procedure Overview

- **Diagnosis:**
- Clinical examination identifies tenderness, swelling, and pain localized at the heel.
- Imaging, such as ultrasound or MRI, confirms inflammation of the retrocalcaneal bursa and evaluates the condition of the Achilles tendon.
- **Conservative Management:**
- Rest, ice application, and anti-inflammatory medications.
- Physical therapy, including stretching and strengthening exercises.
- Orthotics, such as heel lifts, to reduce tension on the Achilles tendon.
- **Surgical Intervention:** In refractory cases, endoscopic bursectomy or debridement of the inflamed bursa is performed to relieve symptoms and restore function.

Results and Interpretation

- **Conservative Treatment:** Many patients experience significant relief with non-invasive measures, including pain reduction and improved mobility.
- **Surgical Outcomes:** Endoscopic techniques have a high success rate, with minimal scarring and a quicker return to

activity compared to open surgery.

- **Prognosis:** With appropriate treatment, most patients recover fully; however, recurrence is possible if contributing factors (e.g., improper footwear, overuse) are not addressed.

Physiological Basis

- The *retrocalcaneal bursa* serves as a cushion between the Achilles tendon and the calcaneus, reducing friction during movement.
- Inflammation of this bursa, caused by overuse, repetitive stress, or biomechanical abnormalities, results in pain and swelling.
- Prolonged inflammation can lead to changes in the tendon, such as *tendinosis*, or complications like a tendon rupture.

Clinical Applications

- **Orthopedics and Sports Medicine:** Management of Albert's disease in athletes and active individuals to restore performance and prevent long-term disability.
- **Rehabilitation:** Designing individualized therapy plans to address biomechanical issues and prevent recurrence.
- **Surgical Techniques:** Advancements in endoscopic surgery have improved outcomes for patients with chronic or severe cases.

Limitations and Technical Considerations

- **Conservative Treatment:** While effective for most, it may not resolve symptoms in severe or chronic cases.
- **Surgical Risks:** Although minimally invasive, endoscopic procedures carry risks such as infection, nerve damage, or incomplete symptom resolution.
- **Rehabilitation Challenges:** Non-compliance with physical therapy and improper post-treatment care can lead to recurrence or delayed recovery.

Modern Relevance

- The condition remains common, particularly in individuals engaging in repetitive or high-impact activities.
- *Imaging advancements* such as high-resolution ultrasound and MRI enable more accurate diagnosis and tailored treatment plans.
- *Minimally invasive surgical techniques* have made refractory cases of Albert's disease more manageable, improving patient satisfaction and recovery times.

Associated Conditions

- **Achillodynia:** A broader term encompassing pain in the Achilles region, often overlapping with Albert's disease.
- **Achilles Tendinitis:** Inflammation of the Achilles tendon itself, frequently co-occurring with bursitis.
- **Haglund's Deformity:** A bony prominence on the calcaneus that predisposes individuals to retrocalcaneal bursitis.
- **Plantar Fasciitis:** Occasionally associated due to overlapping mechanical stresses in the foot.

Clinical Importance

- **Functional Recovery:** Early diagnosis and treatment of Albert's disease are essential for maintaining mobility and quality of life.
- **Preventing Chronic Complications:** Untreated retrocalcaneal bursitis can lead to tendon degeneration, rupture, or persistent pain, impacting daily activities.
- **Interdisciplinary Care:** Collaboration among orthopedic surgeons, physical therapists, and sports medicine specialists ensures comprehensive care for patients with Albert's disease.

Bibliography

E. Albert: Achillodynie. Wiener medizinische Presse, 1893, 34: 41-43.

Leitze Z, Sella EJ, Aversa JM. Endoscopic decompression of the retrocalcaneal space. J Bone Joint Surg Am 2003; 85–A: 1488–96.

Mosby C. Mosby medical encyclopedia. Middlesex: Signet, 1996.

Albers-Schönberg's disease

Overview

Albers-Schönberg's disease, also known as osteopetrosis or marble bone disease, is a rare genetic condition characterized by abnormal bone density due to defective osteoclast-mediated bone resorption. This results in excessively calcified, brittle bones that are prone to fractures. The disease presents in two primary forms: an autosomal dominant form, which is usually benign, and an autosomal recessive form, which can be severe and often fatal in infancy. Associated complications include anemia, hepatomegaly, and various cranial nerve disorders.

Historical Background

- The disease was first described by *Heinrich Ernst Albers-Schönberg* in 1904, following radiographic observations of unusually dense bones.
- Subsequent work by *Herbert Assmann* and others expanded understanding of the clinical spectrum, linking it to fractures, hematological abnormalities, and other systemic effects.
- *Philip Showalter Hench*, a Nobel laureate, further contributed to understanding the disease's genetic underpinnings and metabolic implications, cementing its place in medical literature.

Purpose

- **Diagnosis:** To identify and distinguish between the benign and severe forms of osteopetrosis through clinical, radiological, and genetic evaluation.

- **Management:** To address complications such as fractures, anemia, and cranial nerve dysfunction, while improving the patient's quality of life.
- **Genetic Counseling:** To inform affected families about inheritance patterns and risks for future offspring.

Procedure Overview

Diagnosis:

- Radiographs reveal dense, "marble-like" bones with increased skeletal radiodensity.
- Genetic testing confirms mutations in genes such as CLCN7 and TCIRG1, associated with autosomal dominant and recessive forms, respectively.
- **Management of Symptoms:**
- Treatment focuses on mitigating fractures, anemia, and nerve compression syndromes.
- Bisphosphonates, interferon gamma-1b, and bone marrow transplantation are used in severe cases to improve bone remodeling.
- **Supportive Care:** Includes management of secondary complications, such as poor dentition, hearing loss, or recurrent infections (e.g., osteomyelitis).

Results and Interpretation

- **Benign (Autosomal Dominant) Form:** Often asymptomatic or associated with mild fractures, incidental findings on imaging, and minimal systemic complications.
- **Severe (Autosomal Recessive) Form:** Presents early in infancy with severe anemia, hepatosplenomegaly, cranial nerve dysfunction, and a high risk of fatal complications.
- **Prognosis:** Autosomal dominant cases have a good prognosis with supportive care, while the recessive form often requires aggressive treatment, such as hematopoietic stem cell transplantation, for survival.

Physiological Basis

- **Bone Remodeling Defect:** Osteopetrosis results from defective osteoclast activity, leading to inadequate bone resorption and excessive calcification.
- **Hematological and Neurological Impact:** Bone marrow space reduction causes anemia and immune deficiency.
- Cranial nerve compression leads to visual, auditory, and facial dysfunction due to narrowed foramina.
- **Electrolyte Imbalance:** Reduced bone turnover disrupts calcium-phosphorus metabolism, resulting in hypocalcemia and elevated serum phosphorus levels.

Clinical Applications

- **Orthopedic Management:** Surgical intervention for fractures and deformities, as well as careful monitoring of bone health.
- **Hematological Treatment:** Blood transfusions and erythropoiesis-stimulating agents for anemia.
- **Neurological Interventions:** Addressing cranial nerve compression through decompression surgeries, where possible.

- **Transplantation:** Hematopoietic stem cell transplantation offers a potential cure for the autosomal recessive form by introducing functional osteoclast precursors.

Limitations and Technical Considerations

- **Diagnostic Challenges:** Differentiating between autosomal dominant and recessive forms requires genetic confirmation and detailed clinical evaluation.
- **Treatment Risks:** Bone marrow transplantation is risky, with potential for graft-versus-host disease and high mortality rates.
- **Recurrent Complications:** Chronic issues, such as fractures, infections, and cranial nerve dysfunction, require ongoing management and multidisciplinary care.

Modern Relevance

- **Advances in** *genetic testing* have improved the diagnosis and classification of Albers-Schönberg's disease.
- Modern therapies, including *hematopoietic stem cell transplantation*, bisphosphonates, and interferon gamma-1b, have expanded treatment options for severe cases.
- The condition underscores the importance of *osteoclast function* in bone health and provides insights into other skeletal disorders.

Associated Conditions

- **Anemia and Hepatosplenomegaly:** Result from bone marrow compression and compensatory extramedullary hematopoiesis.
- **Cranial Nerve Disorders:** Compression of nerves causes visual impairment, hearing loss, and facial paralysis.
- **Osteomyelitis:** Frequent infections of the mandible and maxilla due to poor blood supply and dental complications.
- **Hypocalcemia:** Often associated with the metabolic derangements of impaired bone resorption.

Clinical Importance

- **Differentiating Benign and Severe Forms:** Early diagnosis allows for tailored treatment strategies, improving outcomes and reducing morbidity.
- **Insights into Bone Biology:** The study of Albers-Schönberg's disease has advanced understanding of bone remodeling and the role of osteoclasts.
- **Multidisciplinary Approach:** Effective management requires collaboration among orthopedists, hematologists, geneticists, and neurologists to address the disease's multisystemic effects.

References

H. E. Albers-Schönberg: Projektions-Röntgenbilder einer seltenen Erkrankung. Fortschritte auf dem Gebiete der Röntgenstrahlen, Hamburg, 1903-1904, 7: 158-

Röntgenbilder einer seltenen Knochenerkrankung. Münchener medizinische Wochenschrift, 1904, 51: 365.

Albright-Hadorn Syndrome

Overview

Albright-Hadorn syndrome is a rare clinical condition characterized by episodes of paroxysmal hypokalemic muscular paralysis associated with osteomalacia, often secondary to renal tubular acidosis (RTA). This syndrome highlights the interplay between metabolic abnormalities in renal function, bone metabolism, and neuromuscular health.

Historical Background

- *Fuller Albright*, an American endocrinologist, and *Walter Hadorn*, a Swiss physician, were key figures in elucidating the relationship between renal tubular acidosis, bone demineralization, and muscle dysfunction.
- Their work laid the foundation for understanding how systemic electrolyte disturbances can affect skeletal integrity and neuromuscular function, leading to the identification of this syndrome.
- The eponym honors their contributions to recognizing the clinical interplay of hypokalemia, osteomalacia, and renal dysfunction.

Purpose

- **Diagnosis and Management:** To identify and treat the underlying causes of hypokalemia, osteomalacia, and muscular paralysis in the context of renal tubular acidosis.
- **Preventing Long-Term Complications:** To address metabolic and skeletal abnormalities early, minimizing the risk of chronic bone fragility and recurrent muscle weakness.

Procedure Overview

Diagnosis:

- Clinical suspicion arises from episodes of muscle weakness or paralysis, bone pain, and laboratory findings of hypokalemia.
- Blood tests often reveal low serum potassium, metabolic acidosis, and signs of vitamin D deficiency or bone demineralization.
- Imaging studies, including X-rays or bone scans, confirm osteomalacia.
- Testing for renal tubular function identifies renal tubular acidosis (RTA) as the underlying cause.
- **Management:**
- **Potassium Replacement:** Immediate correction of hypokalemia with oral or intravenous potassium.
- **Alkalization Therapy:** Administration of bicarbonate or citrate to correct acidosis.
- **Vitamin D and Calcium Supplementation:** To improve bone mineralization and treat osteomalacia.
- **Addressing Underlying RTA:** Treating primary or secondary renal tubular acidosis to prevent recurrence.

Results and Interpretation

- **Symptom Relief:** Effective potassium replacement alleviates muscular paralysis and weakness during acute episodes.
- **Bone Health Improvement:** Long-

term supplementation with calcium and vitamin D improves bone density and reduces symptoms of osteomalacia.

- **Prognosis:** With proper management, patients experience significant improvement in symptoms; however, recurrent hypokalemia and acidosis may occur if underlying RTA remains uncontrolled.

Physiological Basis

- **Hypokalemic Paralysis:** Low serum potassium impairs nerve conduction and muscle contractility, leading to episodic paralysis or profound muscle weakness.
- **Osteomalacia:** Chronic acidosis and renal tubular dysfunction disrupt calcium-phosphate metabolism, impairing bone mineralization.
- **Renal Tubular Dysfunction:** Renal tubular acidosis results in systemic metabolic acidosis, further aggravating hypokalemia and osteomalacia.

Clinical Applications

- **Endocrinology and Nephrology:** Management of Albright-Hadorn syndrome involves addressing renal tubular acidosis and its systemic complications.
- **Bone Health Monitoring:** Regular assessment of bone density and mineralization to prevent fractures and deformities.
- **Acute and Chronic Care:** Emergency treatment for hypokalemic paralysis and long-term metabolic correction for osteomalacia.

Limitations and Technical Considerations

- **Diagnostic Challenges:** The syndrome's symptoms are nonspecific, requiring a high index of suspicion and comprehensive metabolic workup.
- **Recurrent Hypokalemia:** Frequent episodes of muscle weakness may persist if renal tubular dysfunction is not adequately managed.
- **Complications of Therapy:** Overcorrection of potassium or bicarbonate can lead to other metabolic disturbances, requiring careful monitoring.

Modern Relevance

- **Advances in** *renal function testing* and *imaging techniques* have improved the diagnosis and management of Albright-Hadorn syndrome.
- The recognition of this syndrome highlights the need for a *multidisciplinary approach*, involving nephrology, endocrinology, and orthopedics.
- Modern treatment options, including tailored supplementation and acid-base correction, have significantly reduced morbidity associated with this condition.

Associated Conditions

- **Renal Tubular Acidosis (RTA):** A primary feature of the syndrome, leading to systemic acidosis and electrolyte imbalances.
- **Osteomalacia:** Chronic bone demineralization due to disrupted calcium-phosphate homeostasis.
- **Hypokalemic Paralysis:** Episodic muscle weakness or paralysis due to

severe potassium deficiency.

Clinical Importance

- **Timely Diagnosis:** Early identification and treatment prevent long-term complications like skeletal deformities and chronic muscle weakness.
- **Interdisciplinary Management:** Successful outcomes require coordination between specialists to address the syndrome's systemic manifestations.
- **Understanding Metabolic Interplay:** The syndrome underscores the intricate connections between renal function, electrolyte balance, and skeletal health.

References

F. Albright, et al: Osteomalacia and late rickets. The various etiologies met in the United States with emphasis on that resulting from a specific form of renal acidosis, the therapeutic indications of each etiological sub-group, and the relationship between osteomalacia and Milkman's syndrome. Medicine, Baltimore, 1946, 25: 399-479.

W. Hadorn: Osteomalacie mit paroxysmaler hypokalämischer Muskellähmung; ein neues Syndrom. Schweizerische medizinische Wochenschrift, Basel, 1948, 78: 1328-1241.

Allison's Syndrome

Overview

Allison's syndrome refers to bone demineralization that occurs following extended periods of immobilization. The condition can range from being asymptomatic to causing generalized weakness and articular pain during motion, depending on the severity of the demineralization and the duration of immobilization. This syndrome highlights the relationship between mechanical loading of bones and bone density, emphasizing the critical role of physical activity in maintaining skeletal health.

Historical Background

- Named after *Nathaniel Allison*, an early 20th-century physician who described the phenomenon of bone weakening and demineralization resulting from prolonged immobilization.
- Allison's work demonstrated the physiological impact of reduced mechanical stress on bone structure, contributing to the understanding of conditions like disuse osteoporosis.
- The syndrome's recognition prompted significant advancements in rehabilitative practices and preventive measures for immobility-related bone loss.

Purpose

- **Diagnosis:** To identify early signs of bone demineralization in patients subjected to prolonged immobilization, reducing the risk of fractures and long-term skeletal weakness.

- **Management:** To restore bone density and prevent complications such as fractures and joint pain through appropriate therapeutic interventions.
- **Prevention:** To develop strategies that mitigate the effects of immobilization on bone health in at-risk populations.

Procedure Overview

Diagnosis:

- **Clinical Evaluation:** Assessment of symptoms such as generalized weakness, joint pain, or limited mobility.
- **Imaging Studies:** X-rays or dual-energy X-ray absorptiometry (DXA) scans to measure bone density and confirm demineralization.
- **Blood Tests:** Monitoring markers of bone turnover, such as calcium, phosphorus, and alkaline phosphatase levels.

Treatment:

- **Physical Rehabilitation:** Gradual reintroduction of weight-bearing exercises to stimulate bone remodeling.
- **Nutritional Support:** Adequate calcium and vitamin D intake to promote bone health.
- **Pharmacological Intervention:** Bisphosphonates or other bone-strengthening medications may be used in severe cases.
- **Monitoring:** Periodic assessment of bone density and functional mobility to evaluate the effectiveness of interventions.

Results and Interpretation

- **Positive Outcomes:** Early intervention often leads to gradual restoration of bone density and reduction in symptoms.
- **Variable Severity:** Asymptomatic cases resolve with simple activity resumption, while severe cases may require intensive rehabilitation and pharmacological treatment.
- **Prognosis:** Recovery depends on the duration of immobilization, the extent of demineralization, and the timeliness of treatment.

Physiological Basis

- **Bone Remodeling and Mechanical Stress:** Bones require regular mechanical loading to maintain density and strength. Immobilization disrupts this balance, leading to increased bone resorption and decreased bone formation.
- **Calcium and Collagen Loss:** Prolonged inactivity reduces calcium deposition in bones and collagen matrix maintenance, leading to structural weakening.
- **Articular Pain:** Joint pain results from increased mechanical strain on weakened bone structures during motion.

Clinical Applications

- **Orthopedics and Rehabilitation:** Addressing bone health in patients recovering from fractures, surgeries, or prolonged bed rest.
- **Geriatric Medicine:** Managing immobilization-related bone loss in

elderly patients with limited mobility.

- **Sports Medicine:** Preventing and managing bone density loss in athletes recovering from injuries requiring prolonged rest.

Limitations and Technical Considerations

- **Diagnostic Challenges:** Mild cases may go undetected without routine bone density screening.
- **Delayed Recovery:** Severe demineralization can take months to years to fully recover, requiring patient adherence to long-term therapy.
- **Risk of Recurrence:** Without sustained mobility and proper bone health maintenance, patients remain at risk for recurrent episodes of demineralization.

Modern Relevance

- **Advances in** *bone imaging* techniques, such as DXA and quantitative computed tomography, have improved the early detection of bone loss in immobilized patients.
- *Preventive strategies*, such as early physical therapy and nutritional optimization, have reduced the incidence of severe cases of Allison's syndrome.
- The condition underscores the importance of *multidisciplinary care*, integrating orthopedics, nutrition, and physical therapy for effective management.

Associated Conditions

- **Disuse Osteoporosis:** A broader term for bone loss due to inactivity or reduced mechanical loading.
- **Post-Surgical Bone Loss:** Occurs after orthopedic surgeries requiring prolonged immobilization.
- **Chronic Pain Syndromes:** Joint pain and weakness related to persistent skeletal demineralization.
- **Immobilization-Related Fractures:** Increased risk of fractures in weakened bones subjected to minimal stress.

Clinical Importance

- **Early Intervention:** Timely diagnosis and management can prevent complications such as fractures, chronic pain, and prolonged disability.
- **Holistic Care:** Combines physical therapy, nutritional support, and pharmacological treatment to ensure optimal recovery.
- **Awareness and Prevention:** Educating at-risk populations, including post-operative and elderly patients, about maintaining bone health during periods of immobilization.

References

N. Allison, B. Brooks: Bone atrophy; a clinical study of the changes in bone which result from nonuse. Archives of Surgery, Chicago, 1922, 5: 499-526.

André's Syndrome

Overview

André's syndrome is a rare genetic disorder characterized by peculiar facial features (orofacial anomalies) and skeletal defects. It includes abnormalities such as hypertelorism, cleft palate, and retrognathia, coupled with osseous defects like faulty cranial ossification, rib malformations, and long bone deformities. The condition is believed to follow an X-linked inheritance pattern and is often lethal within weeks after birth due to severe structural and functional abnormalities.

Historical Background

- Named after *M. André*, who first described the syndrome and its distinct combination of craniofacial and skeletal defects.
- The identification of André's syndrome advanced the understanding of congenital disorders involving multiple systems and their genetic inheritance patterns.
- Early studies highlighted the syndrome's high mortality rate and severe phenotypic presentation, emphasizing the need for prenatal detection and genetic counseling.

Purpose

- **Diagnosis:** To identify the syndrome in affected neonates based on its characteristic orofacial and skeletal features.
- **Genetic Counseling:** To inform families about the X-linked inheritance and risks of recurrence in future pregnancies.
- **Management:** Although the condition is typically lethal, supportive care can aim to improve quality of life during the short survival period.

Procedure Overview

Diagnosis:

- **Clinical Examination:** Identifying facial anomalies, such as hypertelorism, low-set ears, and Robin's anomaly.
- **Imaging Studies:** Radiographs or CT scans to assess skeletal abnormalities, including broad cranial sutures, long bone deformities, and rib anomalies.
- **Genetic Testing:** Confirmation of X-linked inheritance and identification of specific mutations, where possible.

Management:

- **Supportive Care:** Addressing feeding difficulties due to cleft palate and retrognathia.
- Managing respiratory issues associated with craniofacial abnormalities.
- **Parental Support:** Providing emotional and psychological support to families.
- **Palliative Approaches:**
- Focused on comfort care given the high mortality rate and lack of curative treatment.

Results and Interpretation

- **Phenotypic Features:** Facial and skeletal anomalies are distinct and identifiable shortly after birth.
- **Prognosis:** The condition is typically fatal within the first few weeks of life

due to respiratory complications, feeding difficulties, and other systemic challenges.

- **Clinical Challenges:** The syndrome's severity and rapid progression limit the scope of therapeutic interventions.

Physiological Basis

- **Craniofacial Development:** Abnormal ossification and fusion processes result in hypertelorism, retrognathia, and broad cranial sutures.
- **Skeletal Defects:** Faulty ossification and hyperostosis disrupt the structural integrity of long bones, ribs, and vertebrae, contributing to systemic instability.
- **X-Linked Inheritance:** The condition's genetic transmission affects males more severely, with mutations impairing critical developmental pathways.

Clinical Applications

- **Prenatal Diagnosis:** High-resolution ultrasound and genetic testing in at-risk pregnancies allow for early detection.
- **Genetic Counseling:** Helps families understand recurrence risks and explore reproductive options.
- **Postnatal Care:** Although limited by the syndrome's lethality, supportive measures address immediate challenges, such as feeding and respiratory difficulties.

Limitations and Technical Considerations

- **Diagnostic Challenges:** Overlap with other congenital syndromes can complicate diagnosis without genetic confirmation.
- **Therapeutic Limitations:** The lack of curative treatment underscores the need for Advances in genetic and prenatal interventions.
- **Emotional Burden:** Families face significant psychological distress due to the syndrome's prognosis, requiring robust emotional support systems.

Modern Relevance

- **Advances in Genetics:** Improvements in molecular diagnostics have enhanced the ability to detect and understand X-linked conditions like André's syndrome.
- **Prenatal Screening:** Techniques such as non-invasive prenatal testing (NIPT) and targeted genetic analysis provide early risk assessment.
- **Focus on Supportive Care:** Enhanced neonatal care and palliative approaches aim to improve the short lifespan and comfort of affected infants.

Associated Conditions

- **Robin's Anomaly:** A component of the syndrome, involving micrognathia, glossoptosis, and airway obstruction.
- **Craniosynostosis:** Abnormal cranial suture development, contributing to facial deformities and potential intracranial pressure issues.
- **Long Bone Dysplasia:** Abnormal bowing, hyperostosis, and ossification defects of the limbs.
- **Respiratory and Feeding Difficulties:** Secondary to craniofacial abnormalities and structural instability.

Clinical Importance

- **Multisystem Disorder:** Highlights the complexity of congenital syndromes involving craniofacial and skeletal anomalies.
- **Genetic Implications:** Emphasizes the importance of understanding X-linked inheritance patterns in family planning.
- **Educational Value:** Serves as a critical example in medical genetics, pediatrics, and neonatology for diagnosing and managing rare congenital conditions.

References

M. André, et al: Abnormal facies, cleft palate, and generalized dysostosis: A lethal X-linked syndrome. Journal of Pediatrics, St. Louis, 1981, 98: 747-752.

Antley-Bixler Syndrome

Overview

Antley-Bixler syndrome (ABS) is a rare congenital disorder characterized by bone and cartilage maldevelopment, leading to a combination of craniofacial abnormalities, skeletal malformations, and joint anomalies. These include craniosynostoses, midface hypoplasia, and limb defects such as humeroradial synostosis and femoral bowing. ABS is associated with frequent bone fractures and other systemic complications. It can occur sporadically or follow an autosomal recessive inheritance pattern, with cases appearing in both sexes.

Historical Background

- The syndrome was first described in *1975* by *Ray M. Antley* and *David Bixler*, based on a single case demonstrating severe craniofacial and skeletal abnormalities.
- Their work established ABS as a distinct dysmorphic syndrome, providing the foundation for subsequent studies on its genetic basis and clinical variability.
- Later investigations identified mutations in the *FGFR2* gene and *POR (P450 oxidoreductase)*, linking ABS to defects in steroidogenesis and bone development pathways.

Purpose

- **Clinical Identification:** To diagnose ABS based on characteristic craniofacial, skeletal, and systemic features, enabling early intervention and management.

- **Genetic Counseling:** To understand inheritance patterns and assess recurrence risks in families with autosomal recessive cases.
- **Management:** To address multisystem complications, including respiratory, musculoskeletal, and endocrine issues, to improve survival and quality of life.

Procedure Overview

Diagnosis:

- **Clinical Evaluation:** Identification of hallmark features such as craniosynostoses, midface hypoplasia, and limb deformities.
- **Imaging:** X-rays or CT scans to confirm cranial, skeletal, and joint anomalies.
- **Genetic Testing:** Detection of FGFR2 or POR mutations to confirm the diagnosis and differentiate ABS from similar syndromes.

Treatment:

- **Surgical Interventions:** Corrective surgeries for craniosynostoses and midface hypoplasia to prevent intracranial pressure and improve appearance.
- **Orthopedic Management:** Addressing limb deformities, joint synostosis, and frequent fractures.
- **Endocrine Therapy:** Hormonal treatments in cases linked to POR mutations, addressing adrenal insufficiency or disordered steroidogenesis.
- **Monitoring:** Ongoing surveillance for complications such as respiratory issues, fractures, and developmental delays.

Results and Interpretation

- **Variable Presentation:** The severity of ABS varies, with some cases presenting mild skeletal deformities and others experiencing life-threatening complications at birth.
- **Prognosis:** Outcomes depend on the extent of craniofacial and skeletal involvement, as well as access to multidisciplinary care.
- **Genetic Insights:** Identification of causative mutations helps tailor management and provide reproductive counseling.

Physiological Basis

- **Craniofacial and Skeletal Development:** Mutations in FGFR2 disrupt fibroblast growth factor signaling, critical for bone and cartilage formation.
- **Steroidogenesis Defects:** POR mutations impair adrenal and gonadal steroid synthesis, leading to potential endocrine abnormalities in some cases.
- **Bone Fragility:** Abnormal ossification contributes to increased susceptibility to fractures, often present at birth.

Clinical Applications

- **Surgical and Orthopedic Care:** Management of craniosynostoses, limb deformities, and fractures through multidisciplinary approaches.
- **Endocrinology:** Addressing hormone imbalances in patients with POR mutations, especially during critical growth periods.
- **Genetic Testing and Counseling:** Providing families with a comprehensive

understanding of ABS, including recurrence risks and prenatal diagnostic options.

Limitations and Technical Considerations

- **Diagnostic Overlap:** ABS shares features with other syndromes (e.g., Crouzon or Pfeiffer syndrome), necessitating genetic confirmation.
- **Surgical Risks:** Corrective surgeries, particularly for craniosynostoses, carry risks such as infection, incomplete correction, or neurological complications.
- **Recurrent Fractures:** Bone fragility complicates long-term management, requiring vigilant monitoring and preventive care.

Modern Relevance

- **Advances in** *genetic testing* have clarified the molecular basis of ABS, distinguishing it from phenotypically similar syndromes.
- Improved *surgical techniques* and multidisciplinary care have enhanced outcomes, particularly for craniofacial abnormalities.
- Research into *FGFR2* and *POR pathways* offers potential targets for novel therapies addressing both skeletal and endocrine abnormalities.

Associated Conditions

- **Craniosynostoses:** Premature fusion of cranial sutures, leading to abnormal skull shapes and potential intracranial pressure issues.
- **Humeroradial Synostosis:** Fusion of the humerus and radius, impairing arm movement.
- **Endocrine Abnormalities:** Steroidogenesis defects in cases linked to POR mutations, potentially causing adrenal insufficiency or ambiguous genitalia.
- **Bone Fragility:** Increased fracture risk due to abnormal bone development and ossification.

Clinical Importance

- **Early Diagnosis:** Recognizing ABS at birth enables timely interventions, particularly for life-threatening complications such as respiratory distress.
- **Multisystem Management:** Effective treatment requires collaboration among surgeons, endocrinologists, geneticists, and orthopedic specialists.
- **Advancing Genetic Knowledge:** ABS serves as a model for understanding disorders of FGFR2 signaling and steroidogenesis, with implications for broader applications in genetics and developmental biology.

References

R. M. Antley, D. Bixler: X-trapezoidocephaly, midfacial hypoplasia and cartilage abnormalities with multiple synostoses and skeletal fractures. Birth Defects Original Article Series, New York, XI(2), 1975: 397-401.

D. Bixler, R.M. Antley: Development in trapezoidocephaly-multiple synostosis syndrome. American Journal of Medical Genetics, New York, 1983, 14: 149-150.

Ashley's Syndrome

Overview

Ashley's syndrome is a rare congenital disorder characterized by multiple anomalies, including distinctive facial features, musculoskeletal deformities, and orthopedic abnormalities such as hip dislocation, scoliosis, and vertical talus. Additional features include hand malformations, short stature, poor wound healing, and dental crowding. These findings suggest a complex interplay of genetic and developmental disruptions affecting multiple systems.

Historical Background

- Named after *R. K. Ashley*, who first described the syndrome, highlighting its distinct combination of musculoskeletal and craniofacial abnormalities.
- Early studies of Ashley's syndrome emphasized its clinical variability and the need for early recognition to manage orthopedic and systemic complications effectively.
- Research into its genetic underpinnings remains ongoing, though no definitive causative mutations have been universally identified.

Purpose

- **Diagnosis:** To identify key features of Ashley's syndrome for early intervention and management of its associated complications.
- **Multidisciplinary Care:** To address the diverse manifestations, including orthopedic, dental, and growth abnormalities, through coordinated specialist care.
- **Understanding Developmental Pathways:** To explore the genetic and developmental basis for the syndrome to guide future therapies and preventative strategies.

Procedure Overview

Diagnosis:

- **Clinical Examination:** Identification of hallmark features such as unusual facies, musculoskeletal anomalies, and hand abnormalities.
- **Imaging Studies:** X-rays, MRI, or CT scans to evaluate hip dislocation, scoliosis, and other skeletal abnormalities.
- **Genetic Testing:** While no specific gene is currently linked, genetic analysis may identify underlying mutations or syndromic associations.

Treatment:

- **Orthopedic Interventions:** Management of hip dislocations, scoliosis, and vertical talus through surgical or non-surgical means.
- **Growth and Development Support:** Addressing short stature through growth hormone therapy or other supportive measures.
- **Dental Care:** Orthodontic interventions for crowded teeth and associated dental issues.
- **Monitoring:** Regular follow-ups to track skeletal development, wound healing, and overall growth.

Results and Interpretation

- **Variable Presentation:** The severity of anomalies and their impact on daily functioning vary widely among individuals.
- **Prognosis:** With timely intervention, many complications can be mitigated, though some features, such as short stature and poor wound healing, may persist.
- **Outcomes:** Multidisciplinary care significantly improves quality of life and reduces the impact of associated complications.

Physiological Basis

- **Musculoskeletal Development:** Anomalies in cartilage and bone formation likely underlie features such as hip dislocation, scoliosis, and vertical talus.
- **Facial and Dental Development:** Disruptions in craniofacial growth contribute to unusual facies and dental crowding.
- **Wound Healing:** Impaired tissue repair mechanisms may account for poor wound healing, posing additional challenges during surgical interventions.

Clinical Applications

- **Orthopedic Surgery:** Surgical corrections for hip dislocations, scoliosis, and foot deformities to improve mobility and reduce pain.
- **Growth Monitoring:** Ensuring optimal management of growth delays and addressing underlying causes of short stature.
- **Dental and Craniofacial Care:** Comprehensive orthodontic management and treatment of craniofacial anomalies.

Limitations and Technical Considerations

- **Diagnostic Challenges:** The syndrome's features overlap with other congenital disorders, requiring careful differentiation.
- **Surgical Risks:** Poor wound healing increases the risk of complications following surgical interventions.
- **Long-Term Care Needs:** Patients often require lifelong follow-up to manage recurring orthopedic issues and systemic complications.

Modern Relevance

- **Advances in** *orthopedic and craniofacial surgery* have significantly improved outcomes for patients with Ashley's syndrome.
- *Genomic technologies* continue to enhance diagnostic precision, helping distinguish Ashley's syndrome from similar conditions.
- Multidisciplinary approaches highlight the importance of integrating orthopedic, dental, and genetic care in rare syndromes.

Associated Conditions

- **Scoliosis:** Common in Ashley's syndrome, requiring monitoring and potential surgical intervention.
- **Vertical Talus:** A congenital foot deformity that may necessitate early corrective measures.
- **Dental Anomalies:** Crowding and misalignment of teeth are prominent features requiring orthodontic care.

- **Growth Delays:** Short stature often accompanies the syndrome and requires supportive interventions.

Clinical Importance

- **Early Intervention:** Prompt diagnosis and management of orthopedic deformities improve mobility and quality of life.
- **Comprehensive Care:** Multidisciplinary approaches ensure holistic management of the syndrome's diverse manifestations.
- **Research Implications:** Ongoing investigations into the genetic basis of Ashley's syndrome may lead to improved diagnostic and therapeutic options.

References

R. K. Ashley, et al: Congenital matacarpotalar syndrome. Annals of the Academy of Medicine, Singapore, 1981, 10: 434-441.

Atlas

Overview

The Atlas is the first cervical vertebra (C1), named after the Titan of Greek mythology, who was condemned to hold the heavens aloft. It plays a critical role in the articulation between the skull and the spine, allowing for the nodding and rotational movements of the head. The Atlas vertebra, along with the Axis (C2), forms the atlanto-occipital and atlantoaxial joints, essential for head mobility and spinal alignment.

Historical Background

- The term "Atlas" originates from *Greek mythology*, where *Atlas*, the son of the Titan Iapetus, was condemned to carry the heavens as a punishment for warring against Zeus.
- The association of Atlas with the vertebra stems from its role in supporting the *head*, likened to Atlas bearing the heavens.
- Anatomical descriptions of the Atlas date back to early anatomical studies, with its unique structure and functional significance emphasized by anatomists during the Renaissance.

Purpose

- **Structural Support:** The Atlas serves as the primary support for the skull, enabling the head's articulation with the spine.
- **Head Mobility:** Its articulation with the occipital condyles facilitates nodding movements (flexion and extension of the head).

- **Neurological Protection:** The Atlas forms part of the bony ring protecting the spinal cord at the junction between the brainstem and cervical spine.

Procedure Overview (Clinical Context)

- **Evaluation of Atlas-Related Conditions:** Imaging studies, such as X-rays, CT scans, or MRI, are used to assess fractures, misalignments, or degenerative changes in the Atlas.
- **Surgical and Non-Surgical Management:** Non-Surgical: Physical therapy and cervical orthoses are used for minor misalignments or injuries.
- **Surgical:** Spinal stabilization procedures may be required in cases of fractures, dislocations, or instability.
- **Rehabilitation:** Focuses on restoring neck mobility and reducing pain while preventing further complications.

Results and Interpretation

- **Functional Integrity:** The Atlas's bony ring and articulation points are critical for maintaining head and neck mobility.
- **Injury Outcomes:** Fractures or dislocations of the Atlas can lead to severe complications, including spinal cord injury or reduced head mobility.
- **Prognosis:** Early diagnosis and treatment result in favorable outcomes, with most patients regaining full functionality.

Physiological Basis

- **Anatomical Structure:** The Atlas is unique among vertebrae, lacking a body and spinous process. It forms a bony ring with anterior and posterior arches, lateral masses, and large transverse processes.
- **Articulation:** The superior articular facets of the Atlas articulate with the occipital condyles of the skull, enabling nodding motions.
- **The inferior articular facets articulate with the Axis (C2), allowing for head rotation.**
- **Neurological Considerations:** The Atlas's vertebral foramen houses the spinal cord and vertebral arteries, playing a vital role in protecting these critical structures.

Clinical Applications

- **Trauma Management:** Addressing fractures or dislocations, such as Jefferson fractures, caused by axial loading or blunt trauma.
- **Neurological Assessments:** Diagnosing conditions like cervical myelopathy or vertebral artery compression, which can arise from Atlas anomalies.
- **Chiropractic Care:** Focused adjustments of the Atlas vertebra to address alignment and improve overall cervical spine function.

Limitations and Technical Considerations

- **Vulnerability to Injury:** The Atlas's unique structure makes it susceptible to fractures and misalignments under axial load or sudden trauma.
- **Surgical Challenges:** Stabilization procedures require precision to avoid compromising the spinal cord or vertebral arteries.

- **Long-Term Management:** Chronic conditions affecting the Atlas, such as degenerative arthritis or congenital anomalies, require ongoing care and monitoring.

Modern Relevance

- **Advances in** *spinal imaging* have improved the diagnosis of Atlas-related injuries and anomalies.
- Surgical techniques, including *minimally invasive procedures*, have enhanced outcomes for patients with severe Atlas injuries or instability.
- Increased awareness of *Atlas misalignments* has led to greater integration of chiropractic and physical therapy approaches in managing cervical spine conditions.

Associated Conditions

- **Atlantoaxial Instability:** A condition involving excessive movement at the junction of the Atlas and Axis, often associated with congenital disorders or trauma.
- **Jefferson Fracture:** A burst fracture of the Atlas caused by axial compression forces.
- **Congenital Anomalies:** Conditions such as fusion of the Atlas to the occipital bone (occipitalization) or incomplete development of its arches.
- **Degenerative Disorders:** Arthritis or spondylosis affecting the Atlas and its articulations, leading to pain and reduced mobility.

Clinical Importance

- **Head and Neck Mobility:** The Atlas is essential for enabling a wide range of head movements, including nodding and rotation.
- **Neurological Protection:** Its role in safeguarding the spinal cord and vertebral arteries underscores its significance in overall neurological health.
- **Structural Integrity:** Maintaining the alignment and function of the Atlas is crucial for spinal health and preventing secondary complications.

Aviator Astragalus

Overview

Aviator Astragalus refers to a historical term describing isolated fracture or fracture-dislocation injuries of the talus, particularly the talar neck, resulting from high-energy trauma such as aviation crashes or falls. This injury pattern is associated with severe complications, including avascular necrosis and post-traumatic arthritis.

Historical Background

- **1608:** Fractures and dislocations of the talus were first documented.

1919:

- The term "Aviator Astragalus" was introduced by Henry Graeme Anderson to describe injury patterns observed in pilots involved in low-velocity plane crashes during the early days of aviation.
- The term is now obsolete, as aviation-related talus injuries are no longer common.

Purpose

- **Primary Objective:** To identify and appropriately manage talus fractures and dislocations, ensuring anatomical realignment and minimizing complications like avascular necrosis.
- **Clinical Relevance:** Effective management helps prevent long-term morbidity, including joint dysfunction and osteoarthritis.

Procedure Overview

Diagnosis:

- Begins with a detailed history and physical examination, focusing on trauma mechanisms.
- Radiographic imaging (AP, lateral, and oblique X-rays) is essential, with CT scans recommended for occult or complex fractures.
- **Treatment Options:** Nondisplaced Fractures: Managed conservatively with immobilization and limited weight-bearing.
- **Displaced Fractures:** Require surgical intervention, typically through open reduction and internal fixation (ORIF).
- **Surgical Techniques:** Depending on the fracture type and displacement, approaches may include medial or lateral incisions, with or without malleolar osteotomy.
- External fixation may be required for complex dislocations.

Results and Interpretation

- **Expected Outcomes:** Timely and anatomically accurate fracture reduction minimizes the risk of avascular necrosis (AVN) and post-traumatic arthritis.
- Successful management restores joint stability and function.
- **Radiographic Findings:** Fracture lines or displacement, often in the talar neck or body.
- CT scans can reveal subtle injuries, especially compression fractures.

Physiological Basis

- **Bone Characteristics:** The talus has over 60% cartilaginous coverage, with no muscle insertions, making it vulnerable to dislocation and AVN.

- **Vascular Supply:** Blood supply is primarily from the posterior tibial artery, dorsalis pedis artery, and perforating peroneal artery, making the talar neck particularly susceptible to AVN when disrupted.

Clinical Applications

- **Trauma Management:** Used to address high-impact injuries involving the ankle and foot, such as car accidents or falls.
- **Orthopedic Surgery:** Guiding surgical decisions in complex talar fractures or fracture-dislocations.
- **Postoperative Rehabilitation:** Focused on restoring mobility, minimizing weight-bearing stress, and monitoring for AVN or arthritis.

Limitations and Technical Considerations

- **Challenges in Diagnosis:** Radiographically occult fractures can be misdiagnosed as sprains; advanced imaging (CT or MRI) may be required.
- **Surgical Complications:** Improper reduction or delayed intervention increases the risk of AVN and joint dysfunction.
- **Patient Factors:** Healing may be prolonged in patients with poor vascular health or systemic conditions.

Modern Relevance

- **Refined Imaging and Techniques:** Improved imaging modalities, including 3D CT, allow for better visualization and classification of talus injuries.
- **Surgical Advances:** Enhanced fixation techniques reduce the risk of long-term complications.
- **Interprofessional Care:** Management involves a team approach, including orthopedic surgeons, radiologists, and rehabilitation specialists.

Associated Conditions

- **Avascular Necrosis (AVN):** A common complication due to compromised blood supply.
- **Post-Traumatic Arthritis:** Results from articular surface disruption.
- **Osteomyelitis:** Potential risk in open fractures.

Clinical Importance

- **Diagnostic Vigilance:** Early recognition and appropriate imaging are critical to preventing misdiagnosis.
- **Treatment Goals:** Achieving anatomical reduction and joint stability to preserve function and prevent complications.
- **Comprehensive Care:** Effective management requires collaboration among orthopedic surgeons, radiologists, and rehabilitation teams for optimal patient outcomes.

The Aviator Astragalus remains a compelling example of early trauma management linked to the history of aviation, and while the term is no longer widely used, the injury pattern and its management continue to be clinically significant.

Baby Car Injuries

Overview

*Baby Car Injuries (also known as sideswipe injuries or traffic elbow injuries) are complex, high-energy trauma cases often involving the elbow. These injuries occur when an individual's arm, typically resting on a vehicle window, is struck by an obje*CT **or** *another vehicle. Common in areas with open-window vehicles, these injuries often involve polytrauma, including head and chest injuries. They are associated with significant complications and require multidisciplinary management for optimal outcomes.*

Historical Background

- The term "sideswipe injuries" emerged from the nature of the trauma mechanism, although it is insufficient in describing the injury's complexity.
- The phenomenon has been documented more frequently in regions where vehicles with open windows or buses are prevalent, but no specific originating year or individual associated with its naming has been noted.

Purpose

- **Primary Objective:** To prevent loss of limb and ensure the maximum possible functional recovery in patients.
- **Secondary Objective:** To address polytrauma, mitigate complications, and achieve stable fixation and mobility.

Procedure Overview

- **Initial Assessment:** Patients often present with multiple injuries requiring immediate triage. A detailed evaluation, including imaging studies, is critical for assessing fractures, soft tissue damage, and vascular compromise.
- **Staged Surgical Protocol:**
- **Step 1:** Initial soft tissue debridement to prevent infection and prepare for further reconstruction.
- **Step 2:** Fracture stabilization using internal or external fixation, depending on the nature and severity of the injury.
- **Step 3:** Vascular repair if needed, often performed alongside fracture management.
- **Step 4:** Soft tissue reconstruction or coverage through skin grafts or flaps in cases with significant tissue loss.
- **Rehabilitation:** Postoperative therapy aims to restore function, manage pain, and prevent stiffness or contractures.

Results and Interpretation

- **Expected Outcomes:** Successful limb salvage and functional restoration when a structured treatment algorithm is followed.
- Outcomes depend on injury severity, timely intervention, and adherence to multidisciplinary management.
- **Complications:** Stiffness, nonunion, deformity, infection, and chronic pain are common if not managed effectively.

Physiological Basis

- **Trauma Mechanism:** High-energy impact results in a combination of bone fractures, soft tissue damage, and vascular compromise, particularly around the elbow.
- **Affected Structures:** Frequent involvement of supracondylar humerus fractures with intraarticular extension and fractures of the radius and ulna. Damage to nearby arteries and nerves exacerbates the complexity.

Clinical Applications

- **Trauma Management:** Immediate stabilization and vascular repair are priorities in life- or limb-threatening cases.
- **Surgical Intervention:** Internal fixation is preferred in most fractures; external fixation is reserved for severe comminution, open fractures, and polytrauma.
- **Rehabilitation:** Early physiotherapy helps regain mobility and prevent long-term stiffness or functional loss.

Limitations and Technical Considerations

- **Complexity of Injury:** Variability in fracture patterns and soft tissue damage complicates standard treatment protocols.
- **Risk of Infection:** Open fractures are highly susceptible to contamination and require meticulous debridement and infection control measures.
- **Challenges in Fixation:** Severe comminution or bone loss may necessitate external fixation or staged surgeries.

Modern Relevance

- **Trauma Care Protocols:** Algorithmic approaches to trauma management and advancements in surgical techniques have improved outcomes.
- **Education and Prevention:** Raising awareness about the dangers of resting limbs on vehicle windows is critical in preventing such injuries.
- **Multidisciplinary Management:** Collaborative care involving orthopedic, vascular, and plastic surgeons ensures comprehensive treatment.

Associated Conditions

- **Polytrauma:** Frequently associated with head and chest injuries due to the high-energy nature of the trauma.
- **Vascular Compromise:** Risk of ischemia and limb loss without timely vascular repair.
- **Soft Tissue Loss:** Often necessitates advanced reconstruction techniques like flap surgery.

Clinical Importance

- **Prevention:** Educating the public about the risks of keeping limbs outside vehicles can significantly reduce incidence rates.
- **Aggressive Treatment:** Early and comprehensive management is crucial to minimizing disability and achieving functional recovery.
- **Rehabilitation:** Postoperative care focusing on range-of-motion exercises and strength training plays a vital role in long-term outcomes.

The term "Baby Car Injuries" highlights the preventable nature of this trauma, emphasizing the importance of awareness and safety measures. However, the injury's complexity underscores the need for a structured, multidisciplinary approach to optimize recovery.

Baker's Cyst

Overview

Baker's cyst, also known as a popliteal cyst, is a fluid-filled sac that forms in the synovial membrane of the knee joint, typically as a result of synovial fluid leaking through a natural channel or hernial opening. It is often associated with limited knee extension, aching, and stiffness. While Baker's cysts can occur at any age, they are most commonly observed in males aged 15–30 years. The exact etiology remains unclear, but familial cases suggest a possible genetic predisposition.

Historical Background

- The condition was first described by *William Morrant Baker*, a 19th-century British surgeon, who noted the formation of synovial cysts in the knee joint and their association with joint dysfunction.
- Baker's observations highlighted the relationship between excessive synovial fluid production, joint pathologies, and cyst development.
- Over time, the term "Baker's cyst" became widely recognized in clinical practice, emphasizing its role as a diagnostic marker for underlying joint disorders.

Purpose

- **Diagnosis:** To identify Baker's cysts and differentiate them from other causes of knee pain and swelling, such as deep vein thrombosis or soft tissue tumors.
- **Treatment:** To alleviate symptoms

such as knee stiffness, pain, and reduced mobility, and to address any underlying joint pathology.

- **Prevention of Complications:** To minimize risks such as cyst rupture, infection, or compression of nearby neurovascular structures.

Procedure Overview

Diagnosis:

- **Clinical Examination:** Palpation of a soft, bulging mass in the popliteal fossa, often noticeable during knee extension.
- **Imaging:** Ultrasound or MRI to confirm the presence of a cyst, assess its size, and identify underlying joint pathology (e.g., arthritis or meniscal tears).
- **Joint Aspiration:** In some cases, synovial fluid may be aspirated to rule out infection or inflammatory conditions.

Treatment:

- **Conservative Management:** Rest, ice application, and nonsteroidal anti-inflammatory drugs (NSAIDs) to reduce swelling and pain.
- Physical therapy to improve knee function and reduce joint stress.
- **Aspiration:** Needle aspiration of the cyst to relieve discomfort, often combined with corticosteroid injections to reduce inflammation.
- **Surgical Intervention:** Reserved for recurrent or symptomatic cysts, involving excision of the cyst and repair of any underlying joint defect.
- **Follow-Up:** Regular monitoring to detect recurrence or complications.

Results and Interpretation

- **Clinical Improvement:** Most patients experience symptom relief with conservative measures, although recurrence is common if underlying joint pathology is not addressed.
- **Prognosis:** The condition is generally benign, but untreated cases may lead to complications such as cyst rupture or chronic knee dysfunction.
- **Complication Management:** Early intervention minimizes risks of rupture, which can mimic deep vein thrombosis with calf swelling and pain.

Physiological Basis

- **Synovial Fluid Dynamics:** Excess synovial fluid, often due to joint inflammation or injury, escapes into the popliteal fossa through weakened or herniated areas of the synovial membrane.
- **Cyst Formation:** The accumulation of synovial fluid within a closed sac creates a palpable mass, leading to symptoms of pain, stiffness, and restricted knee mobility.
- **Knee Biomechanics:** Increased intra-articular pressure contributes to cyst formation, especially in individuals with predisposing joint conditions like osteoarthritis or meniscal tears.

Clinical Applications

- **Orthopedic Management:** Addressing Baker's cysts as part of the treatment plan for underlying joint disorders, such as arthritis or ligament injuries.
- **Sports Medicine:** Preventing recurrence in athletes by addressing mechanical stress and optimizing joint function

through rehabilitation.

- **Differential Diagnosis:** Distinguishing Baker's cysts from other causes of posterior knee swelling, such as deep vein thrombosis or tumors.

Limitations and Technical Considerations

- **Recurrent Cysts:** Even with treatment, cysts may recur if underlying joint issues are not resolved.
- **Risk of MisDiagnosis:** Cyst rupture can mimic other conditions like deep vein thrombosis, requiring careful clinical and imaging assessment.
- **Invasive Treatments:** Surgical excision carries risks, including infection, nerve damage, and postoperative stiffness.

Modern Relevance

- **Advances in** *imaging techniques*, such as high-resolution ultrasound and MRI, have improved the diagnosis and characterization of Baker's cysts.
- *Minimally invasive procedures*, such as ultrasound-guided aspiration and arthroscopic repair, have enhanced treatment outcomes.
- Increased awareness of *underlying joint pathologies* has emphasized the need for comprehensive management rather than isolated cyst treatment.

Associated Conditions

- **Osteoarthritis:** A common underlying cause of Baker's cysts, contributing to synovial fluid overproduction.
- **Rheumatoid Arthritis:** Chronic inflammation of the joint lining can predispose to cyst formation.
- **Meniscal Tears:** Joint injuries that disrupt normal synovial fluid dynamics, leading to cyst development.
- **Cyst Rupture:** A complication where cyst contents leak into surrounding tissues, causing pain and swelling resembling thrombophlebitis.

Clinical Importance

- **Symptom Relief:** Effective management alleviates discomfort and restores knee mobility, improving quality of life.
- **Underlying Joint Health:** Treating Baker's cysts provides an opportunity to address broader joint issues, preventing further complications.
- **Education and Prevention:** Raising awareness about risk factors and early symptoms helps reduce the impact of Baker's cysts and associated joint conditions.

References

W. M. Baker: The formation of abnormal synovial cysts in connection with the joints. St.Bartholomew's Hospital Reports, London, 1885, 21: 177-190.

Bakwin-Eiger Syndrome

Overview

Bakwin-Eiger syndrome, also known as Juvenile Paget's disease, is a rare hereditary skeletal dysplasia characterized by cortical hyperplasia, macrocrania, and hyperphosphatasia, along with elevated biochemical markers such as uric acid, aminopeptidase, and urinary peptide-bound hydroxyproline. Symptoms typically manifest in late infancy and include growth deficiency, cranial enlargement, hearing loss, osteoporosis, and occasional multiple fractures. This condition follows an autosomal recessive inheritance pattern with significant variability in expression, even within families.

Historical Background

- The syndrome is named after *Harry Bakwin* and *Marvin S. Eiger*, who contributed to its characterization, as well as *Sir James Paget*, who first described a similar form of bone disease in adults.
- Initially recognized as a distinct condition from adult Paget's disease, *Juvenile Paget's disease* was linked to hereditary causes and distinct clinical manifestations.
- Research into Bakwin-Eiger syndrome has advanced understanding of skeletal dysplasias and bone remodeling disorders.

Purpose

- **Diagnosis:** To identify and differentiate Bakwin-Eiger syndrome from other skeletal dysplasias and metabolic bone diseases.
- **Management:** To address growth deficiencies, bone deformities, and systemic complications like hypertension and hearing loss.
- **Genetic Counseling:** To inform families about the autosomal recessive inheritance and assess recurrence risks in future generations.

Procedure Overview

Diagnosis:

- **Clinical Examination:** Identification of characteristic skeletal deformities, macrocrania, and blue sclerae.
- **Imaging:** X-rays to reveal cortical hyperplasia, bone bowing, and severe osteoporosis or demineralization.
- **Laboratory Testing:** Elevated markers including serum alkaline phosphatase, uric acid, and urinary hydroxyproline.
- **Genetic Testing:** Confirmatory testing for mutations associated with autosomal recessive inheritance.

Treatment:

- **Bone-Targeted Therapies:** Bisphosphonates to improve bone density and reduce fracture risk.
- **Hearing Support:** Management of hearing loss through assistive devices or surgical interventions.
- **Nutritional and Hormonal Support:** Adequate calcium and vitamin D supplementation, along with growth hormone therapy in some cases.
- **Orthopedic Surgery:** Correction of severe deformities or fractures.

- **Monitoring:** Regular assessment of bone density, growth parameters, and systemic complications like optic atrophy and hypertension.

Results and Interpretation

- **Variable Severity:** Presentation ranges from mild osteoporosis and occasional fractures to severe skeletal deformities and systemic complications.
- **Treatment Outcomes:** Bisphosphonate therapy has significantly improved bone density and reduced fracture rates in affected individuals.
- **Prognosis:** While the condition is chronic, most patients maintain normal intelligence and, with appropriate management, can lead productive lives.

Physiological Basis

- **Bone Remodeling Defect:** The syndrome involves excessive bone turnover, leading to weakened and deformed bones despite cortical hyperplasia.
- **Skeletal Deformities:** Bowing of long bones and cranial enlargement arise from abnormal osteoblast and osteoclast activity.
- **Neurological and Sensory Impact:** Compression of cranial nerves and optic pathways causes hearing loss, optic atrophy, and associated sensory deficits.

Clinical Applications

- **Pediatric Management:** Early diagnosis and intervention prevent complications like severe deformities, fractures, and sensory loss.
- **Endocrinology:** Monitoring and managing metabolic abnormalities, including hyperphosphatasia and elevated uric acid levels.
- **Orthopedics:** Addressing structural deformities and fractures through medical and surgical interventions.

Limitations and Technical Considerations

- **Diagnostic Challenges:** The syndrome's symptoms overlap with other skeletal dysplasias, necessitating detailed biochemical and genetic evaluations.
- **Treatment Limitations:** Bisphosphonates improve bone density but may not fully prevent deformities or fractures.
- **Long-Term Monitoring:** Continuous care is required to manage systemic complications like hypertension, dental caries, and sensory deficits.

Modern Relevance

- **Advances in** *bone-targeted therapies*, including second-generation bisphosphonates, have improved outcomes for Bakwin-Eiger syndrome.
- Genetic research has enhanced understanding of autosomal recessive inheritance and the variability of phenotypic expression within families.
- Increased awareness and early screening in at-risk populations have improved early diagnosis and management.

Associated Conditions

- **Osteoporosis and Demineralization:** Severe reduction in bone density, predisposing to fractures and deformities.
- **Hearing Loss:** Caused by cranial nerve

compression or structural abnormalities in the auditory pathways.

- **Hypertension and Retinal Abnormalities:** Complications include optic atrophy and angioid streaks in the retina.
- **Bone Deformities:** Bowing of long bones, cranial enlargement, and fusiform swelling are hallmark features.

Clinical Importance

- **Holistic Management:** Effective care integrates orthopedic, endocrinological, and sensory rehabilitation strategies.
- **Genetic Insights:** Understanding the hereditary nature of the syndrome aids in family counseling and reproductive planning.
- **Improving Quality of Life:** Advances in therapy and supportive care have significantly enhanced the prognosis and daily functioning of affected individuals.

References

H. Bakwin, M. Eiger: Fragile bones and macrocranium. Journal of Pediatrics, St. Louis, 1956, 49: 558-564.

Ballard's Syndrome

Overview

Ballard's syndrome is a rare condition of unknown etiology characterized by hepatomegaly, splenomegaly, and pathologic fractures. The syndrome affects both sexes and presents with systemic involvement, particularly of the liver, spleen, and skeletal system. The condition's exact pathophysiological mechanisms and genetic underpinnings remain unclear, and it is primarily identified by its clinical features and systemic manifestations.

Historical Background

- Named after *H. S. Ballard*, who first described the syndrome based on its characteristic combination of systemic and skeletal abnormalities.
- Ballard's observations emphasized the unique combination of visceral enlargement (hepatosplenomegaly) and skeletal fragility, prompting further research into its unknown etiology.
- The syndrome remains poorly understood, with limited cases reported, highlighting the need for further investigation into its causes and management.

Purpose

- **Diagnosis:** To identify the syndrome through its hallmark features, particularly hepatosplenomegaly and pathologic fractures, and rule out other systemic or metabolic conditions.
- **Management:** To alleviate symptoms and prevent complications such as recurrent fractures and organ dysfunction.

- **Research:** To explore potential genetic, infectious, or metabolic causes and improve understanding of its etiology.

Procedure Overview

Diagnosis:

- **Clinical Examination:** Detection of hepatomegaly and splenomegaly through palpation and imaging.
- **Imaging:** X-rays to identify fractures or bone abnormalities and ultrasound or CT to assess liver and spleen enlargement.
- **Laboratory Tests:** Blood tests to evaluate liver function, bone metabolism markers, and exclude other systemic conditions.

Treatment:

- **Supportive Care:** Pain management and physical support for fractures.
- **Orthopedic Interventions:** Stabilization of fractures using casts, splints, or surgical fixation if needed.
- **Monitoring of Organ Function:** Regular follow-ups to assess liver and spleen size and functionality.
- **Monitoring:** Long-term follow-up to identify complications and assess disease progression.

Results and Interpretation

- **Systemic Manifestations:** Hepatosplenomegaly is a consistent feature, often accompanied by functional impairment.
- **Skeletal Fragility:** Pathologic fractures are indicative of underlying bone weakness or metabolic abnormalities.
- **Variable Prognosis:** The prognosis depends on the severity of systemic involvement and the management of complications.

Physiological Basis

- **Visceral Enlargement:** Hepatomegaly and splenomegaly suggest an underlying systemic disorder, possibly linked to metabolic dysfunction or infiltration.
- **Bone Fragility:** Pathologic fractures point to defects in bone remodeling or structural integrity, potentially due to secondary metabolic bone disease or an unknown primary defect.
- **Unknown Etiology:** The syndrome's cause is yet to be elucidated, leaving room for speculation regarding genetic, infectious, or systemic metabolic pathways.

Clinical Applications

- **Orthopedic Management:** Addressing pathologic fractures through stabilization and rehabilitation to restore mobility and reduce pain.
- **Hepatology and Hematology:** Monitoring and managing potential complications from liver and spleen involvement, such as portal hypertension or splenic rupture.
- **Multisystem Approach:** Collaborative care involving orthopedists, hepatologists, and internists to address the diverse manifestations of the syndrome.

Limitations and Technical Considerations

- **Diagnostic Challenges:** The absence of specific biomarkers or known etiologies complicates diagnosis and differentiation from other systemic conditions.

- **Treatment Limitations:** Management remains largely supportive, with no definitive therapy available due to the lack of understanding of the syndrome's underlying mechanisms.
- **Long-Term Complications:** Recurrent fractures and progressive organ enlargement pose significant challenges in disease management.

Modern Relevance

- **Advances in** *imaging* and *biochemical testing* have improved the detection of hepatosplenomegaly and fractures, aiding in diagnosis.
- Research into systemic disorders of unknown etiology may eventually provide insights into the mechanisms underlying Ballard's syndrome.
- The syndrome underscores the need for comprehensive, multidisciplinary care for rare diseases with systemic manifestations.

Associated Conditions

- **Metabolic Bone Disorders:** The skeletal fragility seen in Ballard's syndrome shares features with osteoporosis or other conditions affecting bone density.
- **Hepatic and Splenic Diseases:** Conditions involving organomegaly, such as Gaucher's disease or other infiltrative disorders, may present similarly.
- **Systemic Disorders:** Hepatosplenomegaly and fractures raise considerations for underlying systemic or genetic syndromes.

Clinical Importance

- **Early Recognition:** Identifying the syndrome early allows for symptom management and prevention of complications, particularly recurrent fractures.
- **Holistic Care:** Multidisciplinary management is crucial to address both systemic and skeletal aspects of the disease.
- **Research Potential:** Ballard's syndrome highlights the need for continued research into rare syndromes of unknown etiology, with the hope of finding specific causes and targeted treatments.

References

H. S. Ballard, L. M. Hamilton, A. J. Mazcus: A new variant of heavy chain disease (μ chain disease). New England Journal of Medicine, Boston, 1970, 282: 1060-1062.

Bankart's Operation

Overview

Bankart's operation is a surgical technique developed to repair recurrent anterior shoulder instability caused by a Bankart lesion, which is an anteroinferior detachment of the glenoid labrum. Bankart lesions, commonly seen in 85–97% of first-time traumatic anterior shoulder dislocations, can involve soft tissue only (soft Bankart) or include a bony Bankart, where part of the glenoid bone is fractured. This condition is frequently associated with a Hill-Sachs lesion, as both share a common mechanism of injury. The goal of Bankart's operation is to restore stability to the shoulder joint, preventing further dislocations and improving function.

Historical Background

- The procedure is named after *Arthur Sydney Blundell Bankart*, a renowned English orthopedic surgeon who first described it in the early 20th century.
- Earlier contributions by *Auguste Broca* and *Georg Clemens Perthes* laid the groundwork for understanding labral injuries and their role in shoulder instability.
- Bankart's operation became a cornerstone in orthopedic surgery, evolving over time to include arthroscopic techniques and bone reconstruction options for more severe injuries.

Purpose

- **Stabilization of the Shoulder:** To repair and restore the stability of the shoulder joint after a Bankart lesion, addressing recurrent dislocations.
- **Prevention of Long-Term Damage:** To minimize secondary complications, such as arthritis, that can arise from repeated shoulder instability.
- **Functional Restoration:** To improve range of motion, strength, and confidence in shoulder movements, especially in athletes and active individuals.

Procedure Overview

- **Preoperative Evaluation:** Imaging, such as MRI or CT scans with 3D reconstructions, to confirm the presence of a Bankart lesion and assess bone loss.
- Assessment for concomitant injuries, such as a Hill-Sachs lesion, which may influence surgical planning.

Surgical Approach:

- **Soft Bankart Repair:** Involves reattachment of the detached labrum to the anterior glenoid using sutures or anchors.
- **Bony Bankart Repair:** If significant bone loss is present, bone grafts or implants may be used to reconstruct the glenoid rim.
- Techniques can be performed via open surgery or arthroscopically, with arthroscopy being the preferred method for most cases due to reduced invasiveness and quicker recovery.
- **Postoperative Care:** Immobilization of the shoulder in a sling for 4–6 weeks, followed by gradual physiotherapy to regain strength and range of motion.

Results and Interpretation

- **Success Rates:** Bankart's operation has high success rates, with most patients achieving stable shoulders and reduced risk of recurrence.
- **Functional Outcomes:** Improved strength and mobility, enabling patients to resume normal activities, including sports.
- **Complications:** While rare, complications may include nerve injury, stiffness, or failure of repair, leading to continued instability.

Physiological Basis

- **Labrum Function:** The glenoid labrum deepens the shoulder joint and provides stability by creating a suction-like seal. Damage to the labrum disrupts this stability.
- **Bankart Lesions:** Soft Bankart lesions involve the fibrocartilaginous labrum, while bony Bankart lesions involve fractures of the anterior-inferior glenoid rim, compromising the structural integrity of the joint.
- **Joint Instability:** The detachment of the labrum predisposes the shoulder to recurrent dislocations, particularly during overhead or high-impact activities.

Clinical Applications

- **Sports Medicine:** Particularly relevant for athletes involved in contact sports (e.g., rugby, football) or overhead sports (e.g., tennis, baseball), where shoulder stability is crucial.
- **Orthopedic Surgery:** A key procedure for managing traumatic anterior shoulder dislocations and preventing recurrent instability.
- **Rehabilitation:** Postoperative physical therapy is essential for restoring joint function and preventing stiffness.

Limitations and Technical Considerations

- **Recurrent Dislocations:** While highly effective, failure rates increase if the patient resumes high-risk activities prematurely or has significant bone loss.
- **Surgical Complexity:** Arthroscopic repair requires technical precision, particularly in cases with complex or extensive lesions.
- **Bone Loss:** Severe glenoid bone loss may necessitate more invasive procedures, such as bone block surgery, which carries additional risks.

Modern Relevance

- **Advances in** *arthroscopic techniques* have made Bankart's operation less invasive, with shorter recovery times and improved cosmetic outcomes.
- Enhanced imaging modalities, such as 3D CT scans, have improved preoperative planning and identification of coexisting injuries like Hill-Sachs lesions.
- **Tailored Approaches:** Combining Bankart repair with bone reconstruction techniques allows for effective management of severe cases with substantial bone loss.

Associated Conditions

- **Hill-Sachs Lesion:** A compression fracture of the humeral head caused by impaction against the glenoid during dislocation.

- **Recurrent Shoulder Dislocations:** Often the result of untreated Bankart lesions, leading to chronic instability and secondary complications.
- **Post-Traumatic Arthritis:** Can develop over time due to repeated instability and joint damage if the condition is not properly managed.

Clinical Importance

- **Restoring Stability:** Bankart's operation remains a gold standard for managing anterior shoulder instability, especially in young and active patients.
- **Preventing Long-Term Damage:** Early intervention reduces the risk of recurrent dislocations, joint degeneration, and secondary injuries.
- **Improved Quality of Life:** Effective repair allows patients to return to their desired level of activity with reduced pain and increased confidence in shoulder stability.

References

G. C. von Perthes: Über operationen bei habitueller Schulterluxation. Deutsche Zeitschrift für Chirurgie, Leipzig, 1906, 85: 199-227.

A. S. B. Bankart: Recurrent or habitual dislocation of the shoulder. British Medical Journal, London, 1923, 2: 1132-1133.

Sheehan SE, Gaviola G, Gordon R, Sacks A, Shi LL, Smith SE. Traumatic shoulder injuries: a force mechanism analysis-glenohumeral dislocation and instability. AJR Am J Roentgenol. 2013;201(2):378–93.

The pathology and treatment of recurrent dislocation of the shoulder-joint. British Journal of Surgery, London, 1938, 26: 23-29.

H. Osmond-Clarke: Habitual dislocation of the shoulder-joint. Journal of Bone and Joint Surgery, British Volume, London, 1948, 30: 19-25.

Broca A, Hartman H. Contribution à l'étude des luxations de l'épaule (luxations anciennes, luxations recidivantes). Bulletins de La Société Anatomique de Paris 5, serie IV, 312-336. June 1890.

Barton Fracture

Overview

A Barton fracture is an intra-articular fracture of the distal radius associated with subluxation or dislocation of the radiocarpal joint. This "shear-type" fracture involves the articular surface of the radius, with either the ventral (anterior) or dorsal (posterior) aspect fractured. The dorsal type, originally described by John Rhea Barton, is considered the classic Barton fracture, while the volar (anterior) variant, also known as a reverse Barton fracture, is more commonly seen today. These injuries are uncommon but require precise diagnosis and management due to their involvement of the joint surface and potential for instability.

Historical Background

- *John Rhea Barton*, an American surgeon, first described the posterior marginal fracture of the distal radius with dislocation in the early 19th century. His original focus was on dorsal injuries.
- Later, the anterior variant, now termed the *volar Barton fracture*, was recognized as a distinct but related injury.
- Barton faced criticism from contemporaries like *Joseph François Malgaigne* and *Lewis Atterbury Stimson*, who questioned his reliance on clinical observation without corroboration from autopsy specimens. Despite this, his work remains foundational in the understanding of intra-articular fractures of the distal radius.

- Contributions from *Lorenz Böhler*, an Austrian surgeon, further refined the classification and management of these fractures.

Purpose

- **Diagnosis:** To accurately identify Barton fractures and distinguish between the dorsal and volar variants for appropriate treatment.
- **Restoration of Joint Function:** To achieve anatomical reduction of the fracture and prevent long-term complications such as arthritis or joint instability.
- **Prevention of Recurrence:** To stabilize the radiocarpal joint and prevent further dislocation or subluxation.

Procedure Overview

Diagnosis:

- **Clinical Examination:** Patients typically present with wrist pain, swelling, and deformity following trauma.
- **Imaging:** X-rays confirm the fracture and joint involvement. CT scans may be necessary for detailed assessment of the articular surface and fracture alignment.

Treatment:

- **Non-Surgical Management:** Reserved for non-displaced fractures, involving closed reduction and casting.
- **Surgical Intervention:** Common for displaced or unstable fractures.
- **Techniques include:** Open Reduction and Internal Fixation (ORIF): Using plates and screws to stabilize the fracture.
- **External Fixation:** Occasionally used for comminuted fractures or cases with significant soft tissue injury.
- **Postoperative Care:** Immobilization in a splint or cast followed by structured physical therapy to restore range of motion and strength.

Results and Interpretation

- **Surgical Outcomes:** ORIF has a high success rate in achieving stable fixation and restoring wrist function.
- **Complications:** Improper reduction or fixation can result in joint instability, malunion, or post-traumatic arthritis.
- **Prognosis:** With timely and appropriate treatment, most patients regain good wrist function, although recovery may vary depending on the severity of the fracture and associated injuries.

Physiological Basis

- **Shear-Type Fracture:** Barton fractures occur due to high-energy forces that shear the articular surface of the distal radius, disrupting the radiocarpal joint.
- **Joint Instability:** The dislocation or subluxation of the radiocarpal joint results from ligamentous and bony disruption, necessitating precise alignment for restoration of function.
- **Dorsal vs. Volar Injury:** Dorsal Barton Fracture: Affects the posterior aspect of the distal radius and is less common.
- **Volar Barton Fracture:** Involves the anterior margin and is more frequently encountered in clinical practice.

Clinical Applications

- **Orthopedic Surgery:** Management of Barton fractures is a cornerstone in orthopedic trauma care, particularly for wrist injuries.
- **Sports and Trauma Medicine:** Commonly seen in high-energy trauma, such as falls on an outstretched hand or motor vehicle accidents.
- **Rehabilitation:** Postoperative physiotherapy is essential for restoring full wrist function and preventing stiffness.

Limitations and Technical Considerations

- **Diagnostic Challenges:** Distinguishing Barton fractures from similar injuries, such as Colles fractures, requires detailed imaging and careful clinical evaluation.
- **Surgical Risks:** Open reduction may involve risks of infection, hardware failure, or nerve damage.
- **Functional Recovery:** Regaining full range of motion and strength can be challenging, especially in cases with delayed treatment or poor compliance with rehabilitation.

Modern Relevance

- **Advances in** *imaging techniques*, such as high-resolution CT scans, have improved diagnostic accuracy and surgical planning.
- *Minimally invasive surgical techniques* have reduced recovery times and complications associated with Barton fractures.
- Ongoing research into *biomechanical fixation methods* has enhanced the stability of surgical repairs, particularly for complex intra-articular injuries.

Associated Conditions

- **Hill-Sachs Lesion:** Often co-occurs with high-energy injuries, leading to additional challenges in joint stability.
- **Colles Fracture:** A more common extra-articular distal radius fracture that may resemble Barton fractures on initial examination.
- **Post-Traumatic Arthritis:** A long-term complication resulting from inadequate reduction or stabilization of the joint.

Clinical Importance

- **Precision in Diagnosis:** Differentiating Barton fractures from other distal radius injuries ensures appropriate treatment and avoids long-term complications.
- **Restoration of Function:** Timely surgical intervention minimizes the risk of chronic wrist instability and arthritis, improving patient outcomes.
- **Historical and Clinical Significance:** The evolution of Barton's concepts reflects the advancement of orthopedic knowledge and its application to modern trauma care.

References

Barton, JR. Views and treatment of an important injury of the wrist. Medical Examiner. 1838;1:365–368.

Nickson C. Stairs versus Wrist. LITFL 2018

Thompson GH, Grant TT. Barton's fractures-reverse Barton's fractures. Confusing eponyms. Clin Orthop Relat Res. 1977 Jan-Feb;(122):210-21 [PMID 837611]

Jupiter JB, Fernandez DL. Comparative classification for fractures of the distal end of the radius. J Hand Surg Am. 1997;22(4):563-571. [PMID 9260608]

Fernandez DL, Jupiter JB. The Fracture of the Distal End of the Radius: An Historical Perspective. In: Fractures of the

Distal Radius: A Practical Approach to Management. Springer. 2002:1-21

Malgaigne J. A Treatise on Fractures. [Translated by John Packard] Philadelphia: Lippincott. 1859:53

Beals' Syndrome

Overview

Beals' syndrome is a rare bone dysplasia characterized by short stature, skeletal anomalies such as hypoplasia of the capitellum, broad shoulders, horizontal clavicles, and unique ear morphology with elongated attached lobules. The condition is also associated with limitation of elbow motion and, in some cases, limping. It affects both sexes and follows an autosomal dominant inheritance pattern, with considerable variability in expression among individuals.

Historical Background

- *Rodney Kenneth Beals*, an American orthopedist, first described the syndrome, identifying its distinct skeletal and physical features.
- Beals' observations highlighted the genetic basis of the condition, contributing to the understanding of heritable skeletal dysplasias and their clinical presentations.
- The syndrome remains an important example in orthopedic and genetic research, particularly for its autosomal dominant inheritance and unique skeletal characteristics.

Purpose

- **Diagnosis:** To identify Beals' syndrome based on its characteristic skeletal and physical anomalies, differentiating it from other bone dysplasias.
- **Management:** To address limitations in mobility and skeletal deformities, improving quality of life for affected

individuals.

- **Genetic Counseling:** To inform families about the autosomal dominant inheritance and recurrence risks in future offspring.

Procedure Overview

Diagnosis:

- **Clinical Examination:** Identification of hallmark features such as short stature, abnormal clavicle alignment, and unique ear morphology.
- **Imaging:** X-rays to evaluate hypoplasia of the capitellum, radial dislocation, and clavicular anomalies.
- **Genetic Testing:** Identification of mutations confirming autosomal dominant inheritance.

Treatment:

- **Orthopedic Management:** Addressing skeletal deformities, including radial dislocation and limitations in elbow mobility, through physical therapy or surgical intervention when necessary.
- **Mobility Support:** Providing braces or orthotic devices for individuals with limping or other gait abnormalities.
- **Follow-Up:** Regular monitoring of growth, joint function, and mobility to manage progressive symptoms.

Results and Interpretation

- **Physical Characteristics:** Short stature, broad shoulders, horizontal clavicles, and ear anomalies are consistent features.
- **Skeletal Anomalies:** Hypoplasia of the capitellum and limited elbow motion are common, but severity varies among individuals.
- **Prognosis:** Most individuals lead functional lives, although mobility issues may require ongoing management.

Physiological Basis

- **Bone Dysplasia:** Beals' syndrome results from mutations affecting bone growth and development, particularly in the upper limbs and shoulders.
- **Joint Abnormalities:** Hypoplasia of the capitellum and radial dislocation contribute to limited elbow motion and mobility challenges.
- **Morphological Features:** The distinctive ear shape and clavicular alignment are hallmark physical manifestations, reflecting developmental abnormalities.

Clinical Applications

- **Orthopedic Surgery:** Surgical intervention may be necessary for severe radial dislocation or other deformities affecting mobility and function.
- **Physical Therapy:** Targeted exercises can improve joint motion and alleviate mobility restrictions.
- **Genetic Counseling:** Assisting families in understanding inheritance patterns and planning for future pregnancies.

Limitations and Technical Considerations

- **Diagnostic Challenges:** Variability in symptom expression can complicate early diagnosis and differentiation from other skeletal dysplasias.

- **Management of Joint Limitations:** Elbow motion restriction and mobility issues may persist despite therapy, necessitating lifelong care.

- **Surgical Risks:** Interventions to correct skeletal deformities carry risks, including infection, joint stiffness, or incomplete correction.

Modern Relevance

- **Advances in** *genetic research* have improved the understanding of Beals' syndrome, enhancing diagnostic accuracy and family counseling.

- *Imaging technologies* allow for earlier and more detailed identification of skeletal anomalies, facilitating prompt intervention.

- The condition remains an important focus in studies of autosomal dominant skeletal dysplasias, providing insights into bone development and inheritance patterns.

Associated Conditions

- **Radial Dislocation:** A common feature, often associated with limited elbow motion.

- **Short Stature:** Reflects the underlying dysplasia, typically present from early childhood.

- **Mobility Challenges:** Limping and gait abnormalities are reported in some individuals, requiring orthopedic support.

Clinical Importance

- **Early Recognition:** Identifying Beals' syndrome early enables timely interventions, particularly for mobility and joint limitations.

- **Multidisciplinary Care:** Effective management requires collaboration among orthopedists, geneticists, and physical therapists.

- **Educational Value:** Beals' syndrome serves as an example of the variability and impact of autosomal dominant skeletal disorders, informing research and clinical practice.

References

R. K. Beals: Auriculo-osteodysplasia: A syndrome of multiple osseous dysplasia, ear anomaly, and short stature. Journal of Bone and Joint Surgery, Boston, 1967, 49: 1541-1550.

Béclard's Core of Bone

Overview

Béclard's core of bone refers to the ossification center of the distal epiphysis of the femur, an important developmental landmark in the human skeletal system. This ossification core is particularly significant in forensic medicine as it aids in determining the age or developmental stage of a fetus or infant, especially in cases where skeletal age assessment is required. It serves as a critical indicator of normal or delayed skeletal maturation.

Historical Background

- Named after *Pierre Augustin Béclard*, a renowned French anatomist and surgeon of the 19th century, who made significant contributions to the study of human anatomy and developmental biology.
- Béclard's observations highlighted the role of ossification centers in the growth and development of bones, particularly the femur.
- His work laid the foundation for the use of skeletal ossification patterns in both clinical and forensic settings, emphasizing the core's importance in age estimation.

Purpose

- **Forensic Applications:** To estimate the age of a fetus or infant by examining the ossification center of the distal femoral epiphysis.
- **Developmental Assessment:** To evaluate skeletal maturation and identify abnormalities in bone growth or delayed development.
- **Research:** To study the timeline and process of ossification in human skeletal development.

Procedure Overview

Examination in Forensic or Clinical Contexts:

- **Radiographic Imaging:** X-rays or ultrasound are used to identify the presence, size, and development of Béclard's core.
- **Skeletal Analysis:** In forensic cases, the distal femoral ossification core is analyzed in skeletal remains or fetuses.
- **Correlation with Developmental Age:** The size and presence of the ossification center are compared to established age-based standards to estimate the developmental stage.
- **Interpretation:** Determining whether the ossification corresponds to the expected age, indicating normal or delayed skeletal growth.

Results and Interpretation

- **Developmental Milestones:** Béclard's core typically appears between 32 and 36 weeks of gestation, making it a reliable marker for late fetal development.
- **Forensic Utility:** The ossification core can accurately estimate gestational age or infant age in forensic cases.
- **Clinical Relevance:** Deviations from the normal development timeline may indicate skeletal disorders, growth delays, or other congenital abnormalities.

Physiological Basis

- **Bone Ossification:** Ossification begins in the distal femoral epiphysis during late gestation as part of endochondral bone formation, where cartilage is replaced by bone tissue.
- **Growth Plate Role:** The presence and size of the ossification center are critical markers of skeletal maturity and the activity of the growth plate.
- **Developmental Indicators:** The timing and progression of Béclard's core development correlate closely with the overall maturation of the fetal skeleton.

Clinical Applications

- **Forensic Medicine:** Used to determine the age of skeletal remains in medico-legal cases involving fetuses or infants.
- **Pediatrics and Neonatology:** Assessment of skeletal age in preterm infants or those with suspected growth abnormalities.
- **Developmental Biology:** A key marker in studying the progression of skeletal development and bone maturation.

Limitations and Technical Considerations

- **Variability in Development:** The timing of ossification can vary slightly between individuals, potentially complicating age estimation in borderline cases.
- **Imaging Challenges:** Small ossification centers in early stages may be difficult to visualize, requiring advanced imaging techniques.
- **Differential Diagnosis:** Delayed or absent ossification must be differentiated from congenital or metabolic disorders affecting skeletal development.

Modern Relevance

- **Advances in** *imaging modalities*, such as high-resolution ultrasound and MRI, have improved the detection and measurement of Béclard's core, enhancing accuracy in age estimation.
- The ossification center remains an essential tool in forensic investigations, particularly in identifying remains or estimating gestational age in legal cases.
- Continued research in *skeletal biology* provides deeper insights into the factors influencing ossification and its role in diagnosing developmental disorders.

Associated Conditions

- **Delayed Ossification:** May occur in conditions such as rickets, osteogenesis imperfecta, or intrauterine growth restriction (IUGR).
- **Skeletal Dysplasias:** Congenital disorders affecting bone growth may alter the appearance or development of Béclard's core.
- **Growth Plate Disorders:** Conditions such as epiphyseal dysplasia can impact the ossification process.

Clinical Importance

- **Forensic Significance:** Béclard's core is a critical marker for estimating fetal and infant age, aiding in legal and investigative processes.
- **Developmental Monitoring:** Its presence and progression provide valuable information about skeletal maturity

and overall growth.

- **Diagnostic Marker:** Identifying abnormalities in the development of Béclard's core can lead to early intervention for skeletal disorders or growth delays.

Beemer's Syndrome

Overview

Beemer's syndrome is a rare congenital skeletal dysplasia characterized by dwarfism, hydrops fetalis, median cleft of the upper lip, bulbous nose, broad nasal bridge, narrow chest, protuberant abdomen, and short, bowed limbs. Additional anomalies include brachydactyly, malformed ears, omphalocele, ambiguous genitalia, intestinal malrotation, and congenital heart defects such as a double-outlet right ventricle. The condition follows an autosomal recessive inheritance pattern, and its etiology remains unknown. The syndrome was first described in two unrelated infants who succumbed shortly after birth.

Historical Background

- *Frederikus Antonius Beemer*, a Dutch geneticist, described this syndrome, noting its constellation of severe congenital abnormalities and its fatal outcome in the neonatal period.
- The initial reports highlighted the syndrome's genetic basis, emphasizing its rarity and the challenges in diagnosing and managing affected infants.
- Since its identification, Beemer's syndrome has remained an enigmatic condition with only a few reported cases, limiting the understanding of its pathophysiology.

Purpose

- **Clinical Recognition:** To identify Beemer's syndrome based on its distinct combination of craniofacial, skeletal, and systemic anomalies.
- **Genetic Counseling:** To inform families about the autosomal recessive inheritance and recurrence risks in subsequent pregnancies.
- **Research:** To investigate the genetic and molecular basis of the syndrome for improved diagnosis and potential interventions.

Procedure Overview

Diagnosis:

- **Prenatal Ultrasound:** Detects features such as hydrops, narrow chest, omphalocele, and bowed limbs during fetal development.
- **Postnatal Examination:** Identification of craniofacial anomalies (cleft lip, bulbous nose), skeletal abnormalities, and systemic defects.
- **Imaging and Tests:** X-rays for skeletal dysplasia, echocardiography for cardiac defects, and abdominal imaging for intestinal malrotation.
- **Genetic Testing:** Analysis to confirm autosomal recessive inheritance and identify potential causative mutations.

Management:

- **Supportive Care:** Neonatal resuscitation and management of severe anomalies, such as omphalocele and cardiac defects, during the immediate postnatal period.
- **Palliative Measures:** In cases with poor prognosis, focus shifts to comfort care and family support.

Results and Interpretation

- **Physical Anomalies:** The combination of craniofacial, skeletal, and systemic abnormalities is diagnostic of Beemer's syndrome.
- **Prognosis:** The condition is typically fatal shortly after birth due to the severity of associated anomalies, including cardiac defects and respiratory compromise.
- **Diagnostic Challenges:** Rare occurrence and overlapping features with other syndromes make diagnosis complex without comprehensive evaluation.

Physiological Basis

- **Skeletal Dysplasia:** Short stature and bowed limbs result from abnormal bone development and growth plate dysfunction.
- **Cardiac and Systemic Defects:** The double-outlet right ventricle leads to cyanosis and circulatory compromise, contributing to the poor prognosis.
- **Multisystem Involvement:** The constellation of anomalies reflects disruptions in early embryonic development affecting multiple organ systems.

Clinical Applications

- **Prenatal Diagnosis:** Early detection of Beemer's syndrome through detailed fetal ultrasound enables informed decision-making and genetic counseling.
- **Neonatal Care:** Immediate interventions for life-threatening anomalies, though the prognosis remains grim in most cases.

- **Genetic Counseling:** Essential for families with affected children to understand inheritance patterns and recurrence risks.

Limitations and Technical Considerations

- **Diagnostic Limitations:** The syndrome's rarity and similarity to other conditions complicate early and definitive diagnosis.
- **Management Challenges:** The severe nature of the anomalies limits therapeutic options, often requiring a palliative approach.
- **Genetic Insights:** The lack of identified causative mutations impedes targeted research and potential therapeutic developments.

Modern Relevance

- **Advances in** *genomic technologies*, such as whole-exome sequencing, offer hope for identifying the genetic basis of Beemer's syndrome.
- Improved *prenatal imaging techniques* allow for earlier detection of fetal anomalies associated with the syndrome.
- Research into similar syndromes and skeletal dysplasias contributes to understanding the broader spectrum of congenital disorders.

Associated Conditions

- **Hydrops Fetalis:** Common in Beemer's syndrome and a marker of poor prognosis due to widespread edema.
- **Omphalocele:** A congenital abdominal wall defect frequently observed in affected infants.
- **Congenital Heart Defects:** Including double-outlet right ventricle, significantly impacting survival.
- **Intestinal Malrotation:** A common gastrointestinal anomaly in the syndrome, complicating neonatal care.

Clinical Importance

- **Early Recognition:** Timely diagnosis through prenatal imaging and postnatal assessment is critical for appropriate family counseling.
- **Multidisciplinary Care:** Managing Beemer's syndrome requires a collaborative approach involving neonatologists, geneticists, and surgeons.
- **Research Potential:** Understanding Beemer's syndrome provides insights into the mechanisms of skeletal dysplasias and multisystem developmental disorders.

References

F. A. Beemer, L. O. Langer, J. M. Klep-de-Pater, A. M. Hemmes, J. B. Bylsma, R. M. Pauli, T. L. Myers, C. C. Haw: A new short rib syndrome: report of two cases. American Journal of Medical Genetics, New York, 1983, 14: 115-123.

L. O. Langer is the U. S. radiologist Leonard O. Langer, born 1928. He is eponymously associated with Langer's mesomelic dwarfism, and Langer's syndrome (Léri-Weill syndrome).

F. Beemer, I. Ertbruggen: Peculiar facial appearance, hydrocephalus, double-outlet right ventricle, genital anomalies and dense bones with lethaloutcome. American Journal of Medical Genetics, New York, 1984, 19: 391-394.

Bennett Fracture

Overview

The Bennett fracture, also known as Bennett fracture-dislocation, is an intra-articular two-part fracture involving the base of the first metacarpal. It occurs at the carpometacarpal (CMC) joint of the thumb and is typically caused by forced abduction of the first metacarpal, such as during a fall or high-impact trauma to the thumb. The fracture is characterized by an oblique fracture line and dislocation or subluxation of the metacarpal, leading to thumb instability.

Historical Background

- Named after *Edward Hallaran Bennett*, an Irish surgeon who first described the fracture in detail in 1880, focusing on its mechanics and treatment challenges.
- During his presentation, *Sir William Stokes* proposed that the fracture be named in honor of Bennett due to his significant contributions to the understanding of this injury.
- The injury is distinct from the *Rolando fracture*, a more complex comminuted fracture of the first metacarpal base, also associated with the thumb but with a poorer prognosis.

Purpose

- **Restoration of Thumb Function:** To stabilize the first metacarpal and restore normal motion and strength in the thumb, essential for grip and fine motor tasks.
- **Prevention of Long-Term Complications:** To avoid post-traumatic arthritis, persistent instability, and deformity of the CMC joint.
- **Anatomical Reduction:** To achieve proper alignment of the fracture and maintain joint congruency.

Procedure Overview

Diagnosis:

- **Clinical Examination:** Observation of pain, swelling, deformity, and limited motion at the base of the thumb.
- **Imaging:** X-rays confirm the fracture and subluxation. A lateral and oblique view helps evaluate the extent of the intra-articular involvement and displacement.

Treatment:

- **Non-Surgical Management:** For minimally displaced fractures, closed reduction followed by immobilization with a thumb spica cast may suffice.

Surgical Intervention:

- **Closed Reduction and Percutaneous Pinning:** Pins are used to stabilize the fracture fragment and metacarpal.
- **Open Reduction and Internal Fixation (ORIF):** Necessary for severely displaced or unstable fractures to restore alignment and stability.
- **Rehabilitation:** Following immobilization or surgery, physical therapy is critical for regaining motion and strength.

Results and Interpretation

- **Short-Term Outcomes:** With proper treatment, most patients regain functional use of the thumb.
- **Complications:** Delayed or improper

treatment may result in persistent instability, deformity, or arthritis of the CMC joint.

- **Prognosis:** Surgical repair generally leads to better outcomes, particularly in unstable fractures.

Physiological Basis

- **Mechanism of Injury:** Forced abduction of the first metacarpal applies stress to the CMC joint, causing the oblique fracture.
- **Instability:** The strong pull of the abductor pollicis longus tendon causes displacement of the metacarpal shaft, resulting in subluxation or dislocation.
- **Thumb Function:** The CMC joint is crucial for thumb opposition, grasp, and dexterity, making stabilization of this fracture essential.

Clinical Applications

- **Orthopedic Management:** Bennett fractures are a common injury in sports or trauma involving high-impact forces to the hand.
- **Hand Surgery:** Surgical intervention ensures joint stability and prevents deformity in cases of displacement.
- **Rehabilitation:** Post-treatment therapy focuses on regaining mobility and preventing stiffness.

Limitations and Technical Considerations

- **Challenges in Non-Surgical Management:** Closed reduction is often inadequate due to the strong pull of the abductor pollicis longus, necessitating surgical intervention.
- **Surgical Risks:** Complications such as infection, nerve damage, or hardware failure can arise from surgical fixation.
- **Long-Term Outcomes:** Even with treatment, some patients may develop post-traumatic arthritis in the CMC joint.

Modern Relevance

- **Advances in** *imaging techniques* and surgical tools have improved the accuracy of diagnosis and treatment.
- *Minimally invasive techniques*, such as percutaneous pinning, reduce recovery time and complications compared to traditional open surgery.
- Emphasis on *early rehabilitation* has improved functional outcomes for patients recovering from Bennett fractures.

Associated Conditions

- **Rolando Fracture:** A comminuted intra-articular fracture of the base of the first metacarpal, more complex than the Bennett fracture.
- **CMC Joint Arthritis:** A potential long-term complication resulting from untreated or improperly managed Bennett fractures.
- **Thumb Instability:** Chronic instability may occur without proper anatomical reduction and fixation.

Clinical Importance

- **Critical for Thumb Function:** The injury affects the CMC joint, which is essential for thumb opposition and grip strength.
- **Prompt Diagnosis and Treatment:**

Early intervention prevents complications like arthritis, deformity, and loss of thumb function.

- **Legacy in Orthopedics:** Bennett's contributions continue to influence the diagnosis and management of thumb injuries, ensuring better outcomes for patients.

References

Bennett EH. Fractures of the metacarpal bones. Dublin J Med Sci 1882;73:72-75

Bennett EH. On fracture of the metacarpal bone of the thumb. Br Med J 1886;2:12-13 [PMC2257374]

Bennett EH. Report of a Meeting of the Royal Academy of Medicine in Ireland 14 May 1897. Br Med J 1897;1:1479

Blount Staple

Overview

The Blount staple is a surgical technique used to correct limb length discrepancies by temporarily inhibiting bone growth at the epiphyseal plates. Metal staples are strategically placed around the epiphyseal disks of the tibia or other long bones, allowing controlled growth modification. This method provides an effective way to manage discrepancies in lower extremity length by permitting subsequent correction as the staples can be removed once the desired growth is achieved.

Historical Background

- The technique is named after *Walter Putnam Blount*, an American orthopedic surgeon, who pioneered the use of metallic staples for temporary epiphyseal growth inhibition.

- Before Blount's innovation, growth inhibition methods were largely permanent, such as epiphyseodesis, which irreversibly fused the growth plates. Blount's method offered a *reversible solution*, improving outcomes and reducing the need for complex corrective surgeries.

- Introduced in the mid-20th century, the *Blount staple* revolutionized the management of limb length discrepancies, becoming a cornerstone in pediatric orthopedics.

Purpose

- **Growth Modulation:** To temporarily inhibit growth at the epiphyseal plate of the longer limb, allowing the shorter limb to "catch up."

- **Correction of Limb Length Discrepancies:** To manage conditions like congenital limb inequality, post-traumatic growth disturbances, and idiopathic discrepancies.

- **Preservation of Future Options:** Unlike permanent growth-inhibiting methods, Blount staples allow for later removal and potential resumption of normal growth.

Procedure Overview

Preoperative Planning:

- **Imaging:** X-rays or CT scans are used to measure limb length discrepancies and identify the optimal placement for the staples.

- **Timing:** Surgery is typically performed in children or adolescents who have substantial growth potential remaining.

Surgical Technique:

- **Staple Placement:** Metal staples are inserted around the epiphyseal disk of the tibia or other affected bones.

- **Temporary Fixation:** The staples inhibit growth in the selected area, allowing the contralateral limb or untreated bone to equalize in length.

- **Postoperative Care:** Monitoring for staple position and bone growth progression is critical.

Follow-Up:

- **Staple Removal:** Once the desired correction is achieved, the staples are removed to allow normal growth to resume.

Results and Interpretation

- **Effective Growth Modulation:** Blount staples successfully induce temporary growth inhibition, enabling the correction of limb length discrepancies in growing children.

- **Reversibility:** Unlike permanent methods, the technique preserves the potential for normal growth after staple removal.

- **Prognosis:** Most patients achieve satisfactory correction with minimal complications if the procedure is performed and monitored properly.

Physiological Basis

- **Epiphyseal Growth Modulation:** Growth occurs at the epiphyseal plates, where cartilage is converted into bone. Staples disrupt this process temporarily by exerting mechanical pressure on the growth plate.

- **Equalization Mechanism:** By slowing growth in the longer limb, the untreated shorter limb continues to grow, gradually equalizing limb lengths.

- **Reversibility:** The staples do not cause permanent damage to the growth plate, allowing it to resume function once they are removed.

Clinical Applications

- **Pediatric Orthopedics:** Widely used in children with limb length discrepancies caused by congenital conditions, trauma, or disease.

- **Correction of Angular Deformities:** In some cases, Blount staples are also applied to manage angular deformities by selectively inhibiting growth on one side of a bone.

- **Growth-Dependent Treatments:** The method is particularly effective in patients with significant remaining growth potential.

Limitations and Technical Considerations

- **Timing Sensitivity:** The procedure must be carefully timed to coincide with periods of active growth, as delayed intervention may limit its effectiveness.
- **Monitoring Requirements:** Frequent follow-ups are necessary to monitor growth and ensure the staples are functioning as intended.
- **Complications:** Risks include staple migration, overcorrection, or incomplete correction if growth stops prematurely or the timing of removal is misjudged.

Modern Relevance

- **Advances in** *implant design* have improved the safety and efficacy of growth modulation techniques, with modern staples offering greater durability and reduced risk of migration.
- Blount staples are still widely used, but they have been supplemented by newer techniques like *eight-plate growth modulation*, which offer more flexibility in certain cases.
- The procedure remains a key option in managing pediatric limb discrepancies due to its reliability, reversibility, and cost-effectiveness.

Associated Conditions

- **Congenital Limb Length Discrepancies:** Conditions such as hemihypertrophy or fibular hemimelia often necessitate growth modulation.
- **Post-Traumatic Growth Disturbances:** Growth plate injuries can lead to asymmetric limb growth, correctable with Blount staples.
- **Angular Deformities:** In addition to length discrepancies, angular deformities like genu valgum or genu varum may benefit from similar growth modulation techniques.

Clinical Importance

- **Minimally Invasive Correction:** Blount staples offer a straightforward, reversible approach to managing limb discrepancies, avoiding the need for more invasive or permanent solutions.
- **Preservation of Growth Potential:** By maintaining the integrity of the growth plate, the procedure allows for natural growth after correction.
- **Advancing Pediatric Orthopedics:** The technique has paved the way for modern growth modulation methods, contributing significantly to the treatment of skeletal abnormalities in children.

References

W. P. Blount, George R. Clarke: Control of bone growth by epiphyseal stapling: A preliminary report. Journal of Bone and Joint Surgery, Boston, 1949, 31-A: 464-478.

Blount's Splint

Overview

Blount's splint is a specialized orthopedic device used for the fixation of bone ends following osteotomies, providing stability and promoting proper alignment during the healing process. It is commonly employed to manage fractures and deformities of long bones, particularly in pediatric patients. The splint is designed to maintain immobilization while allowing some degree of functional movement, depending on the location and purpose of the osteotomy.

Historical Background

- Named after *Walter Putnam Blount*, an influential American orthopedic surgeon, who contributed extensively to the development of treatments for skeletal deformities and injuries.
- Blount's innovations emphasized practical, durable, and adjustable solutions for managing bone fractures and post-surgical fixation.
- The splint represents an evolution in orthopedic care, improving outcomes by stabilizing bones while accommodating natural growth and healing.

Purpose

- **Stabilization:** To ensure proper alignment and immobilization of bone ends after osteotomies or corrective procedures.
- **Facilitation of Healing:** By maintaining the correct positioning, the splint supports bone healing and reduces the risk of complications such as malunion or nonunion.
- **Adjustability:** To provide flexibility for postoperative adjustments without compromising stability, particularly important in pediatric cases.

Procedure Overview

- **Application:** The splint is fitted immediately following the osteotomy or corrective surgery to stabilize the bone ends.
- Customization ensures proper alignment of the bone segments while accommodating the patient's anatomy and specific surgical outcomes.
- **Adjustment and Monitoring:** Regular follow-up visits are necessary to adjust the splint as required, ensuring it continues to provide optimal support throughout the healing period.
- **Removal:** The splint is removed once sufficient bone healing has occurred, allowing for progression to physical therapy or other rehabilitation strategies.

Results and Interpretation

- **Enhanced Healing:** The controlled immobilization provided by the splint facilitates effective bone regeneration and alignment.
- **Improved Outcomes:** Proper splint application reduces the risks of malalignment and postoperative complications.
- **Patient-Specific Benefits:** The splint's design allows for adjustments to accommodate growth or changing needs during the recovery period.

Physiological Basis

- **Bone Healing:** Following an osteotomy, the splint stabilizes the bone ends to enable the natural healing processes of callus formation and bone remodeling.
- **Joint Preservation:** Proper immobilization ensures that nearby joints remain aligned and functional during and after the healing process.
- **Load Distribution:** The splint distributes mechanical forces evenly, preventing excessive stress on the healing bone.

Clinical Applications

- **Post-Osteotomy Management:** Commonly used following surgical procedures to correct bone deformities or length discrepancies.
- **Fracture Fixation:** Provides stability for fractures that require precise alignment, especially in pediatric patients.
- **Growth-Related Adjustments:** Particularly useful in children, where the splint can be adjusted to accommodate ongoing growth during recovery.

Limitations and Technical Considerations

- **Skill-Dependent Application:** Proper fitting and adjustment require experienced practitioners to avoid complications such as pressure sores or misalignment.
- **Restricted Mobility:** Although functional splints allow some movement, prolonged use can lead to stiffness or muscle atrophy if not complemented with rehabilitation.
- **Monitoring Requirements:** Regular follow-ups are essential to ensure the splint maintains proper alignment and support throughout the healing process.

Modern Relevance

- **Advances in** *splint materials and design* have improved the comfort and effectiveness of devices like Blount's splint, making them lighter and more adaptable.
- The splint remains widely used, particularly in *pediatric orthopedic surgery*, where its adjustability is critical for growing bones.
- Its role has evolved alongside new technologies, such as 3D imaging and custom-molded splints, to enhance precision and patient outcomes.

Associated Conditions

- **Tibial Osteotomies:** Commonly used in corrective procedures for conditions like Blount's disease or other angular deformities of the tibia.
- **Fractures Requiring External Stabilization:** Ideal for complex fractures where internal fixation may not be suitable or where temporary immobilization is needed.
- **Growth Plate Disorders:** Applied in cases where surgical intervention affects the epiphyseal plates, requiring controlled immobilization.

Clinical Importance

- **Enhanced Recovery:** Blount's splint supports a controlled and effective healing process, minimizing complications.
- **Pediatric Adaptability:** Its adjustability makes it particularly valuable in children, where growth and bone remod-

eling are critical factors.

- **Historical and Practical Significance:** Blount's splint represents a milestone in orthopedic innovation, bridging traditional methods and modern surgical care to ensure better outcomes for patients with skeletal injuries or deformities.

Bosworth Fracture

Overview

A Bosworth fracture, first described by David Marsh Bosworth in 1947, is a rare injury involving a fracture of the distal fibula with a fixed posterior dislocation of the proximal fibular fragment. The proximal fragment becomes trapped behind the posterior tibial tubercle, causing significant instability and mechanical obstruction to reduction. This injury represents a variation of the entrapment mechanism described by Ashhurst and Bromer in 1922, which involved the displacement of an intact fibula.

Historical Background

- *David Marsh Bosworth* provided the first detailed account of this fracture-dislocation, emphasizing its unique pathophysiology and challenges in management.
- Earlier, in *1922, Ashhurst and Bromer* described the entrapment of an intact fibula behind the tibia, setting the stage for understanding variations of fibular entrapment injuries.
- The Bosworth fracture gained recognition for its rarity and complexity, requiring advanced imaging and precise surgical techniques for effective treatment.

Purpose

- **Stabilization of the Ankle Joint:** To restore normal alignment of the fibula and tibia, ensuring functional stability of the ankle.
- **Reduction of Dislocation:** To free

the proximal fibular fragment from its entrapment behind the posterior tibial tubercle.

- **Prevention of Long-Term Complications:** To avoid joint instability, chronic pain, and post-traumatic arthritis associated with untreated or mismanaged injuries.

Procedure Overview

Diagnosis:

- **Clinical Assessment:** Presentation includes severe pain, swelling, deformity, and an inability to bear weight on the affected limb.

- **Imaging:** X-rays often reveal the fracture and dislocation. CT scans provide a more detailed view of the trapped fibular fragment and associated joint injuries.

Treatment:

- **Closed Reduction:** Initial attempts to reduce the dislocation are often unsuccessful due to mechanical entrapment.

Surgical Intervention:

- **Open Reduction and Internal Fixation (ORIF):** A common approach involving the release of the fibular fragment, reduction of the dislocation, and stabilization of the fracture with plates or screws.

- **Soft Tissue Repair:** Addressing ligamentous injuries to restore overall joint stability.

- **Postoperative Care:** Immobilization in a cast or brace followed by gradual weight-bearing and physical therapy.

Results and Interpretation

- **Reduction and Stabilization:** Surgical management typically restores proper alignment and function of the ankle joint.

- **Prognosis:** Outcomes are favorable with timely diagnosis and appropriate treatment, though recovery may take months.

- **Complications:** Delayed or inadequate treatment can lead to chronic instability, deformity, and post-traumatic arthritis.

Physiological Basis

- **Entrapment Mechanism:** The proximal fibular fragment is displaced posteriorly and becomes wedged behind the posterior tibial tubercle, preventing natural reduction.

- **Ankle Instability:** The fracture and dislocation disrupt the syndesmotic and lateral ligamentous structures, impairing joint stability.

- **Mechanical Block:** The trapped fibular fragment acts as a physical barrier, necessitating surgical release for successful reduction.

Clinical Applications

- **Orthopedic Trauma Management:** The Bosworth fracture exemplifies the need for specialized techniques to manage rare but complex ankle injuries.

- **Surgical Expertise:** Successful treatment requires skilled surgical intervention, particularly for releasing the fibular fragment and stabilizing the joint.

- **Rehabilitation:** Postoperative therapy focuses on restoring mobility, strength, and preventing stiffness.

Limitations and Technical Considerations

- **Diagnostic Challenges:** Initial imaging may fail to identify the fibular entrapment, necessitating advanced modalities like CT scans for confirmation.
- **Surgical Complexity:** The entrapment often requires meticulous dissection and release, increasing the difficulty and duration of surgery.
- **Postoperative Risks:** Risks include infection, hardware-related issues, or incomplete recovery of joint function.

Modern Relevance

- **Advances in** *imaging technologies* and *surgical techniques* have improved the diagnosis and treatment of Bosworth fractures, reducing complication rates.
- The injury serves as a model for understanding complex ankle trauma and the importance of early, accurate intervention.
- Ongoing research in *biomechanics* and *implant technology* continues to enhance outcomes for patients with similar high-energy injuries.

Associated Conditions

- **Ashhurst-Bromer Injury:** Entrapment of an intact fibula behind the tibia, a precursor to the understanding of Bosworth fractures.
- **Syndesmotic Injuries:** Commonly associated with Bosworth fractures, requiring concurrent management for joint stability.
- **Post-Traumatic Arthritis:** A potential long-term complication if the joint surfaces are not adequately restored.

Clinical Importance

- **Complex Injury Pattern:** The Bosworth fracture highlights the challenges of managing high-energy trauma to the ankle, requiring advanced diagnostic and surgical skills.
- **Timely Intervention:** Early recognition and treatment are critical to preventing long-term disability and ensuring optimal recovery.
- **Educational Significance:** The fracture is frequently discussed in orthopedic education as an example of rare but severe ankle trauma requiring specialized care.

References

ASHHURST APC, BROMER RS. CLASSIFICATION AND MECHANISM OF FRACTURES OF THE LEG BONES INVOLVING THE ANKLE: BASED ON A STUDY OF THREE HUNDRED CASES FROM THE EPISCOPAL HOSPITAL. Arch Surg 1922; 4: 51.

BOSWORTH DM. Fracture-dislocation of the ankle with fixed displacement of the fibula behind the tibia. J Bone Joint Surg Am 1947; 29: 130–5.

Bosworth DM. Fracture-dislocation of the ankle with fixed displacement of the fibula behind the tibia. J Bone Joint Surg Am. 1947 Jan;29(1):130-5. [PMID 20284692]

Yeoh CSN, Tan GMJ. Bosworth fracture-dislocation of the ankle: a case report. Journal of Orthopaedic Surgery 2013;21(2):249-52

Silverio A et al. Bosworth Ankle Fracture-Dislocation. The Orthopod

Boxer's Fracture

Overview

Boxer's Fracture refers to a fracture of the 5th metacarpal bone of the hand, near the knuckle, though it can occasionally include the 4th metacarpal. It is a common injury, especially among individuals who strike an object with a closed fist. Symptoms include pain, swelling, and a depressed or misaligned knuckle, often accompanied by bruising and limited finger movement. These fractures constitute about 20% of hand fractures, primarily affecting males.

Historical Background

- The colloquial term *"Boxer's Fracture"* emerged from the association of this injury with inexperienced fighters or individuals punching improperly.
- Early medical references emphasized its differentiation from other metacarpal fractures, such as *"bar room fractures"*, which involve the 4th and 5th metacarpals. Over time, the distinction has blurred, and many clinicians use "Boxer's Fracture" to describe fractures of any metacarpal bone resulting from punching injuries.

Purpose

- To identify and manage fractures of the metacarpal bones, particularly those caused by blunt trauma to the hand.
- Ensure proper alignment and stabilization to restore hand function and prevent long-term deformities or complications.

Procedure Overview

- **Clinical Examination:** Symptoms such as swelling, pain, and a depressed knuckle guide initial suspicion.
- The injured hand is assessed for misalignment, tenderness, and functional impairment.
- **Imaging:** X-rays are the primary diagnostic tool to confirm the fracture and evaluate its angulation or displacement.
- In rare cases, CT scans may be used for detailed evaluation.
- **Management:**
- **Conservative Treatment:** Buddy taping and tensor bandaging are effective for fractures with <70° angulation.
- **Reduction and Splinting:** Recommended for fractures with >70° angulation or rotational deformities.
- **Surgical Intervention:** Indicated for severe deformities or open fractures.
- **Rehabilitation:** Physical therapy is often initiated after stabilization to restore strength, motion, and dexterity.

Results and Interpretation

- **Short-Term Outcomes:** Most patients experience pain relief and functional improvement within weeks with appropriate treatment.
- **Long-Term Outcomes:** Residual knuckle deformities are common but rarely impair function significantly.
- **Physiological Basis:**
- The *4th and 5th metacarpals* are less robust than the 2nd and 3rd, making

them prone to fractures during improper punching.

- Misalignment during impact creates dorsal bending forces, leading to fractures when the bone exceeds its stress tolerance.

Clinical Applications

- **Orthopedic Management:** Treatment focuses on restoring alignment and preventing complications like stiffness or malunion.
- **Prevention:** Education on proper punching techniques can reduce incidence.
- **Rehabilitation:** Focused physiotherapy ensures recovery of hand function.

Limitations and Technical Considerations

- **High-Angulation Fractures:** Require careful reduction and stabilization to avoid chronic deformity or dysfunction.
- **Delayed Diagnosis:** Misdiagnosis as a simple hand sprain can lead to complications.
- **Surgical Complexity:** Severe comminution or open fractures may necessitate advanced surgical intervention.

Modern Relevance

- **Improved Treatment Protocols:** Advances in imaging and fixation techniques have optimized outcomes for these injuries.
- **Awareness Campaigns:** Increased emphasis on hand protection in sports and occupational safety has reduced prevalence.
- **Technological Aids:** Portable imaging devices and telemedicine consultations enable rapid diagnosis in remote settings.

Associated Conditions

- **Bar Room Fractures:** Differentiated as fractures of the 4th and 5th metacarpals caused by improper punching.
- **Tendon Injuries:** Soft tissue damage around the fracture site is common.
- **Joint Dislocations:** Rare but possible in severe trauma cases.

Clinical Importance

- **Prevention of Long-Term Disability:** Prompt and appropriate treatment minimizes risks of malunion or chronic pain.
- **Restoration of Hand Function:** Ensures the individual can resume daily activities and, in some cases, professional or athletic pursuits.
- **Public Awareness:** Reinforces the importance of avoiding high-risk behavior, such as punching without proper training or protection.

A Boxer's Fracture exemplifies how an injury stemming from a seemingly common activity can pose significant challenges if improperly managed. Early diagnosis and adherence to treatment protocols are vital for optimal recovery.

Brodie's Abscess

Overview

Brodie's abscess is a chronic metaphyseal abscess that presents as a pus-filled cavity within a bone, surrounded by a wall of dense fibrous tissue. It typically occurs in the metaphyses of long bones, such as the tibia, and is often asymptomatic for years before manifesting as intermittent pain or localized discomfort. The abscess contains necrotic debris, inflammatory cells, and sometimes bacteria, which may lead to osteomyelitis if untreated. The term initially referred to a tuberculous abscess of the tibial head but is now associated with various bacterial infections.

Historical Background

- Named after *Sir Benjamin Collins Brodie*, a British surgeon and pathologist, who first described the condition in a 24-year-old patient in the 19th century.
- Brodie's landmark case involved a chronic abscess in the tibia. He proposed *trephination* (surgical removal of bone tissue) as an alternative to amputation, which was the prevailing treatment of the time.
- His work contributed significantly to the understanding of *chronic osteomyelitis* and its management, emphasizing the need for early diagnosis and intervention to preserve the limb.

Purpose

- **Diagnosis:** To identify and differentiate Brodie's abscess from other conditions like tumors or cysts that may present with similar radiographic features.
- **Prevention of Osteomyelitis:** To manage the abscess effectively before it leads to more severe infections or systemic complications.
- **Limb Preservation:** To treat the condition with minimally invasive techniques, avoiding aggressive procedures like amputation.

Procedure Overview

Diagnosis:

- **Clinical Examination:** Patients often present with intermittent pain near the end of a long bone, localized tenderness, and occasional low-grade fever.
- **Imaging:** X-rays typically show a well-defined radiolucent lesion surrounded by sclerotic bone. MRI or CT scans provide better visualization of the abscess cavity and surrounding tissue.
- **Biopsy:** Confirmatory testing involves sampling the abscess content to identify the presence of bacteria or necrotic material.

Treatment:

Surgical Management:

- **Curettage:** The abscess cavity is surgically opened and cleared of pus and necrotic material.
- **Debridement:** In cases with significant infection or osteomyelitis, extensive cleaning of infected bone is performed.
- **Antibiotic Therapy:** Broad-spectrum antibiotics are started, often tailored after bacterial culture results.
- **Follow-Up:** Regular imaging and clinical assessments ensure the resolution of the abscess and monitor for recurrence.

Results and Interpretation

- **Short-Term Outcomes:** Early surgical intervention combined with antibiotics typically resolves the infection and alleviates symptoms.
- **Prognosis:** Most cases have favorable outcomes if treated promptly. However, delayed diagnosis may lead to osteomyelitis or chronic bone damage.
- **Complications:** Inadequate treatment may result in persistent infection, pathological fractures, or systemic spread of bacteria.

Physiological Basis

- **Pathogenesis:** Brodie's abscess often results from a localized infection within the bone, caused by organisms like Staphylococcus aureus.
- **Immune Response:** The body attempts to contain the infection by forming a dense fibrous wall around the abscess, preventing systemic spread but creating a chronic reservoir for bacteria.
- **Chronic Pain and Inflammation:** Intermittent symptoms arise due to fluctuating bacterial activity and inflammatory responses in the surrounding bone.

Clinical Applications

- **Orthopedic Surgery:** Treating Brodie's abscess is a cornerstone of managing localized bone infections and preventing osteomyelitis.
- **Infectious Disease Management:** Antibiotic therapy plays a critical role in eradicating bacterial infections associated with the abscess.
- **Forensic and Diagnostic Imaging:** Identifying Brodie's abscess is important in differentiating it from malignancies or benign bone lesions in diagnostic evaluations.

Limitations and Technical Considerations

- **Diagnosis Challenges:** The asymptomatic nature of early-stage abscesses can delay detection, and imaging findings may mimic tumors or cysts.
- **Surgical Risks:** Curettage and debridement carry risks such as bone weakening, incomplete abscess removal, or reinfection.
- **Recurrence:** Insufficient treatment or incomplete antibiotic therapy may result in relapse, necessitating further intervention.

Modern Relevance

- **Advances in** *imaging modalities*, such as MRI, have improved early detection and differentiation of Brodie's abscess from other bone pathologies.
- Modern *antibiotic regimens* tailored to culture results have reduced the need for aggressive surgical interventions.
- The condition remains a key topic in the study of *chronic osteomyelitis* and localized bone infections, providing insights into their management.

Associated Conditions

- **Osteomyelitis:** Brodie's abscess often precedes or accompanies chronic bone infections if left untreated.
- **Tuberculous Bone Abscess:** Initially described in tuberculosis cases, the abscess may mimic other granulomatous diseases in imaging and pathology.

- **Pathological Fractures:** Weakened bone surrounding the abscess cavity increases the risk of fractures.

Clinical Importance

- **Early Diagnosis and Treatment:** Prompt intervention prevents the progression to osteomyelitis, systemic infection, or irreversible bone damage.
- **Multidisciplinary Approach:** Effective management requires collaboration between orthopedic surgeons, infectious disease specialists, and radiologists.
- **Historical Significance:** Brodie's abscess underscores the evolution of surgical and medical approaches to bone infections, bridging historical methods with modern innovations.

References

B. C. Brodie: An account of some cases of chronic abscess of the tibia. Medico-Chirurgical Transactions, London, 1832, 17: 239-249

Brodie's Knee

Overview

Brodie's knee refers to a condition characterized by chronic inflammation or hypertrophic synovitis of the knee joint, resulting in stiffness, swelling, and pain. Initially associated with hysterical patients in historical medical literature, the term now primarily describes a pathological condition involving chronic synovial thickening and inflammation in the knee. This condition can cause functional impairment and is distinct from acute inflammatory processes or mechanical knee injuries.

Historical Background

The condition was named after Sir Benjamin Collins Brodie, a 19th-century British surgeon and pathologist, who documented cases of stiff knees in patients presenting with psychological symptoms, initially attributing the condition to hysteria.

- **As understanding of joint pathology advanced, the term evolved to describe a more specific entity:** chronic hypertrophic synovitis, a persistent inflammation of the knee joint unrelated to psychological factors.
- Brodie's observations highlighted the interplay between physical and psychological health in the historical context of medical practice.

Purpose

- **Diagnosis:** To identify Brodie's knee as a form of chronic inflammation distinct from acute arthritis, traumatic injury, or other joint conditions.

- **Treatment Planning:** To address the chronic synovitis and improve knee function through medical or surgical interventions.
- **Functional Restoration:** To alleviate symptoms such as pain and stiffness, restoring mobility and quality of life.

Procedure Overview

Diagnosis:

- **Clinical Examination:** Key findings include joint swelling, limited range of motion, and tenderness.
- **Imaging:** X-rays and MRI are used to detect synovial thickening, effusion, or joint degeneration.
- **Arthroscopy:** Direct visualization of the joint may confirm hypertrophic synovitis and rule out other intra-articular pathologies.

Treatment:

- **Conservative Management:** Anti-inflammatory medications (NSAIDs) and corticosteroid injections to reduce inflammation.
- Physical therapy to restore range of motion and strengthen surrounding muscles.

Surgical Intervention:

- **Arthroscopic Synovectomy:** Removal of the inflamed synovial tissue for cases resistant to conservative treatment.
- **Open Surgery:** In rare cases, open synovectomy or joint reconstruction may be required.
- **Rehabilitation:** Post-treatment physiotherapy focuses on improving mobility, strength, and joint function.

Results and Interpretation

- **Improvement of Symptoms:** Conservative and surgical treatments effectively reduce pain and swelling, improving mobility.
- **Chronic Nature:** Without treatment, Brodie's knee may lead to progressive joint damage and functional limitations.
- **Prognosis:** With timely intervention, patients can achieve significant symptom relief and functional recovery.

Physiological Basis

- **Synovial Inflammation:** Chronic irritation of the synovium leads to hypertrophy, effusion, and joint stiffness.
- **Hypertrophic Changes:** Persistent inflammation results in thickening of the synovial membrane, impairing normal joint function.
- **Pain and Stiffness:** Inflammatory mediators and mechanical obstruction from hypertrophic tissue contribute to symptoms.

Clinical Applications

- **Orthopedic and Rheumatologic Care:** Brodie's knee serves as a diagnostic consideration in cases of chronic knee pain and stiffness not attributable to trauma or systemic inflammatory diseases.
- **Minimally Invasive Surgery:** Arthroscopy allows for targeted removal of hypertrophic synovium with minimal disruption to surrounding tissues.
- **Rehabilitation Medicine:** Comprehensive care involving physiotherapy

ensures optimal recovery of joint mobility and strength.

Limitations and Technical Considerations

- **Chronicity:** Late diagnosis or inadequate treatment may lead to irreversible joint damage or secondary osteoarthritis.
- **Differential Diagnosis:** Conditions such as rheumatoid arthritis, gout, or septic arthritis must be excluded before confirming Brodie's knee.
- **Surgical Risks:** Arthroscopic or open procedures carry risks of infection, stiffness, or incomplete symptom resolution.

Modern Relevance

- **Advances in** *imaging* and *arthroscopic techniques* have improved the diagnosis and treatment of Brodie's knee, minimizing recovery times and enhancing outcomes.
- The condition serves as a reminder of the importance of recognizing chronic inflammatory processes in joint pathology, distinct from acute or systemic disorders.
- Brodie's knee is now better understood in the context of *synovial pathologies*, shedding its historical association with hysteria.

Associated Conditions

- **Chronic Hypertrophic Synovitis:** The primary pathology underlying Brodie's knee, marked by persistent synovial inflammation and thickening.
- **Osteoarthritis:** Chronic synovitis may accelerate joint degeneration, leading to secondary osteoarthritis.
- **Joint Effusion:** Associated swelling and fluid accumulation in the knee joint.

Clinical Importance

- **Early Recognition:** Identifying Brodie's knee early enables prompt treatment, preventing joint deterioration and maintaining function.
- **Multidisciplinary Approach:** Collaboration between orthopedic surgeons, rheumatologists, and physical therapists ensures comprehensive care.
- **Historical and Clinical Significance:** The evolution of Brodie's knee from a psychosomatic association to a recognized chronic inflammatory condition underscores the progress in understanding joint pathology.

References

B. C. Brodie: Pathological researches respecting the diseases of the joints. Medico-Chirurgical Transactions, London, 1813, 4: 207-277.

Bryant's Triangle

Overview

Bryant's triangle is a hypothetical geometric construct used in clinical orthopedics to assess upward displacement of the trochanter in cases of suspected fractures of the neck of the femur or other hip deformities. It consists of three lines drawn on the body, forming a triangle, to measure displacement and identify deviations that suggest pathological conditions. This surgical marking is crucial in diagnosing femoral neck fractures and provides a straightforward method to detect abnormalities in alignment and bone positioning.

Historical Background

- Named after *Sir Thomas Bryant*, an eminent British surgeon of the 19th century, who developed the triangle to facilitate the *diagnosis of hip and femoral deformities.*
- Bryant's work emphasized the need for practical, visual tools in orthopedic diagnosis, making his triangle a foundational concept in clinical examination.
- The method has remained relevant over time due to its simplicity and effectiveness, particularly before the advent of advanced imaging technologies.

Purpose

- **Fracture Diagnosis:** To identify upward displacement of the femoral trochanter in suspected fractures of the neck of the femur.
- **Assessment of Deformities:** To detect deviations in bone alignment in various hip and pelvic conditions.
- **Surgical Planning:** To guide surgical intervention by accurately determining the extent and nature of the displacement.

Procedure Overview

Constructing the Triangle:

- **Line 1:** Drawn horizontally from the anterior superior iliac spine (ASIS) toward the body midline.
- **Line 2:** Drawn vertically from the greater trochanter to intersect the horizontal line at a right angle.
- **Line 3:** The hypotenuse, connecting the ASIS to the tip of the greater trochanter.
- **Analysis:** Normal alignment forms a predictable triangle.
- Any deviation in these lines suggests displacement of the femoral head or trochanter, indicative of fractures or other abnormalities.
- **Clinical Correlation:** The observations are combined with physical examination findings, such as limb shortening or external rotation, to confirm the diagnosis.

Results and Interpretation

- **Normal Alignment:** The triangle appears symmetric and proportional, ruling out significant displacement.
- **Pathological Deviations:** Upward displacement of the greater trochanter results in an asymmetrical triangle, strongly suggesting a femoral neck fracture or hip deformity.

- **Clinical Accuracy:** While simple and reliable, the method is often supplemented with imaging to confirm findings.

Physiological Basis

- **Anatomical Landmarks:** The ASIS and the greater trochanter serve as fixed bony points for constructing the triangle, reflecting changes in femoral positioning.
- **Femoral Neck Fractures:** These injuries result in the upward migration of the trochanter due to muscular traction, disrupting the geometric relationship of Bryant's triangle.
- **Biomechanical Insight:** The triangle highlights misalignment caused by fractures or dislocations, aiding in understanding the mechanical impact of these injuries.

Clinical Applications

- **Orthopedic Diagnosis:** Bryant's triangle remains a valuable tool in bedside assessment of hip injuries, particularly in resource-limited settings without access to imaging.
- **Pre-Surgical Evaluation:** Guides surgical decision-making by estimating the severity and direction of displacement.
- **Teaching and Training:** The concept is a fundamental part of medical education, emphasizing basic clinical diagnostic techniques.

Limitations and Technical Considerations

- **Subjectivity:** Accurate construction of the triangle depends on the examiner's skill, introducing potential variability.
- **Complementary Role:** While useful, Bryant's triangle should be used alongside imaging for a definitive diagnosis.
- **Restricted Applicability:** The method is less reliable in patients with atypical anatomy, such as obesity or congenital deformities.

Modern Relevance

- Though modern imaging modalities like *X-rays* and *MRI* have largely replaced clinical geometric constructs, Bryant's triangle retains its value in *preliminary assessments* and *clinical teaching*.
- It serves as a reminder of the importance of physical examination in diagnosing fractures and deformities, even in the era of advanced diagnostics.
- **Advances in** *3D imaging* and *computer modeling* can incorporate Bryant's triangle principles into surgical simulation and planning.

Associated Conditions

- **Femoral Neck Fractures:** The primary condition assessed using Bryant's triangle, characterized by displacement of the greater trochanter.
- **Hip Dislocations:** May also disrupt the geometry of the triangle due to misalignment of the femoral head and trochanter.
- **Pelvic Asymmetry:** Conditions causing asymmetry in pelvic landmarks can also alter the triangle's alignment.

Clinical Importance

- **Practical Diagnostic Tool:** Bryant's triangle offers a quick and non-invasive method for assessing hip and femoral injuries.

- **Educational Value:** Its simplicity makes it a fundamental concept in orthopedic training, demonstrating the integration of anatomy and clinical diagnosis.

- **Historical Significance:** The technique underscores the evolution of diagnostic methods in orthopedics, bridging traditional examination tools with modern imaging.

References

T. Bryant: Clinical lectures on the diagnostic value of the iliofemoral triangle in cases of injury to the hip-point, more particularly of impacted fracture. The Lancet, London, 1876, 1: 119-120.

Bucket Handle Fracture

Overview

Bucket Handle Fractures (also known as metaphyseal corner fractures or classical metaphyseal lesions, CML) are fractures of the metaphysis observed almost exclusively in children under the age of These fractures are highly suggestive of non-accidental injury (NAI), particularly in cases of child abuse. They occur due to shearing or whiplash forces applied to the immature bone during shaking or other traumatic manipulations.

Historical Background

- **Early Identification:** The term and recognition of metaphyseal corner fractures emerged in the context of child abuse diagnostics.

- Over time, the link between these fractures and *non-accidental injury* was highlighted through studies in pediatric trauma radiology.

- Modern understanding incorporates biomechanics and forensic investigation into the causative mechanisms of these injuries.

Purpose

- **Primary Objective:** To diagnose metaphyseal fractures accurately and distinguish between accidental and non-accidental causes.

- **Forensic Application:** Used as a critical indicator in suspected cases of child abuse to protect vulnerable children.

- **Treatment and Management:** Ensuring appropriate care for affected children while identifying and mitigating further risks.

Procedure Overview

- **Clinical Assessment:** Examination for tenderness, swelling, or bruising, though external symptoms may be minimal.
- Detailed history-taking to identify potential inconsistencies or concerns about trauma mechanisms.
- **Imaging Studies:**
- **X-rays:** The primary tool to identify radiolucent areas perpendicular to the bone axis and fractures across the metaphysis.
- **Scintigraphy:** Can detect abnormal technetium-99m uptake, though increased uptake may also be physiological in young children.
- **MRI or CT scans:** Useful for identifying subtle fractures and related injuries.
- **Diagnosis:** Requires correlation between clinical findings, imaging results, and context of trauma.

Results and Interpretation

- **Radiographic Findings:** Bucket handle fractures appear as radiolucent bands at the metaphysis, often perpendicular to the bone axis.
- **Confirmation:** Evidence of incomplete or complete fractures with minimal external symptoms supports the diagnosis.
- **Challenges:** Distinguishing fractures from normal developmental variants can be difficult.

Physiological Basis

The metaphysis is a growth plate consisting of immature, mineralized cartilage, which is structurally vulnerable to shearing forces.

- **Biomechanics:** Repeated microfractures occur when forces such as shaking or twisting create perpendicular stress on the metaphysis.
- **Developmental Context:** This type of injury is specific to young children due to the fragility of their developing skeletal structures.

Clinical Applications

- **Child Abuse Diagnostics:** A critical marker in determining non-accidental trauma.
- **Differentiation:** Helps in distinguishing between accidental fractures and abuse-related injuries.
- **Multidisciplinary Care:** Requires collaboration between radiologists, pediatricians, and social services.

Limitations and Technical Considerations

- **Subtle Presentation:** Bucket handle fractures are often occult, with minimal external clinical symptoms.
- **Diagnostic Challenges:** Differentiating true fractures from normal anatomical variants.
- Accurately dating the fracture due to a lack of callus formation.
- **Legal Implications:** Diagnosis carries significant weight in legal and social contexts, requiring rigorous investigation and evidence.

Modern Relevance

- **Improved Forensic Analysis:** Advances in imaging technology and forensic radiology have enhanced diagnostic accuracy.
- **Awareness Campaigns:** Increased understanding among clinicians has improved early detection of child abuse.
- **Evolving Definitions:** The shift from "twist and pull" to "twist or pull" reflects ongoing refinement in understanding fracture mechanisms.

Associated Conditions

- **Traumatic Delivery:** In neonates, these fractures may result from breech presentations or delivery trauma.
- **Accidental Injuries:** Rare but possible in contexts such as falls.
- **Polytrauma:** Other injuries may coexist, necessitating comprehensive evaluation.

Clinical Importance

- **Child Protection:** Early identification prevents further harm and aids in legal proceedings against abusers.
- **Forensic Clarity:** Ensures that innocent caregivers are not falsely implicated in cases of accidental injury.
- **Standardized Care:** Promotes the development of specific algorithms for diagnosing and managing metaphyseal fractures.

Bucket handle fractures are emblematic of the intersection of medicine, law, and ethics, demanding careful diagnostic scrutiny and interdisciplinary collaboration to safeguard the well-being of children.

Bumper Fracture

Overview

Bumper Fracture, also known as tibial plateau fracture, refers to a fracture of the proximal tibia often associated with high-energy trauma, such as impact with a vehicle bumper or falls from height. These injuries involve one or both tibial condyles and are often accompanied by soft tissue and ligamentous damage. While the term "bumper fracture" originated from the prevalence of automobile accidents, only 25% of tibial plateau fractures result from this mechanism.

Historical Background

- The term "bumper fracture" was first used to describe tibial plateau fractures linked to vehicle collisions.
- Over time, improved diagnostic imaging and classification systems, such as the *Schatzker classification* (introduced in 1979), refined the understanding and management of these fractures.

Purpose

- **Primary Objective:** To accurately diagnose and classify tibial plateau fractures for appropriate treatment, minimizing complications such as post-traumatic arthritis and compartment syndrome.
- **Secondary Goals:** To restore joint congruity, maintain knee stability, and preserve long-term functionality.

Procedure Overview

- **Initial Evaluation:** Assessment begins with a detailed history of the trauma, focusing on the mechanism of injury.
- Physical examination includes inspection for deformity, swelling, and ecchymosis, as well as assessment of vascular and neurological status.
- **Imaging Modalities:**
- **X-rays:** Anteroposterior, lateral, and oblique views are standard for initial evaluation.
- **CT scans:** Essential for understanding complex fracture patterns and planning surgical interventions.
- **MRI:** Used to evaluate associated soft tissue injuries, including meniscal and ligamentous tears.
- **Management:**
- Non-operative management includes immobilization for stable fractures without displacement or minimal articular involvement.
- Surgical intervention, typically open reduction and internal fixation (ORIF), is required for displaced or unstable fractures.

Results and Interpretation

- Imaging reveals fracture patterns, articular depression, or comminution.
- Evaluation of ligamentous and vascular integrity guides surgical planning and prognostication.
- The *three-column theory* aids in categorizing the fracture as purely articular, single-column, or multi-column involvement.

Physiological Basis

- The *tibial plateau* bears significant weight and serves as the articulation point for the femur.
- The medial plateau is thicker and bears a higher percentage of weight (60%), while the lateral plateau is thinner and more prone to injury.
- Associated ligamentous and vascular injuries are common due to the proximity of structures such as the *popliteal artery* and the anterior cruciate ligament (ACL).

Clinical Applications

- **Orthopedic Management:** Ensuring joint stability, alignment, and functionality post-injury.
- **Trauma Surgery:** Addressing associated injuries, such as vascular compromise or compartment syndrome.
- **Rehabilitation:** Physical therapy for restoring strength, mobility, and range of motion.

Limitations and Technical Considerations

Complications:

- **Immediate:** Compartment syndrome, vascular injury, and infection.
- **Long-term:** Post-traumatic arthritis, knee stiffness, and delayed union or non-union.
- **Challenges in Diagnosis:** Occult fractures may require advanced imaging for detection.
- Subtle ligamentous injuries are often underdiagnosed without MRI.

- **Surgical Risks:** Infection and hardware-related complications can occur, particularly in complex fractures.

Modern Relevance

- Improved imaging modalities, such as CT and MRI, have enhanced diagnostic accuracy and preoperative planning.
- The *Schatzker classification* remains widely used but is complemented by other advanced systems for specific injury patterns.
- Multidisciplinary trauma care and advanced fixation techniques have significantly improved outcomes.

Associated Conditions

- **Ligamentous Injuries:** Commonly involve the ACL, PCL, and menisci.
- **Compartment Syndrome:** High suspicion in cases of severe swelling or vascular compromise.
- **Vascular Injury:** Schatzker Type IV fractures are particularly prone to popliteal artery injury.

Clinical Importance

- **Restoration of Functionality:** Proper treatment minimizes the risk of chronic pain, instability, and degenerative changes.
- **Multidisciplinary Management:** Effective outcomes require collaboration among orthopedic surgeons, physical therapists, and trauma specialists.
- **Patient Education:** Patients should understand the importance of adherence to rehabilitation protocols and follow-up care.

Tibial plateau fractures, though rare, pose significant challenges due to their complexity and potential for complications. Modern surgical techniques and multidisciplinary care have improved prognosis, but patient-specific treatment plans remain critical for optimal outcomes.

Büngner's Point

Overview

Büngner's point is a clinically significant anatomical landmark identified as the most favorable site for a sagittal puncture of the hip joint. This point allows for safe and effective access to the hip joint cavity, facilitating diagnostic and therapeutic procedures such as joint aspiration, intra-articular injections, or synovial fluid analysis. Named after Otto von Büngner, this concept underscores the importance of precise anatomical understanding for invasive interventions.

Historical Background

- *Otto von Büngner*, a prominent figure in orthopedic surgery and anatomy, identified this specific point based on his studies of the hip joint's anatomical structure.
- Büngner emphasized the need for a *consistent, reproducible access point* for joint puncture to reduce complications and improve procedural outcomes.
- The concept of Büngner's point gained traction in the early 20th century, providing a standardized approach for accessing the hip joint, which was particularly useful before imaging-guided techniques became widespread.

Purpose

- **Safe Joint Access:** To identify an optimal site for puncturing the hip joint, minimizing the risk of injury to surrounding structures.
- **Diagnostic Use:** To facilitate the extraction of synovial fluid for analysis in conditions such as infections, inflammation, or joint effusions.
- **Therapeutic Applications:** To enable precise delivery of medications, such as corticosteroids or anesthetics, directly into the joint cavity.

Procedure Overview

- **Locating Büngner's Point:** The point is identified on the sagittal plane, based on anatomical landmarks of the hip joint. The exact position may vary slightly depending on patient anatomy and positioning.
- **Joint Puncture:** Using aseptic technique, a needle is introduced perpendicularly to the skin at Büngner's point, directed toward the joint capsule.
- **Fluid Aspiration or Injection:** Synovial fluid is aspirated for diagnostic purposes, or medications are injected for therapeutic interventions.
- **Post-Procedure:** The site is cleaned, and the patient is monitored for signs of complications, such as infection or bleeding.

Results and Interpretation

- **Accuracy of Access:** Utilizing Büngner's point improves the likelihood of successful entry into the hip joint without damage to surrounding tissues.
- **Clinical Outcomes:** Proper access ensures effective fluid aspiration or drug delivery, contributing to better diagnostic and therapeutic results.
- **Complications:** Incorrect technique or deviation from the anatomical landmark may result in failed access or injury to nearby structures.

Physiological Basis

- **Anatomical Precision:** Büngner's point leverages the natural alignment of the hip joint's anatomical features, providing a clear path to the joint cavity.
- **Joint Structure:** The sagittal puncture targets the capsule of the hip joint, avoiding critical structures such as blood vessels, nerves, and tendons.
- **Minimization of Risk:** The point reduces the likelihood of complications by avoiding highly vascularized or innervated areas near the hip joint.

Clinical Applications

- **Arthrocentesis:** Aspiration of synovial fluid for diagnosing infections, gout, or inflammatory arthritis.
- **Intra-Articular Injections:** Delivery of medications for conditions such as osteoarthritis, rheumatoid arthritis, or hip joint pain.
- **Therapeutic Drainage:** Relieving joint effusion or hemarthrosis through precise puncture and fluid removal.

Limitations and Technical Considerations

- **Patient Variation:** Anatomical differences between individuals may require slight adjustments in locating Büngner's point.
- **Skill Dependency:** Success relies heavily on the practitioner's familiarity with hip joint anatomy and proper technique.
- **Imaging-Guided Alternatives:** Modern imaging techniques, such as ultrasound or fluoroscopy, have reduced reliance on anatomical landmarks for joint punctures.

Modern Relevance

- **Advances in** *imaging-guided procedures* have supplemented the use of Büngner's point, though the landmark remains relevant for clinicians in resource-limited settings or when imaging is unavailable.
- Büngner's work continues to inform the practice of *manual arthrocentesis* and *joint injections*, ensuring precision in invasive hip joint procedures.
- Educational programs for orthopedic surgeons and rheumatologists still emphasize Büngner's point as a critical anatomical reference.

Associated Conditions

- **Osteoarthritis:** Joint injections at Büngner's point provide pain relief and reduce inflammation in affected patients.
- **Septic Arthritis:** Aspiration of purulent synovial fluid aids in diagnosing and managing infections within the hip joint.
- **Traumatic Effusions:** The landmark is used to relieve fluid buildup caused by injuries to the hip joint.

Clinical Importance

- **Practical Diagnostic and Therapeutic Tool:** Büngner's point simplifies access to the hip joint, enhancing the accuracy and safety of invasive procedures.
- **Historical and Educational Value:** The landmark serves as a bridge between traditional anatomical knowledge and modern interventional techniques.
- **Support in Low-Resource Settings:** In the absence of imaging guidance,

Büngner's point remains a vital tool for orthopedic and rheumatologic interventions.

References

O. von Büngner: Zur Wahl der Einstichstelle bei der Jodoforminjektion in das tuberkulös erkrankte Hüftgelenk. Centralblatt für Chirurgie, Leipzig, 1882, 9: 1057-1064.

Burgio's Pseudodiastrophic Dwarfism

Overview

Burgio's pseudodiastrophic dwarfism is a rare hereditary skeletal dysplasia characterized by short-limb dwarfing, brevicollis (short neck), clubfoot, joint contractures and dislocations, cleft palate, and distinct facial features. It is considered a congenital bone disorder with probable autosomal recessive inheritance. The syndrome manifests at birth or early in infancy, and the combination of skeletal, joint, and craniofacial abnormalities results in significant functional and developmental challenges.

Historical Background

- Named after *G. R. Burgio*, who first described the condition in association with its hallmark features of dwarfism and skeletal anomalies.
- Burgio's work highlighted the syndrome as distinct from other forms of dwarfism, such as diastrophic dysplasia, based on its unique constellation of features.
- The term "pseudodiastrophic" reflects its resemblance to diastrophic dysplasia while indicating differences in etiology, inheritance, and clinical manifestations.

Purpose

- **Diagnosis:** To distinguish Burgio's pseudodiastrophic dwarfism from other skeletal dysplasias with overlapping features, such as diastrophic or achondroplastic dwarfism.

- **Management Planning:** To provide a comprehensive care plan addressing skeletal deformities, joint abnormalities, and craniofacial issues.
- **Genetic Counseling:** To inform affected families about the hereditary nature of the condition and the associated recurrence risks.

Procedure Overview

Diagnosis:

- **Clinical Examination:** Identification of short-limb dwarfism, characteristic facies, clubfoot, and cleft palate.
- **Imaging:** X-rays reveal shortened long bones, spinal anomalies, and joint deformities.
- **Genetic Testing:** Confirmatory analysis to identify mutations associated with the syndrome.

Treatment:

- **Orthopedic Interventions:** Management of joint dislocations, contractures, and clubfoot through splinting, casting, or surgery.
- **Surgical Correction:** Repair of cleft palate and correction of skeletal deformities as needed.
- **Physical Therapy:** Ongoing rehabilitation to improve mobility and reduce functional limitations.
- **Supportive Care:** Multidisciplinary management involving orthopedic surgeons, geneticists, and speech therapists to address the spectrum of clinical challenges.

Results and Interpretation

- **Physical and Functional Improvement:** Surgical and therapeutic interventions improve mobility, joint function, and quality of life.
- **Long-Term Challenges:** Despite treatment, affected individuals may continue to experience growth limitations, joint stiffness, and craniofacial abnormalities.
- **Prognosis:** The condition is not typically life-threatening but requires lifelong management to optimize function and address complications.

Physiological Basis

- **Skeletal Dysplasia:** Mutations affecting cartilage and bone development lead to shortened limbs, joint abnormalities, and spinal deformities.
- **Connective Tissue Abnormalities:** Dysfunction in connective tissue contributes to joint contractures, dislocations, and craniofacial anomalies.
- **Growth Restriction:** Impaired endochondral ossification and abnormal growth plate activity result in the characteristic short stature.

Clinical Applications

- **Pediatric Orthopedics:** Early intervention in joint and skeletal deformities minimizes long-term functional impairments.
- **Craniofacial Surgery:** Repair of cleft palate improves feeding, speech, and overall quality of life.
- **Rehabilitation Medicine:** Tailored physical therapy programs enhance mobility and prevent further joint stiffness.

Limitations and Technical Considerations

- **Diagnostic Challenges:** Overlap with other skeletal dysplasias may delay diagnosis, necessitating genetic confirmation.
- **Surgical Risks:** Orthopedic and craniofacial surgeries carry risks of infection, incomplete correction, or recurrence of deformities.
- **Functional Limitations:** Despite treatment, some individuals may face lifelong challenges related to mobility, dexterity, and physical development.

Modern Relevance

- **Advances in** *genetic research* have improved the identification of mutations associated with Burgio's pseudodiastrophic dwarfism, aiding in early and accurate diagnosis.
- Development of *minimally invasive surgical techniques* has enhanced outcomes for joint and craniofacial abnormalities.
- Multidisciplinary approaches emphasize comprehensive care, improving quality of life for affected individuals and their families.

Associated Conditions

- **Diastrophic Dysplasia:** A related form of skeletal dysplasia with overlapping features but differing genetic and clinical profiles.
- **Clubfoot:** A hallmark feature requiring early intervention to prevent lifelong deformity and gait issues.
- **Cleft Palate:** A craniofacial anomaly necessitating surgical correction to address feeding and speech difficulties.

Clinical Importance

- **Early Identification:** Prompt diagnosis enables timely intervention, reducing the severity of deformities and functional impairments.
- **Genetic Counseling:** Families benefit from understanding inheritance patterns and the risk of recurrence in future pregnancies.
- **Multidisciplinary Care:** Effective management requires collaboration among specialists, highlighting the importance of integrated care for rare skeletal dysplasias.

References

G. R. Burgio, et al: Nanisme pseudodiastrophique. Étude de deux soeurs nouveau-nées. Archives francaises de pédiatrie, Paris, 1974, 31: 681.

Burst Fracture

Overview

Burst Fracture refers to a severe and often comminuted vertebral body fracture where bone fragments "burst" out in multiple directions, frequently impinging on the spinal canal and causing potential spinal cord injury. This injury commonly results from high-energy axial trauma, such as motor vehicle accidents or falls from significant heights, and is considered a critical orthopedic emergency.

Historical Background

- The understanding of spinal fractures and their mechanics dates back centuries, with substantial advances made in the 20th century.
- In 1983, Denis introduced the *Three-Column Theory*, which remains a cornerstone in classifying spinal fractures, including burst fractures. This theory provides a framework for understanding fracture stability and guiding treatment.

Purpose

- **Primary Goal:** To stabilize the spine, prevent neurological deficits, and maintain spinal alignment.
- **Secondary Objectives:** To alleviate pain, restore function, and minimize the risk of long-term complications, such as kyphotic deformity and chronic pain.

Procedure Overview

- **Initial Evaluation:** History of the trauma and physical examination to assess neurological function, spinal tenderness, and associated injuries.
- Use of the Thoracolumbar Injury Classification and Severity Score (TLICS) to guide management decisions.
- **Imaging Studies:**
- **X-rays:** For initial assessment, focusing on vertebral alignment and height loss.
- **CT scans:** Essential for evaluating fracture patterns, retropulsion of fragments, and canal compromise.
- **MRI:** For soft tissue evaluation, including ligamentous injury and spinal cord compromise.
- **Management:**
- **Non-operative Treatment:** Indicated for stable fractures without neurological deficits, involving bracing and physical therapy.
- **Surgical Intervention:** Required for unstable fractures, significant canal compromise, or neurological deficits. Common procedures include posterior or anterior fixation, laminectomy, or decompression.

Results and Interpretation

- Imaging findings confirm vertebral height loss, fragment retropulsion into the canal, and disruption of the posterior ligamentous complex (PLC) in severe cases.
- Stability and neurological integrity are assessed to determine the need for surgical intervention.
- Postoperative imaging is used to evaluate fracture reduction, alignment, and hardware placement.

Physiological Basis

- The vertebrae act as load-bearing structures in the spine, with the cancellous bone in the vertebral body absorbing axial forces.
- Burst fractures occur when high-energy axial loading exceeds the bone's capacity, leading to comminution and fragment displacement.
- The involvement of the posterior ligamentous complex can result in instability, necessitating surgical stabilization.

Clinical Applications

- **Orthopedic Surgery:** Stabilization and reconstruction of spinal fractures to restore function.
- **Neurology:** Assessment and management of spinal cord injuries caused by retropulsed fragments.
- **Rehabilitation Medicine:** Physical therapy to improve mobility and reduce long-term disability.

Limitations and Technical Considerations

- **Non-operative Challenges:** Conservative treatment risks kyphotic deformity and delayed healing.
- **Surgical Risks:** Hardware failure, infection, and potential neurological deterioration are concerns.
- **Imaging Limitations:** Subtle ligamentous injuries may require advanced imaging techniques like MRI for accurate diagnosis.
- **Postoperative Care:** Ensuring proper rehabilitation and avoiding complications like deep vein thrombosis (DVT) or chronic pain.

Modern Relevance

- **Advances in** surgical techniques, including minimally invasive procedures, have improved outcomes for burst fractures.
- Enhanced imaging modalities, such as high-resolution CT and functional MRI, aid in precise diagnosis and planning.
- Multidisciplinary care teams, including orthopedic surgeons, neurosurgeons, and rehabilitation specialists, play critical roles in patient management.

Associated Conditions

- **Neurological Deficits:** Spinal cord injury or nerve root compression can result from retropulsed fragments.
- **Compartment Syndrome:** Rare but severe, particularly in high-energy trauma cases.
- **Post-Traumatic Kyphosis:** Progressive deformity resulting from untreated or inadequately managed fractures.

Clinical Importance

- **Timely Diagnosis and Management:** Critical to prevent neurological deficits and deformities.
- **Interprofessional Care:** Collaboration between orthopedic, neurological, and rehabilitation teams ensures comprehensive management.
- **Patient Education:** Informing patients about the importance of lifestyle modifications, including osteoporosis prevention and fall risk reduction.

Burst fractures represent a challenging orthopedic emergency with potential for significant morbidity. Timely diagnosis, appropriate classification, and tailored treatment plans are essential for optimizing outcomes and minimizing long-term disability.

Calvé's Syndrome

Overview

Calvé's syndrome refers to aseptic epiphyseal necrosis that leads to the flattening of vertebral bodies in children. The condition, which can present acutely or insidiously, most commonly affects boys. It results from diminished blood supply to the vertebral epiphyses, leading to fragmentation and collapse of the affected vertebrae. In some cases, eosinophilic granulomas are implicated as the underlying cause, though the exact pathogenesis varies.

Historical Background

- Named after *Jacques Calvé*, a French orthopedic surgeon who described the condition in detail.
- Calvé's pioneering work on vertebral diseases in children contributed to the understanding of epiphyseal necrosis as a distinct pathological process.
- The syndrome is now recognized as part of the spectrum of disorders affecting bone growth and vascular supply, emphasizing the importance of early detection and management.

Purpose

- **Diagnosis:** To identify vertebral epiphyseal necrosis in children, distinguishing it from other causes of vertebral flattening such as trauma or infection.
- **Management:** To prevent further vertebral collapse and associated deformities through early intervention.
- **Understanding Etiology:** To explore underlying causes such as eosinophilic

granulomas or vascular compromise for targeted treatment.

Procedure Overview

Diagnosis:

- **Clinical Examination:** Common findings include back pain, restricted mobility, and kyphotic posturing in severe cases.
- **Imaging:** X-rays show characteristic vertebral flattening (vertebra plana) and fragmentation. MRI may reveal reduced blood supply and soft tissue involvement.
- **Biopsy (if needed):** Performed to confirm eosinophilic granulomas or rule out malignancies.

Treatment:

- **Conservative Management:** Rest, bracing, and physical therapy to alleviate symptoms and reduce spinal stress.
- **Surgical Intervention:** Reserved for severe cases with instability or progressive deformity, involving spinal fusion or vertebral body reconstruction.
- **Targeted Therapy:** Corticosteroids or radiation therapy for eosinophilic granulomas, if identified.
- **Follow-Up:** Regular monitoring with imaging to assess vertebral healing and detect complications.

Results and Interpretation

- **Healing and Recovery:** With proper treatment, most children achieve stabilization of the vertebrae and symptom relief.
- **Residual Deformities:** Vertebral collapse may leave lasting kyphotic or scoliotic deformities in untreated or severe cases.
- **Prognosis:** Generally good if managed early, though long-term follow-up is required to monitor spinal alignment and growth.

Physiological Basis

- **Vascular Compromise:** Reduced blood flow to the vertebral epiphysis leads to ischemic necrosis, initiating the process of fragmentation and collapse.
- **Mechanical Stress:** The weight-bearing nature of the spine exacerbates the damage to necrotic vertebral bodies.
- **Eosinophilic Granulomas:** In cases linked to this condition, the granulomas disrupt normal bone remodeling, contributing to vertebral damage.

Clinical Applications

- **Pediatric Orthopedics:** Early recognition and management are essential to prevent deformities and ensure normal spinal growth.
- **Radiology:** Imaging plays a critical role in diagnosing vertebral necrosis and monitoring the progression of the disease.
- **Multidisciplinary Care:** Collaboration between pediatricians, orthopedists, and radiologists ensures comprehensive management.

Limitations and Technical Considerations

- **Delayed Diagnosis:** Insidious onset and nonspecific symptoms may delay diagnosis, leading to advanced vertebral collapse.

- **Surgical Risks:** Spinal surgeries carry risks such as infection, neurological damage, and failure of hardware.
- **Long-Term Monitoring:** Lifelong follow-up may be necessary to detect late-onset complications such as scoliosis or chronic pain.

Modern Relevance

- **Advances in** *imaging techniques*, such as MRI, have improved early detection of Calvé's syndrome and its differentiation from other spinal disorders.
- Improved surgical tools and techniques have enhanced outcomes in cases requiring intervention for deformities.
- Continued research into the role of *eosinophilic granulomas* has provided new insights into the condition's pathogenesis and management.

Associated Conditions

- **Eosinophilic Granuloma:** Frequently implicated in cases of vertebral necrosis associated with Calvé's syndrome, representing a localized form of Langerhans cell histiocytosis.
- **Vertebra Plana:** The hallmark radiographic feature of the syndrome, characterized by complete flattening of the vertebral body.
- **Spinal Deformities:** Untreated or severe cases may lead to kyphosis, scoliosis, or chronic spinal instability.

Clinical Importance

- **Early Intervention:** Timely diagnosis and management prevent progression to severe deformities and chronic complications.
- **Educational Value:** Calvé's syndrome highlights the importance of vascular health in bone development and the role of imaging in pediatric orthopedics.
- **Integrated Care:** Effective treatment requires a multidisciplinary approach to address both the immediate and long-term challenges posed by the condition.

References

J. Calvé: Sur une affection particulière de la colonne vertébrale chez l'enfant simulant le mal de Pott. Ostéo-chondrite vertébrale infantile. Journal de radiologie, d'électrologie, 1925, 9: 22-27.

A localized affection of the spine suggesting osteochondritis of the vertebral body, with the clinical aspect of Pott's disease. Journal of Bone Surgery, 1925, 7: 41-46.

Calvé-Legg-Perthes Disease

Overview

Calvé-Legg-Perthes disease, also known as Legg-Calvé-Perthes disease, is a childhood disorder characterized by aseptic necrosis of the femoral head epiphysis. It results from an insufficient blood supply to the femur, leading to the death of bone tissue (necrosis). The disease progresses through distinct stages, including revascularization, mottling, fragmentation, and eventual reossification of the femoral head. This process can span several years. It presents with hip pain, stiffness, restricted movement, and a limp. The condition is most common in boys aged 5 to 10 years and can be unilateral or bilateral, depending on whether it is sporadic or hereditary.

Historical Background

- **The condition is associated with several prominent figures:** Karel Maydl: Credited with the first description in 1897.
- **Jacques Calvé, Arthur Thornton Legg, and Georg Clemens Perthes:** Provided detailed clinical characterizations, leading to the eponymous name.
- **Johann Henning Waldenström:** Made further contributions to understanding the disease's pathophysiology.

Historically, the disease was a mystery due to its spontaneous occurrence and progression through necrosis and repair phases. It represents a milestone in pediatric orthopedics for its recognition as a vascular disorder of the hip.

Purpose

- **Diagnosis:** To identify the disease in its early stages, enabling timely intervention to minimize joint damage and deformity.
- **Management:** To relieve symptoms, maintain joint function, and support the reossification process of the femoral head.
- **Prognosis Assessment:** To predict long-term outcomes based on the extent of femoral head involvement and response to treatment.

Procedure Overview

Diagnosis:

- **Clinical Examination:** Identifying hip pain, stiffness, and a limp as key symptoms.
- **Imaging:** X-rays show stages of necrosis, fragmentation, and reossification. MRI and bone scans can detect early vascular compromise before radiographic changes appear.
- **Differential Diagnosis:** Rule out other conditions, such as slipped capital femoral epiphysis or infections.

Treatment:

- **Conservative Management:** Rest, activity restriction, and physical therapy to reduce joint stress and improve mobility.
- **Bracing:** Use of abduction braces to ensure proper joint alignment during reossification.
- **Surgical Intervention:** Osteotomy or femoral head containment procedures for severe cases to preserve joint congruency.

- **Follow-Up:** Regular monitoring with imaging and clinical assessments to track disease progression and response to treatment.

Results and Interpretation

- **Progression of Disease:** The condition evolves over several years, with stages of necrosis, fragmentation, revascularization, and reossification.
- **Outcomes:** Younger children (under 6 years) typically have better outcomes due to greater remodeling potential.
- **Older children or those with extensive involvement of the femoral head may experience residual deformity or early-onset arthritis.**
- **Complications:** Long-term issues include femoral head flattening, leg-length discrepancy, and hip arthritis.

Physiological Basis

- **Vascular Insufficiency:** Disruption of blood flow to the femoral epiphysis causes ischemia and necrosis of bone tissue.
- **Bone Remodeling:** The natural process of revascularization brings new blood supply, leading to gradual bone regeneration and replacement of necrotic tissue.
- **Joint Mechanics:** During fragmentation and reossification, the shape and congruency of the femoral head are critical for preserving hip function.

Clinical Applications

- **Pediatric Orthopedics:** The disease underscores the importance of early detection and tailored treatment to prevent deformities.
- **Imaging Diagnostics:** Advanced imaging technologies, such as MRI, enhance early diagnosis and treatment planning.
- **Rehabilitation Medicine:** Physical therapy plays a vital role in maintaining mobility and preventing joint stiffness.

Limitations and Technical Considerations

- **Late Diagnosis:** Early stages can be difficult to detect without advanced imaging, delaying intervention.
- **Treatment Challenges:** Conservative methods may not fully prevent femoral head deformities in severe cases, necessitating surgery.
- **Long-Term Monitoring:** Lifelong follow-up may be required for patients with residual deformities or early joint degeneration.

Modern Relevance

- **Advances in** *early detection* and *surgical techniques* have improved outcomes for children with Calvé-Legg-Perthes disease.
- Research into the genetic and vascular mechanisms underlying the disease has expanded understanding of its etiology and inheritance patterns.
- The condition remains a key area of focus in pediatric orthopedics, serving as a model for managing ischemic bone diseases.

Associated Conditions

- **Eosinophilic Granuloma:** Rarely associated with similar femoral head necrosis.

- **Slipped Capital Femoral Epiphysis (SCFE):** A differential diagnosis that can mimic some symptoms of the disease.
- **Developmental Dysplasia of the Hip (DDH):** Structural hip abnormalities may complicate or coexist with the condition.

Clinical Importance

- **Early Intervention:** Prompt diagnosis and management are crucial to minimize joint damage and long-term disability.
- **Multidisciplinary Care:** Collaboration among pediatricians, orthopedic surgeons, radiologists, and physical therapists ensures comprehensive management.
- **Educational Significance:** The condition illustrates the interplay between vascular supply, bone growth, and joint function, making it a cornerstone topic in pediatric orthopedics.

References

Karel Maydl in: Wiener klinische Rundschau, 1897, 11: 153.

A. T. Legg: The cause of atrophy in joint disease. American Journal of Orthopedic Surgery, 1908-1909, 6: 84-90.

An obscure affection of the hip-joint. Boston Medical and Surgical Journal, 1910, 162: 202-204.

H. Waldenström: Der obere tuberkulöse Cullumherd. Zeitschrift für Orthopädische Chirurgie, Stuttgart, 1909, 24: 487-512.

J. Calvé: Sur une forme particulière de pseudo-coxalgie greffée sur des déformations caractéristiques de l'extrémité supérieure du fémur. Revue de chirurgie, Paris, 1910, 42: 54-84.

G. Perthes: Über Arthritis deformans juvenilis. Deutsche Zeitschrift für Chirurgie, Leipzig, 1910, 107: 111-159.

Campanacci's Syndrome

Overview

Campanacci's syndrome refers to osteofibrous dysplasia of the tibia and fibula, characterized by antero-lateral bowing of the shins, along with osteolytic and sclerotic changes in the cortical bone. The condition is a rare, non-neoplastic lesion that typically presents during childhood. Mario Campanacci, an Italian orthopedic surgeon, introduced the term in 1976, highlighting its congenital origin and its histological similarity to fibrous dysplasia. While the pathogenesis remains unclear, it is thought to be a localized developmental disorder of bone growth.

Historical Background

- First systematically described by *Mario Campanacci* in 1976, who noted its exclusive occurrence in the tibia and fibula and its resemblance to fibrous dysplasia.
- Campanacci, along with *Laus*, expanded on the syndrome in a landmark 1981 report that analyzed *35 cases*, establishing key clinical and radiological features of the condition.
- The syndrome's characterization as *osteofibrous dysplasia* differentiated it from other bone dysplasias, contributing to advancements in diagnostic and therapeutic approaches.

Purpose

- **Accurate Diagnosis:** To identify osteofibrous dysplasia of the tibia and fibula, distinguishing it from conditions like fibrous dysplasia, osteosarcoma, or other congenital tibial abnormalities.

- **Management of Symptoms:** To alleviate the antero-lateral bowing and prevent complications such as pathological fractures.
- **Preservation of Function:** To maintain the structural integrity and functionality of the lower limbs in affected individuals.

Procedure Overview

Diagnosis:

- **Clinical Presentation:** Children typically present with visible bowing of the shins, localized swelling, or pain.
- **Imaging:** X-rays reveal cortical thinning, osteolytic lesions, and sclerotic changes. CT and MRI may provide detailed visualization of the lesion's extent.
- **Histological Examination:** Biopsy confirms the diagnosis, showing fibro-osseous tissue and areas resembling fibrous dysplasia.

Treatment:

- **Conservative Management:** Observation for asymptomatic cases or mild deformities.
- **Orthopedic Interventions:** Corrective osteotomy and internal fixation for significant bowing or functional impairment.
- **Bone Grafting:** Used to stabilize weakened bone and prevent recurrence of lesions.
- **Follow-Up:** Regular imaging and clinical assessments are critical to monitor disease progression and detect potential complications.

Results and Interpretation

- **Natural Course:** The condition often stabilizes after skeletal maturity, with lesions becoming less active.
- **Treatment Outcomes:** Surgical correction generally improves limb alignment and functionality, although recurrence of lesions is possible.
- **Prognosis:** Good long-term outcomes are achievable with appropriate management, but severe deformities may result in chronic discomfort or gait abnormalities.

Physiological Basis

- **Bone Dysplasia:** Osteofibrous dysplasia involves disorganized growth of fibrous tissue and bone within the cortical layer, leading to structural weakness and deformity.
- **Cortical Changes:** The interplay of osteolytic (bone resorption) and sclerotic (bone hardening) processes results in the characteristic radiological appearance.
- **Localized Nature:** Unlike fibrous dysplasia, Campanacci's syndrome is limited to the tibia and fibula, suggesting a site-specific developmental anomaly.

Clinical Applications

- **Orthopedic Management:** Campanacci's syndrome is a critical consideration in the differential diagnosis of tibial and fibular deformities in pediatric patients.
- **Reconstructive Surgery:** Techniques like osteotomy and bone grafting are essential for correcting deformities and restoring functionality.

- **Diagnostic Imaging:** Radiological features are pivotal for early identification and monitoring of disease progression.

Limitations and Technical Considerations

- **Diagnostic Challenges:** The condition may be misdiagnosed as fibrous dysplasia or malignant bone tumors due to overlapping radiological and histological features.
- **Surgical Risks:** Procedures such as osteotomy carry risks of infection, nonunion, or recurrence of lesions.
- **Recurrence Potential:** Lesions may persist or recur, particularly in younger patients with significant growth potential remaining.

Modern Relevance

- **Advances in** *imaging modalities*, including high-resolution CT and MRI, have enhanced the accuracy of diagnosing Campanacci's syndrome.
- Improved surgical techniques, such as minimally invasive osteotomies and advanced bone grafting, have optimized treatment outcomes.
- Ongoing research into the *molecular basis* of the syndrome may yield insights into its pathogenesis and potential targeted therapies.

Associated Conditions

- **Fibrous Dysplasia:** Shares histological features with Campanacci's syndrome but differs in its widespread distribution and genetic underpinnings.
- **Congenital Tibial Bowing:** A differential diagnosis requiring exclusion based on radiological and clinical findings.
- **Pathological Fractures:** A potential complication of untreated or severe osteofibrous dysplasia.

Clinical Importance

- **Early Detection:** Prompt diagnosis and monitoring are essential to prevent severe deformities and functional limitations.
- **Multidisciplinary Approach:** Effective management requires collaboration among orthopedic surgeons, radiologists, and pathologists.
- **Historical Significance:** Campanacci's syndrome highlights the evolution of diagnostic frameworks for bone dysplasias and emphasizes the importance of histopathological correlation in orthopedic disorders.

References

M. Campanacci: Osteofibrous dysplasia of long bones. A new clinical entity. Italian Journal of Orthopaedics and Traumatology, 2: 221-237, 1976.

M. Campanacci, M. Laus: Osteofibrous dysplasia of the tibia and fibula. The Journal of Bone and Joint Surgery, Boston, 1981, 63A (3): 367-375.

Chance Fracture

Overview

A Chance fracture, also known as a seatbelt fracture, is a transverse fracture involving the vertebral body and the neural arch, typically occurring at the thoracolumbar junction. It is most commonly associated with motor vehicle accidents where abrupt deceleration causes hyperflexion of the spine against a fixed fulcrum, such as a lap belt. Initially described as a purely osseous injury, the term has since expanded to include ligamentous, disc, and mixed injuries. Chance fractures are unstable injuries and carry a significant risk of associated abdominal organ damage, particularly to the bowel.

Historical Background

- First described by *George Quentin Chance* in *1948*, the fracture was initially characterized as an *osseous injury* resulting from extreme spinal flexion.
- The term *"Chance fracture"* was popularized by Nicoll in 1949, cementing its association with seatbelt injuries.
- **Advances in** automotive safety, including lap and shoulder restraints, have reduced the incidence of these injuries, although they remain a notable concern in high-speed vehicular trauma.

Purpose

- **Diagnosis:** To identify the fracture and differentiate it from other spinal injuries to guide appropriate management.
- **Stabilization:** To ensure spinal stability and prevent neurological compromise in patients with Chance fractures.
- **Detection of Associated Injuries:** To address accompanying abdominal or thoracic organ damage, which frequently coexists with this fracture pattern.

Procedure Overview

Diagnosis:

- **Clinical Examination:** Patients often present with mid-back or lower-back pain following trauma, coupled with possible abdominal tenderness.

Imaging:

- **X-rays:** Lateral views show the classic horizontal splitting of the vertebral body and posterior elements.
- **CT scans:** Provides detailed visualization of the fracture, including ligamentous or mixed patterns.
- **MRI:** Essential for evaluating ligamentous and disc injuries and for ruling out spinal cord involvement.

Treatment:

- **Conservative Management:** Immobilization with a thoracolumbosacral orthosis (TLSO) for stable fractures without neurological deficits.
- **Surgical Intervention:** Required for unstable fractures or those with significant neurological compromise. Techniques include posterior fixation with pedicle screws or combined anterior and posterior approaches for severe injuries.
- **Monitoring for Associated Injuries:** Regular abdominal imaging and monitoring are critical to detect bowel perforations or other visceral damage.

Results and Interpretation

- **Stabilization of the Spine:** Conservative or surgical management usually restores spinal stability, preventing progressive deformities.
- **Complications:** Neurological compromise or visceral injuries, if untreated, can lead to significant morbidity.
- **Prognosis:** Outcomes are generally good with timely intervention, although recovery may be prolonged in cases with severe associated injuries.

Physiological Basis

- **Mechanism of Injury:** The flexion-distraction force causes a "splitting" of the vertebral body and posterior elements, with the injury severity dependent on the force and extent of ligamentous involvement.
- **Column Involvement:** The injury disrupts the posterior and middle columns of the spine, and in severe cases, the anterior column may also be affected, leading to instability.
- **Visceral Risks:** The flexion force transmitted to the abdominal cavity often causes compression or tearing of bowel or mesenteric structures, necessitating vigilant monitoring.

Clinical Applications

- **Trauma Management:** Chance fractures highlight the importance of a multidisciplinary approach to spinal and abdominal trauma.
- **Orthopedic and Neurosurgical Care:** Surgical techniques ensure spinal stabilization in unstable or complex cases.
- **Emergency Medicine:** Recognition of this fracture pattern in trauma patients facilitates early intervention and prevents secondary complications.

Limitations and Technical Considerations

- **Diagnostic Challenges:** Ligamentous and mixed injuries may be missed on plain X-rays, requiring advanced imaging modalities like MRI or CT.
- **Surgical Risks:** Surgery carries risks of infection, hardware failure, and incomplete restoration of stability.
- **Associated Injuries:** The high likelihood of visceral injury complicates the treatment course, requiring coordinated care.

Modern Relevance

- **Advances in** *seatbelt design*, such as three-point restraints, have significantly reduced the incidence of Chance fractures.
- Improved *imaging technologies* enable earlier and more accurate diagnosis of osseous and ligamentous injuries.
- Surgical innovations, including minimally invasive techniques, have enhanced outcomes for unstable fractures while reducing recovery times.

Associated Conditions

- **Bowel and Mesenteric Injuries:** Commonly associated with Chance fractures due to the forceful compression of the abdomen.
- **Fracture-Dislocations:** Severe variants involving anterior column disruption increase the risk of spinal instability and neurological injury.

- **Spinal Cord Injury:** Rare but possible in high-energy trauma, especially with fracture-dislocations.

Clinical Importance

- **Comprehensive Trauma Care:** Recognizing Chance fractures ensures early intervention for spinal and associated visceral injuries, reducing mortality and morbidity.
- **Multidisciplinary Approach:** Effective management requires collaboration among trauma surgeons, orthopedic specialists, neurosurgeons, and radiologists.
- **Educational Significance:** The fracture serves as a classic example of flexion-distraction spinal injuries, reinforcing the importance of mechanism-of-injury assessment in trauma care.

References

Chance GQ. Note on a type of flexion fracture of the spine. Br J Radiol. 1948 Sep;21(249):452. [PMID 18878306]

Bernstein MP, Mirvis SE, Shanmuganathan K. Chance-type fractures of the thoracolumbar spine: imaging analysis in 53 patients. AJR Am J Roentgenol. 2006 Oct;187(4):859-68. [PMID 16985126]

Nicoll EA. Fractures of the dorso-lumbar spine. J Bone Joint Surg Br. 1949 Aug;31B(3):376-94. [PMID 18148776]

Hunter TB, Peltier LF, Lund PJ. Radiologic History Exhibit Musculoskeletal Eponyms: Who Are Those Guys? Radiographics. 2000 May-Jun;20(3):819-36.[Full text]

Chalk Stick Fractures

Overview

Chalk Stick Fractures, also referred to as Carrot Stick Fractures, are fractures of the fused spine that typically occur in patients with Ankylosing Spondylitis (AS) or other conditions causing spinal fusion, such as Diffuse Idiopathic Skeletal Hyperostosis (DISH) or surgical spine fusions. These fractures are named for their resemblance to a piece of chalk breaking under pressure and are indicative of significant spinal instability.

Historical Background

- The term *chalk stick fracture* emerged to describe the unique morphology of fractures in fused spines, initially observed in patients with ankylosing spondylitis.
- **Advances in** imaging techniques, particularly in the mid-to-late 20th century, helped elucidate the pathophysiology of such fractures, distinguishing them from fractures in otherwise healthy spines.

Purpose

- **Primary Goal:** To stabilize the spine and prevent neurological damage by identifying and managing these fractures promptly.
- **Secondary Objectives:** To minimize pain, restore function, and reduce the likelihood of complications, such as progressive kyphosis or spinal cord injury.

Procedure Overview

- **Initial Assessment:** History of conditions such as ankylosing spondylitis or DISH, coupled with clinical symptoms of severe pain or deformity.
- Neurological assessment to evaluate motor, sensory, and reflex functions.
- **Imaging:**
- **X-rays:** Initial screening to identify fracture lines in the fused spine.
- **CT scans:** Gold standard for detecting the exact location, extent, and alignment of the fracture.
- **MRI:** To evaluate associated soft tissue and spinal cord injuries.
- **Management:**
- **Non-Surgical:** Stabilization with orthotics for patients with stable fractures and no neurological deficits.
- **Surgical:** Indicated for unstable fractures or when neurological impairment is present. Techniques include spinal fixation and decompression.

Results and Interpretation

- Imaging typically reveals a transverse fracture pattern at the disco-vertebral junction, often in the lower cervical or upper thoracic spine.
- Fractures in these conditions demonstrate reduced flexibility and increased fragility due to excessive and abnormal bone formation.

Physiological Basis

- In *Ankylosing Spondylitis*, the inflammatory process leads to new bone formation, resulting in spinal fusion (bamboo spine). However, this new bone is structurally abnormal and prone to fracture under minimal trauma.
- The rigidity of the fused spine transfers stress to a localized area during trauma, leading to transverse fractures resembling the breakage of a chalk stick.

Clinical Applications

- **Orthopedic Care:** Stabilization and realignment of the spine to ensure functional outcomes.
- **Neurological Management:** Addressing any associated spinal cord compression to prevent long-term neurological deficits.
- **Rehabilitation Medicine:** Focus on mobility and strength restoration through physical therapy post-stabilization.

Limitations and Technical Considerations

- **Non-Surgical Management:** Risks include delayed union, poor alignment, and progressive kyphotic deformity.
- **Surgical Management:** Challenges include difficulty accessing the fracture site in fused spines, risk of neurological complications, and postoperative infections.
- **Imaging Limitations:** Subtle fractures may be missed on initial X-rays, necessitating advanced imaging modalities like CT or MRI.

Modern Relevance

- **Advances in** minimally invasive spine surgery and improved imaging modalities have enhanced diagnostic accuracy and surgical outcomes for chalk stick fractures.
- Greater awareness of these fractures in patients with AS or DISH has led to earlier intervention, reducing the risk of complications.

Associated Conditions

- **Ankylosing Spondylitis (AS):** The most common underlying condition, characterized by inflammation and subsequent fusion of the spine.
- **Diffuse Idiopathic Skeletal Hyperostosis (DISH):** Involves excessive calcification and ossification of spinal ligaments, increasing fracture risk.
- **Osteoporosis:** May coexist, further weakening the spine and predisposing it to fractures.

Clinical Importance

- **Early Recognition:** Prompt identification of chalk stick fractures in patients with AS or DISH is critical to prevent catastrophic neurological outcomes.
- **Comprehensive Management:** Requires a multidisciplinary approach involving orthopedic surgeons, neurologists, and rehabilitation specialists.
- **Patient Education:** Patients with conditions predisposing them to chalk stick fractures should be counseled on injury prevention and the importance of regular follow-ups.

Chalk stick fractures highlight the fragility of fused spines in conditions like ankylosing spondylitis and necessitate a detailed and strategic approach to diagnosis and treatment. Early intervention and a multidisciplinary care plan are pivotal for ensuring optimal patient outcomes.

Charcot's Disease

Overview

Charcot's disease, commonly referred to as amyotrophic lateral sclerosis (ALS) or Lou Gehrig's disease, is a rare neurodegenerative disorder characterized by progressive degeneration of motor neurons. This leads to muscle weakness, spasticity, cramps, and atrophy, eventually impairing voluntary muscle control. The disease typically affects adults over 50 years, although cases have been reported in younger individuals. The condition progresses rapidly, with about 50% of patients succumbing within three years of symptom onset. The male-to-female ratio is approximately 2:1, and while sporadic cases predominate, familial forms with autosomal dominant inheritance have been observed.

Historical Background

- *Jean-Martin Charcot*, a French neurologist, first described the clinical and pathological features of ALS in the late *19th century*, coining the term "amyotrophic lateral sclerosis."
- *Henry Louis Gehrig*, a famous American baseball player, brought public awareness to the disease when he succumbed to it in *1941*, leading to its colloquial name, "Lou Gehrig's disease."
- In *1993*, researchers identified a mutation in the *SOD1 gene* as a cause of some familial cases, advancing the understanding of its genetic basis.

Purpose

- **Diagnostic Clarity:** To identify ALS through clinical features, electrophysiological testing, and exclusion of other neurodegenerative disorders.
- **Symptom Management:** To alleviate muscle weakness, spasticity, and other symptoms to improve the patient's quality of life.
- **Research Focus:** To investigate the genetic and molecular mechanisms of ALS for potential therapies.

Procedure Overview

Diagnosis:

- **Clinical Assessment:** Early signs include asymmetric muscle weakness, fatigue, cramps, and spasticity.
- **Electromyography (EMG):** Detects denervation and reinnervation in affected muscles, confirming motor neuron involvement.
- **MRI and Laboratory Testing:** Rule out other conditions, such as cervical spondylosis or multiple sclerosis.
- **Genetic Testing:** Identifies mutations in familial ALS cases, including the SOD1, C9orf72, or TDP-43 genes.

Treatment:

- **Pharmacotherapy:** Riluzole and edaravone are FDA-approved drugs that modestly slow disease progression.
- **Supportive Care:** Multidisciplinary approaches including physical therapy, speech therapy, and nutritional support.
- **Ventilatory Assistance:** Non-invasive ventilation for respiratory muscle weakness.

- **Palliative Care:** Focuses on symptom relief and psychosocial support as the disease progresses.

Results and Interpretation

- **Disease Course:** Progresses from localized muscle weakness to widespread atrophy and paralysis, with respiratory failure being the most common cause of death.
- **Prognosis:** Median survival time is 2–5 years, though some patients survive for decades with supportive care.
- **Variability:** Familial cases may progress differently from sporadic forms, influenced by genetic and environmental factors.

Physiological Basis

- **Motor Neuron Degeneration:** ALS primarily affects upper motor neurons in the cerebral cortex and lower motor neurons in the brainstem and spinal cord, disrupting signal transmission to muscles.
- **Muscle Atrophy:** Denervation leads to muscle wasting, weakness, and the hallmark fasciculations.
- **Genetic Influence:** Mutations in genes like SOD1 and C9orf72 disrupt cellular processes, including oxidative stress management, RNA metabolism, and autophagy.

Clinical Applications

- **Neurology:** ALS remains a key focus in understanding neurodegenerative processes and developing interventions.
- **Genetics:** Advances in genetic testing have improved familial ALS diagnosis and counseling.
- **Rehabilitation Medicine:** Tailored physical and occupational therapy programs support functional independence for as long as possible.

Limitations and Technical Considerations

- **Diagnostic Challenges:** Early symptoms overlap with other neuromuscular disorders, often delaying diagnosis.
- **Lack of Curative Treatments:** Current therapies only modestly slow progression; there is no cure for ALS.
- **Rapid Progression:** The swift decline in function limits the effectiveness of late-stage interventions.

Modern Relevance

- **Advances in** *genomic research* have uncovered numerous genetic mutations implicated in ALS, opening avenues for targeted therapies.
- *Clinical trials* are ongoing to explore novel approaches, including stem cell therapy, gene editing (e.g., CRISPR), and neuroprotective agents.
- The disease has gained public attention through campaigns like the *Ice Bucket Challenge*, boosting research funding and awareness.

Associated Conditions

- **Frontotemporal Dementia (FTD):** Approximately 15–20% of ALS patients have comorbid FTD due to shared genetic and pathological mechanisms.
- **Primary Lateral Sclerosis (PLS):** A related condition involving only upper motor neurons, with slower progression.

- **Spinal Muscular Atrophy (SMA):** Another motor neuron disorder, but with distinct genetic and clinical features.

Clinical Importance

- **Public Awareness:** ALS's association with Lou Gehrig has heightened global recognition and support for research and patient care.
- **Multidisciplinary Care:** Effective management involves neurologists, physiotherapists, speech therapists, and palliative care specialists.
- **Research Implications:** Understanding ALS has broader implications for other neurodegenerative diseases, including Parkinson's and Alzheimer's.

References

J. M. Charcot, Alexis Joffroy: Deux cas d'atrophie musculaire progressive avec lésions de la substance grise et des faiseaux antérolatéraux de la moelle épinière. Archives de physiologie normale et pathologique, Paris, 1869, 2: 354-367, 629-649, 744-760.

J. M. Charcot: Des amyotrophies spinales chroniques. Progrés médical, Paris, 1874, 2: 573-574.

J. M. Charcot, P.Marie: Deux nouveaux cas de sclérose latérale amyotrophique suivi d'autopsie. Archives de Neurologie, 1885.

Charcot's Syndrome I

Overview

Charcot's Syndrome I, now considered an outdated term, referred to an intermittent gait disturbance caused by obliterating angiopathy, leading to reduced blood circulation in the leg muscles. Symptoms included pain, cramps, tension, and weakness in the legs, which typically occurred after physical activity and resolved with rest. The syndrome was a symptom of underlying vascular diseases, including Buerger disease, and closely resembled conditions like dysbasia angiosclerotica. It was most commonly observed in the elderly and those with advanced vascular compromise.

Historical Background

- The syndrome is named after *Jean-Martin Charcot*, a pioneering neurologist and pathologist, whose contributions to medical science included the study of multiple neurological and vascular conditions.
- During the late 19th century, Charcot's work in understanding vascular diseases linked *intermittent claudication* to impaired blood flow, forming the basis for the description of Charcot's Syndrome I.
- Over time, **Advances in** vascular pathology and terminology have rendered the term obsolete, with modern medicine now describing such conditions under broader terms like *peripheral artery disease (PAD)* or *Buerger disease.*

Purpose

- **Identification of Vascular Impairments:** To diagnose and describe the intermittent symptoms of poor blood circulation in the lower limbs.
- **Symptom Management:** To address pain, weakness, and functional limitations caused by the reduced blood supply.
- **Guidance for Treatment:** To prompt investigation into underlying vascular conditions and initiate appropriate interventions.

Procedure Overview

Diagnosis:

- **Clinical Examination:** Symptoms of pain, cramping, and weakness in the legs appearing after exertion and relieved by rest.
- **Doppler Ultrasound:** Non-invasive imaging to detect blood flow abnormalities in the lower limbs.
- **Angiography:** Gold-standard imaging to identify arterial blockages or obliterating angiopathy.Laboratory Tests:
- Assess risk factors such as hyperlipidemia, diabetes, or smoking-related vascular damage.

Treatment:

- **Conservative Measures:** Smoking cessation, exercise therapy, and dietary changes to improve circulation and reduce vascular risk factors.
- **Pharmacotherapy:** Antiplatelet agents, vasodilators, or anticoagulants to enhance blood flow and prevent clot formation.
- **Surgical Intervention:** Bypass surgery or angioplasty for severe cases with significant arterial obstruction.
- **Follow-Up:** Regular monitoring of vascular health and symptom progression to adjust treatment as needed.

Results and Interpretation

- **Improvement in Symptoms:** Successful management often alleviates intermittent pain and cramping, improving walking distance and quality of life.
- **Underlying Conditions:** Diagnosis often uncovers systemic vascular diseases requiring long-term care and lifestyle modifications.
- **Prognosis:** Outcomes depend on the severity of vascular impairment and adherence to treatment protocols.

Physiological Basis

- **Reduced Circulation:** Obliterating angiopathy narrows or blocks arteries supplying the leg muscles, limiting oxygen delivery during physical exertion.
- **Ischemic Pain:** Accumulation of metabolic byproducts due to inadequate blood supply causes pain, cramps, and tension, relieved by rest.
- **Chronic Vascular Damage:** Conditions like atherosclerosis and thromboangiitis obliterans (Buerger disease) progressively impair blood flow, worsening symptoms over time.

Clinical Applications

- **Peripheral Artery Disease (PAD):** Modern diagnosis and management of intermittent claudication as part of systemic vascular disease.

- **Vascular Rehabilitation:** Exercise programs to improve circulation and promote collateral vessel formation.
- **Risk Factor Management:** Smoking cessation, lipid-lowering therapies, and diabetes management to prevent progression of vascular diseases.

Limitations and Technical Considerations

- **Diagnostic Challenges:** Similar symptoms can occur in other conditions, such as neurogenic claudication or muscular disorders, complicating diagnosis.
- **Progressive Nature:** Without early intervention, vascular diseases often progress, leading to critical limb ischemia or amputation.
- **Obsolete Terminology:** Charcot's Syndrome I is no longer used in clinical practice, with its symptoms now described under broader vascular pathologies.

Modern Relevance

- **Advances in** *vascular imaging* and *endovascular therapies* have improved the diagnosis and treatment of conditions resembling Charcot's Syndrome I.
- The understanding of intermittent claudication as a symptom of systemic vascular disease has reinforced the need for holistic cardiovascular care.
- Modern terminology, such as *PAD*, emphasizes the systemic nature of vascular diseases, integrating Charcot's early observations into contemporary frameworks.

Associated Conditions

- **Buerger Disease:** A specific type of obliterating angiopathy linked to tobacco use, presenting with similar symptoms.
- **Atherosclerosis:** A common underlying cause of obliterating angiopathy, contributing to intermittent claudication.
- **Diabetic Vascular Disease:** Diabetes-associated microvascular and macrovascular complications often exacerbate symptoms of reduced blood flow.

Clinical Importance

- **Early Recognition:** Identifying intermittent gait disturbance as a vascular symptom can prevent progression to critical ischemia or amputation.
- **Holistic Vascular Care:** Management of underlying systemic conditions, such as diabetes or hyperlipidemia, is crucial for overall cardiovascular health.
- **Educational Significance:** Charcot's work underscores the importance of clinical observation in linking symptoms to underlying pathophysiology, laying the groundwork for modern vascular medicine.

References

J. M. Charcot: Sur la claudication intermittente observé dans un cas d'obliteration complète des artères iliaques primitives. Comptes rendus des seances de la Société de biologie, Paris, 1858; Mémoires, 1859, 2nd series; 5: 225-258.

Chopart Fracture Dislocation

Overview

Chopart fracture-dislocation refers to a rare but severe injury involving the Chopart joint, which connects the hindfoot (calcaneus and talus) to the midfoot (navicular and cuboid). It typically occurs as a dislocation through the talonavicular and calcaneocuboid joints, often with associated fractures. This injury disrupts the structural integrity of the longitudinal arch of the foot, resulting in significant instability and impaired weight-bearing. Due to the high-energy trauma required to produce this injury, associated soft tissue damage and fractures are common.

Historical Background

- Named after *François Chopart*, a renowned French surgeon who detailed the *Chopart joint* and its clinical significance in the late 18th century.
- In *1792*, Lafiteau described *Chopart's method* of partial foot amputation through this joint, published in Fourcroy's *La médecine éclairée par les sciences physiques*.
- Over time, the joint has become a focal point for understanding midfoot injuries, with its complex anatomy and biomechanical role in the foot's stability.

Purpose

- **Stabilization of the Foot:** To restore the alignment and stability of the Chopart joint and prevent long-term functional impairment.
- **Preservation of Arch Integrity:** To maintain the structural integrity of the longitudinal arch, essential for normal gait mechanics.
- **Prevention of Complications:** To mitigate risks such as chronic pain, joint degeneration, and post-traumatic arthritis.

Procedure Overview

Diagnosis:

- **Clinical Signs:** Pain, swelling, deformity, and inability to bear weight on the foot.
- **Imaging:**
- **X-rays:** Disruption of the cyma line, indicating misalignment of the talonavicular and calcaneocuboid joints.
- Identification of associated fractures.
- **CT Scan:** Provides detailed visualization of fractures and joint dislocation.
- **MRI:** Assesses ligamentous injuries and soft tissue involvement.

Treatment:

- **Closed Reduction:** Attempted initially for dislocations without severe fractures.
- **Surgical Intervention:** Open reduction and internal fixation (ORIF) is the standard for unstable injuries or those with significant fractures.
- **Ligament repair or augmentation may be required.**
- **Postoperative Care:** Immobilization in a cast or boot, followed by progressive weight-bearing and physical therapy.
- **Rehabilitation:** Focus on restoring mobility, strength, and proper gait mechanics over several months.

Results and Interpretation

- **Reduction Success:** Accurate realignment and stabilization of the Chopart joint lead to better functional outcomes.
- **Prognosis:** Early intervention and effective rehabilitation can prevent long-term complications, but outcomes depend on the severity of the initial injury.
- **Complications:** Risks include chronic pain, stiffness, post-traumatic arthritis, and deformities, particularly if the injury is mismanaged or diagnosis is delayed.

Physiological Basis

- **Biomechanical Role of the Chopart Joint:** The joint facilitates foot flexibility and load distribution during gait, acting as a fulcrum between the hindfoot and midfoot.
- **Disruption of the Longitudinal Arch:** Injury to the talonavicular and calcaneocuboid joints compromises the foot's ability to bear weight and absorb shock.
- **Soft Tissue Involvement:** The bifurcate ligament (calcaneonavicular and calcaneocuboid ligaments) is critical for joint stability and is often damaged in Chopart injuries.

Clinical Applications

- **Trauma Management:** The Chopart fracture-dislocation is a key consideration in high-energy foot injuries, requiring prompt and precise management.
- **Reconstructive Surgery:** Advanced techniques in ORIF and ligament repair have improved outcomes for these complex injuries.
- **Rehabilitation Medicine:** Physical therapy tailored to restoring the foot's biomechanical function is essential for recovery.

Limitations and Technical Considerations

- **Diagnostic Challenges:** Subtle misalignments may be missed on initial imaging, requiring high-resolution CT or MRI for accurate diagnosis.
- **Surgical Complexity:** Reconstructing the Chopart joint demands meticulous attention to alignment and stabilization, with a risk of soft tissue complications.
- **Delayed Recovery:** The injury often necessitates prolonged rehabilitation, with residual stiffness or discomfort common even after successful treatment.

Modern Relevance

- **Advances in** *diagnostic imaging* and *surgical techniques* have enhanced the management of Chopart injuries, leading to better functional outcomes.
- Awareness of the *cyma line* and other radiological markers aids in early and accurate diagnosis.
- Improved understanding of the joint's biomechanical role has informed rehabilitation strategies, emphasizing arch stability and joint mobility.

Associated Conditions

- **Post-Traumatic Arthritis:** Common in untreated or poorly managed cases, leading to chronic pain and functional impairment.
- **Soft Tissue Injuries:** Ligament tears, particularly of the bifurcate ligament, frequently accompany Chopart disloca-

tions.

- **Fracture-Dislocation Syndromes:** Often associated with calcaneal or navicular fractures, further complicating treatment.

Clinical Importance

- **Early Diagnosis:** Prompt recognition of Chopart injuries prevents complications such as joint degeneration and deformity.
- **Multidisciplinary Approach:** Collaboration between trauma surgeons, orthopedic specialists, and rehabilitation therapists ensures comprehensive care.
- **Educational Value:** The injury highlights the importance of understanding joint anatomy, biomechanics, and the role of advanced imaging in trauma care.

References

Lafiteau. "Observation sur une amputation partielle du pied" In: Antoine François Fourcroy. La médecine éclairée par les sciences physiques, ou Journal des découvertes relatives aux différentes parties de l'art de guéri. Paris, chez Buisoon, 1792. Volume IV p85-88.

Main BJ, Jowett RL. Injuries of the midtarsal joint. J Bone Joint Surg Br. 1975 Feb;57(1):89-97. [PMID 234971]

Klaue K. Chopart fractures. Injury. 2004 Sep;35 Suppl 2:SB64-70. [PMID 15315880]

Ip KY, Lui TH. Isolated dorsal midtarsal (Chopart) dislocation: a case report. J Orthop Surg (Hong Kong). 2006 Dec;14(3):357-9. [PMID 17200547]

Swords MP, Schramski M, Switzer K, Nemec S. Chopart fractures and dislocations. Foot Ankle Clin. 2008 Dec;13(4):679-93, viii. [PMID 19013402]

van Dorp KB, de Vries MR, van der Elst M, Schepers T. Chopart joint injury: a study of outcome and morbidity. J Foot Ankle Surg. 2010 Nov-Dec;49(6):541-5. [PMID 21035040]

Chauffeur's Fracture

Overview

Chauffeur's Fracture is an intra-articular fracture of the radial styloid, a bony prominence of the distal radius near the wrist. It commonly results from trauma, often involving a fall on an outstretched hand (FOOSH). This injury frequently involves ligamentous damage and can lead to instability in the wrist joint. Historically associated with hand-crank car engines, this fracture earned its name due to its frequent occurrence among early chauffeurs.

Historical Background

- The term *Chauffeur's Fracture* originates from the late 19th and early 20th centuries when drivers were injured while starting vehicles with a hand crank. The crank would sometimes backfire, causing sudden forceful dorsiflexion of the wrist, leading to a fracture.
- This mechanism of injury has become rare due to technological **Advances in** automobile ignition systems, but the term persists in clinical practice.

Purpose

- **Primary Objective:** Stabilize the fractured radial styloid to prevent wrist instability and preserve joint function.
- **Secondary Goal:** Address associated ligament injuries, including those of the radioscaphocapitate and scapholunate ligaments, to avoid long-term complications like chronic pain and arthritis.

Procedure Overview

- **Initial Assessment:** Clinical signs include wrist pain, swelling, tenderness, and limited motion.
- Radiological confirmation via X-rays and, if necessary, CT scans for detailed visualization.
- **Treatment Approaches:**
- **Non-Surgical:** Splinting or casting for small, stable fractures without displacement.
- **Surgical:** Open reduction and internal fixation (ORIF) for displaced fractures or those associated with ligamentous instability.

Results and Interpretation

- X-rays reveal an avulsion or intra-articular fracture of the radial styloid.
- Advanced imaging may show additional injuries, such as scapholunate dissociation or lunate dislocation, particularly in severe cases.

Physiological Basis

- The radial styloid provides attachment for the *radioscaphocapitate ligament*, which stabilizes the scaphoid and lunate. Trauma leading to a Chauffeur's Fracture often disrupts these ligamentous attachments.
- The scaphoid's compression against the styloid during dorsiflexion and abduction transmits excessive force, resulting in a fracture.

Clinical Applications

- Restoring joint stability is critical to preventing chronic wrist pain and functional impairment.
- Early detection and appropriate management minimize the risk of post-traumatic arthritis.

Limitations and Technical Considerations

- **Non-Surgical Treatment:** Suitable only for non-displaced fractures, but carries the risk of delayed complications if ligament injuries are overlooked.
- **Surgical Management:** Requires precise alignment of fracture fragments and careful evaluation of ligament injuries to prevent long-term instability.

Modern Relevance

- Chauffeur's Fracture remains clinically significant, especially in high-energy trauma scenarios or FOOSH injuries.
- **Advances in** imaging and surgical techniques have improved the prognosis for patients with this injury, but early diagnosis and treatment remain critical.

Associated Conditions

- **Scapholunate Dissociation:** Frequently associated due to ligament disruption during injury.
- **Lunate Dislocation:** May occur if ligament damage is extensive.
- **Post-Traumatic Arthritis:** A common complication if the fracture or ligament injury is not adequately addressed.

Clinical Importance

- **Diagnosis:** Prompt identification of Chauffeur's Fracture is crucial to avoid missed ligament injuries, which can significantly affect wrist function.
- **Multidisciplinary Approach:** Optimal outcomes are achieved through coordination between emergency physicians, orthopedic surgeons, and rehabilitation specialists.
- **Patient Education:** Patients should be informed about the importance of adhering to follow-up and rehabilitation plans to restore wrist function and avoid long-term complications.

Chauffeur's Fracture exemplifies the complexity of distal radial injuries, requiring a thorough evaluation of both bony and ligamentous structures to ensure comprehensive care and successful recovery.

Chopart Fracture

Overview

Chopart fracture-dislocation refers to an injury involving the midtarsal joints of the foot, specifically the talonavicular and calcaneocuboid joints. This injury often results from high-energy trauma, such as falls from height or road traffic accidents, and frequently involves fractures of surrounding bones such as the calcaneus, cuboid, talus, or navicular. It is associated with significant long-term morbidity, including stiffness and osteoarthritis if not appropriately managed.

Historical Background

- Named after *François Chopart (1743–1795)*, a renowned French surgeon, who identified the midtarsal joint as an anatomical point for amputation in the treatment of distal foot tumors.
- Chopart first introduced the concept of the *Chopart joint* and its utility in amputation procedures, emphasizing its central role in foot articulation.

Purpose

- **Primary Objective:** Restore anatomical alignment of the midtarsal joint to maintain foot functionality and prevent complications such as arthritis or compartment syndrome.
- **Secondary Goals:** Address associated fractures to preserve the medial and lateral foot arches.
- Prevent long-term morbidity by achieving congruent joint surfaces and ligament stability.

Procedure Overview

- **Initial Assessment:** Clinical examination reveals pain, swelling, and deformity in the midfoot region.
- Radiographic imaging, including X-rays and CT scans, helps identify fractures and dislocations.

Treatment:

- **Non-Surgical:** Closed reduction may be attempted for simple dislocations without significant soft tissue or bony injury.
- **Surgical:** Open reduction and internal fixation (ORIF) for complex injuries involving fractures.
- Fusion of joints (e.g., talonavicular or calcaneocuboid) in cases of severe joint destruction.
- **Postoperative Care:** Immobilization followed by structured rehabilitation for recovery of foot function.

Results and Interpretation

- Proper alignment of the *talonavicular and calcaneocuboid joints* is critical for preserving the *medial and lateral foot arches.*
- Imaging post-reduction or surgery is necessary to confirm successful realignment and evaluate the efficacy of treatment.

Physiological Basis

- The *Chopart joint* plays a key role in foot mobility, providing a pivot for *inversion and eversion.*
- Traumatic forces during plantar flexion and inversion or eversion often cause midtarsal dislocation or associated fractures.
- Injuries to the surrounding ligaments compromise joint stability, necessitating anatomical reconstruction.

Clinical Applications

- Appropriate management can restore *foot alignment and functionality*, preventing complications like *chronic pain*, *stiffness*, or *arthritis.*
- Timely intervention reduces the risk of secondary complications such as *compartment syndrome* or *amputation* in severe cases.

Limitations and Technical Considerations

- Misdiagnosis or delayed treatment is common, with up to *41% of cases* being missed on initial evaluation.
- Closed reduction may fail in cases of *severe joint disruption*, necessitating open surgical intervention.
- External fixation, while useful, often results in *residual stiffness.*

Modern Relevance

- Chopart fracture-dislocations remain a diagnostic and therapeutic challenge, particularly in *polytrauma patients.*
- **Advances in** imaging and surgical techniques have improved outcomes, though long-term follow-up is essential to monitor for *post-traumatic arthritis.*

Associated Conditions

- **Compartment Syndrome:** Risk increases in high-energy injuries, requiring urgent intervention to prevent permanent tissue damage.

- **Post-Traumatic Arthritis:** Degenerative changes are common due to disruption of joint congruity.
- **Fractures:** Frequently involves the navicular, cuboid, talus, or calcaneus, complicating treatment.

Clinical Importance

- **Diagnosis:** Early recognition and treatment are critical to preventing long-term complications.
- **Multidisciplinary Approach:** Requires collaboration between orthopedic surgeons, radiologists, and rehabilitation specialists for optimal outcomes.
- **Patient Education:** Patients must be informed about the complexity of the injury and the importance of compliance with follow-up care and rehabilitation.

Chopart fracture-dislocations highlight the intricate relationship between midtarsal joint stability and foot functionality. Effective management demands timely diagnosis, meticulous surgical intervention, and long-term care to ensure successful recovery and mobility.

Clay-Shoveler Fracture

Overview

Clay-shoveler's fracture is a stable fracture involving the spinous process of the lower cervical or upper thoracic vertebrae, most commonly at C6 or C7. It typically results from a sudden, forceful muscle pull or reflex transmitted through the supraspinous ligaments, often during activities requiring intense upper body exertion. These fractures are generally stable and do not compromise spinal cord integrity, but they may cause localized pain and limited mobility.

Historical Background

- The term *Clay-shoveler's fracture* originated in *1930s Australia*, where laborers digging deep ditches with long-handled shovels would experience fractures in their cervical spinous processes. This injury occurred due to the sudden snapping of the sticky clay on their shovels during repetitive, forceful movements.
- Although first identified in manual laborers, this fracture now serves as a reminder of the biomechanical stresses placed on the cervical spine.

Purpose

- **The primary goal of managing a Clay-shoveler's fracture is to:** Relieve pain and inflammation caused by the fracture.
- Ensure proper spinal alignment to facilitate healing.
- Prevent further injury or complications, such as chronic pain or reduced range of

motion.

Procedure Overview

Diagnosis:

- Symptoms include localized pain at the site of the fracture, swelling, and tenderness.
- Plain film radiographs are typically sufficient for diagnosing this fracture, revealing an avulsion of the spinous process.
- CT scans may be used to assess adjacent injuries or ensure no additional instability.

Treatment:

- **Conservative Management:** Immobilization with a soft cervical collar, rest, and physical therapy are often sufficient for healing.
- **Pain Management:** NSAIDs and muscle relaxants may be prescribed for pain relief.
- Surgical intervention is rarely required as this is a stable fracture with no direct risk to the spinal cord.

Results and Interpretation

- Proper immobilization and adherence to treatment result in complete healing of the fracture without lasting deformities.
- Functional outcomes are typically favorable, with most individuals regaining full range of motion and returning to normal activities after adequate rest and rehabilitation.

Physiological Basis

- The fracture occurs due to extreme tension applied to the *supraspinous ligament*, which transmits the force to the spinous process.
- This avulsion is more common in individuals performing repetitive, forceful movements involving the upper body, as these actions place significant biomechanical stress on the cervical vertebrae.

Clinical Applications

- **Orthopedic and Rehabilitation Management:** Ensures the patient achieves pain relief, regains mobility, and prevents recurrent injuries.
- **Occupational Medicine:** Highlights the need for ergonomic interventions in high-risk professions to minimize repetitive stress injuries.

Limitations and Technical Considerations

- The fracture may occasionally be confused with *other cervical spine injuries* or conditions, necessitating careful imaging and evaluation.
- Although rare, concurrent injuries such as ligamentous tears or other vertebral fractures may occur and require additional management.

Modern Relevance

- With the decline of manual labor involving clay shoveling, these fractures are now commonly seen in *high-energy sports* or activities requiring repetitive upper-body force.
- **Advances in** diagnostic imaging ensure that the condition is identified early and managed appropriately.

Associated Conditions

- **Vertebral Artery Injury:** Fractures extending into the foramina transversarium should be evaluated for vascular compromise.
- **Cervical Muscle Strain:** Often accompanies the fracture, contributing to pain and restricted movement.

Clinical Importance

- **Stable Nature:** The fracture is generally non-threatening to the spinal cord, making conservative management highly effective.
- **Awareness in Diagnosis:** Early recognition prevents misdiagnosis or unnecessary interventions.
- **Occupational Insight:** This condition underscores the importance of proper technique and ergonomics in physical labor and sports to prevent similar injuries.

Clay-shoveler's fracture exemplifies how specific occupational activities can influence medical conditions, reinforcing the need for preventive measures and targeted rehabilitation to optimize recovery.

Codman's Exercises

Overview

Codman's exercises are a series of gentle pendulum movements of the upper extremities, designed to restore or maintain the range of motion in the shoulder joint following injury, fracture, or surgery. These exercises emphasize controlled, passive motion, allowing for gradual mobilization of the joint while minimizing stress on healing tissues. They are particularly effective during the early stages of rehabilitation for conditions such as rotator cuff injuries or shoulder fractures.

Historical Background

- Named after *Ernest Armory Codman*, an American orthopedic surgeon and pioneer in shoulder surgery, who introduced these exercises as part of his broader contributions to orthopedic care.
- Codman was also an early advocate for *outcome-based medicine*, emphasizing the importance of rehabilitation and functional recovery in his practice.
- His pendulum exercises remain widely used as a foundational technique in shoulder rehabilitation, reflecting their simplicity and effectiveness.

Purpose

- **Restoration of Mobility:** To facilitate a gradual return to normal range of motion (ROM) in the shoulder joint without stressing healing tissues.
- **Pain Relief:** The gentle motion helps reduce stiffness and improve circulation,

alleviating discomfort.

- **Prevention of Adhesions:** Early mobilization minimizes the risk of scar tissue formation, particularly in conditions like adhesive capsulitis (frozen shoulder).

Procedure Overview

- **Preparation:** The patient leans forward, allowing the arm to dangle freely with minimal effort.
- The body provides stability, typically with support from the unaffected arm resting on a surface like a table.
- **Pendulum Movements:** The patient uses body momentum to generate small circular or side-to-side movements of the affected arm.
- Movements are passive, with no active muscle engagement from the shoulder.
- **Progression:** As pain decreases and mobility improves, the range and intensity of movements can be gradually increased.
- Active-assisted or resistance exercises may be introduced later in rehabilitation.
- **Post-Exercise Immobilization:** Following the exercises, the shoulder may be immobilized to support healing and minimize strain.

Results and Interpretation

- **Improved Mobility:** Regular performance of Codman's exercises enhances shoulder joint flexibility and reduces stiffness.
- **Pain Reduction:** Gentle mobilization alleviates pain associated with immobility or post-injury inflammation.
- **Healing Support:** Early controlled movement promotes circulation, aiding tissue repair and recovery.

Physiological Basis

- **Passive Movement:** By relying on gravitational forces and body momentum, the exercises minimize strain on healing tissues while promoting joint mobilization.
- **Circulation and Lymphatic Flow:** Movement improves blood and lymphatic flow to the shoulder, reducing swelling and supporting recovery.
- **Joint Capsule Stretching:** Pendulum motions gently stretch the joint capsule, reducing stiffness and preventing contracture formation.

Clinical Applications

- **Post-Surgical Rehabilitation:** Commonly used after procedures like rotator cuff repair, shoulder arthroscopy, or fracture fixation.
- **Frozen Shoulder (Adhesive Capsulitis):** Effective in reducing stiffness and gradually restoring ROM in early-stage adhesive capsulitis.
- **Post-Fracture Mobilization:** Particularly valuable after humeral or clavicular fractures to maintain shoulder mobility during healing.

Limitations and Technical Considerations

- **Limited Applicability in Severe Cases:** Patients with severe pain or unstable fractures may be unable to perform these exercises initially.

- **Requires Guidance:** Proper technique is critical to avoid unintended strain or improper movement, necessitating supervision by a physical therapist in early stages.
- **Gradual Progression:** Overzealous progression or excessive ROM can jeopardize healing, underscoring the need for cautious implementation.

Modern Relevance

- Codman's exercises remain a cornerstone of *shoulder rehabilitation*, thanks to their simplicity, safety, and effectiveness.
- **Advances in** physical therapy and biomechanics have further refined their application, integrating them into broader rehabilitation protocols.
- Despite modern innovations, the fundamental principles of Codman's exercises - gentle, passive mobilization - are still highly relevant in clinical practice.

Associated Conditions

- **Rotator Cuff Injuries:** Enhances recovery and prevents stiffness post-surgery or injury.
- **Shoulder Impingement Syndrome:** Provides pain relief and promotes mobility in cases of impingement.
- **Adhesive Capsulitis:** Facilitates early mobilization, reducing the risk of long-term stiffness and disability.

Clinical Importance

- **Foundational Rehabilitation Technique:** Codman's exercises are often the first step in shoulder rehabilitation, enabling safe and controlled reintroduction of movement.
- **Accessible and Effective:** Their simplicity makes them easily teachable and applicable across a wide range of patients, from athletes to elderly individuals.
- **Historical and Practical Significance:** The exercises exemplify Ernest Codman's enduring contributions to orthopedic medicine and emphasize the importance of functional recovery in clinical care.

Codman's Sign

Overview

Codman's sign is a clinical indicator of rotator cuff dysfunction, most commonly associated with a rupture of the supraspinatus tendon. It is characterized by the ability to passively abduct the arm without pain, but upon releasing support, the contraction of the deltoid muscle causes pain, leading the patient to hunch their shoulder and drop the arm. This sign helps clinicians identify rotator cuff tears and assess shoulder stability and functionality.

Historical Background

- Named after *Ernest Armory Codman*, a pioneering orthopedic surgeon known for his groundbreaking work in shoulder pathology and rehabilitation.
- Codman's meticulous study of the *shoulder anatomy and function* laid the foundation for understanding rotator cuff injuries and associated diagnostic techniques.
- His description of Codman's sign has since become a classic clinical tool for diagnosing supraspinatus tendon injuries and rotator cuff tears.

Purpose

- **Diagnostic Clarity:** To detect the absence of rotator cuff function, particularly in cases of supraspinatus tendon rupture.
- **Assessment of Shoulder Stability:** To evaluate the ability of the shoulder musculature, especially the rotator cuff, to maintain joint alignment during movement.
- **Differentiation of Shoulder Pathologies:** To distinguish between rotator cuff injuries and other causes of shoulder pain or dysfunction.

Procedure Overview

- **Positioning the Patient:** The patient is seated or standing with their arm in a neutral position.
- **Passive Abduction:** The clinician passively abducts the patient's arm to about 90 degrees, ensuring minimal pain during this movement.
- **Releasing Support:** The arm is released, and the patient attempts to hold it in the abducted position using their deltoid muscle.
- **Observation:** If the supraspinatus tendon is ruptured, the patient will experience pain, causing them to hunch the shoulder and drop the arm.

Results and Interpretation

- **Positive Codman's Sign:** Pain upon deltoid contraction with an inability to maintain arm abduction indicates a ruptured supraspinatus tendon or severe rotator cuff dysfunction.
- **Negative Codman's Sign:** Smooth movement and maintained abduction without pain suggest an intact rotator cuff.
- **Additional Findings:** Observing shoulder compensation or scapular dyskinesis during the test may reveal concurrent shoulder instability or muscular imbalance.

Physiological Basis

- **Supraspinatus Tendon Function:** The supraspinatus initiates arm abduction and stabilizes the humeral head in the glenoid cavity. A rupture disrupts this function, shifting the load to the deltoid.
- **Deltoid Contraction:** Without rotator cuff stabilization, deltoid contraction causes superior migration of the humeral head, resulting in pain and an inability to maintain abduction.
- **Compensatory Mechanisms:** Patients hunch their shoulders or drop the arm to avoid pain caused by mechanical stress on the shoulder joint.

Clinical Applications

- **Rotator Cuff Tear Diagnosis:** Codman's sign is a reliable bedside tool for identifying tears or dysfunction in the supraspinatus tendon.
- **Pre-Surgical Assessment:** Helps determine the severity of rotator cuff injuries, guiding the decision for conservative versus surgical intervention.
- **Rehabilitation Monitoring:** Tracking improvements in Codman's sign during therapy provides insights into recovery and muscle function restoration.

Limitations and Technical Considerations

- **Subjectivity:** Pain tolerance and patient cooperation can influence the results, making the test less reliable in certain populations.
- **Adjunct Testing Required:** While Codman's sign suggests rotator cuff injury, confirmation with imaging (e.g., MRI or ultrasound) is necessary for a definitive diagnosis.
- **Non-Specificity:** Positive findings may overlap with other shoulder conditions, such as impingement syndrome or biceps tendon pathology.

Modern Relevance

- Despite **Advances in** imaging and diagnostics, *Codman's sign* remains a fundamental clinical tool due to its simplicity and effectiveness in initial evaluations.
- Modern understanding of *shoulder biomechanics* has reinforced the value of Codman's insights, especially in resource-limited settings where imaging may not be immediately available.
- The sign is now integrated into broader clinical protocols for assessing rotator cuff tears and guiding rehabilitation.

Associated Conditions

- **Rotator Cuff Tear:** Most commonly detected by Codman's sign, particularly supraspinatus tendon injuries.
- **Impingement Syndrome:** Can present with overlapping symptoms, necessitating further diagnostic workup.
- **Frozen Shoulder (Adhesive Capsulitis):** Reduced shoulder mobility may mimic Codman's sign but without the characteristic pain pattern.

Clinical Importance

- **Early Detection:** Codman's sign aids in the early diagnosis of rotator cuff injuries, allowing timely intervention to prevent further degeneration or shoulder instability.

- **Educational Value:** The test remains a cornerstone of clinical training in orthopedics and physical therapy, emphasizing functional assessment of the shoulder.
- **Historical Significance:** Reflects Codman's broader contributions to shoulder surgery and rehabilitation, demonstrating the enduring relevance of his work in modern medicine.

References

E. A. Codman: The Shoulder: Rupture of the Supraspinatus Tendon and Other Lesions in or about the Subacromial Bursa.

Boston : Privately printed, 1934. Reprint, Malabar, Florida : Krieger, 1965.

Codman's Triangle

Overview

Codman's triangle is a radiological sign observed in conditions such as osteosarcoma, characterized by an incomplete triangular shadow between a growing bone tumor and the surrounding normal bone. It is formed when the periosteum is lifted by the tumor but remains attached at the edges, creating a triangular appearance on imaging. While characteristic of aggressive bone lesions, Codman's triangle is not exclusive to osteosarcoma and can appear in other pathological conditions involving periosteal elevation.

Historical Background

- Named after *Ernest Armory Codman*, a pioneering orthopedic surgeon, whose work extended to bone tumors and radiological interpretation.
- Although *Codman's triangle* is strongly associated with *osteosarcoma*, it has also been observed in other aggressive bone lesions, reflecting its diagnostic value in orthopedic oncology.
- Codman's contributions to clinical orthopedics, including this radiological sign, highlight his lasting impact on musculoskeletal medicine.

Purpose

- **Radiological Identification:** To recognize Codman's triangle as an indicator of aggressive bone pathology, prompting further investigation.
- **Differentiation of Tumors:** To distinguish between benign and malignant

bone lesions based on the presence of periosteal reactions.

- **Guiding Clinical Management:** To support decisions regarding biopsy, surgical intervention, or additional imaging studies in suspected bone malignancies.

Procedure Overview

Imaging Techniques:

- **X-ray:** The primary modality for identifying Codman's triangle, typically seen as a triangular area of periosteal elevation.
- **CT Scan:** Offers detailed visualization of the lesion, aiding in the evaluation of tumor margins and bone destruction.
- **MRI:** Assesses soft tissue involvement, vascular invasion, and the extent of the periosteal reaction.
- **Bone Scintigraphy:** Used to detect metastatic spread or additional sites of bone involvement.
- **Histological Confirmation:** A biopsy is performed to confirm the diagnosis, particularly when osteosarcoma is suspected.
- **Follow-Up Imaging:** Regular monitoring through imaging assesses the response to treatment or progression of the disease.

Results and Interpretation

- **Presence of Codman's Triangle:** Indicates an aggressive bone lesion with rapid periosteal reaction, often associated with osteosarcoma but not pathognomonic.
- **Additional Findings:** Frequently accompanies other signs of malignancy, such as bone lysis, soft tissue mass, and irregular periosteal reactions.
- **Diagnostic Implications:** While suggestive, Codman's triangle must be interpreted alongside clinical and histological findings for definitive diagnosis.

Physiological Basis

- **Periosteal Reaction:** Codman's triangle forms as the periosteum attempts to regenerate in response to rapid tumor growth, leading to localized elevation and detachment.
- **Aggressive Bone Lesions:** The rapid pace of tumor expansion outstrips the periosteum's ability to adapt, resulting in incomplete ossification and the characteristic triangular shadow.
- **Underlying Pathology:** Conditions causing Codman's triangle often involve high levels of bone destruction and replacement by malignant or infectious tissue.

Clinical Applications

- **Oncology:** A critical feature in diagnosing primary bone tumors like osteosarcoma and aiding in tumor staging and planning.
- **Infectious Diseases:** Can be observed in osteomyelitis, where periosteal elevation occurs due to infection-induced bone destruction.
- **Trauma and Fractures:** In cases of stress fractures or healing periosteal reactions, Codman's triangle may appear, though its context differs significantly from malignancy.

Limitations and Technical Considerations

- **Non-Specificity:** While characteristic, Codman's triangle is not exclusive to osteosarcoma and can appear in other conditions, including infections and trauma.
- **Dependency on Imaging Quality:** Poor-quality X-rays or inappropriate imaging angles may obscure the periosteal reaction.
- **Requirement for Adjunct Testing:** Further diagnostic tools like biopsies are essential to confirm the underlying pathology.

Modern Relevance

- **Advances in** *imaging modalities*, including high-resolution CT and MRI, have improved the identification and characterization of Codman's triangle, enhancing diagnostic accuracy.
- The radiological sign remains a cornerstone in *oncological diagnostics*, particularly for early recognition of aggressive bone tumors.
- Modern understanding of periosteal biology has expanded its diagnostic scope to include other conditions, such as *eosinophilic granuloma* and *metastatic disease.*

Associated Conditions

- **Osteosarcoma:** The most common malignancy associated with Codman's triangle, typically affecting adolescents and young adults.
- **Ewing Sarcoma:** Another aggressive bone tumor where Codman's triangle may be observed.
- **Osteomyelitis:** Severe infections causing rapid periosteal elevation can mimic the radiological appearance of Codman's triangle.
- **Stress Fractures:** In cases of rapid bone remodeling, periosteal elevation may produce a similar radiological pattern.

Clinical Importance

- **Early Detection of Malignancies:** Recognizing Codman's triangle on imaging prompts timely investigation and intervention in potentially life-threatening conditions like osteosarcoma.
- **Differential Diagnosis:** Its presence aids in distinguishing between benign and aggressive lesions, influencing treatment strategies.
- **Educational Value:** Codman's triangle remains a key teaching point in radiology and orthopedic oncology, emphasizing the integration of imaging findings with clinical and histological data.

Codman's Tumour

Overview

Codman's tumour, also known as a chondroblastoma, is a rare, benign tumor of cartilage-forming connective tissue. It primarily occurs in the epiphyses of long bones such as the femur, humerus, and tibia. Patients typically present with localized pain and limited joint motion in the affected area. While benign, these tumors may cause functional limitations due to their proximity to joints. They predominantly affect adolescent and young adult males, and the condition is rarely associated with malignant transformation. The exact etiology remains unknown.

Historical Background

- The tumor is associated with *Ernest Armory Codman*, an early pioneer in orthopedic surgery, who contributed significantly to the understanding of musculoskeletal tumors.
- Codman described the tumor in detail as a distinct pathological entity, highlighting its unique localization to the epiphyses and its cartilage-forming nature.
- Over time, Codman's tumor has become recognized as a rare but important diagnosis in orthopedic oncology due to its implications for joint function and mobility.

Purpose

- **Early Detection:** To identify the tumor in its early stages to prevent joint damage and associated complications.
- **Differentiation:** To distinguish Codman's tumor from malignant bone lesions, such as osteosarcoma or chondrosarcoma, through imaging and histopathology.
- **Management:** To alleviate symptoms and preserve joint functionality through surgical intervention or other treatments.

Procedure Overview

Diagnosis:

- **Clinical Examination:** Patients present with pain, swelling, and restricted joint movement localized to the affected bone.
- **Imaging:**
- **X-rays:** Show a well-demarcated lytic lesion in the epiphysis with thin sclerotic borders.
- **MRI:** Provides detailed visualization of tumor extent and its relationship with surrounding soft tissue and cartilage.
- **CT Scan:** Useful for assessing bone involvement and calcifications within the lesion.
- **Biopsy:** Confirmatory diagnosis through histological examination of tumor tissue.

Treatment:

- **Curettage:** The primary treatment involves surgical removal of the tumor through curettage, often followed by bone grafting.
- **Adjuvant Therapy:** Local adjuvants, such as phenol or cryotherapy, may be used to reduce recurrence risk.
- **Rehabilitation:** Physical therapy post-surgery to restore joint mobility

and function.

- **Follow-Up:** Regular imaging is required to monitor for recurrence, which is uncommon but possible.

Results and Interpretation

- **Benign Nature:** Codman's tumor is a benign lesion with a low risk of malignant transformation.
- **Functional Recovery:** With proper treatment, most patients regain joint function and mobility.
- **Prognosis:** Excellent in the majority of cases, provided the tumor is treated early to minimize joint damage.

Physiological Basis

- **Cartilage Formation:** Codman's tumor originates from cartilage-forming connective tissue in the epiphyses, disrupting normal bone and cartilage growth.
- **Localized Effects:** The tumor's proximity to the joint capsule causes pain, swelling, and restricted motion due to mechanical and inflammatory factors.
- **Benign Behavior:** Despite its aggressive appearance on imaging, the tumor seldom metastasizes or undergoes malignant transformation.

Clinical Applications

- **Orthopedic Oncology:** Codman's tumor is an important consideration in the differential diagnosis of epiphyseal lesions in young adults.
- **Surgical Management:** Advances in curettage and adjuvant therapies have improved outcomes and reduced recurrence rates.
- **Rehabilitation:** Comprehensive post-surgical rehabilitation ensures restoration of joint mobility and function.

Limitations and Technical Considerations

- **Diagnostic Challenges:** Radiological overlap with other bone lesions, such as osteoid osteoma or chondrosarcoma, can complicate diagnosis.
- **Recurrence Risk:** Incomplete removal during curettage may lead to recurrence, necessitating close follow-up.
- **Surgical Risks:** Potential complications include joint instability, infection, or damage to surrounding structures.

Modern Relevance

- **Advances in** *imaging techniques* have enhanced early detection and characterization of Codman's tumor, aiding in precise surgical planning.
- *Adjuvant therapies*, such as cryotherapy and phenol application, have reduced recurrence rates, improving long-term outcomes.
- The condition remains a focus of interest in pediatric and adolescent orthopedics due to its age-specific prevalence and impact on joint health.

Associated Conditions

- **Epiphyseal Lesions:** Includes other benign tumors like giant cell tumors or chondromyxoid fibroma, which share similar anatomical localization.
- **Osteoarthritis:** Joint involvement by Codman's tumor can lead to secondary degenerative changes if untreated.
- **Osteochondritis Dissecans:** A differ-

ential diagnosis in cases of joint pain and swelling in adolescents.

Clinical Importance

- **Preservation of Joint Function:** Early detection and management are crucial to prevent irreversible joint damage and ensure optimal mobility.
- **Differential Diagnosis:** Codman's tumor must be distinguished from malignant bone tumors to avoid unnecessary aggressive treatments.
- **Historical Significance:** Codman's contributions to the understanding of benign bone tumors underscore the importance of accurate diagnosis and individualized treatment in orthopedic oncology.

References

E. A. Codman: Epiphyseal chondromatous giant cell tumours of the upper end of the humerus. Surgery, Gynecology and Obstetrics, Chicago, 1931, 32: 543-548.

Colles Fracture

Overview

A Colles fracture is an extra-articular fracture of the distal radius characterized by dorsal angulation of the distal fragment. It often occurs about 1.5 inches above the carpal extremity of the radius and is frequently associated with a styloid fracture of the ulna and volar angulation of the fracture apex. This type of fracture is most commonly caused by a fall onto an outstretched hand (FOOSH) and is often observed in older adults, particularly postmenopausal women with osteoporosis. Clinical presentation includes wrist deformity, pain, and swelling with a characteristic "dinner fork" deformity on examination.

Historical Background

- *Abraham Colles*, an Irish surgeon, first described the fracture in *1814*, meticulously detailing its anatomical and clinical features.
- Earlier descriptions were noted by *Jean-Louis Petit* and *Claude Pouteau*, but Colles is credited with distinguishing this specific fracture type.
- Contributions from others, including *Robert William Smith* and *Ernest Amory Codman*, further refined the understanding and treatment of distal radius fractures, particularly in differentiating articular from extra-articular injuries.

Purpose

- **Accurate Diagnosis:** To identify the fracture pattern and assess the alignment of the distal radius and ulna.

- **Restoration of Wrist Function:** To reduce the fracture and stabilize the joint, ensuring proper healing and preventing long-term complications.
- **Preventing Deformities:** To address and correct the dorsal angulation to avoid permanent dinner fork deformity and loss of wrist mobility.

Procedure Overview

Diagnosis:

- **Clinical Signs:** Pain, swelling, and deformity at the wrist with tenderness over the distal radius.

Imaging:

- **X-rays:** Confirm the diagnosis, showing dorsal angulation, fracture line, and potential involvement of the ulna styloid.
- **CT or MRI:** May be required to assess associated soft tissue injuries or comminution in complex cases.

Treatment:

- **Closed Reduction and Casting:** Performed under local anesthesia to restore alignment, followed by immobilization in a plaster cast for 4–6 weeks.
- **Surgical Intervention:** Open reduction and internal fixation (ORIF) with plates and screws are used for unstable or comminuted fractures.
- **Physiotherapy:** Rehabilitation to restore strength, range of motion, and functionality after cast removal or surgery.
- **Follow-Up:** Regular X-rays to monitor fracture alignment and healing progress.

Results and Interpretation

- **Fracture Healing:** Most fractures heal within 6–8 weeks, provided adequate reduction and immobilization are achieved.
- **Functional Recovery:** Early physiotherapy ensures better outcomes in terms of wrist strength and mobility.
- **Complications:** Malunion or dorsal displacement may occur if reduction is inadequate, leading to persistent deformity and dysfunction.

Physiological Basis

- **Mechanism of Injury:** A fall onto an outstretched hand (FOOSH) transmits force through the wrist, causing the distal radius to fracture under axial compression.
- **Bone Weakness:** Osteoporosis, particularly in postmenopausal women, increases susceptibility to distal radius fractures.
- **Joint Biomechanics:** The dorsal displacement disrupts wrist biomechanics, requiring precise reduction to restore function.

Clinical Applications

- **Trauma Management:** Colles fracture is a cornerstone diagnosis in orthopedic and emergency medicine, emphasizing the importance of early recognition and management.
- **Rehabilitation Medicine:** Post-treatment physiotherapy is critical to regain wrist function and prevent stiffness.
- **Geriatric Care:** Highlighting the role of bone health in fracture prevention, particularly in populations at risk of

osteoporosis.

Limitations and Technical Considerations

- **Complications of Reduction:** Inadequate reduction or fixation can lead to malunion, chronic pain, and reduced wrist functionality.
- **Associated Injuries:** Ligamentous injuries or fractures of the ulna styloid may complicate treatment and require additional intervention.
- **Bone Quality:** Poor bone quality in elderly or osteoporotic patients may necessitate specific surgical techniques for stabilization.

Modern Relevance

- **Advances in** *surgical techniques*, including volar plating and external fixation, have improved outcomes for complex Colles fractures.
- *Imaging technologies* such as CT and 3D reconstruction aid in detailed fracture assessment, enhancing treatment planning.
- Preventive strategies like *bone health optimization* (e.g., calcium and vitamin D supplementation) play a critical role in reducing the incidence of Colles fractures in high-risk populations.

Associated Conditions

- **Osteoporosis:** A major risk factor, particularly in elderly women, leading to fragility fractures like the Colles fracture.
- **Scaphoid Fractures:** May occur concurrently in high-energy trauma to the wrist.
- **Carpal Tunnel Syndrome:** Swelling and displacement in Colles fractures can compress the median nerve, necessitating careful monitoring.

Clinical Importance

- **Early Intervention:** Prompt reduction and immobilization minimize deformity and optimize recovery.
- **Comprehensive Care:** The fracture highlights the need for multidisciplinary approaches, including orthopedic care, physiotherapy, and geriatric management.
- **Historical and Educational Value:** Colles fracture serves as a classic example in orthopedic education, emphasizing the interplay between anatomy, biomechanics, and clinical management.

References

Petit JL. L'art de guérir les maladies des os Traité des maladies des os. Paris: Cavellier 1705 [A treatise of the diseases of the bones – translated 1726] Commentary on distal radius fractures [1705;X:126-140]

Pouteau C. Mélanges de chirurgie. Paris. 1760

Colles A. On the fracture of the carpal extremity of the radius. The Edinburgh medical and surgical journal. 1814;10:182-186. [Clin Orthop Relat Res. 2006;445:5-7. PMID 16601406]

Smith RW. On Fractures of the Bones of the Fore-arm in the Vicinity of the Wrist Joint. In: A Treatise on Fractures in the Vicinity of Joint and on Certain Forms of Accidental and Congenital Dislocations. Dublin: Hodges Smith. 1847:129-175

Cotton Fracture

Overview

A Cotton fracture, also known as a trimalleolar fracture, is a severe ankle injury involving fractures of the lateral malleolus, medial malleolus, and the posterior malleolus of the distal tibia. This fracture pattern results in significant instability of the ankle joint, often accompanied by posterior dislocation or subluxation. Cotton fractures typically occur due to high-energy rotational forces applied to the ankle, such as during sports injuries, falls, or accidents.

Historical Background

- Named after *Frederic Jay Cotton*, who detailed the fracture in his seminal textbook *Dislocations and Joint-Fractures* (1910) and in a series of case studies published in *JAMA in 1915.*
- Cotton expanded on the work of *Percivall Pott*, who had earlier described bimalleolar fractures in detail.
- Cotton's contributions provided a deeper understanding of the mechanism, reduction techniques, and operative management of trimalleolar fractures, laying the foundation for modern treatment approaches.

Purpose

- **Stabilization of the Ankle Joint:** To restore joint congruity and prevent chronic instability, which can lead to arthritis and functional impairment.
- **Alignment Restoration:** To ensure proper alignment of the malleoli and articular surface of the tibia, critical for weight-bearing and motion.
- **Functional Recovery:** To enable patients to regain mobility and return to daily activities or sports.

Procedure Overview

Diagnosis:

- **Clinical Assessment:** Symptoms include severe ankle pain, swelling, deformity, and inability to bear weight.

Imaging:

- **X-rays:** Identify fractures of the lateral, medial, and posterior malleoli, along with any dislocation.
- **CT Scan:** Used for complex cases to assess the extent of posterior malleolar involvement and joint surface disruption.
- **MRI:** Evaluates soft tissue injuries, such as ligament tears or syndesmotic disruptions.

Treatment:

- **Non-Surgical Management:** Rarely appropriate; reserved for non-displaced fractures in patients with low activity levels.
- **Surgical Intervention:** Open reduction and internal fixation (ORIF) is the standard treatment, addressing each fractured component:
- **Plates and screws for the lateral malleolus.**
- **Screws or tension band wiring for the medial malleolus.**
- **Posterior malleolus fixation if fragment size exceeds 25% of the articular surface or if instability persists.**

- **Rehabilitation:** Early motion exercises followed by progressive weight-bearing to restore function.
- **Post-Treatment Monitoring:** Regular imaging to confirm healing and assess alignment.
- Rehabilitation progress monitoring to ensure functional recovery.

Results and Interpretation

- **Successful Healing:** Proper reduction and fixation typically result in stable healing and good functional outcomes.
- **Complications:** Delayed or improper treatment may lead to malunion, chronic instability, or post-traumatic arthritis.
- **Prognosis:** Most patients achieve full recovery, although recovery times may vary depending on injury severity and adherence to rehabilitation.

Physiological Basis

- **Rotational Force Mechanism:** High-energy rotational forces cause fractures of the medial, lateral, and posterior malleoli, disrupting the stability of the ankle mortise.
- **Joint Instability:** The involvement of the posterior malleolus compromises the articular surface and posterior tibiofibular ligament, necessitating surgical correction.
- **Soft Tissue Involvement:** Syndesmotic ligament injuries often accompany the fracture, further contributing to instability.

Clinical Applications

- **Trauma Orthopedics:** A critical condition requiring prompt diagnosis and intervention to restore joint function and prevent complications.
- **Reconstructive Surgery:** Techniques developed for Cotton fractures are applicable to other complex fractures involving weight-bearing joints.
- **Rehabilitation Medicine:** Emphasizes the importance of physical therapy in regaining ankle strength, mobility, and proprioception after injury.

Limitations and Technical Considerations

- **Delayed Presentation:** Untreated or mismanaged fractures can result in poor outcomes, necessitating revision surgeries.
- **Surgical Complexity:** Fixation of the posterior malleolus requires precise alignment to restore articular congruity, often requiring advanced imaging for intraoperative guidance.
- **Post-Traumatic Arthritis:** Even with successful reduction, articular surface involvement increases the risk of long-term arthritis.

Modern Relevance

- **Advances in** *imaging techniques* have improved the diagnosis and classification of Cotton fractures, aiding in tailored treatment plans.
- Modern surgical tools and techniques, including minimally invasive approaches, have enhanced outcomes and reduced recovery times.
- Greater emphasis on *functional*

rehabilitation has improved long-term mobility and quality of life for patients.

Associated Conditions

- **Syndesmotic Injury:** Commonly accompanies trimalleolar fractures and requires surgical stabilization.
- **Post-Traumatic Arthritis:** A long-term complication due to articular surface damage.
- **Osteoporosis:** In elderly patients, reduced bone density may complicate fracture fixation and healing.

Clinical Importance

- **Early Intervention:** Prompt and accurate treatment ensures better outcomes, minimizing the risk of deformity or chronic pain.
- **Comprehensive Management:** Cotton fractures emphasize the need for multidisciplinary care involving trauma surgeons, radiologists, and rehabilitation specialists.
- **Educational Significance:** The condition serves as a classic example of complex joint injuries, highlighting the importance of anatomical understanding and precise surgical intervention.

References

Cotton FJ. A new type of ankle fracture. JAMA. 1915;64:318–321.

Cushing's Symphalangism

Overview

Cushing's symphalangism is a rare hereditary condition characterized by fusion of the midphalangeal joints, as well as fusion of elbow, carpal, and tarsal bones. The absence of normal articular folds leads to restricted joint mobility and an abnormal gait. A distinctive feature of this syndrome is conductive deafness, caused by the fusion of the ossicles in the middle ear. Additional features include brachydactyly, cutaneous syndactyly, and a peculiar facial morphology marked by hypoplasia of the alae nasi, a long narrow face, a thin upper lip, and a broad nasal bridge. The syndrome follows an autosomal dominant inheritance pattern with variable expression.

Historical Background

- *Georg Joachimsthal* first described the condition in 1900, emphasizing the skeletal abnormalities.
- In *1906*, *Harvey Williams Cushing* encountered a patient with a brain tumor and rigid fingers at Johns Hopkins Hospital. Over the next decade, Cushing, in collaboration with *Professor Samuel Growe*, studied the condition in detail, documenting the genetic basis through *seven generations* of a single family.
- In *1965*, the condition was revisited by *Strasburger and colleagues*, who highlighted the syndromic inclusion of *conductive deafness* and traced the genetic lineage to *William Brown*,

a Scottish immigrant from the 18th century.

Purpose

- **Understanding Genetic Inheritance:** To explore the autosomal dominant transmission and variability of expression in affected families.
- **Early Diagnosis and Management:** To identify and address functional limitations and associated conductive hearing loss early in life.
- **Preservation of Mobility:** To manage joint stiffness and promote mobility, preventing secondary complications.

Procedure Overview

Diagnosis:

- **Clinical Examination:** Observing features such as rigid fingers, limited motion in the elbows, wrists, and ankles, and characteristic facial morphology.
- **Radiological Assessment:** X-rays to confirm fusion of midphalangeal, carpal, and tarsal bones, as well as elbow joint involvement.
- **Audiological Testing:** Evaluating conductive hearing loss through audiometry and middle ear imaging.
- **Genetic Testing:** Confirming autosomal dominant inheritance and identifying gene mutations associated with the condition.

Management:

- **Physical Therapy:** Focused on maintaining joint mobility and minimizing functional impairment.
- **Surgical Interventions:** Possible correction for severe syndactyly or joint contractures to improve hand functionality.
- **Hearing Aids:** Addressing conductive hearing loss with amplification devices or surgical options, such as ossicular chain reconstruction.
- **Long-Term Monitoring:** Regular follow-ups to assess mobility, hearing, and potential secondary complications.

Results and Interpretation

- **Functional Impairment:** Joint fusions lead to stiffness and restricted movement, particularly in the hands and lower limbs, which can affect daily activities and gait.
- **Hearing Loss:** Conductive hearing loss significantly impacts communication and quality of life but is manageable with appropriate interventions.
- **Variable Expression:** The severity of skeletal abnormalities and hearing loss varies widely, even within the same family.

Physiological Basis

- **Skeletal Development:** Fusion of the midphalangeal joints and absence of articular folds are due to disrupted endochondral ossification.
- **Conductive Deafness:** The ossicles' fusion in the middle ear prevents efficient sound conduction, leading to hearing loss.
- **Facial Morphology:** The distinct facial features result from congenital developmental anomalies affecting cartilage and soft tissues.

Clinical Applications

- **Orthopedic and Rehabilitation Medicine:** Focuses on managing joint stiffness and improving mobility in affected individuals.
- **Audiology:** Early detection and management of conductive hearing loss enhance communication and social functioning.
- **Genetic Counseling:** Assists families in understanding inheritance patterns, risks, and options for managing the condition.

Limitations and Technical Considerations

- **Diagnostic Challenges:** Variability in expression may delay diagnosis, particularly in mild cases.
- **Surgical Risks:** Corrective procedures for joint fusion or syndactyly carry risks of infection, scarring, or limited improvement in function.
- **Hearing Aid Limitations:** While effective, hearing aids do not fully address the underlying ossicular fusion, necessitating lifelong management.

Modern Relevance

- **Advances in** *genetic testing* have improved diagnostic accuracy and the ability to predict variability within families.
- *Imaging technologies*, such as CT and MRI, have enhanced the ability to detect skeletal and auditory abnormalities, leading to earlier and more effective interventions.
- Research into *osseous and cartilage formation pathways* may lead to targeted therapies for syndromes like Cushing's symphalangism.

Associated Conditions

- **Symphalangism:** Fusion of interphalangeal joints is a hallmark feature of the syndrome.
- **Brachydactyly and Syndactyly:** Additional skeletal anomalies often seen in affected individuals.
- **Congenital Hearing Loss:** Conductive deafness due to ossicular fusion is a consistent feature.
- **Gait Abnormalities:** Restricted lower limb joint mobility leads to difficulty in walking.

Clinical Importance

- **Multisystem Involvement:** The syndrome's combination of skeletal, auditory, and facial abnormalities requires a multidisciplinary approach to management.
- **Genetic Insights:** Cushing's symphalangism is a classic example of autosomal dominant inheritance with variable expression, valuable in genetic education and research.
- **Functional Impacts:** Early diagnosis and intervention significantly improve quality of life, highlighting the importance of integrating orthopedic, audiological, and rehabilitative care.

References

G. Joachimsthal: Die angeborenen Verbildungen der oberen Extremitäten. Hamburg, 1900.

H. W. Cushing: Hereditary anchylosis of proximal phalangeal joints (symphalangism). Genetics, Austin, Texas, 1916, 1: 90-106.

E. S. Vessel: Symphalangism, strabism and hearing loss in mother and daughter. New England Journal of Medicine, Boston, 1960, 263: 839-842.

li>A. K. Strasburger, M. R. Hawkins, R. Eldridge, R. L. Hargrave,

V. A. McKusick: Symphalangism: genetic and clinical aspects. Bulletin of the Johns Hopkins Hospital, Baltimore, 1965, 117: 108-127.

P. Maroteaux, J. P. Bouvet, M. L. Briard: La maladie des synostose multiples. La presse médicale, Paris, 1972, 1: 3041-3047.

Crescent Pelvic Fracture

Overview

Crescent pelvic fracture is a type of pelvic ring injury resulting from high-energy lateral compression trauma. It involves a partial dislocation of the sacroiliac (SI) joint and a fracture of the posterior iliac crest. This condition leads to a rotationally unstable but vertically stable hemipelvis. Accurate reduction and fixation are critical to ensure proper alignment and to avoid complications such as malunion and arthritis.

Historical Background

- Pelvic fractures have been recognized for centuries as significant injuries often associated with trauma.
- Crescent pelvic fractures, as a specific subtype, were better characterized with the advent of advanced imaging techniques and classification systems, such as the *Day classification system*, in the late 20th century.

Purpose

- **The goal in managing crescent pelvic fractures is to:** Stabilize the pelvic ring.
- Restore the anatomical alignment of the sacroiliac joint.
- Prevent complications such as chronic pain, malunion, and post-traumatic arthritis.

Procedure Overview

Diagnosis:

- Clinical examination often reveals pain, instability, and possible deformity of the pelvis.
- Imaging modalities such as X-rays, CT scans, and sometimes MRI are used to evaluate fracture patterns and sacroiliac joint involvement.
- **Surgical Intervention:**
- **Type I fractures:** Often treated with minimally invasive percutaneous iliosacral screws for stabilization.
- **Type II and III fractures:** Require open reduction and fixation with reconstruction plates and/or iliosacral screws to restore stability and alignment.
- **Post-operative Care:** Early mobilization and rehabilitation are critical to regain functionality and prevent long-term complications.

Results and Interpretation

- **Successful treatment of crescent pelvic fractures leads to:**
- Restored pelvic stability.
- Pain relief.
- Prevention of long-term complications such as malalignment and arthritis.
- Outcomes depend on the quality of reduction and fixation as well as the timeliness of intervention.

Physiological Basis

- The pelvis, being a ring-like structure, distributes weight and stabilizes the axial skeleton with the lower extremities.
- Crescent fractures occur due to *lateral compression forces*, which disrupt the *inferior portion of the sacroiliac joint* while sparing the posterior ligamentous attachments.
- This results in rotational instability of the hemipelvis, requiring surgical fixation to maintain proper load distribution.

Clinical Applications

- **Emergency Management:** In polytrauma patients, addressing pelvic stability is crucial for overall survival and recovery.
- **Surgical Planning:** Understanding the fracture type (Day classification) helps guide the choice of surgical approach and fixation techniques.

Limitations and Technical Considerations

- **These fractures are complex and require:** Accurate imaging to assess fracture configuration and joint congruency.
- Skilled surgical intervention to avoid complications such as nerve injury or fixation failure.
- Late presentation or delay in surgical management increases the risk of *malunion*, chronic pain, and reduced functional outcomes.

Modern Relevance

- **Advances in** *percutaneous fixation techniques* and imaging modalities have improved outcomes and minimized soft tissue disruption.
- The condition remains relevant due to its association with *high-energy trauma*,

such as motor vehicle accidents, and its complexity in polytrauma patients.

Associated Conditions

- **Sacral fractures:** Often co-exist with crescent fractures.
- **Anterior pelvic ring injuries:** Frequently accompany posterior crescent fractures, requiring comprehensive management.
- **Compartment syndrome:** A rare but serious complication of pelvic fractures.

Clinical Importance

- **Timely Diagnosis:** Early identification and management are crucial to preventing debilitating complications.
- **Multidisciplinary Approach:** Collaboration between orthopedic surgeons, radiologists, and trauma specialists ensures optimal care.
- **Rehabilitation:** Post-surgical rehabilitation is vital to regain mobility and prevent complications such as stiffness or seating obliquity.Crescent pelvic fractures, while rare, represent a significant challenge in trauma care and necessitate a structured, evidence-based approach to achieve the best patient outcomes.

Danis-Weber Classification

Overview

The Danis-Weber classification is a widely used system for categorizing ankle fractures based on the location of the fibular fracture relative to the distal tibiofibular syndesmosis. The classification includes three types:

- **Type A:** Fracture of the fibula distal to the syndesmosis.
- **Type B:** Fracture of the fibula at the level of the syndesmosis.
- **Type C:** Fracture of the fibula proximal to the syndesmosis.

This system emphasizes the importance of the syndesmosis in ankle stability, guiding treatment decisions. It was first introduced by Robert Danis in 1949 and later modified and popularized by Bernhard Georg Weber in 1972, becoming the Weber classification.

Historical Background

- **1949:** Robert Danis described the system in his publication *Théorie et pratique de l'ostéosynthèse*, establishing a foundation for classifying fibular fractures.
- **1972:** Bernhard Weber refined and popularized the classification, simplifying it for practical use in clinical settings.
- **Lauge-Hansen Classification (1950):** A contemporary rotational classification of ankle fractures based on the mechanism of injury, which complements the Danis-Weber system.

Purpose

- **Simplified Fracture Description:** To provide a clear and concise method for categorizing fibular fractures in relation to the syndesmosis.
- **Guiding Treatment:** To differentiate between stable and unstable fractures, helping determine the need for surgical intervention.
- **Predicting Outcomes:** To assess the likelihood of associated injuries, such as syndesmotic instability or ligamentous disruption.

Procedure Overview

Diagnosis:

- **Clinical Evaluation:** Pain, swelling, deformity, and inability to bear weight on the ankle.
- **Imaging:** X-rays: Standard imaging to classify fractures into Type A, B, or C.
- **Lateral and AP views assess alignment and fracture location.**
- **CT or MRI:** Used for complex fractures or when syndesmotic injury is suspected.

Classification:

- **Type A:** Fibula fracture below the syndesmosis, often stable.
- **May include an oblique medial malleolus fracture.**
- **Type B:** Fibula fracture at the syndesmosis level.
- **Stability depends on associated ligament injuries or medial malleolus fractures.**
- **Type C:** Fibula fracture above the syndesmosis, typically unstable.
- Associated with syndesmotic injuries and possible medial malleolus fractures or deltoid ligament rupture.

Treatment:

- **Type A:** Conservative management with casting or bracing.
- **Type B:** Conservative treatment for stable fractures; surgical fixation for unstable injuries.
- **Type C:** Requires surgical intervention (e.g., open reduction and internal fixation [ORIF]) to restore syndesmotic stability.

Results and Interpretation

- **Accurate Fracture Classification:** Determines fracture stability and the likelihood of associated ligamentous injuries.
- **Guided Treatment:** Type A fractures typically respond to conservative treatment, whereas Types B and C often require surgical management.
- **Prognostic Value:** Higher classifications (Type C) are associated with greater instability and worse outcomes without appropriate intervention.

Physiological Basis

- **Role of the Syndesmosis:** The syndesmosis stabilizes the ankle mortise; fractures at or above its level often disrupt joint integrity.
- **Fracture Mechanics:** Rotational forces, combined with axial loading, determine the location and severity of the fracture.
- **Stability and Associated Injuries:** Displacement of the fibula alters ankle

biomechanics, often causing medial ligament tears or malleolar fractures.

Clinical Applications

- **Trauma Classification:** A critical tool in orthopedic and emergency medicine for systematically describing ankle fractures.
- **Surgical Planning:** Differentiating between fracture types helps guide decisions on conservative versus surgical management.
- **Teaching Tool:** The simplicity of the Danis-Weber system makes it an excellent resource for educating medical students and trainees.

Limitations and Technical Considerations

- **Exclusivity to Fibular Fractures:** The system focuses solely on fibular fractures and does not directly address associated ligamentous or bony injuries.
- **Stability Assessment:** While useful, the classification does not always reliably predict syndesmotic stability or the need for fixation.
- **Complementary Use:** Often used in conjunction with the Lauge-Hansen classification for a more comprehensive understanding of the injury.

Modern Relevance

- The Danis-Weber classification remains a cornerstone in ankle fracture management due to its simplicity and effectiveness.
- **Advances in** *imaging techniques* (e.g., 3D CT) have enhanced the system's application by providing detailed views of fracture patterns and associated injuries.
- Its widespread use in trauma registries and research has standardized reporting and facilitated comparison of outcomes across studies.

Associated Conditions

- **Syndesmotic Injuries:** Particularly common in Type B and C fractures, requiring additional surgical fixation.
- **Deltoid Ligament Rupture:** Commonly associated with Type B and C fractures, often leading to instability.
- **Medial Malleolus Fractures:** Frequently accompany higher-grade fractures, complicating management.

Clinical Importance

- **Standardized Communication:** The classification provides a common language for healthcare providers to describe and discuss ankle fractures.
- **Improved Outcomes:** By guiding treatment, the classification helps ensure appropriate management, reducing complications such as chronic instability or arthritis.
- **Historical and Educational Significance:** A testament to the evolution of trauma classification systems, the Danis-Weber framework reflects decades of refinement in understanding ankle fractures.

References

Danis R. Theorie et pratique de l'osteosynthese. Paris: Masson&Cie, 1949.

Weber BG. Die Verletzungen des oberen Sprunggelenkes, 2nd edn. Bern: Huber, 1972.

Danis R. Les fractures malleolaires. In: Danis R (ed). Theorie et pratique de l'osteosynthese. Masson et Cie, Paris, pp 296. 1949.

Weber BG. Die Verletzungen des oberen Sprunggelenkes (The injuries of the upper ankle), 2nd edition. Huber 1972

Lauge-Hansen N. Fractures of the ankle. II. Combined experimental-surgical and experimental-roentgenologic investigations. Arch Surg. 1950 May;60(5):957-85. [PMID 15411319]

Bugler KE, White TO, Thordarson DB. Foot & Ankle: Focus On Ankle fractures. JBJS. 2012;94;1107 [Full Text]

Hughes JL, Weber H, Willenegger H, Kuner EH. Evaluation of ankle fractures: non-operative and operative treatment. Clin Orthop Relat Res. 1979 Jan-Feb;(138):111-9. [PMID 445892]

Dancer's Fracture

Overview

Dancer's fracture is an avulsion fracture at the base of the fifth metatarsal, often caused by twisting injuries. Commonly referred to as a "pseudo-Jones fracture," it typically responds well to non-operative treatment, distinguishing it from the more serious Jones fracture. These fractures are common in athletes and individuals engaged in high-impact physical activities.

Historical Background

- Fractures of the fifth metatarsal were first described extensively by Sir Robert Jones in 190 He identified fractures specific to the base of the fifth metatarsal that demonstrated poor healing tendencies.
- The term "dancer's fracture" emerged due to its prevalence among dancers, whose lateral forefoot is prone to stress from repetitive motions.

Purpose

- **The main goals in managing dancer's fractures are:** Ensuring proper bone alignment and healing.
- Preventing complications such as non-union or malunion.
- Restoring functional mobility without long-term pain or disability.

Procedure Overview

Diagnosis:

- **Clinical Presentation:** Pain and tenderness on the lateral forefoot.
- Swelling and bruising at the injury site.

- Difficulty bearing weight and pain during foot eversion.
- **Imaging:** X-rays confirm fracture location and type. In some cases, MRI or CT scans may be used to evaluate associated injuries like stress fractures or Lisfranc injuries.

Treatment:

- **Non-operative:** Most zone 1 and pseudo-Jones fractures are treated with immobilization in a walking boot or cast, with weight-bearing as tolerated.
- **Surgical:** Indicated for fractures with significant displacement or if complications like nonunion occur. Techniques include intramedullary screw fixation or planar plating, especially in athletes.
- **Rehabilitation:** Gradual reintroduction of weight-bearing activities.
- Physical therapy to restore range of motion and strengthen the foot.

Results and Interpretation

- Most patients with dancer's fractures recover fully with conservative treatment, achieving union rates of up to *97%*.
- Early surgical intervention in complicated cases can significantly reduce long-term complications and restore pre-injury levels of activity.

Physiological Basis

- The *fifth metatarsal* is structurally important for lateral foot stability and weight distribution.
- Avulsion fractures occur when the peroneus brevis tendon exerts excessive force on the *tuberosity* during sudden inversion or twisting of the foot.
- Vascular supply to the fifth metatarsal, particularly in zone 2, contributes to a higher risk of nonunion in fractures.

Clinical Applications

- **Sports Medicine:** Recognizing and managing dancer's fractures is crucial in athletes to ensure timely recovery and return to activity.
- **Emergency Medicine:** Prompt identification in acute trauma settings prevents delays in treatment.

Limitations and Technical Considerations

- The vascular watershed in zone 2 complicates healing and increases the risk of *nonunion*.
- Surgical fixation with screws requires precise technique; improper screw length or diameter can lead to *malreduction* or *fixation failure*.
- Misdiagnosis or delayed treatment may result in chronic pain or deformity.

Modern Relevance

- Dancer's fractures remain a frequent injury in active populations, with **Advances in** minimally invasive surgical techniques improving outcomes.
- Growing participation in organized sports and physical activities has led to increased awareness and better management strategies.

Associated Conditions

- **Jones fracture:** Fractures involving the metaphyseal-diaphyseal junction.
- **Stress fractures:** Repetitive

microtrauma leading to chronic injuries of the fifth metatarsal.

- **Ankle sprains:** Often occur concurrently, necessitating careful examination of ligamentous structures.

Clinical Importance

- **Timely Management:** Early identification and appropriate treatment ensure optimal healing and prevent long-term disability.
- **Interprofessional Care:** Effective treatment involves collaboration among orthopedic surgeons, nurses, physical therapists, and radiologists.
- **Patient Education:** Patients must understand the importance of adherence to weight-bearing restrictions and rehabilitation protocols to avoid complications.

Dancer's fracture, though typically straightforward to manage, requires careful attention to prevent complications and ensure a full recovery, especially in active individuals.

Dashboard Fracture

Overview

Dashboard fracture, also referred to as an acetabular fracture, is a traumatic injury to the acetabulum caused by a forceful impact, typically during a high-speed automobile accident. The injury occurs when the femoral head is driven into the pelvis, usually following a direct blow to the knee against a dashboard, hence the name. This injury may result in hip dislocation and other associated complications.

Historical Background

- **1964:** French surgeons Robert Judet, Jean Judet, and Emile Letournel provided the first detailed classification, mechanism, and treatment strategies for acetabular fractures. Their work emphasized the distinction between elementary (simple) and associated (complex) fractures.
- The term "dashboard fracture" became popularized with the rise of automobile-related trauma as a distinct clinical presentation of acetabular fractures.

Purpose

- **The management of dashboard fractures aims to:** Achieve stable reduction of the acetabulum and femoral head.
- Preserve the function of the hip joint.
- Prevent long-term complications such as avascular necrosis, sciatic nerve injury, and post-traumatic arthritis.

Procedure Overview

- **Diagnosis:** Clinical examination may reveal pain, deformity, and restricted movement of the hip.
- **Imaging studies include:**
- **X-rays:** To identify fracture type and displacement.
- **CT scans:** For a detailed understanding of the fracture configuration and associated injuries.

Management:

- **Non-Surgical Treatment:** Reduction of the dislocated hip under anesthesia.
- **Application of skeletal traction to maintain alignment.**
- **Suitable for minimally displaced fractures or patients unfit for surgery.**
- **Surgical Treatment:** Open reduction and internal fixation (ORIF) are recommended for displaced fractures.
- Specialized techniques may involve reconstructive plates or screws to stabilize the acetabulum.
- **Rehabilitation:** Gradual weight-bearing after 6–12 weeks.
- Physical therapy to restore joint mobility and muscle strength.

Results and Interpretation

- Successful treatment restores the congruity of the hip joint, preventing complications like *osteonecrosis* or *chronic arthritis*.
- Outcomes are highly dependent on the fracture type, the adequacy of reduction, and early intervention.

Physiological Basis

- The acetabulum is a crucial weight-bearing structure that articulates with the femoral head to form the hip joint.
- High-energy trauma, such as a dashboard impact, drives the femoral head into the acetabulum, causing fractures or dislocation.
- Potential injury to the *sciatic nerve* and disruption of the vascular supply to the femoral head further complicates the management.

Clinical Applications

- **Trauma Surgery:** Essential in managing high-energy trauma cases associated with motor vehicle accidents.
- **Orthopedic Rehabilitation:** Plays a vital role in ensuring functional recovery of the hip joint post-treatment.

Limitations and Technical Considerations

- Associated complications like *sciatic nerve injury*, *vascular disruption*, and *heterotopic ossification* require careful intraoperative and postoperative management.
- Late diagnosis or inadequate reduction can result in poor joint function and chronic pain.
- Non-surgical management is limited to specific fracture patterns and requires prolonged immobilization.

Modern Relevance

- The incidence of dashboard fractures has declined in regions with advanced automobile safety measures, including airbags and improved vehicle designs.

- However, they remain a significant concern in areas with high rates of road traffic accidents or poor vehicle safety standards.

Associated Conditions

- **Hip Dislocation:** Frequently accompanies dashboard fractures and requires urgent reduction.
- **Avascular Necrosis:** A potential consequence of vascular disruption to the femoral head.
- **Post-traumatic Arthritis:** A long-term complication due to joint incongruity or cartilage damage.

Clinical Importance

- **Early Diagnosis and Management:** Prompt identification of dashboard fractures ensures timely intervention, reducing the risk of complications.
- **Team-based Care:** Effective management requires collaboration between emergency physicians, trauma surgeons, orthopedic specialists, and physical therapists.
- **Education and Prevention:** Emphasizing vehicle safety measures, such as seatbelt use and proper sitting posture, can prevent dashboard injuries.

Dashboard fractures represent a complex and potentially debilitating injury that necessitates a multidisciplinary approach for optimal outcomes. Early intervention and adherence to rehabilitation protocols are crucial in restoring joint function and minimizing long-term complications.

Didiee View

Overview

The Didiee view is a specialized radiographic technique used to evaluate the glenoid rim, particularly for detecting osseous Bankart defects on the anteroinferior portion of the glenoid. This view is most commonly employed in cases of shoulder instability or trauma. By utilizing a specific positioning of the patient and the X-ray beam, the Didiee view provides detailed visualization of the glenoid rim, optimizing the diagnosis of fractures and other abnormalities that might not be evident in standard radiographic projections.

Historical Background

The Didiee view does not have a widely attributed historical origin or specific named individual, unlike the West Point view, which is another similar imaging technique.

Its utility in shoulder radiography, particularly for detecting glenoid rim fractures, has become more prominent with the increasing focus on shoulder instability and Bankart lesions in orthopedic and sports medicine.

Purpose

- **Diagnosis of Glenoid Rim Fractures:** To accurately identify osseous Bankart defects, ensuring proper diagnosis and management of shoulder instability.
- **Enhanced Radiographic Visualization:** Provides a clear view of the anteroinferior glenoid rim, an area difficult

to assess in standard projections.

- **Complementary Role:** Used in conjunction with other views (e.g., internal rotation, Stryker notch) to maximize diagnostic accuracy while minimizing costs, time, and radiation exposure.

Procedure Overview

- **Patient Positioning:**
- The patient is positioned prone with the affected shoulder over a cassette placed beneath the shoulder.
- The arm is positioned parallel to the table with a 7.5 cm pad under the elbow.
- The dorsum of the hand is placed on the ipsilateral hip with the thumb directed upward.
- **Beam Angulation:** The X-ray beam is angled at 45 degrees, targeting the glenoid rim for optimal visualization.
- **Imaging Technique:** A focused radiograph of the glenoid rim is captured, providing a detailed view of the anteroinferior glenoid area.
- **Complementary Views:** Often combined with internal rotation, Stryker notch, or West Point views to ensure comprehensive evaluation of shoulder injuries.

Results and Interpretation

- **Osseous Bankart Defects:** The Didiee view provides a clear image of fractures or lesions on the anteroinferior glenoid rim.
- **Fracture Identification:** Enhances detection of small or subtle glenoid fractures that may not be visible on standard shoulder X-rays.
- **Clinical Utility:** Improves diagnostic accuracy for unstable shoulders, aiding in surgical planning or conservative management.

Physiological Basis

- **Glenoid Anatomy:** The glenoid rim plays a critical role in shoulder stability, with fractures or defects (e.g., Bankart lesions) leading to recurrent dislocations or instability.
- **Specific Angulation:** The 45-degree beam angle and precise positioning align the X-ray beam with the anteroinferior glenoid, minimizing overlap of surrounding structures and enhancing visualization.
- **Mechanism of Injury:** Traumatic shoulder dislocations often result in damage to the anteroinferior glenoid rim, necessitating targeted imaging like the Didiee view.

Clinical Applications

- **Shoulder Instability:** Used to evaluate structural damage in cases of recurrent shoulder dislocations.
- **Sports Injuries:** Commonly employed in athletes with anterior shoulder instability or post-traumatic shoulder injuries.
- **Pre-Surgical Assessment:** Assists in planning surgical interventions, such as Bankart repair or glenoid reconstruction, by delineating the extent of bone loss or fractures.

Limitations and Technical Considerations

- **Technical Skill Required:** Proper positioning of the patient and accurate beam angulation are essential for obtaining diagnostic-quality images.
- **Radiation Exposure:** While minimized, the cumulative exposure from multiple views (Didiee, West Point, Stryker notch) must be considered.
- **Limited Availability:** May not be readily available in all clinical settings, requiring familiarity with alternative views.
- **Complementary Role:** Should be used alongside other imaging modalities, such as CT scans, for comprehensive assessment of complex injuries.

Modern Relevance

- **Advances in Imaging:** Although CT and MRI provide superior detail, the Didiee view remains relevant for its cost-effectiveness and utility in initial evaluations.
- **Increased Awareness of Shoulder Pathologies:** The growing recognition of shoulder instability in sports and trauma medicine has highlighted the value of specialized radiographic techniques like the Didiee view.
- **Surgical Planning:** Its ability to clearly visualize glenoid rim defects aids in decision-making for both conservative and surgical treatments.

Associated Conditions

- **Osseous Bankart Lesions:** A fracture or defect of the anteroinferior glenoid rim, often associated with anterior shoulder dislocations.
- **Hill-Sachs Lesions:** Frequently co-occurs with Bankart lesions, necessitating complementary imaging to evaluate humeral head damage.
- **Recurrent Shoulder Dislocations:** Chronic instability due to glenoid or ligamentous damage often requires imaging via Didiee or similar views.

Clinical Importance

- **Enhanced Diagnostic Accuracy:** By focusing on the anteroinferior glenoid rim, the Didiee view reduces the risk of missed diagnoses, particularly in subtle fractures.
- **Cost-Effective Imaging:** Provides detailed information at a fraction of the cost of advanced imaging techniques like CT or MRI.
- **Educational Value:** Emphasizes the importance of targeted imaging in musculoskeletal radiology and orthopedic trauma.

References

Pavlov H, Warren RF, Weiss CB Jr, et al. The roentgenographic evaluation of anterior shoulder instability. Clin Orthop Relat Res. 1985; (194):153-8.

Jacobson JA, Lin J, Jamadar DA et al.Aids to Successful Shoulder Arthrography Performed with a Fluoroscopically Guided Anterior Approach.Radiographics 2003; 23(2):373-378.

De Quervain's Fracture

Overview

De Quervain's fracture is a transscaphoid perilunate fracture-dislocation of the wrist. This injury involves the lunate and the proximal pole of the scaphoid dislocating palmarward, while the distal pole of the scaphoid and the remaining carpal bones retain their usual alignment. This complex wrist injury results from high-energy trauma, often seen in falls onto an outstretched hand or motor vehicle accidents. The condition is challenging to manage due to the risk of delayed union or nonunion of the scaphoid, leading many surgeons to favor open reduction and internal fixation (ORIF).

Historical Background

Fritz de Quervain, a Swiss surgeon, described various wrist and hand pathologies, contributing significantly to the understanding of scaphoid injuries.

While the exact description of de Quervain's fracture as a distinct entity was not detailed by de Quervain himself, his work on the wrist laid the groundwork for its recognition.

The understanding of this injury has evolved with **Advances in** *imaging and surgical techniques, emphasizing its complex nature and need for precise management.*

Purpose

- **Restoration of Wrist Alignment:** To realign the dislocated lunate and scaphoid fragments, restoring normal wrist biomechanics.
- **Stabilization of the Scaphoid:** To promote healing and prevent complications like nonunion or delayed union of the scaphoid.
- **Prevention of Long-Term Dysfunction:** To reduce the risk of chronic pain, arthritis, or loss of wrist motion.

Procedure Overview

Diagnosis:

- **Clinical Examination:** Symptoms include severe wrist pain, swelling, deformity, and restricted motion.

Imaging:

- **X-rays:** Lateral and PA views reveal the transscaphoid fracture and perilunate dislocation.
- **CT Scan:** Provides detailed visualization of fracture patterns and dislocation severity.
- **MRI:** Evaluates ligamentous damage and vascular supply to the scaphoid.

Treatment:

- **Closed Reduction:** Attempted in acute cases, but may not provide stable alignment or address scaphoid fracture risks.
- **Open Reduction and Internal Fixation (ORIF):** Preferred for achieving anatomical reduction and secure fixation of the scaphoid and lunate.
- **Fixation is achieved using screws or pins, often with ligamentous repair if necessary.**
- **Postoperative Management:** Immobilization in a cast or splint for 6–12 weeks, followed by progressive rehabilitation.

Results and Interpretation

- **Immediate Realignment:** Successful reduction restores the normal relationship between the carpal bones.
- **Healing of the Scaphoid:** ORIF improves the likelihood of scaphoid union and minimizes the risk of nonunion.
- **Functional Recovery:** With appropriate treatment, patients can regain wrist strength and mobility, though prolonged recovery is common.

Physiological Basis

- **Mechanism of Injury:** High-energy trauma forces the lunate and proximal scaphoid palmarward while the distal scaphoid and other carpal bones remain relatively stationary.
- **Scaphoid Blood Supply:** The precarious vascularity of the scaphoid predisposes it to nonunion or avascular necrosis, particularly when fractured.
- **Wrist Biomechanics:** Disruption of the scaphoid and lunate alignment compromises wrist stability and motion, emphasizing the need for anatomical reduction.

Clinical Applications

- **Trauma Surgery:** De Quervain's fracture represents a critical condition requiring expertise in wrist and hand trauma management.
- **Orthopedic Rehabilitation:** Postoperative care and physical therapy are essential to restore wrist function and prevent stiffness.
- **Diagnostic Imaging:** Advanced imaging techniques have improved the early recognition and detailed assessment of this complex injury.

Limitations and Technical Considerations

- **Complexity of Reduction:** Closed reduction may be inadequate for maintaining stability, necessitating surgical intervention.
- **Risk of Nonunion:** The scaphoid's vascular anatomy complicates healing, requiring vigilant monitoring and possible secondary interventions.
- **Delayed Diagnosis:** Subtle dislocations or fractures may be overlooked on initial X-rays, emphasizing the need for advanced imaging in high-risk injuries.

Modern Relevance

- **Advances in Fixation Techniques:** Modern screw designs and minimally invasive approaches have improved outcomes for scaphoid and perilunate injuries.
- **Enhanced Imaging:** CT and MRI enable precise diagnosis and surgical planning, minimizing the risk of missed injuries.
- **Focus on Long-Term Outcomes:** Increased awareness of post-traumatic arthritis and chronic instability has led to more aggressive treatment strategies.

Associated Conditions

- **Scapholunate Dissociation:** Commonly accompanies perilunate dislocations, requiring simultaneous repair.
- **Avascular Necrosis:** Particularly in the proximal pole of the scaphoid, due to disrupted blood supply.
- **Post-Traumatic Arthritis:** A long-

term complication of inadequately treated or malaligned fractures.

Clinical Importance

- **High-Stakes Injury:** De Quervain's fracture represents a severe wrist injury requiring prompt and precise management to prevent lifelong disability.
- **Multidisciplinary Approach:** Successful outcomes rely on coordination between trauma surgeons, radiologists, and rehabilitation specialists.
- **Educational Value:** The injury highlights the complexity of wrist biomechanics and the importance of timely and accurate intervention in orthopedic trauma.

References

de Quervain F. Spezielle chirurgische Diagnostik fur Studierende und Aerzte. Leipzig: FCW Vogel, 1907.

de Quervain F. Clinical surgical diagnosis for students and practitioners, 4th ed. Snowman J, translator. New York: William Wood, 1913.

Die-Punch Fracture

Overview

Die-punch fractures are intra-articular fractures of the lunate fossa of the distal radius caused by an axial loading force. The term "die-punch" reflects the depressed or impacted nature of the fracture, likened to the indentation created by a mechanical die tool. This fracture type commonly results from vertical loading injuries and is often associated with instability and significant joint depression, necessitating surgical intervention.

Historical Background

- **1962:** The term "die-punch fracture" was first introduced by Scheck et al. as a specific dorsal fracture fragment of the lunate fossa of the distal radius.
- The term is derived from machining terminology, where a die punch creates an impression or depression, mirroring the fracture mechanics.

Purpose

- **The treatment aims to:** Restore the articular surface of the distal radius.
- Re-establish wrist stability and function.
- Prevent post-traumatic arthritis and deformity.

Procedure Overview

Diagnosis:

- **Clinical Examination:** Patients present with swelling, pain, and limited wrist movement.
- Examination often reveals tenderness at the distal radius.

Imaging:

- **X-rays:** Initial modality to identify the fracture and assess depression.
- **CT scans:** Gold standard for determining the exact location, severity, and complexity of the fracture.

Management:

- **Non-Surgical Treatment:** Reserved for minimally displaced fractures.
- Immobilization with a cast or splint for up to 6 weeks.

Surgical Treatment:

- **Open Reduction and Internal Fixation (ORIF):** The most common approach, using locking plates and screws.
- **Achieves anatomical reduction and stable fixation.**
- **Volar or Dorsal Approach:** Chosen based on the fracture location and surgeon preference.
- **Adjunct Techniques:** Use of K-wires, mini-external fixators, or arthroscopic assistance in complex cases.
- **Postoperative Care:**
- Early mobilization with physiotherapy is critical for regaining function.
- Radiographic follow-ups ensure fracture healing and alignment.

Results and Interpretation

- Surgical intervention typically yields good outcomes when anatomic reduction is achieved.
- Poorly managed or untreated fractures can result in long-term complications such as stiffness, pain, or arthritis.

Physiological Basis

- The lunate fossa of the distal radius is a key articular surface that articulates with the lunate bone of the wrist joint.
- Axial loading injuries drive the lunate into the fossa, causing depression fractures.
- Disruption of the articular surface compromises wrist biomechanics and can lead to long-term joint degeneration if untreated.

Clinical Applications

- **Orthopedic Surgery:** Essential for managing unstable or complex die-punch fractures to restore wrist function.
- **Wrist Arthroscopy:** Useful for assessing joint congruity and addressing associated soft tissue injuries.

Limitations and Technical Considerations

- Accurate diagnosis can be challenging in subtle cases; *CT imaging* is often required for precise evaluation.
- **Surgical complexity increases with:** Severe comminution (multiple bone fragments).
- Involvement of both volar and dorsal surfaces.
- No consensus on the optimal surgical approach or fixation technique, leading to variability in outcomes.

Modern Relevance

- The classification of die-punch fractures has evolved, with contemporary systems offering better guidance for treatment and prognosis.

- **Advances in** imaging and surgical techniques, such as arthroscopy and locking plate technology, have improved management outcomes.

Associated Conditions

- **Post-Traumatic Arthritis:** A common sequela of poorly managed intra-articular fractures.
- **Wrist Instability:** Resulting from disrupted alignment or ligament injury.
- **Median Nerve Compression:** Due to swelling or fracture displacement. Clinical Importance
- **Timely Diagnosis and Treatment:** Early recognition and intervention are critical to prevent joint dysfunction and chronic pain.
- **Multidisciplinary Approach:** Collaboration between radiologists, orthopedic surgeons, and physical therapists ensures optimal outcomes.
- **Patient Education:** Informing patients about rehabilitation and potential complications improves compliance and recovery.

Die-punch fractures represent a challenging subset of distal radius fractures, demanding precise diagnosis and tailored treatment strategies to restore wrist function and minimize long-term disability.

Duchenne's Sign

Overview

Duchenne's sign is a claw deformity of the ring and small fingers, characterized by the inability to adduct the small finger to the ring finger. This classic sign is indicative of ulnar nerve palsy and results from the paralysis of the intrinsic hand muscles, with preserved function of the extrinsic extensors and flexors. The deformity is marked by hyperextension of the proximal phalanx and flexion of the interphalangeal joints, creating a claw-like appearance. The inability to play high notes on a violin, as described in historical accounts, is due to the combined loss of ulnar nerve functions necessary for proper finger positioning and control.

Historical Background

- Named after *Guillaume-Benjamin-Amand Duchenne*, a French neurologist renowned for his pioneering work in the study of muscular dystrophy and neuromuscular conditions.
- Duchenne was instrumental in identifying various signs and syndromes associated with peripheral nerve injuries, including *Duchenne's sign*, as a hallmark of *ulnar nerve dysfunction.*
- The sign has remained a cornerstone in diagnosing ulnar neuropathies and understanding the interplay of intrinsic and extrinsic hand muscle mechanics.

Purpose

- **Diagnosis of Ulnar Nerve Palsy:** To identify ulnar nerve dysfunction by assessing claw deformity and loss of finger adduction.

- **Functional Assessment:** To evaluate the degree of motor impairment in the intrinsic muscles of the hand, particularly in the third palmar interosseous and other ulnar-innervated muscles.
- **Differentiating Nerve Lesions:** To distinguish between high and low ulnar nerve lesions based on the severity and presentation of the claw deformity.

Procedure Overview

Clinical Examination:

- **Observation:** Look for claw deformity of the ring and small fingers, characterized by hyperextension of the metacarpophalangeal joints and flexion of the interphalangeal joints.
- **Adduction Test:** Assess the ability of the patient to adduct the small finger toward the ring finger.
- **Functional Tasks:** Test fine motor tasks, such as the ability to grasp small objects or play high notes on a violin, for further assessment of ulnar nerve functionality.

Associated Signs:

- **Andre-Thomas Sign:** An unconscious effort to extend the fingers by palmar flexion of the wrist, which exaggerates the claw deformity.
- **Froment's Sign:** Indicates weakness of the adductor pollicis muscle during tasks requiring thumb adduction.

Imaging and Electrophysiology:

- **Electromyography (EMG):** Confirms denervation of the intrinsic muscles.
- **Nerve Conduction Studies (NCS):** Identifies ulnar nerve compression or damage, distinguishing high versus low lesions.

Results and Interpretation

- **Classic Claw Deformity:** Hyperextension of the proximal phalanges and flexion of the interphalangeal joints indicate intrinsic muscle paralysis.
- **Inability to Adduct the Small Finger:** Denervation of the third palmar interosseous muscle results in the hallmark loss of finger adduction.
- **Loss of Fine Motor Skills:** Tasks like playing high notes on a violin reveal the extent of functional loss in the ulnar-innervated muscles.

Physiological Basis

- **Intrinsic Muscle Paralysis:** Loss of function in the lumbricals and palmar interossei, which normally flex the metacarpophalangeal joints and extend the interphalangeal joints, leads to unopposed action of the extensor digitorum and flexor muscles, resulting in the claw deformity.
- **Denervation of Key Muscles:** The opponens digiti minimi and flexor carpi ulnaris are crucial for fine motor control, and their paralysis contributes to the inability to position fingers for activities like playing the violin.
- **Proximal vs. Distal Lesions:** High ulnar nerve lesions, affecting the flexor digitorum profundus, may diminish the claw deformity, as these muscles are responsible for flexing the distal interphalangeal joints.

Clinical Applications

- **Neurological Assessment:** Duchenne's sign is a key diagnostic tool for identifying and assessing the severity of ulnar nerve injuries.
- **Rehabilitation Planning:** Understanding the extent of intrinsic muscle paralysis helps in devising targeted physical therapy and splinting strategies.
- **Surgical Consideration:** In cases of severe ulnar nerve damage, the sign guides decisions for nerve repair or tendon transfer surgeries.

Limitations and Technical Considerations

- **Subjective Assessment:** The evaluation of claw deformity and fine motor skills relies on clinical observation, which may vary among examiners.
- **Compensation Mechanisms:** Patients may unconsciously compensate for motor deficits, masking the true extent of dysfunction.
- **Overlap with Other Conditions:** Similar claw deformities can occur in combined nerve injuries or other peripheral neuropathies, necessitating careful differential diagnosis.

Modern Relevance

- **Electrophysiological Advancements:** Modern techniques like EMG and high-resolution ultrasound enhance the diagnostic accuracy of ulnar neuropathies associated with Duchenne's sign.
- **Focus on Functional Outcomes:** Rehabilitation now incorporates advanced splinting and neurostimulation techniques to mitigate functional losses and improve quality of life.
- **Surgical Innovations:** Advances in nerve transfer and tendon repair have improved outcomes for patients with severe ulnar nerve injuries.

Associated Conditions

- **Ulnar Nerve Palsy:** Most common cause, often resulting from compression at the elbow (cubital tunnel syndrome) or wrist (Guyon's canal syndrome).
- **Claw Hand:** A broader term encompassing deformities caused by both ulnar and median nerve injuries.
- **Peripheral Neuropathies:** Conditions like leprosy or diabetes may produce similar signs due to diffuse nerve involvement.

Clinical Importance

- **Early Diagnosis:** Recognizing Duchenne's sign allows for prompt identification of ulnar nerve injuries, preventing further functional decline.
- **Guidance for Treatment:** The sign directs interventions, ranging from conservative management to surgical repair, depending on the severity and duration of the nerve lesion.
- **Educational Value:** The sign is a fundamental teaching point in neurology and orthopedics, illustrating the interplay between intrinsic and extrinsic hand muscle function in ulnar nerve pathology.

References

Duchenne GBA. Physiology of motion [Physiologie des movements demontree a l'aide de l'experimentation electrique et de l'oberservation clinique et applicable a l'etude des paralysies et des degenerations. 1867.]. Kaplan EB, translator and ed. Philadelphia: WB Saunders, 1959.

Dunn View

Overview

The Dunn view is a specialized radiographic technique designed for the evaluation of the femoral head and neck, particularly in cases of suspected femoroacetabular impingement (FAI). This view provides detailed visualization of the articular space in the anterior and posterior compartments of the hip joint, enabling the assessment of femoral head sphericity and neck anteversion. Originally introduced to measure femoral neck anteversion in children, the Dunn view is now extensively used in young adults to detect cam-type FAI and associated hip pathologies.

Historical Background

- **1952:** Dennis M. Dunn described the view in his seminal work published in the *Journal of Bone and Joint Surgery* titled "Anteversion of the Neck of the Femur: A Method of Measurement."
- Initially developed to measure *femoral neck anteversion in pediatric patients*, its utility has since expanded to include *morphological abnormalities of the femoral head-neck junction.*
- The Dunn view remains an essential tool in modern orthopedic imaging, particularly with the increasing recognition of *FAI syndrome.*

Purpose

- **Evaluation of Femoral Head Sphericity:** To detect subtle abnormalities such as cam deformities that may predispose patients to FAI.
- **Measurement of Femoral Neck Anteversion:** To quantify the alignment of the femoral neck relative to the acetabulum, critical for surgical planning.
- **Assessment of Articular Space:** To evaluate the integrity of the hip joint's anterior and posterior compartments, aiding in the diagnosis of early hip joint degeneration.

Procedure Overview

- **Patient Positioning:**
- The patient is placed in a supine position on the radiographic table.
- The hip of interest is aligned parallel to the X-ray chassis, and the patient's trunk is tilted at a 65° angle from the horizontal plane.
- The contralateral hip is flexed and abducted out of the field of view to avoid overlap.
- **Radiographic Technique:**
- The X-ray beam is centered on the femoral head, ensuring clear visualization of the femoral neck and acetabulum.
- Proper positioning ensures a gap between the femoral heads, confirming correct alignment.
- **Post-Imaging Verification:** The image is reviewed for appropriate visualization of the femoral head-neck junction, acetabulum, and articular spaces.

Results and Interpretation

- **Cam Deformities:** The Dunn view is highly sensitive for detecting cam lesions, characterized by loss of sphericity at the femoral head-neck junction.

- **Femoral Neck Anteversion:** Accurate measurements of femoral neck alignment help in diagnosing structural abnormalities and planning corrective surgeries.
- **Joint Space Assessment:** Reduced joint space in the anterior or posterior compartments may indicate early degeneration or cartilage loss.

Physiological Basis

- **Femoral Head-Neck Morphology:** Cam-type FAI results from abnormal femoral head-neck morphology, leading to impingement during hip flexion and rotation.
- **Articular Space Integrity:** Changes in the anterior or posterior joint space often signify cartilage wear or labral damage.
- **Alignment and Function:** The femoral neck anteversion angle affects hip stability and range of motion, with deviations contributing to abnormal joint mechanics.

Clinical Applications

- **Femoroacetabular Impingement (FAI):** The Dunn view is a cornerstone for diagnosing cam-type FAI, aiding in early detection and intervention to prevent osteoarthritis.
- **Pre-Surgical Planning:** Precise measurements of femoral neck anteversion and joint morphology guide procedures such as hip arthroscopy or osteotomies.
- **Pediatric Orthopedics:** Initially developed for assessing femoral neck anteversion in children, it retains value in pediatric cases involving structural hip abnormalities.

Limitations and Technical Considerations

- **Patient Positioning:** Accurate positioning is critical; improper alignment can obscure diagnostic findings or lead to incorrect measurements.
- **Radiation Exposure:** Though minimal, repeated imaging for bilateral assessment increases cumulative exposure.
- **Limited Soft Tissue Visualization:** The Dunn view primarily evaluates bony structures; additional imaging (e.g., MRI) is needed for detailed assessment of soft tissue injuries like labral tears.

Modern Relevance

- **Focus on FAI:** The rise in recognition of FAI as a cause of early hip arthritis has made the Dunn view a standard in orthopedic diagnostics.
- **Advances in Imaging:** High-resolution X-rays and digital imaging enhance the accuracy of this view, complementing other modalities like CT or MRI.
- **Integration in Multimodal Protocols:** The Dunn view is now part of comprehensive imaging protocols for evaluating young adults with hip pain and suspected structural abnormalities.

Associated Conditions

- **Cam-Type Femoroacetabular Impingement:** The most common application, characterized by loss of femoral head sphericity visible on the Dunn view.
- **Pincer-Type FAI:** While primarily bony, some cases may benefit from Dunn view imaging to evaluate co-existing joint space narrowing.
- **Developmental Dysplasia of the**

Hip (DDH): Can be used in certain cases to assess femoral neck alignment and acetabular morphology.

Clinical Importance

- **Early Detection:** The Dunn view allows for the identification of FAI and other structural abnormalities before significant joint degeneration occurs.
- **Guidance for Intervention:** Measurements obtained from the Dunn view support targeted surgical and non-surgical interventions, improving patient outcomes.
- **Educational Value:** A fundamental technique in orthopedic radiology, the Dunn view teaches the importance of precision in imaging and the interplay between anatomy and pathology.

References

Pavlov H, Warren RF, Weiss CB Jr, et al. The roentgenographic evaluation of anterior shoulder instability. Clin Orthop Relat Res. 1985; (194):153-8.

Jacobson JA, Lin J, Jamadar DA et al.Aids to Successful Shoulder Arthrography Performed with a Fluoroscopically Guided Anterior Approach.Radiographics 2003; 23(2):373-378.

Dupuytren Fracture

Overview

The Dupuytren fracture refers to a fracture of the fibula that occurs either low (approximately 1 inch above the tibiofibular syndesmosis) or high (2.5 to 3 inches above the syndesmosis). This type of injury often involves disruption of the ankle joint stability, making it clinically significant in orthopedic trauma. Named after Guillaume Dupuytren, a prominent French surgeon, this fracture remains an important diagnostic consideration in ankle trauma.

Historical Background

- **Guillaume Dupuytren (1777–1835):** Dupuytren was a distinguished surgeon and anatomist in early 19th-century France, renowned for his work at the Hôtel-Dieu Hospital in Paris, where he served as chief surgeon for over 20 years.
- His meticulous surgical techniques, diagnostic acumen, and contributions to orthopedic conditions, including the eponymous Dupuytren's contracture and Dupuytren fracture, have cemented his legacy in medical history.
- Despite his brilliance, Dupuytren's perfectionist and demanding personality earned him controversial nicknames like "Napoleon of surgery." His relentless dedication to medical education and innovation, however, remains universally respected.

Purpose

- **Evaluation of Ankle Stability:** To assess whether the fracture has disrupted the syndesmosis or the surrounding ligamentous structures, as these factors influence treatment decisions.

- **Classification of Fibular Fractures:** Differentiating between low Dupuytren and high Dupuytren fractures is essential for determining the severity and treatment strategy.
- **Facilitation of Treatment Planning:** To guide the choice between conservative management (e.g., casting) or surgical intervention (e.g., fixation).

Procedure Overview

Diagnosis:

- **Clinical Signs:** Pain, swelling, and tenderness over the fibula, often associated with an inability to bear weight.
- Ankle instability may be evident in cases of syndesmotic disruption.

Imaging:

- **X-rays:** Standard anteroposterior, lateral, and mortise views to localize the fracture and assess alignment.
- **Stress Radiographs:** Used to evaluate syndesmotic integrity in suspected unstable injuries.
- **CT Scan:** Provides detailed assessment of fracture pattern and associated syndesmotic injuries.

Treatment:

- **Conservative Management:** For stable fractures without significant displacement or syndesmotic injury, immobilization with a cast or boot is sufficient.
- **Surgical Intervention:** Open reduction and internal fixation (ORIF) is required for unstable or displaced fractures, especially those involving syndesmotic disruption.
- **Rehabilitation:** Weight-bearing is typically restricted for 6–8 weeks, followed by physiotherapy to restore strength and range of motion.

Results and Interpretation

- **Stable Fractures:** Low Dupuytren fractures without syndesmotic involvement often heal well with conservative management.
- **Unstable Fractures:** High Dupuytren fractures or those with syndesmotic injury require surgical fixation to restore stability and prevent long-term complications.
- **Prognostic Indicators:** Proper alignment and stabilization during treatment are crucial for achieving good functional outcomes.

Physiological Basis

- **Role of the Syndesmosis:** The syndesmotic ligaments stabilize the distal tibiofibular joint, and their integrity is critical for normal ankle function.
- **Fracture Biomechanics:** The location of the fracture (low or high) and the involvement of associated structures like the deltoid ligament affect joint stability and dictate treatment strategy.
- **Healing and Remodeling:** The fibula's vascular supply and alignment significantly impact fracture healing and the risk of complications such as malunion or nonunion.

Clinical Applications

- **Trauma Management:** The Dupuytren fracture is a cornerstone in orthopedic trauma care, emphasizing the importance of recognizing syndesmotic injuries.

- **Sports Medicine:** Commonly encountered in athletes, this injury highlights the need for precise diagnosis and management to ensure full recovery and prevent recurrence.
- **Rehabilitation and Recovery:** An essential focus in ensuring long-term joint function and preventing complications like stiffness or instability.

Limitations and Technical Considerations

- **Diagnostic Challenges:** Low Dupuytren fractures may be easily missed on initial X-rays, especially if subtle syndesmotic involvement is not evaluated with stress radiographs.
- **Surgical Risks:** ORIF carries potential complications such as infection, hardware irritation, or inadequate reduction of the syndesmosis.
- **Patient Compliance:** Successful outcomes depend on adherence to weight-bearing restrictions and rehabilitation protocols.

Modern Relevance

- **Advances in Imaging:** High-resolution CT and MRI have improved the ability to detect subtle syndesmotic injuries and fracture details, optimizing treatment planning.
- **Evolution of Fixation Techniques:** Modern surgical tools, including syndesmotic screws and suture-button devices, have enhanced the stabilization of complex fractures.
- **Increased Awareness of Long-Term Outcomes:** Emphasis on early detection and appropriate management has reduced the incidence of post-traumatic arthritis and chronic instability.

Associated Conditions

- **Syndesmotic Injuries:** Frequently accompany Dupuytren fractures, especially in high variants, necessitating careful evaluation and stabilization.
- **Deltoid Ligament Damage:** Rupture of the deltoid ligament can contribute to medial ankle instability, complicating the treatment.
- **Post-Traumatic Arthritis:** A potential long-term complication if the fracture or syndesmosis is inadequately treated.

Clinical Importance

- **Early Intervention:** Timely diagnosis and treatment are critical to prevent chronic instability, pain, and long-term joint degeneration.
- **Educational Value:** The Dupuytren fracture serves as an educational model for understanding the interplay between fractures, syndesmotic stability, and ankle biomechanics.
- **Historical and Clinical Relevance:** Named after one of the most influential surgeons in medical history, this fracture reflects the enduring importance of precise anatomical understanding in orthopedic care.

References

Gilgenkrantz S. [The Baron Guillaume Dupuytren]. Med Sci (Paris) 2006; 22: 771–2.

Dupuytren G. Memoire sur la fracture de l'extrémité inferieure du peroné, les luxations et les accidents qui en sont la suite. Ann Med Chir Hop Paris 1819; 1: 2–212.

Nélaton A. Elémens de pathologie chirurgicale, 2nd edn. Paris: Germer-Bailliere, 1874.

Dupuytre's Contracture

Overview

Dupuytren's contracture is a chronic condition characterized by thickening and fibrosis of the palmar and digital fascia, leading to the formation of nodules and fibrous cords. This results in progressive flexion contracture of the fingers, most commonly affecting the ring and little fingers, with significant loss of hand function over time. Palmar and digital fasciectomy or minimally invasive techniques, such as needle aponeurotomy, are commonly performed to restore hand mobility and improve quality of life.

Historical Background

- Guillaume Dupuytren, a prominent French surgeon, first described the condition in 183 He linked the contracture to pathologic changes in the palmar fascia and demonstrated the effectiveness of surgical intervention to release the tension.
- Dupuytren's keen observational skills and pioneering work at the Hôtel-Dieu Hospital in Paris contributed to the establishment of the condition as a distinct clinical entity.
- Though surgical techniques have evolved since Dupuytren's time, his emphasis on treating the functional limitations of this condition remains relevant.

Purpose

- **Restoration of Hand Function:** To release contractures and restore full extension and mobility of the affected fingers.
- **Prevention of Progression:** To address the condition early before severe contractures and secondary complications arise.
- **Improvement of Quality of Life:** To enable patients to perform daily activities without restrictions caused by finger contractures.

Procedure Overview

Diagnosis:

- **Clinical Examination:** Palpation of thickened palmar fascia, nodules, and cords.
- Assessing range of motion and extent of contractures, often using the tabletop test (inability to lay the hand flat on a surface).
- **Imaging:** Rarely required, but ultrasonography or MRI can evaluate soft tissue involvement in complex cases.

Treatment Options:

- **Non-Surgical Management:** Collagenase injections (e.g., Clostridium histolyticum) to enzymatically break down the fibrous cords.
- Needle aponeurotomy for minimally invasive cord release.

Surgical Intervention:

- **Partial Fasciectomy:** Removal of the diseased fascia to improve finger extension.
- **Dermofasciectomy:** Excision of both the fascia and overlying skin in severe cases, often requiring skin grafting.
- **Post-Treatment Rehabilitation:**
- Physical therapy to restore strength and mobility.

- Splinting to maintain extension and prevent recurrence.

Results and Interpretation

- **Immediate Improvement:** Patients typically experience a marked increase in finger extension and functional use of the hand following treatment.
- **Recurrence:** The condition has a high recurrence rate, particularly in younger patients or those with a strong family history of Dupuytren's disease.
- **Complications:** Surgical treatments may lead to scarring, nerve injury, or reduced sensitivity in the hand, requiring careful monitoring.

Physiological Basis

- **Pathophysiology:** The condition results from fibroblast proliferation and excessive collagen deposition in the palmar fascia, leading to thickened cords and nodules.
- **Genetic Predisposition:** Dupuytren's contracture has a strong hereditary component, particularly in individuals of Northern European descent.
- **Progression:** The disease progresses from localized nodule formation to cord development, causing flexion contractures that impair finger extension.

Clinical Applications

- **Hand Surgery:** Dupuytren's contracture is a common indication for hand surgeons, requiring a mix of conservative and surgical approaches.
- **Rehabilitation:** Post-treatment physiotherapy plays a crucial role in maximizing outcomes and preventing stiffness or recurrence.
- **Preventive Strategies:** Early identification and minimally invasive treatments reduce the need for extensive surgical procedures.

Limitations and Technical Considerations

- **Recurrence:** Even after successful treatment, recurrence rates are high, with some patients requiring multiple interventions.
- **Complications of Surgery:** Risks include nerve or vessel injury, wound healing issues, and reduced grip strength.
- **Patient Selection:** Aggressive treatment may not be necessary for mild cases that do not impair hand function.

Modern Relevance

- **Advances in Minimally Invasive Techniques:** Innovations like needle aponeurotomy and collagenase injections have provided effective alternatives to traditional surgery, reducing recovery times and costs.
- **Genetic Insights:** Ongoing research into the genetic and molecular pathways of Dupuytren's contracture is opening avenues for targeted therapies.
- **Enhanced Patient Outcomes:** Modern techniques emphasize preserving hand function with fewer complications and quicker recovery.

Associated Conditions

- **Diabetes Mellitus:** A known risk factor, as patients with diabetes are more prone to developing Dupuytren's contracture.

- **Alcoholism:** Associated with a higher prevalence of the condition, though the exact mechanism remains unclear.
- **Frozen Shoulder (Adhesive Capsulitis):** Dupuytren's contracture has been linked to other fibrotic conditions, suggesting shared pathophysiological mechanisms.

Clinical Importance

- **Functional Impact:** Untreated, Dupuytren's contracture can lead to significant disability, emphasizing the importance of early diagnosis and treatment.
- **Multidisciplinary Approach:** Management often involves collaboration between primary care physicians, hand surgeons, and physical therapists.
- **Historical and Educational Significance:** The condition highlights the importance of recognizing progressive, hereditary diseases and their impact on musculoskeletal function.

References

Dupuytren G. De la retraction des doigts par suite d'une affection de l'aponevrose palmaire - description de la maladie - operation chirurgicale qui convient dans ce cas. Compte rendu de la clinique chirurgicale de l'Hotel Dieu par MM les docteurs Alexandre Paillard et Marx. J Univers Hebdom Med Chir Prat Inst Med 5:349–365, 1831.

Egawa Sign

Overview

The Egawa sign is a clinical indicator of ulnar nerve dysfunction, characterized by the inability of the flexed long (middle) finger to abduct radioulnarly or to rotate at the metacarpophalangeal (MCP) joint. This impairment occurs due to the paralysis of the interosseous muscles, which are innervated by the ulnar nerve. The Egawa sign is useful in diagnosing and localizing nerve injuries, particularly involving the ulnar nerve.

Historical Background

- The *Egawa sign* was first described by *Egawa T.*, a physician who identified the relationship between interosseous muscle paralysis and the inability to perform fine motor movements of the fingers.
- Over time, the sign has become an established clinical test for assessing *ulnar nerve function*, complementing other diagnostic maneuvers like *Froment's sign* and *Duchenne's sign*.
- It highlights the early understanding of the intricate interplay between muscle innervation and hand movements.

Purpose

- **Assessment of Ulnar Nerve Dysfunction:** To detect paralysis of the interosseous muscles and confirm involvement of the ulnar nerve.
- **Localization of Nerve Injury:** To differentiate between high and low ulnar nerve lesions based on accompanying signs and symptoms.

- **Functional Evaluation:** To assess the extent of motor impairment in tasks requiring fine finger movements.

Procedure Overview

- **Patient Positioning:** The patient is seated with the hand and fingers relaxed and supported on a flat surface.
- **Test Execution:** The examiner asks the patient to flex the long (middle) finger at the MCP joint.
- The patient is then instructed to move the finger side-to-side (abduct radioulnarly) or rotate it at the MCP joint.
- **Observation:** The inability to perform the movements indicates a positive Egawa sign, suggestive of interosseous muscle paralysis due to ulnar nerve dysfunction.
- **Complementary Tests:** Additional signs like Froment's sign and tests of grip strength can be performed to confirm ulnar nerve involvement.

Results and Interpretation

- **Positive Egawa Sign:** Failure to abduCT or rotate the flexed long finger indicates interosseous muscle weakness or paralysis.
- **Diagnostic Implications:** Confirms ulnar nerve dysfunction and provides insight into the extent and location of the injury.
- **Normal Test:** The ability to perform the required movements rules out significant ulnar nerve impairment.

Physiological Basis

- **Role of Interosseous Muscles:** The dorsal and palmar interosseous muscles, innervated by the ulnar nerve, control finger abduction, adduction, and fine motor adjustments.
- **Impact of Ulnar Nerve Dysfunction:** Loss of interosseous muscle function prevents the flexed long finger from being abducted radioulnarly or rotated, as the unopposed extensor digitorum communis cannot perform these movements effectively.
- **Compensatory Mechanisms:** Other fingers may show signs of compensation through extrinsic muscle activation, but the middle finger's motion remains impaired.

Clinical Applications

- **Peripheral Nerve Injury Diagnosis:** The Egawa sign is a reliable test for identifying ulnar nerve dysfunction in trauma or compression syndromes.
- **Monitoring Neuropathy Progression:** Useful in conditions like cubital tunnel syndrome, where early identification of motor involvement can guide treatment.
- **Post-Surgical Evaluation:** Assess recovery of ulnar nerve function following nerve repair or decompression surgeries.

Limitations and Technical Considerations

- **Subjective Assessment:** The interpretation of the Egawa sign depends on examiner experience, making it prone to variability.
- **Overlap with Other Conditions:**

Similar findings may occur in combined nerve injuries or central nervous system disorders, requiring differential diagnosis.

- **Patient Cooperation:** Accurate results depend on patient compliance and understanding of the test instructions.

Modern Relevance

- **Advances in Neuropathy Management:** While the Egawa sign remains a foundational clinical test, modern imaging (e.g., nerve ultrasound) and electrophysiological studies complement its findings.
- **Focus on Early Detection:** Increased awareness of early signs of ulnar nerve dysfunction has improved the outcomes of conservative and surgical treatments.
- **Educational Importance:** The Egawa sign is routinely taught in medical and physical therapy education as an example of targeted motor testing.

Associated Conditions

- **Ulnar Nerve Palsy:** Commonly results from compression at the cubital tunnel or Guyon's canal, causing paralysis of the interosseous muscles.
- **Claw Hand:** A deformity seen in advanced cases of ulnar nerve dysfunction, often accompanied by a positive Egawa sign.
- **Peripheral Neuropathy:** Conditions like diabetes or leprosy can lead to ulnar nerve involvement and a positive Egawa sign.

Clinical Importance

- **Diagnostic Simplicity:** The Egawa sign is a quick and non-invasive test for assessing ulnar nerve integrity.
- **Functional Insight:** Provides valuable information on the extent of motor impairment, aiding in treatment planning.
- **Integration in Neurological Examination:** Together with other signs, it offers a comprehensive assessment of hand function in peripheral nerve injuries.

References

Egawa T. Electromyographic studies on finger motion. J Osaka Univ Med School 11:1739–1758, 1959.

Mannerelt L. Studies on the hand in ulnar nerve paralysis. Acta Orthop Scand Suppl 87:1–176, 1966.

Ehrenfried's Syndrome

Overview

Ehrenfried's syndrome is a rare bone dysplasia characterized by deformities of the extremities, limited joint movement, and ulnar deviation of the hands. Other notable features include excrescences at the diaphyseal ends of long bones, involvement of the ribs and scapula, and the absence of skull involvement. Patients may experience short stature (variably expressed) and neurological complications due to nerve or spinal cord compression. The condition manifests during the first decade of life and follows an autosomal dominant inheritance pattern, with complete penetrance in males and reduced penetrance in females. The exact etiology remains unknown.

Historical Background

- *Albert Ehrenfried*, an American surgeon and pioneer in the study of skeletal anomalies, first described this syndrome, bringing attention to its distinct combination of skeletal deformities and neurological implications.
- His contributions in the early 20th century to the understanding of bone dysplasias and their genetic inheritance patterns helped pave the way for modern orthopedic and genetic research into skeletal disorders.
- Ehrenfried's syndrome remains an important example of hereditary bone dysplasias in clinical and genetic research.

Purpose

- **Identification of Bone Dysplasia:** To recognize the characteristic skeletal deformities and associated symptoms early for appropriate management.
- **Prevention of Neurological Complications:** To address potential nerve or spinal cord compression, minimizing functional impairments.
- **Understanding Inheritance Patterns:** To provide genetic counseling for affected families.

Procedure Overview

Diagnosis:

- **Clinical Evaluation:** Inspection for extremity deformities, limited joint mobility, ulnar deviation, and evidence of short stature.

Imaging:

- **X-rays:** Visualize excrescences at diaphyseal ends, rib, and scapular involvement.
- Assess skeletal deformities and spinal abnormalities.
- **MRI or CT Scan:** Evaluate nerve or spinal cord compression and assess the extent of bony overgrowth.
- **Genetic Testing:** Confirm autosomal dominant inheritance and assess family history.

Treatment:

- **Orthopedic Interventions:** Corrective surgeries for severe deformities to improve function and appearance.
- **Neurological Management:** Surgical decompression for spinal cord or nerve compression.

- **Physical Therapy:** Focus on maintaining joint mobility and minimizing stiffness.
- **Monitoring:** Regular follow-ups to track progression of skeletal deformities and address emerging complications.

Results and Interpretation

- **Skeletal Features:** Diagnosis is confirmed through characteristic findings on clinical examination and imaging, including diaphyseal excrescences and extremity deformities.
- **Neurological Findings:** Compression-related symptoms such as weakness or sensory deficits highlight the need for urgent intervention.
- **Genetic Insight:** Autosomal dominant inheritance with gender-based penetrance informs family planning and genetic counseling.

Physiological Basis

- **Bone Dysplasia:** The disorder involves abnormal bone remodeling and growth, leading to deformities, diaphyseal overgrowth, and joint restriction.
- **Neurological Complications:** Excess bone growth at diaphyseal ends can compress nerves or the spinal cord, causing neurological symptoms.
- **Variable Stature:** Short stature results from impaired longitudinal bone growth, influenced by genetic factors.

Clinical Applications

- **Orthopedic Management:** Focused on surgical correction of deformities and maintaining mobility through physical therapy.
- **Genetic Counseling:** Provides valuable information on inheritance patterns and recurrence risks for affected families.
- **Neurological Care:** Early detection of compression-related symptoms is critical to prevent long-term complications.

Limitations and Technical Considerations

- **Diagnostic Challenges:** Variability in expression, particularly between males and females, may delay diagnosis.
- **Surgical Risks:** Corrective procedures carry risks of infection, incomplete correction, or recurrence of deformities.
- **Progression Monitoring:** The progressive nature of the disease requires regular follow-ups and imaging studies.

Modern Relevance

- **Advances in Imaging:** High-resolution MRI and CT scans have enhanced the ability to detect and monitor skeletal and neurological complications.
- **Genetic Research:** Ongoing studies aim to identify the genetic mutations responsible for Ehrenfried's syndrome, which could lead to targeted therapies.
- **Improved Surgical Techniques:** Modern orthopedic and neurosurgical interventions have significantly improved outcomes for patients with severe deformities or compression.

Associated Conditions

- **Spinal Cord Compression:** A significant complication caused by excessive bone growth at diaphyseal ends.
- **Neuropathies:** Peripheral nerve com-

pression leading to weakness, sensory deficits, or pain.

- **Joint Contractures:** Progressive stiffness and limited range of motion in affected joints.

Clinical Importance

- **Early Recognition:** Timely diagnosis allows for interventions that can prevent severe deformities and neurological complications.
- **Multidisciplinary Care:** Management requires coordination between orthopedic surgeons, neurologists, geneticists, and physical therapists.
- **Impact on Quality of Life:** Effective treatment and supportive care significantly improve the functional abilities and well-being of affected individuals.

References

R. Virchow: Über multiple Exostosen. Berliner klinische Wochenschrift, 1891, 82: 1082.

A. Ehrenfried: Multiple cartilaginous exostoses hereditary deforming chondrodysplasia. A brief report on a little known disease. Journal of the American Medical Association, Chicago, 1915, 64: 1642-1646.

Elson Test

Overview

The Elson test is a clinical diagnostic tool used to detect early stages of boutonnière deformity, a condition resulting from the rupture of the central slip of the extensor mechanism at the proximal interphalangeal (PIP) joint. The test evaluates the integrity of the central slip by assessing the tone and movement between the PIP and distal interphalangeal (DIP) joints during resisted extension. It is considered the most reliable clinical test for early boutonnière deformity, with particular sensitivity to abnormal mechanical tone in the extensor apparatus.

Historical Background

- *Elson RA* developed the test as a method to diagnose boutonnière deformity in its early stages, improving treatment outcomes by facilitating timely intervention.
- The Elson test has since gained recognition in *orthopedic and hand surgery literature* as a superior diagnostic technique, outperforming other tests like the Boyes test, which becomes positive only in later stages.

Purpose

- **Early Diagnosis:** To detect central slip rupture at an early stage, enabling prompt treatment and preventing progression to fixed deformity.
- **Differentiation of Injuries:** To distinguish between complete and partial ruptures of the central slip, as well as other extensor mechanism injuries.

- **Assessment of Extensor Integrity:** To evaluate the functional contribution of the central slip to the extensor mechanism and lateral bands.

Procedure Overview

- **Positioning:**
- The finger to be examined is flexed at the PIP joint to a right angle (90°) and placed over the edge of a table or a similar stable surface.
- The examiner firmly supports the finger in this position.
- **Testing:**
- The patient is instructed to extend the PIP joint against resistance applied by the examiner to the middle phalanx.
- Simultaneously, the DIP joint is observed for rigidity or movement.
- **Interpretation:**
- **Intact Central Slip:** Pressure is felt over the middle phalanx, and the DIP joint remains flail (unable to extend actively).
- **Central Slip Rupture:** The DIP joint exhibits rigidity and a tendency to extend due to unopposed action of the lateral bands.
- **Confirmation:** If pain impedes testing, a nerve block may be administered to ensure accurate assessment.

Results and Interpretation

- **Positive Test (Central Slip Rupture):** The DIP joint becomes rigid with attempted extension, as the lateral bands compensate for the absent central slip.
- **Negative Test (Intact Central Slip):** The middle phalanx exerts palpable pressure during resisted extension, and the DIP joint remains flail.
- **Limitations:** Partial ruptures may not be detected by the Elson test, requiring additional imaging or diagnostic methods for confirmation.

Physiological Basis

- **Role of the Central Slip:** The central slip inserts into the middle phalanx and extends the PIP joint while restraining the lateral bands from acting distally on the DIP joint.
- **Mechanics of Rupture:** In central slip rupture, the lateral bands become unopposed, causing abnormal extension of the DIP joint and inability to actively extend the PIP joint.
- **Tone Abnormality:** The Elson test leverages the loss of the check-rein effect, where the central slip normally restrains the lateral bands, creating characteristic changes in tone between the PIP and DIP joints.

Clinical Applications

- **Hand and Finger Injuries:** Essential for diagnosing boutonnière deformity in trauma patients, particularly those with PIP joint hyperflexion injuries.
- **Early Detection:** Allows for timely splinting or surgical repair, preventing progression to permanent deformity.
- **Post-Treatment Monitoring:** Used to assess the success of central slip repairs or splinting protocols.

Limitations and Technical Considerations

- **Detection of Partial Ruptures:** The Elson test cannot reliably detect incomplete central slip tears, requiring adjunctive imaging or functional testing.
- **Pain and Cooperation:** Pain or lack of patient cooperation may impede accurate results, necessitating local anesthesia or alternative assessments.
- **Examiner Skill:** The test's accuracy depends on the examiner's ability to assess tone and resistance, making it prone to variability.

Modern Relevance

- **Enhanced Understanding of Extensor Mechanisms:** The Elson test has helped refine our knowledge of finger biomechanics, guiding treatment for extensor injuries.
- **Complementary Diagnostics:** Advances in ultrasound and MRI provide detailed imaging of central slip injuries, supplementing clinical findings from the Elson test.
- **Reliability in Early Detection:** Studies have confirmed its superiority in diagnosing early boutonnière deformity, making it a staple in clinical practice.

Associated Conditions

- **Boutonnière Deformity:** Results from untreated or delayed management of central slip rupture, leading to permanent PIP flexion and DIP hyperextension.
- **Extensor Mechanism Injuries:** Injuries involving the lateral bands, triangular ligament, or extensor hood can mimic central slip dysfunction.
- **Arthritic Conditions:** Rheumatoid arthritis and other inflammatory conditions may cause central slip attenuation, producing similar findings.

Clinical Importance

- **Timely Intervention:** Early detection of central slip rupture via the Elson test facilitates effective treatment, reducing the risk of chronic deformity.
- **Diagnostic Simplicity:** The test provides a quick, non-invasive method for assessing extensor mechanism integrity without requiring advanced imaging.
- **Foundation for Hand Surgery:** The Elson test remains a cornerstone in evaluating PIP joint injuries and extensor dysfunction, reinforcing its value in hand surgery and rehabilitation.

References

Elson RA. Rupture of the central slip of the extensor hood of the finger: a test for early diagnosis. J Bone Joint Surg Br 68:229–231, 1986.

Harris C, Rutledge GL. The functional anatomy of the extensor mechanism of the finger. J Bone Joint Surg Am 54:713–726, 1972.

Rubin J, Bozentka DJ, Bora FW. Diagnosis of closed central slip injuries. J Hand Surg [Br] 21:614–616, 1996.

Engel-von Recklinghausen Syndrome

Overview

Engel-von Recklinghausen syndrome is a historical term describing a generalized rarefying bone disorder associated with advanced hyperparathyroidism. The syndrome is characterized by skeletal deformation, cysts, or brown tumors - deeply pigmented areas of fibrous scarring with pseudocysts, hemorrhages, and collections of osteoclasts. Clinical features include arthralgia, fractures, bowing of long bones, and gross deformities of the spine and chest. Though the term is largely obsolete today, the condition highlights the severe skeletal manifestations of uncontrolled hyperparathyroidism.

Historical Background

- The syndrome was first described by *Gerhard Engel* and *Friedrich Daniel von Recklinghausen*, two prominent physicians who studied bone pathology.
- *Von Recklinghausen* is widely recognized for his contributions to the understanding of *neurofibromatosis* and skeletal disorders, while Engel contributed to defining advanced hyperparathyroidism's effects on the skeleton.
- **Advances in** *biochemistry* and *radiology* have since shifted the terminology, with the condition now recognized as a manifestation of *osteitis fibrosa cystica*, a severe skeletal complication of hyperparathyroidism.

Purpose

- **Diagnosis of Skeletal Abnormalities:** To identify the hallmark features of bone rarefaction, cyst formation, and structural deformities associated with hyperparathyroidism.
- **Understanding Hyperparathyroidism:** To highlight the metabolic and skeletal consequences of parathyroid dysfunction, including excessive bone resorption.
- **Foundation for Treatment:** To emphasize the importance of addressing the underlying parathyroid disorder to prevent or reverse skeletal damage.

Procedure Overview

- **Clinical Evaluation:**
- Patients present with bone pain, joint stiffness, deformities, and fractures.
- Gross deformities, especially of the spine and chest, are examined.

Diagnostic Imaging:

- **X-rays:** Reveal rarefying bone changes, cysts, and bowing of long bones.
- **CT or MRI:** Useful in assessing cystic lesions and spinal deformities.
- **Bone Scans:** Highlight regions of increased metabolic activity due to osteoclastic bone resorption.

Laboratory Tests:

- **Elevated Parathyroid Hormone (PTH):** Confirms hyperparathyroidism.
- **Serum Calcium and Phosphate:** Increased calcium and decreased phosphate levels are typical.

- **Histological Examination:** Biopsy of affected bone shows fibrous tissue, hemorrhages, and osteoclast-rich pseudocysts.

Management:

- **Surgical Parathyroidectomy:** Corrects the underlying hyperparathyroidism, often halting further bone deterioration.
- **Orthopedic Interventions:** Address fractures and deformities.

Results and Interpretation

- **Skeletal Changes:** Cysts or brown tumors, bowing of long bones, and deformities of the spine are classic findings.
- **Bone Biochemistry:** Elevated PTH with associated calcium and phosphate abnormalities confirms metabolic bone disease.
- **Reversal Post-Treatment:** Surgical correction of hyperparathyroidism can lead to significant improvement in bone density and reduction in symptoms.

Physiological Basis

- **Parathyroid Hormone Excess:** Chronic elevation of PTH in hyperparathyroidism stimulates osteoclast activity, leading to excessive bone resorption.
- **Formation of Brown Tumors:** Localized areas of bone resorption filled with fibrous tissue, osteoclasts, and hemosiderin, result in pigmented lesions termed brown tumors.
- **Skeletal Weakening:** Loss of mineralized bone leads to bowing of long bones, fractures, and spinal deformities.

Clinical Applications

- **Management of Hyperparathyroidism:** Recognizing Engel-von Recklinghausen syndrome facilitates early intervention in hyperparathyroid crises.
- **Orthopedic Surgery:** Corrective procedures are often needed to manage structural deformities and fractures.
- **Endocrinology:** Highlights the systemic effects of endocrine disorders on skeletal health.

Limitations and Technical Considerations

- **Historical Context:** The term is rarely used today, with the condition now classified under osteitis fibrosa cystica.
- **Delays in Diagnosis:** Early skeletal manifestations may be subtle, delaying recognition of underlying hyperparathyroidism.
- **Chronic Complications:** Severe deformities, if untreated, may become irreversible, underscoring the need for timely management.

Modern Relevance

- **Reclassification:** The syndrome is now considered part of the spectrum of bone diseases caused by secondary or tertiary hyperparathyroidism.
- **Advanced Imaging:** Modern radiological techniques provide clearer visualization of skeletal deformities and cystic changes.
- **Improved Surgical Outcomes:** Advances in parathyroidectomy and reconstructive surgery have improved patient prognosis.

Associated Conditions

- **Primary Hyperparathyroidism:** Often the underlying cause of Engel-von Recklinghausen syndrome.
- **Renal Osteodystrophy:** Similar skeletal changes may occur in chronic kidney disease with secondary hyperparathyroidism.
- **Neurofibromatosis (von Recklinghausen disease):** Not directly related but historically associated with Friedrich von Recklinghausen's work.

Clinical Importance

- **Historical Significance:** Engel-von Recklinghausen syndrome represents a pivotal chapter in understanding skeletal complications of endocrine disorders.
- **Educational Value:** Highlights the systemic impact of untreated hyperparathyroidism and the importance of multidisciplinary management.
- **Foundation for Modern Endocrinology:** Research into this syndrome contributed to the development of current approaches to diagnosing and managing metabolic bone diseases.

References

G. Engel: Über einen Fall von cystoider Entartung des ganzen Skelettes. Giessen, F. C. Pietsch, 1864.

F. D. von Recklinghausen: Demonstration von Knochen mit Tumor bildender Ostitis deformans.

Tageblatt der Naturforschenden Versammlung 1889. Heidelberg, 1890, p 321. Die fibröse und deformirende Ostitis, die Osteomalacie und die osteoplastische Carcinose in ihren gegenseitigen Beziehungen.

Festschrift für Rudolf Virchow. Georg Reimer Verlag; Berlin, 1891. Untersuchungen über Rachitis und Osteomalacie. Jena, G. Fischer, 1910.

Eeb-Duchenne Palsy

Overview

Erb-Duchenne palsy is a form of upper brachial plexus palsy involving the C5 and C6 nerve roots, and occasionally C7. The condition results in paralysis of key muscles, including the supraspinatus, infraspinatus, rhomboids, deltoid, biceps, and brachialis, with associated weakness in muscles like the pectoralis major, triceps, and extensor carpi radialis longus and brevis. This leads to characteristic functional losses such as impaired shoulder external rotation, elbow flexion, forearm supination, and wrist extension. The affected arm assumes the classic "waiter's tip" position, marked by shoulder adduction and internal rotation, elbow extension, forearm pronation, and wrist flexion.

Historical Background

- *Guillaume Duchenne* and *Wilhelm Erb*, in the 19th century, independently described this form of brachial plexus injury.
- Duchenne's studies on neuromuscular disorders provided critical insights into the relationship between nerve injuries and motor function.
- Erb localized the lesion to the *upper trunk of the brachial plexus*, cementing the condition's name in clinical history.
- The condition is commonly associated with *birth trauma* but is also seen in adults following trauma or excessive stretching of the neck and shoulder.

Purpose

- **Diagnosis of Brachial Plexus Injury:** To identify the level and extent of nerve involvement based on clinical presentation.
- **Functional Assessment:** To evaluate muscle paralysis and weakness in the upper extremity.
- **Guidance for Rehabilitation and Surgical Intervention:** To determine appropriate therapeutic strategies aimed at restoring function and minimizing disability.

Procedure Overview

- **Clinical Examination:**
- Observe for the "waiter's tip" posture of the affected arm.
- Assess muscle strength and movements, focusing on shoulder, elbow, forearm, and wrist function.
- Perform sensory testing for deficits over the lateral upper arm and forearm (C5 and C6 dermatomes).

Diagnostic Imaging:

- **MRI:** Evaluates the brachial plexus for nerve root avulsions or compressions.
- **X-rays:** Rule out fractures or associated skeletal injuries, especially in traumatic cases.
- **Ultrasound:** Used in infants to assess muscle atrophy and nerve continuity.

Electrophysiological Studies:

- **Electromyography (EMG):** Identifies denervation patterns in the affected muscles.
- **Nerve Conduction Studies (NCS):** Evaluates the extent and severity of nerve involvement.

Management:

- **Conservative Treatment:** Physical therapy to maintain range of motion and prevent contractures.
- **Surgical Intervention:** Nerve grafts or transfers for severe cases with poor spontaneous recovery.

Results and Interpretation

- **Classic Presentation:** Paralysis and weakness result in the waiter's tip position, where the arm is adducted and internally rotated, with extended elbow, pronated forearm, and flexed wrist.
- **Muscle Testing:** Significant weakness in muscles innervated by C5-C6, such as the deltoid and biceps, confirms the upper brachial plexus involvement.
- **Prognosis:** Infants with Erb-Duchenne palsy often recover spontaneously with conservative management, whereas adults with severe trauma may require surgical repair.

Physiological Basis

- **Nerve Roots Involved:** Damage to C5 and C6 nerve roots disrupts the function of the upper trunk of the brachial plexus.
- **Muscle Paralysis:** Loss of motor function in muscles primarily innervated by C5 and C6, including:
- **Supraspinatus and infraspinatus (external shoulder rotation).**
- **Deltoid (shoulder abduction).**
- **Biceps and brachialis (elbow flexion and forearm supination).**

- **Sensory Loss:** Sensory deficits occur in the lateral arm and forearm, correlating with C5 and C6 dermatomes.

Clinical Applications

- **Pediatric Neurology:** Commonly diagnosed in neonatal brachial plexus palsy due to traumatic delivery or shoulder dystocia.
- **Trauma and Sports Medicine:** Seen in adults after high-energy trauma or forced neck-shoulder separation, such as during motor vehicle accidents.
- **Rehabilitation Therapy:** Involves passive and active exercises to prevent contractures and maintain joint mobility.

Limitations and Technical Considerations

- **Early Diagnosis Challenges:** Neonatal cases may be difficult to assess due to limited voluntary movements and cooperation.
- **Variable Recovery:** Prognosis depends on the severity of nerve injury (neuropraxia vs. neurotmesis) and timing of intervention.
- **Surgical Complexity:** Nerve grafting and transfers are technically demanding and require precise mapping of functional deficits.

Modern Relevance

- **Advances in Imaging:** High-resolution MRI and ultrasound allow for detailed visualization of brachial plexus injuries, improving diagnostic accuracy.
- **Innovative Surgical Techniques:** Techniques like nerve transfers and functional muscle transfers (e.g., gracilis transfer) have improved outcomes in severe cases.
- **Rehabilitation Focus:** Enhanced physical therapy protocols emphasize early intervention and the use of assistive devices to optimize recovery.

Associated Conditions

- **Klumpke's Palsy:** A lower brachial plexus injury involving C8 and T1, contrasting with the upper plexus injury of Erb-Duchenne palsy.
- **Shoulder Dystocia:** A common cause of neonatal Erb-Duchenne palsy, occurring when the shoulder becomes impacted during delivery.
- **Post-Traumatic Neuropathy:** Adults with severe trauma may experience long-term neuropathy and weakness if untreated.

Clinical Importance

- **Early Intervention:** Prompt recognition and management are critical to preventing secondary complications like contractures and muscle atrophy.
- **Comprehensive Care:** Requires a multidisciplinary approach involving neurologists, orthopedic surgeons, and physical therapists.
- **Educational Significance:** Erb-Duchenne palsy serves as a foundational example of peripheral nerve injuries, highlighting the functional interplay between anatomy and clinical presentation.

References

Duchenne GB. De l'electrisation localisee et de son application a la pathologie et a la therapeutique, 3rd ed. Paris: Bailliere, 1872:357.

Erb W. On a characteristic site of injury in the brachial plexus [translated by Brody and Wilkins]. Arch Neurol 21:443, 1969.

Erdheim's Law

Overview

Erdheim's law is a calcioprotective principle which posits that calcic deposits in bones are largest where static demands from pull and pressure are strongest. This principle emphasizes the relationship between mechanical forces and the distribution of calcium within the skeletal system, aligning with the broader understanding of how stress and strain influence bone density and remodeling. Erdheim's law provides foundational insight into the biomechanical adaptations of bones to their functional demands.

Historical Background

- The law is attributed to *Jakob Erdheim*, an Austrian pathologist renowned for his work in osteology and endocrinology.
- Erdheim's studies in the early 20th century on skeletal pathology laid the groundwork for understanding *how mechanical stresses shape bone physiology*, contributing to modern concepts of *bone remodeling* and *calcium metabolism.*
- The principle resonates with later theories such as *Wolff's law*, which describes the structural adaptation of bone in response to mechanical loads.

Purpose

- **Understanding Bone Adaptation:** To explain how bones allocate calcium deposits in response to mechanical forces, enhancing their strength and durability.
- **Predicting Bone Density:** To identify areas of increased or decreased calcification based on mechanical demands.
- **Guiding Clinical Assessments:** To inform the evaluation of bone health, particularly in conditions involving abnormal stress or calcium metabolism.

Procedure Overview

- **Observation of Bone Calcification:** Radiological or histological examination of bones reveals areas of increased calcification in response to mechanical demands.
- **Mechanical Stress Testing:** Application of controlled loads on bones can simulate the effects of pull and pressure, validating the principle of increased calcification in high-demand areas.
- **Comparative Analysis:** Examination of bones subjected to varying levels of mechanical stress highlights differences in calcic deposition, supporting Erdheim's law.

Results and Interpretation

- **Increased Calcification:** High mechanical demand regions, such as joint surfaces and tendon attachment sites, demonstrate greater calcium deposits.
- **Reduced Calcification:** Areas of low mechanical demand show diminished calcic deposition, reflecting the adaptive economy of bone metabolism.
- **Implications for Bone Health:** Abnormal patterns of calcification may indicate underlying metabolic or mechanical dysfunction.

Physiological Basis

- **Bone Remodeling:** Bone continuously remodels in response to mechanical forces, with osteoblast activity increasing in areas of high stress to enhance mineral density.
- **Calcium Metabolism:** Calcium, a critical component of hydroxyapatite, is deposited where the skeleton needs to resist compressive and tensile forces.
- **Biomechanical Adaptation:** The distribution of calcification aligns with the principle that bones optimize their structure to efficiently bear mechanical loads.

Clinical Applications

- **Orthopedic Assessment:** Guides evaluation of stress-related changes in bones, such as in athletes or individuals with repetitive strain injuries.
- **Bone Health Monitoring:** Used in understanding disorders like osteoporosis or osteomalacia, where calcic deposition is impaired.
- **Rehabilitation Strategies:** Rehabilitation programs leverage the principles of mechanical loading to enhance bone strength and promote healing.

Limitations and Technical Considerations

- **Static vs. Dynamic Loading:** Erdheim's law primarily addresses static mechanical demands, whereas dynamic forces also significantly influence bone remodeling.
- **Variability Among Individuals:** Factors such as age, hormonal status, and systemic conditions affect the application of the law to individual cases.
- **Complex Interactions:** Other biological processes, such as vascularization and nutrient availability, interact with mechanical factors in determining calcification.

Modern Relevance

- **Integration with Wolff's Law:** Erdheim's law complements Wolff's principles, together forming a comprehensive framework for understanding bone adaptation.
- **Advances in Imaging:** Modern imaging techniques, such as DEXA scans and micro-CT, provide precise assessments of calcic deposition in response to mechanical stress.
- **Role in Bone Engineering:** The principle is applied in designing biomaterials and prosthetics that mimic the mechanical properties of natural bone.

Associated Conditions

- **Osteoporosis:** Reduced mechanical stress, such as in immobility, leads to diminished calcification and bone density loss.
- **Stress Fractures:** Imbalances in mechanical loading and bone adaptation can result in microfractures in areas of high demand.
- **Hyperparathyroidism:** Abnormal calcium metabolism affects the distribution of calcic deposits, disrupting the patterns described by Erdheim's law.

Clinical Importance

- **Insight into Bone Physiology:** Erdheim's law underscores the critical interplay between mechanical forces and calcium metabolism in maintaining skeletal integrity.
- **Educational Value:** The principle serves as a foundational concept in orthopedics, pathology, and biomechanics.
- **Guidance for Therapies:** Understanding the calcioprotective effects of mechanical loading aids in developing effective treatments for bone diseases and rehabilitation protocols.

References

J. Erdheim: Rachitis und Epithelkörperchen.

Denkschriften der kaiserlichen Akademie der Wissenschaften in Wien, mathematisch-naturwissenschaftliche Classe, 1914, 90: 363-368. Über das Calcioprotective Gesetz.

Denkschriften der kaiserlichen Akademie der Wissenschaften in Wien, mathematisch-naturwissenschaftliche Classe, 1914, 90: 611-621.

Erdheim's Syndrome

Overview

Erdheim's syndrome is a condition characterized by cervical spondylosis secondary to acromegaly, involving hypertrophy of bone and cartilage in structures such as the clavicle, vertebral bodies, and intervertebral disks. These changes result in clinical manifestations including pain, kyphosis, restricted movement, and chronic discomfort. The syndrome highlights the interplay between endocrine disorders and musculoskeletal changes, particularly the skeletal consequences of excessive growth hormone secretion.

Historical Background

- Erdheim's syndrome is named after *Jakob Erdheim*, an Austrian pathologist known for his extensive work in *bone pathology* and the *systemic effects of endocrine disorders*.
- His contributions, particularly in understanding the skeletal manifestations of *acromegaly*, provided crucial insights into the pathological basis of the condition.
- Acromegaly, recognized as a hormonal disorder caused by excess growth hormone, has long been associated with musculoskeletal complications, with Erdheim's work forming a foundation for their classification and study.

Purpose

- **Recognition of Skeletal Effects:** To identify the structural changes in bones and cartilage caused by chronic growth hormone excess.

- **Diagnosis of Secondary Cervical Spondylosis:** To evaluate and manage spinal complications arising from acromegaly.
- **Guidance for Management:** To address pain, movement impairments, and structural deformities resulting from the syndrome.

Procedure Overview

- **Clinical Evaluation:**
- Assess symptoms such as chronic neck pain, restricted cervical movement, and kyphotic posture.
- Look for signs of acromegaly, including enlarged hands, feet, and facial features.

Imaging Studies:

- **X-rays:** Reveal hypertrophy of vertebral bodies, clavicles, and intervertebral disks.
- **MRI or CT scans:** Provide detailed visualization of spinal cord compression, kyphosis, and soft tissue involvement.
- **Endocrine Assessment:** Growth Hormone and IGF-1 Levels: Elevated levels confirm active acromegaly.
- **Pituitary Imaging:** MRI to detect pituitary adenomas causing growth hormone excess.
- **Management:**
- Address the underlying acromegaly through surgical, medical, or radiation therapies for pituitary adenomas.
- Implement physical therapy, pain management, and orthopedic interventions as needed.

Results and Interpretation

- **Imaging Findings:** Hypertrophy of the clavicle, vertebral bodies, and disks with evidence of kyphosis and narrowing of intervertebral spaces.
- **Endocrine Correlation:** Elevated growth hormone levels and pituitary adenomas confirm the association with acromegaly.
- **Functional Impairment:** Pain and restricted movement significantly impact the patient's quality of life, requiring multidisciplinary management.

Physiological Basis

- **Role of Growth Hormone:** Chronic excess of growth hormone stimulates cartilage and bone growth, leading to structural hypertrophy and deformities.
- **Spinal Changes:** Overgrowth of vertebral bodies and intervertebral disks contributes to cervical spondylosis, with resulting nerve compression and kyphosis.
- **Musculoskeletal Dysfunction:** Abnormal bone and cartilage growth disrupt joint mechanics and spinal alignment, causing movement impairment and pain.

Clinical Applications

- **Orthopedic Management:** Focuses on mitigating structural deformities, improving spinal alignment, and relieving nerve compression.
- **Endocrine Treatment:** Management of acromegaly through growth hormone suppression is critical in halting disease progression.
- **Rehabilitation:** Physical therapy and

pain management improve mobility and enhance quality of life.

Limitations and Technical Considerations

- **Chronic Nature:** The progressive nature of bone and cartilage changes requires ongoing monitoring and treatment adjustments.
- **Complex Management:** Effective treatment often necessitates a multidisciplinary approach, involving endocrinologists, orthopedic surgeons, and physical therapists.
- **Irreversible Changes:** Long-standing hypertrophy and deformities may not fully regress, even with optimal endocrine and orthopedic care.

Modern Relevance

- **Advances in Endocrine Therapy:** Modern treatments, including somatostatin analogs, growth hormone receptor antagonists, and minimally invasive pituitary surgery, have improved outcomes in acromegaly.
- **Improved Imaging:** High-resolution MRI and CT scans provide better visualization of skeletal and spinal changes, aiding diagnosis and treatment planning.
- **Focus on Early Intervention:** Early detection of acromegaly and its complications, including Erdheim's syndrome, prevents severe deformities and functional impairments.

Associated Conditions

- **Acromegaly:** The primary underlying condition, characterized by excess growth hormone and associated systemic effects.
- **Cervical Spondylosis:** Degenerative changes in the cervical spine caused by hypertrophy and disk pathology.
- **Kyphosis:** Spinal curvature and postural abnormalities resulting from structural changes in the vertebral column.

Clinical Importance

- **Integration of Endocrine and Orthopedic Care:** Erdheim's syndrome exemplifies the need for collaborative management of systemic and skeletal disorders.
- **Early Recognition:** Timely diagnosis of acromegaly and its complications prevents irreversible structural deformities and reduces morbidity.
- **Educational Value:** Serves as an example of the systemic impact of endocrine dysfunction on skeletal health, enriching the understanding of bone physiology.

References

J. Erdheim: Rachitis und Epithelkörperchen.

Denkschriften der kaiserlichen Akademie der Wissenschaften in Wien, mathematisch-naturwissenschaftliche Classe, 1914, 90: 363-368. Über das Calcioprotective Gesetz.

Denkschriften der kaiserlichen Akademie der Wissenschaften in Wien, mathematisch-naturwissenschaftliche Classe, 1914, 90: 611-621.

Erlacher-Blount Syndrome

Overview

Erlacher-Blount syndrome is a condition characterized by osteochondrosis affecting the upper tibial epiphysis in children, leading to progressive bowing of one or both legs. It is categorized into two types: the infantile type, presenting before the age of 8 years and typically bilateral, and the adolescent type, occurring after the age of 8 years, usually unilateral. The hallmark deformity is an abrupt angulation with the apex laterally just below the knee. While the condition is often sporadic, familial cases have been noted with an autosomal recessive inheritance pattern.

Historical Background

- *Philipp Erlacher* first documented the syndrome in 1922, coining the term *"tibia vara"* to describe the progressive deformity of the upper tibial epiphysis.
- In 1937, *Walter Putnam Blount* reported 13 cases of bow legs, naming the condition *"osteochondrosis deformans tibiae"*, which highlighted the deformity in the upper medial tibial epiphysis and metaphysis.
- *Carroll Glenn Barber* advanced the understanding of the syndrome through studies in 1939 and 1942, detailing the clinical and pathological findings.
- By the mid-20th century, the syndrome was recognized as a developmental condition affecting growth and development, with significant clinical interest in populations prone to this disorder.

Purpose

- **Early Diagnosis of Tibial Deformity:** To identify the condition in its early stages for effective management and to prevent progression of the bowing deformity.
- **Understanding Etiology and Pathogenesis:** To explore the mechanical, genetic, and environmental factors contributing to the condition.
- **Guidance for Treatment:** To inform orthopedic interventions aimed at correcting the deformity and improving function.

Procedure Overview

- **Clinical Assessment:**
- Evaluate for bowing of the legs, noting the abrupt lateral angulation just below the knee.
- Assess for associated findings, such as overweight in some cases, and the onset age of deformity.

Radiological Examination:

- **X-rays:** Show sloping of the epiphysis, beak-like recurving of the metaphysis, and other characteristic changes.
- **MRI or CT:** May be used to assess cartilage involvement and the extent of deformity.
- **Genetic and Familial Studies:** Analyze family history for patterns of inheritance in familial cases.
- Confirm the autosomal recessive transmission in familial types.

Management Approaches:

- **Conservative Treatment:** Bracing and physiotherapy in mild cases.

- **Surgical Intervention:** Corrective osteotomy for severe deformities, typically reserved for cases unresponsive to conservative measures.

Results and Interpretation

- **Radiographic Findings:** The abrupt angulation of the tibia, with sloping epiphysis and metaphyseal changes, confirms the diagnosis.
- **Clinical Presentation:** Infantile cases are bilateral and evident early, while adolescent cases are unilateral and appear later.
- **Familial Patterns:** Autosomal recessive inheritance is suggested in some cases, with involvement of successive generations.

Physiological Basis

- **Growth Plate Disruption:** Abnormal growth at the medial tibial epiphysis and metaphysis leads to uneven pressure distribution, causing bowing.
- **Mechanical Factors:** Increased weight-bearing stress on the medial tibial growth plate may contribute to deformity progression, especially in overweight children.
- **Genetic Influences:** Familial cases point to a genetic predisposition, influencing the severity and bilateral nature of the condition.

Clinical Applications

- **Orthopedic Management:** Corrective surgeries such as tibial osteotomy are crucial in severe deformities to restore alignment and functionality.
- **Rehabilitation:** Physical therapy helps improve joint mobility and supports postoperative recovery.
- **Public Health Interventions:** Addressing risk factors, such as childhood obesity, may reduce the incidence in susceptible populations.

Limitations and Technical Considerations

- **Variable Progression:** The course of the syndrome differs between individuals, making treatment timing and modality challenging.
- **Surgical Risks:** Osteotomies and other corrective surgeries carry risks of infection, recurrence, or overcorrection.
- **Diagnostic Challenges:** Distinguishing Erlacher-Blount syndrome from other causes of leg bowing, such as rickets, may require thorough evaluation.

Modern Relevance

- **Prevalence in Specific Populations:** The condition is particularly common among certain populations, such as the indigenous population of South Africa, highlighting the importance of regional healthcare strategies.
- **Advances in Imaging:** Modern radiographic and MRI techniques allow earlier detection and more precise evaluation of deformities.
- **Improved Surgical Techniques:** Advances in minimally invasive surgery and postoperative care have enhanced outcomes in severe cases.

Associated Conditions

- **Obesity:** Overweight children are at higher risk due to increased mechanical stress on the medial tibial growth plate.

- **Developmental Disorders:** Conditions affecting skeletal growth may exacerbate the presentation or progression of tibial deformities.
- **Familial Leg Bowing:** Genetic predispositions contribute to the occurrence of similar bowing deformities in families.

Clinical Importance

- **Functional and Cosmetic Concerns:** The deformity significantly impacts walking mechanics and appearance, necessitating timely intervention.
- **Multidisciplinary Approach:** Effective management involves collaboration among orthopedic surgeons, pediatricians, and physical therapists.
- **Educational Value:** The syndrome provides critical insights into the relationship between growth plate mechanics and skeletal deformities, enriching the understanding of pediatric orthopedics.

References

P. Erlacher: Deformierende Prozesse der Epiphysengegend bei Kindern.

Archiv für orthopädische und Unfall-Chirurgie, München, 1922, 20: 81-96.

W. P. Blount: Tibia vara: osteochondrosis deformans tibiae.

Journal of Bone and Joint Surgery, Boston, 1937, 19: 1-29. Tibia vara: osteochondrosis deformans tibiae.

Current Practice of Orthopaedic Surgery, 1966. Volume 3, page 141. Mosby Co., St. Louis, Illinois.

C. G. Barber: Osteochondrosis deformans tibiae. Nonrachitic bow leg in children.

American Journal of Diseases of Children, Chicago, 1942, 64: 831-842.

C. A. Bathfield, P. H. Beighton: Blount disease. A review of etiological factors in 110 patients.

Clinical Orthopaedics and Related Research, Philadelphia, 1978, 135: 29-33.

Essex-Lopresti Fracture

Overview

The Essex-Lopresti fracture-dislocation refers to a rare but clinically significant injury comprising a comminuted radial head fracture, dislocation of the distal radioulnar joint (DRUJ), and disruption of the interosseous membrane (IOM). It typically results from a high-energy axial force applied to the forearm, such as a fall on an outstretched hand. Diagnosis requires thorough evaluation of the forearm, elbow, and wrist to detect associated injuries, particularly DRUJ instability. Treatment often involves open reduction and internal fixation (ORIF) or radial head replacement in cases of severe comminution, with stabilization of the DRUJ via repair of the triangular fibrocartilage complex (TFCC).

Historical Background

- **1930:** Brockman documented two cases of radial head fractures associated with proximal migration of the radius.
- **1946:** Curr and Coe described a case involving a radial head fracture and DRUJ dislocation in a mining accident, managed with traction and closed reduction.
- **1951:** Peter Essex-Lopresti formally identified and described the injury, linking radial head fractures, DRUJ dislocation, and IOM disruption as part of a constellation. He emphasized the importance of preserving the radial head and avoiding excision.
- **1999:** Failla demonstrated the effectiveness of ultrasound imaging

in diagnosing torn interosseous membranes in forearm fractures.

Purpose

- **Early and Accurate Diagnosis:** To ensure timely recognition of the associated DRUJ instability and IOM disruption when a radial head fracture is identified.
- **Comprehensive Injury Management:** To provide appropriate surgical and rehabilitative interventions for restoring function and stability.
- **Preventing Complications:** To avoid long-term issues such as chronic wrist instability, pain, and loss of forearm motion.

Procedure Overview

- **Clinical Examination:**
- Assess for swelling, pain, and limited motion in the elbow, forearm, and wrist.
- Observe for radial deviation of the hand and difficulty with pronation/supination.

Imaging Studies:

- **X-rays:** Detect radial head fractures and DRUJ dislocation.
- **CT scans:** Provide detailed visualization of fracture comminution and DRUJ alignment.
- **Ultrasound or MRI:** Evaluate for IOM disruption and soft tissue injuries.

Management:

- **Open Reduction and Internal Fixation (ORIF):** For repairable radial head fractures.
- **Radial Head Replacement:** Used for severe comminution where ORIF is not feasible.
- **DRUJ Stabilization:** Through TFCC repair to restore joint integrity.
- **Rehabilitation:** Early mobilization protocols to prevent stiffness and enhance recovery of forearm rotation.

Results and Interpretation

- **Positive Findings:** A comminuted radial head fracture with proximal migration of the radius and DRUJ instability confirms the Essex-Lopresti injury pattern.
- **Radiological Correlation:** Imaging findings support the triad of injuries (radial head fracture, DRUJ dislocation, and IOM disruption).
- **Prognosis:** Successful surgical repair can restore forearm stability and function, but delayed or missed diagnosis often results in poor outcomes.

Physiological Basis

- **Interosseous Membrane Function:** The IOM transmits axial loads from the radius to the ulna, stabilizing the forearm. Disruption leads to instability and proximal migration of the radius.
- **DRUJ Disruption:** Radial head fractures destabilize the proximal radius, contributing to DRUJ dislocation and impaired load transmission to the wrist.
- **Radial Head Importance:** The radial head is critical for stabilizing the elbow and transmitting axial forces; its excision without replacement leads to further instability.

Clinical Applications

- **Management of Complex Forearm Injuries:** Helps guide treatment for high-energy trauma with associated soft tissue damage.
- **Surgical Interventions:** Establishes protocols for radial head reconstruction/replacement and DRUJ stabilization.
- **Rehabilitation Focus:** Emphasizes early functional recovery while maintaining stability.

Limitations and Technical Considerations

- **Missed Diagnosis:** Failure to recognize DRUJ instability or IOM disruption can result in poor functional outcomes.
- **Surgical Challenges:** Severe comminution or chronic injuries may complicate repair, requiring advanced reconstructive techniques.
- **Rehabilitation Risks:** Overly aggressive early motion may compromise surgical repairs, while prolonged immobilization risks stiffness.

Modern Relevance

- **Advances in Imaging:** Use of ultrasound and high-resolution MRI enhances early detection of IOM disruptions.
- **Improved Prosthetics:** Modern radial head prostheses allow for better joint restoration in cases requiring replacement.
- **Guidelines for Acute Care:** Emphasizing DRUJ evaluation in all radial head fractures reduces the likelihood of missed injuries.

Associated Conditions

- **Galeazzi Fracture:** Fracture of the distal third of the radius with DRUJ dislocation, often requiring similar surgical stabilization.
- **Monteggia Fracture-Dislocation:** Ulnar fracture with radial head dislocation, highlighting the interplay between forearm bones and joints.
- **Chronic Forearm Instability:** Late complications of untreated Essex-Lopresti injuries, leading to pain and loss of motion.

Clinical Importance

- **Comprehensive Injury Approach:** Essex-Lopresti fractures highlight the importance of evaluating the entire forearm in radial head fractures to prevent missed injuries.
- **Educational Significance:** Serves as a critical example of complex forearm trauma, requiring integrated orthopedic and radiological expertise.
- **Functional Outcomes:** Proper management restores forearm biomechanics, preventing chronic disability and improving quality of life.

References

Essex-Lopresti P. Fractures of the radial head with distal radio-ulnar dislocation; report of two cases. J Bone Joint Surg (Br). 1951;33b(2):244–7.

Dodds SD, Yeh PC, Slade 3rd JF. Essex-Lopresti injuries. Hand Clin. 2008;24(1):125–37.

Wegmann K. The Essex-Lopresti lesion. Strategies in Trauma and Limb Reconstruction. 2012;7(3):131–9.

Brockman EP. Two Cases of Disability at the Wrist-joint following Excision of the Head of the Radius. Proc R Soc Med. 1931 May;24(7):904-5. [PMC2182896]

Curr JF, Coe WA. Dislocation of the inferior radio-ulnar joint. Br J Surg. 1946 Jul;34:74-7. [PMID 20994136]

Essex-Lopresti, P. Fractures of the radial head with distal radio-ulnar dislocation; report of two cases. J Bone Joint Surg Br. 1951 May;33B(2):244-7. [PMID 14832324] [Full Text]

McGlinn EP, Sebastin SJ, Chung KS. A Historical Perspective on the Essex-Lopresti Injury. J Hand Surg Am. 2013 Aug; 38(8): 1599–1606. [PMC4157731]

Wegmann K, Dargel J, Burkhart KJ, Brüggemann GP, Müller LP. The Essex-Lopresti lesion. Strategies Trauma Limb Reconstr. 2012 Nov; 7(3): 131–139. [PMC3482440]

van Riet RP, van Glabbeek F. History of radial head prosthesis in traumatology. Acta Orthop Failla JM, Jacobson J, van Holsbeeck M. Ultrasound diagnosis and surgical pathology of the torn interosseous membrane in forearm fractures/dislocations. J Hand Surg Am. 1999 Mar;24(2):257-66. [PMID 10194008]

Esterly-McKusick Syndrome

Overview

Esterly-McKusick syndrome is a rare inherited disorder characterized by flexion contractures of the fingers and toes, limited motion in other joints, and sclerodermatoid changes of the skin. The syndrome affects both joint mobility and skin texture, presenting as a connective tissue disorder. It has been documented in familial patterns, suggesting an autosomal dominant inheritance.

Historical Background

- First described by *Nancy Burton Esterly* and *Victor Almon McKusick*, who reported the condition in a mother and her two children.
- Their detailed observations highlighted the *familial clustering* of symptoms, which provided early insights into the syndrome's genetic basis.
- McKusick's contributions to the study of inherited diseases further emphasized the importance of understanding this condition within the context of *genetic connective tissue disorders*.

Purpose

- **Diagnostic Understanding:** To identify the clinical and genetic features associated with joint contractures and skin changes.
- **Genetic Counseling:** To provide guidance on inheritance patterns and recurrence risks for affected families.

- **Functional Assessment:** To evaluate joint mobility limitations and their impact on quality of life.

Procedure Overview

- **Clinical Evaluation:**
- Examine for flexion contractures in the fingers and toes.
- Assess joint motion across other affected joints.
- Identify sclerodermatoid changes, including thickened, hardened skin.

Imaging Studies:

- **X-rays:** May reveal joint abnormalities contributing to motion restriction.
- **Ultrasound or MRI:** Useful for assessing soft tissue and connective tissue involvement.
- **Genetic Testing:** Confirm autosomal dominant inheritance patterns in affected families.
- **Management:** Focus on improving joint mobility through physical therapy and, in some cases, surgical intervention for severe contractures.

Results and Interpretation

- **Clinical Findings:** Flexion deformities in digits are prominent, accompanied by limited joint motion and skin changes suggestive of scleroderma.
- **Radiological Correlation:** Imaging supports clinical findings, highlighting structural or connective tissue abnormalities.
- **Genetic Confirmation:** Familial clustering and autosomal dominant patterns strengthen the genetic diagnosis.

Physiological Basis

- **Connective Tissue Changes:** Abnormal connective tissue remodeling leads to contractures and sclerodermatoid skin changes.
- **Joint Involvement:** Limited joint mobility is due to soft tissue fibrosis, affecting tendons and ligaments.
- **Inheritance:** Autosomal dominant mutations likely affect genes involved in connective tissue synthesis and repair.

Clinical Applications

- **Physical Therapy:** Rehabilitation to improve or maintain joint range of motion.
- **Surgical Intervention:** Corrective surgeries for severe contractures to enhance hand or foot function.
- **Dermatological Management:** Addressing skin thickening to prevent complications like ulceration.

Limitations and Technical Considerations

- **Variable Expressivity:** Severity of symptoms may vary significantly, even among affected family members.
- **Challenges in Early Diagnosis:** Subtle initial symptoms may delay recognition, particularly in mild cases.
- **Therapeutic Limitations:** Long-standing contractures and skin fibrosis may not fully respond to therapy or surgery.

Modern Relevance

- **Genetic Advances:** Modern genetic testing has improved the ability to confirm the diagnosis and understand its molecular basis.
- **Enhanced Therapies:** Advances in connective tissue and skin treatments provide new management options for sclerodermatoid changes.
- **Awareness in Familial Disorders:** Increasing awareness of familial connective tissue disorders has led to earlier diagnosis and better outcomes.

Associated Conditions

- **Scleroderma:** The skin changes in Esterly-McKusick syndrome resemble those seen in localized or systemic scleroderma.
- **Dupuytren's Contracture:** The flexion contractures mimic this condition but occur in a different genetic and systemic context.
- **Congenital Contractural Syndromes:** Includes other genetic syndromes with joint contractures as a primary feature.

Clinical Importance

- **Recognition of Rare Disorders:** Awareness of Esterly-McKusick syndrome facilitates early diagnosis and intervention, preventing progression of contractures.
- **Multidisciplinary Management:** Effective care involves collaboration among orthopedic surgeons, physical therapists, and dermatologists.
- **Genetic Counseling:** Crucial for families with affected members, aiding in understanding inheritance patterns and recurrence risks.

References

E. Pichler: Hereditäre Kontrakturen mit sklerodermieartigen Hautveränderungen.

Zeitschrift für Kinderheilkunde, Berlin, 1968, 104: 349-361.

N. B. Esterly, V. A. McKusick: Stiff skin syndrome.

Pediatrics, Evanston, Illinois, 1971, 47: 360-369.

Ewing's sarcoma

Overview

Ewing's sarcoma is a highly malignant primary bone tumor that typically affects the diaphyses (shafts) of long bones in the lower extremities but may also involve the pelvis, ribs, clavicle, and girdles. It is characterized by intermittent pain, slight fever, and destructive tumor growth that spreads rapidly to other parts of the body. Composed of compact, uniform cells with prominent nuclei, the tumor is aggressive and requires radical treatment, though the prognosis remains guarded. It most commonly affects children, adolescents, and young adults, accounting for 10-15% of all primary malignant bone tumors.

Historical Background

- The condition was first extensively described by *James Ewing*, a prominent American pathologist, in the early 20th century.
- Ewing's work in 1920 delineated this tumor from other similar conditions such as *lymphoma* and *neuroblastoma*, establishing its unique identity.
- Earlier descriptions of similar tumors were made by *Georg Albert Lücke* in 1866 and *Otto Hildebrand* in 1890, but Ewing's clinical observations and pathological studies solidified its recognition as a distinct entity.
- The sarcoma is named in honor of Ewing's contributions to its identification and characterization.

Purpose

- **Early Diagnosis:** To detect the tumor at an early stage to improve treatment outcomes and minimize metastasis.
- **Understanding Tumor Pathophysiology:** To study the aggressive nature of the tumor and its rapid dissemination for better therapeutic approaches.
- **Guiding Multimodal Treatment:** To combine surgical, radiological, and chemotherapeutic interventions for comprehensive management.

Procedure Overview

- **Clinical Presentation:**
- Patients present with localized pain in the affected bone, often intermittent initially but intensifying over time.
- Associated symptoms include slight fever, swelling, and tenderness over the involved area.

Diagnostic Imaging:

- **X-rays:** Show a destructive lesion with a characteristic "onion-skin" periosteal reaction.
- **MRI and CT scans:** Provide detailed visualization of soft tissue involvement and tumor extent.
- **PET scans:** Evaluate metastatic spread.
- **Biopsy and Histopathology:**
- A definitive diagnosis is made via biopsy, revealing uniform small round cells with large nuclei and scattered chromatin.
- Immunohistochemistry and molecular testing can confirm specific markers like EWSR1 gene rearrangement.

Management:

- **Chemotherapy:** Used to reduce tumor size and control metastasis.
- **Surgery:** Limb-sparing procedures or amputations depending on tumor extent.
- **Radiation Therapy:** For local control, particularly in non-resectable tumors.

Results and Interpretation

- **Imaging Findings:** Destructive lesions with periosteal reactions confirm aggressive bone involvement.
- **Histopathological Findings:** Compact, uniform tumor cells with mitotic activity and vascular channels differentiate Ewing's sarcoma from other round cell tumors.
- **Treatment Outcomes:** Early-stage localized tumors have better survival rates with multimodal treatment compared to metastatic cases.

Physiological Basis

- **Tumor Origin:** The exact origin remains unclear but is thought to involve neuroectodermal or mesenchymal cells.
- **Aggressive Growth:** The tumor's rapid proliferation leads to bone destruction and systemic spread, often to the lungs, bone marrow, or other skeletal sites.
- **Genetic Marker:** The hallmark genetic abnormality is the EWSR1-FLI1 translocation, aiding diagnosis and understanding of its molecular pathogenesis.

Clinical Applications

- **Early Detection:** Increased awareness and imaging can lead to earlier diagnosis, particularly in pediatric populations.
- **Advancements in Multimodal Treatment:** Use of targeted chemotherapy and improved surgical techniques enhances outcomes.
- **Research into Genetic Therapies:** Exploration of gene-targeted treatments for tumors with EWSR1 translocations offers future potential.

Limitations and Technical Considerations

- **Delayed Diagnosis:** Symptoms are often nonspecific early on, leading to delays in detection and treatment.
- **Treatment Resistance:** The tumor's aggressive nature and potential resistance to therapy can complicate management.
- **High Metastatic Potential:** The rapid spread to distant sites makes prognosis challenging, especially in advanced stages.

Modern Relevance

- **Improved Survival Rates:** Advances in chemotherapy, surgery, and radiation have led to better survival in localized cases, though metastatic disease remains difficult to treat.
- **Genetic and Molecular Insights:** Understanding the EWSR1-FLI1 translocation has paved the way for diagnostic accuracy and targeted research.
- **Multidisciplinary Care:** Effective management requires collaboration across oncology, orthopedics, radiology, and pathology.

Associated Conditions

- **Other Small Round Cell Tumors:** Includes lymphoma, neuroblastoma, and rhabdomyosarcoma, which must be differentiated via histological and genetic studies.
- **Osteosarcoma:** Another primary malignant bone tumor, but distinct in its osteoblastic properties and presentation.

Clinical Importance

- **High Incidence in Young Populations:** Ewing's sarcoma is a significant contributor to morbidity and mortality in children, adolescents, and young adults.
- **Importance of Early Detection:** Early diagnosis is crucial for improving survival rates and preventing extensive metastasis.
- **Educational and Research Value:** The condition provides a model for understanding aggressive malignancies and the role of genetics in oncogenesis.

References

J. Ewing:Diffuse endothelioma of bone. Proceedings of the New York Pathological Society, 1921, 17-24. Review and classification of bone sarcoma.

Archives of Surgery, Chicago, 1922, 4: 485-533. Further report on endothelial endothelioma of bone.

Proceedings of the New York Pathological Society, 1924, 24: 93-101.

Fairbank-Keats Syndrome

Overview

Fairbank-Keats syndrome, also referred to as osteoglophonic dysplasia, is a rare form of bone dysplasia marked by unique bone lesions, disproportionate dwarfism, and craniofacial abnormalities. Clinical features include failure to thrive, craniosynostosis, rhizomelic dwarfism, and multiple metaphyseal defects. The syndrome is characterized radiologically by anterior beaking of the vertebrae and hollowed-out metaphyses, which inspired the term "osteoglophonic." While affected infants often experience early psychomotor retardation and feeding difficulties, these issues may improve, with later normal intelligence and adequate nutrition.

Historical Background

- The syndrome is named after *Harold Arthur Thomas Fairbank*, a British orthopedic surgeon, and *T. E. Keats*, an American radiologist, who contributed to the study and recognition of rare bone dysplasias.
- The term *osteoglophonic dysplasia* is derived from the Greek word meaning *"hollowed out,"* a reference to the characteristic appearance of the metaphyses on radiographic imaging.
- Early reports emphasized the distinctive combination of *craniofacial abnormalities, short stature,* and *metaphyseal defects*, differentiating this condition from other skeletal dysplasias.

Purpose

- **Identification of Rare Bone Dysplasias:** To diagnose and differentiate Fairbank-Keats syndrome from other dwarfing conditions based on its unique clinical and radiological features.
- **Understanding Growth Impairment:** To investigate the underlying pathophysiology of metaphyseal defects and craniosynostosis.
- **Management of Multisystem Involvement:** To address growth abnormalities, respiratory issues, and craniofacial deformities in a holistic manner.

Procedure Overview

- **Clinical Assessment:** Evaluate for growth failure, craniosynostosis, rhizomelic dwarfism, and feeding or respiratory difficulties.
- Document distinctive craniofacial abnormalities, including midface hypoplasia and skull deformities.

Radiological Examination:

- **X-rays:** Highlight the metaphyseal defects and anterior beaking of vertebrae.
- **CT scans:** Detail the severity of craniosynostosis and assess intracranial pressure.
- **MRI:** Rule out complications related to skull or spinal abnormalities.
- **Genetic Testing:** Identify mutations in genes associated with bone growth and craniofacial development, such as FGFR-related mutations.
- **Multidisciplinary Management:** Involve orthopedic surgeons, geneticists, craniofacial specialists, and nutritionists in the care plan.

Results and Interpretation

- **Radiological Findings:** Radiographs reveal hollowed-out metaphyses, anterior vertebral beaking, and rhizomelic shortening of the long bones.
- **Clinical Features:** Disproportionate dwarfism, severe craniofacial abnormalities, and initial feeding or respiratory challenges are key diagnostic clues.
- **Genetic Insights:** FGFR mutations, commonly associated with skeletal dysplasias, may be identified.

Physiological Basis

- **Bone Growth Impairment:** Defective ossification at the metaphyses leads to hollowed-out bone structures and shortened, malformed long bones.
- **Craniofacial Dysmorphology:** Premature fusion of cranial sutures (craniosynostosis) affects skull shape and can increase intracranial pressure.
- **Dwarfism Mechanisms:** Abnormal endochondral ossification disrupts normal growth patterns, leading to rhizomelic dwarfism.

Clinical Applications

- **Craniofacial Surgery:** Surgical correction of craniosynostosis may be necessary to prevent or treat complications such as increased intracranial pressure.
- **Growth Monitoring:** Regular assessment of growth and nutritional status is essential to optimize physical development.
- **Orthopedic Interventions:** Address limb deformities or spinal abnormalities to improve mobility and posture.

Limitations and Technical Considerations

- **Diagnostic Challenges:** The rarity of the syndrome and overlap with other skeletal dysplasias can delay diagnosis.
- **Surgical Risks:** Craniofacial and orthopedic surgeries carry risks, especially in patients with compromised health due to feeding and respiratory issues.
- **Lifelong Monitoring:** The progressive nature of some skeletal abnormalities necessitates ongoing follow-up and multidisciplinary care.

Modern Relevance

- **Advances in Imaging:** High-resolution CT and MRI have enhanced the detection of subtle metaphyseal and craniofacial abnormalities.
- **Genetic Research:** Identification of FGFR mutations has clarified the molecular basis of this syndrome, offering potential for targeted therapies.
- **Improved Outcomes:** Multidisciplinary approaches, including early surgical interventions and nutritional support, have significantly improved patient prognosis.

Associated Conditions

- **Craniosynostosis Syndromes:** Similar cranial deformities are seen in syndromes like Apert or Crouzon syndrome.
- **Skeletal Dysplasias:** Conditions such as achondroplasia or metaphyseal chondrodysplasia share overlapping features but differ in their radiological and clinical presentations.
- **Respiratory Complications:** Airway obstruction due to midface hypoplasia is a common issue in severe craniofacial dysplasias.

Clinical Importance

- **Early Diagnosis and Intervention:** Prompt identification of the syndrome allows for early management of life-threatening complications such as respiratory distress or increased intracranial pressure.
- **Multidisciplinary Approach:** The condition requires input from multiple specialties to address the wide range of clinical manifestations effectively.
- **Educational and Research Value:** Fairbank-Keats syndrome provides valuable insights into the intersection of genetics, bone biology, and craniofacial development.

References

T. Fairbank: An Atlas of General Affections of the Skeleton. Edinburgh, Livingstone, 1951. pp. 181-183.

T. E. Keats, T. H. Smith, D. E. Sweet: Craniofacial dysostosis with fibrous metaphyseal defects. The American Journal of Roentgenology, 1975, 124: 271-275.

R. I. Kelley, P. F. Borns, D. Nichols, E. Zackai: Osteoglophonic dwarfs in two generations. Journal of Medical Genetics, London, 1983, 20: 436-440.

Farber's disease

Overview

Farber's disease, also known as Farber lipogranulomatosis, is a rare, inheritable lysosomal storage disorder caused by a deficiency in the enzyme acid ceramidase, leading to the accumulation of ceramide in various tissues. The condition typically presents at birth or shortly thereafter, with symptoms including failure to thrive, hoarse cry, joint swelling, and skin nodules. The disease follows a progressive course, with severe systemic involvement, leading to cardiac and renal failure, and often results in death during infancy.

Historical Background

- **1952:** Sidney Farber, a renowned American pathologist, first described the disease in a case series, highlighting its unique clinical and pathological features.
- **1957:** Farber further expanded on the clinical findings and proposed the lysosomal enzyme deficiency as the underlying cause.
- *L. Lahut Uzman*, a collaborator, contributed to the understanding of the granulomatous nature of the lesions and their histopathological characteristics.

Purpose

- **Early Diagnosis:** To detect the disease at an early stage through recognition of clinical signs and enzymatic testing.
- **Understanding Pathophysiology:** To elucidate the role of ceramide accumulation in the disease's progression and systemic involvement.
- **Guiding Research:** To explore enzyme replacement or gene therapy as potential treatments.

Procedure Overview

- **Clinical Evaluation:** Assess for characteristic symptoms such as hoarse cry, joint swellings, failure to thrive, and erythematous skin nodules.
- Note systemic manifestations, including recurrent infections and signs of organ failure.
- **Laboratory Testing:** Measure acid ceramidase activity in fibroblasts or leukocytes to confirm the enzyme deficiency.
- Analyze ceramide levels in tissues or bodily fluids.

Imaging Studies:

- **X-rays:** Reveal articular erosion and demineralization, resembling findings in juvenile rheumatoid arthritis.
- **MRI:** May be used to assess organ involvement and granulomatous lesions.
- **Histopathological Analysis:** Biopsy of affected tissues shows granulomatous lesions and ceramide accumulation in the cytoplasm of cells.
- **Genetic Testing:** Confirm autosomal recessive inheritance by identifying mutations in the ASAH1 gene.

Results and Interpretation

- **Clinical Findings:** Nodular plaques in the skin, swollen joints, and systemic signs such as cardiac and renal failure support the diagnosis.
- **Laboratory Results:** Reduced or absent acid ceramidase activity confirms

the lysosomal enzyme deficiency.

- **Histopathological Findings:** Granulomatous lesions with ceramide-laden cells provide definitive pathological evidence.

Physiological Basis

- **Lysosomal Dysfunction:** Acid ceramidase deficiency leads to ceramide accumulation, disrupting normal cellular metabolism and causing tissue damage.
- **Granuloma Formation:** The body's immune response to accumulated ceramide results in granulomatous inflammation, further damaging tissues.
- **Systemic Effects:** Ceramide buildup in joints, skin, and organs leads to multi-organ dysfunction, including cardiac and renal failure.

Clinical Applications

- **Early Interventions:** Early recognition allows for supportive care to address symptoms and prevent complications.
- **Symptom Management:** Treat joint swelling and pain with anti-inflammatory therapies.
- **Palliative Care:** Provide support for feeding difficulties, respiratory distress, and systemic failure in advanced cases.

Limitations and Technical Considerations

- **Diagnostic Challenges:** The rarity of the disease and its resemblance to other conditions like juvenile rheumatoid arthritis can delay diagnosis.
- **Therapeutic Limitations:** No definitive cure exists; current treatments are palliative and focus on symptom management.
- **Progressive Nature:** The rapid progression of systemic complications limits the window for effective intervention.

Modern Relevance

- **Advances in Genetic Testing:** Identification of ASAH1 mutations enables precise genetic counseling and prenatal diagnosis.
- **Research into Enzyme Replacement:** Experimental therapies aim to restore acid ceramidase activity, potentially altering disease progression.
- **Improved Supportive Care:** Advances in managing respiratory, cardiac, and nutritional challenges have improved the quality of life for affected infants.

Associated Conditions

- **Juvenile Rheumatoid Arthritis:** Farber's disease can mimic the articular swelling and erythema seen in JRA, necessitating careful differentiation.
- **Other Lysosomal Storage Disorders:** Conditions like Gaucher's disease and Fabry disease share similar metabolic pathways and systemic effects.
- **Autoimmune-Like Conditions:** The granulomatous inflammation may resemble autoimmune processes, leading to misdiagnosis.

Clinical Importance

- **Awareness of Rare Disorders:** Highlighting Farber's disease ensures earlier recognition and differentiation from more common conditions.
- **Insight into Lysosomal Biology:** The disease provides a model for study-

ing the role of lysosomal dysfunction in systemic pathology.

- **Focus on Genetic Research:** Advances in understanding ASAH1 mutations offer hope for targeted therapies and improved outcomes.

References

S. Farber: A lipid metabolism disorder -disseminated "lipogranulomomatosis" - a syndrome with similarity to, and important difference from Niemann-Pick and Hand-Schüller-Christian disease. American Journal of Diseases of Children, Chicago, 1952, 84: 499-500.

S. Farber, J. Cohen, L. L. Uzman: Lipogranulomatosis: A new lipo-glyco-protein "storage" disease. Journal of the Mount Sinai Hospital, New York, 1957, 24: 816-837.

Ferguson Radiographic View

Overview

The Ferguson radiographic view is a specialized imaging technique used to evaluate the sacroiliac (SI) joints and surrounding pelvic structures. The patient is positioned supine, and the X-ray tube is angled 30–35 degrees cephalically, centered on the midportion of the pelvis. This projection allows the symphysis pubis to overlap the sacrum, enhancing the visualization of the sacroiliac joints. It is particularly useful in assessing inflammatory conditions, arthropathies, and pelvic fractures involving the sacrum, pubis, and ischium.

Historical Background

- Named after *Albert B. Ferguson Jr.*, a pioneering figure in orthopedic radiology, this view was developed to provide a more detailed visualization of the sacroiliac joints and adjacent pelvic structures.
- Initially introduced for diagnosing arthropathies like *ankylosing spondylitis*, the projection became widely adopted for its utility in identifying both inflammatory and traumatic conditions of the pelvis.
- Over time, the Ferguson view has been recognized as a critical diagnostic tool in orthopedic and rheumatologic practices.

Purpose

- **Enhanced Visualization:** To provide a clear and focused view of the sacroiliac joints, minimizing obstructions by the symphysis pubis.

- **Diagnostic Accuracy:** To identify structural abnormalities, including arthropathies, inflammatory changes, and fractures of the pelvic girdle.
- **Guide for Management:** To support the evaluation and monitoring of conditions such as ankylosing spondylitis, psoriatic arthritis, and traumatic injuries.

Procedure Overview

- **Patient Positioning:**
- The patient lies supine on the imaging table.
- Proper alignment ensures that the pelvis is neutral, with no rotation.
- **Radiographic Setup:**
- The X-ray tube is angled 30–35 degrees cephalically.
- The beam is centered on the midportion of the pelvis, ensuring the symphysis pubis overlaps the sacrum.
- **Imaging Parameters:** Ensure appropriate exposure settings to visualize the bony structures without overexposure or loss of detail.
- **Interpretation:** Radiographs are analyzed for joint space irregularities, erosions, sclerosis, or fractures involving the sacrum, pubis, and ischium.

Results and Interpretation

- **Normal Findings:** Symmetric sacroiliac joint spaces with smooth bony margins and no evidence of irregularity or sclerosis.

Pathological Findings:

- **Inflammatory Changes:** Erosions, sclerosis, and narrowing of the SI joint spaces may indicate conditions like ankylosing spondylitis or psoriatic arthritis.
- **Fractures:** Disruption of bony continuity in the sacrum, pubis, or ischium, often associated with trauma.
- **Degenerative Changes:** Irregular joint margins and osteophytes suggest osteoarthritis of the SI joint.

Physiological Basis

- **Sacroiliac Joint:** The SI joint transmits axial loads from the spine to the lower extremities, making it a common site for inflammatory and degenerative changes.
- **Pelvic Anatomy:** The overlap of the pubic symphysis with the sacrum in the Ferguson view eliminates visual obstructions, providing a focused image of the SI joints.
- **Diagnostic Utility:** The angled projection enhances visualization of subtle changes, such as early erosions in arthropathies or minor fractures in trauma cases.

Clinical Applications

- **Evaluation of Arthropathies:** Diagnosis and monitoring of conditions such as ankylosing spondylitis, inflammatory bowel disease-associated arthritis, and psoriatic arthritis.
- **Trauma Assessment:** Identification of fractures involving the sacrum, pubis, or ischium, particularly in complex pelvic injuries.

- **Guidance for Treatment:** Radiographic findings assist in surgical planning or initiation of medical therapies, such as anti-inflammatory agents or physiotherapy.

Limitations and Technical Considerations

- **Radiation Exposure:** The cephalic angulation may require higher doses for adequate imaging, necessitating careful optimization of settings.
- **Positioning Challenges:** Incorrect positioning of the patient or tube can obscure critical structures, leading to diagnostic errors.
- **Overlap of Structures:** Despite its benefits, the Ferguson view may still not provide complete clarity in cases of severe deformity or advanced joint fusion.

Modern Relevance

- **Advances in Imaging:** While CT and MRI are now preferred for detailed evaluation of sacroiliac joints, the Ferguson view remains an important initial diagnostic tool.
- **Integration in Rheumatology:** The projection is routinely used in screening for spondyloarthropathies, aiding early diagnosis and management.
- **Trauma Care:** Rapid and accessible, the Ferguson view remains a cornerstone in evaluating pelvic injuries in acute settings.

Associated Conditions

- **Inflammatory Arthropathies:** Conditions such as ankylosing spondylitis, psoriatic arthritis, and reactive arthritis frequently involve the sacroiliac joints.
- **Pelvic Fractures:** Includes fractures of the sacrum, pubis, and ischium, particularly in high-impact trauma.
- **Degenerative Joint Disease:** Osteoarthritis of the SI joints, presenting with joint space narrowing and osteophyte formation.

Clinical Importance

- **Early Detection of Disease:** The Ferguson view is crucial for identifying early inflammatory changes in the sacroiliac joints, facilitating prompt treatment.
- **Trauma Management:** Provides essential information on pelvic fractures, supporting surgical planning or conservative management.
- **Teaching and Training:** Widely used in medical education to demonstrate the anatomy and pathology of the pelvic girdle.

References

Musculoskeletal Radiographic Views and Eponyms; 10.1594/essr2013/P-0158.

Finkelstein's Test

Overview

Finkelstein's test is a clinical diagnostic maneuver used to evaluate stenosing tenosynovitis of the first dorsal compartment of the wrist, commonly known as de Quervain's tenosynovitis. The test involves stretching the inflamed tendons of the abductor pollicis longus (APL) and extensor pollicis brevis (EPB), with pain over the radial styloid being a hallmark finding. Proper technique is crucial to avoid false-positive results.

Historical Background

- Named after *Harry Finkelstein*, who described the test as a reliable method to diagnose *de Quervain's tenosynovitis.*
- A similar maneuver was described in *1927 by Eichhoff*, which involves placing the thumb inside the palm before wrist abduction. However, this technique was later deemed less specific, often resulting in *false-positive outcomes*, as highlighted by Elliott in 1992.
- Finkelstein's refinement of the test provided a more accurate and reproducible diagnostic tool.

Purpose

- **Identify Tendon Inflammation:** To confirm inflammation or stenosis in the first extensor compartment, particularly in de Quervain's tenosynovitis.
- **Guide Treatment:** Accurate diagnosis supports decisions regarding conservative or surgical management.
- **Differentiate Wrist Pathologies:** To distinguish de Quervain's tenosynovitis from other causes of wrist and radial-sided pain, such as arthritis or scaphoid injury.

Procedure Overview

- **Patient Positioning:** The patient's hand is relaxed, and the forearm is in a neutral position.
- **Execution:** The examiner grasps the patient's thumb and moves the hand ulnarward (toward the ulna), creating a stretch across the first dorsal compartment.
- Alternatively, the thumb may be placed inside the patient's palm with the fingers wrapped around it, followed by wrist ulnar deviation (Eichhoff maneuver).
- **Observation:** The production of pain or discomfort over the radial styloid indicates a positive result.
- **Comparison:** The unaffected wrist should also be tested for baseline comparison.

Results and Interpretation

- **Positive Test:** Pain localized over the radial styloid suggests inflammation or stenosis of the APL and EPB tendons.
- **False Positives:** The Eichhoff maneuver may elicit pain even in normal wrists, reducing specificity.
- **Differential Diagnosis:** Absence of pain suggests alternate conditions like arthritis, ganglion cysts, or radial nerve irritation.

Physiological Basis

- **First Dorsal Compartment Anatomy:** The APL and EPB tendons pass through the first extensor compartment of the wrist. In de Quervain's tenosynovitis, inflammation narrows this space, leading to pain and restricted movement.

- **Mechanism of Pain:** Ulnar deviation stretches these inflamed tendons and their synovial sheath, reproducing characteristic symptoms.

Clinical Applications

- **Diagnosis of de Quervain's Tenosynovitis:** Helps confirm the clinical suspicion of tendon sheath inflammation in patients presenting with radial-sided wrist pain.
- **Treatment Planning:** A positive test guides the initiation of conservative management, such as splinting, NSAIDs, or corticosteroid injections.
- **Post-Treatment Assessment:** Can be used to evaluate the resolution of inflammation after therapeutic interventions.

Limitations and Technical Considerations

- **False Positives:** The Eichhoff maneuver may elicit pain in normal wrists, leading to diagnostic errors.
- **Subjectivity:** The test relies on the patient's pain response, which can vary in intensity and specificity.
- **Alternative Diagnoses:** Conditions such as arthritis, ganglion cysts, or radial styloid fractures may mimic the symptoms of de Quervain's tenosynovitis.

Modern Relevance

- **Widely Used in Clinical Practice:** Despite Advances in imaging, Finkelstein's test remains a cornerstone for diagnosing de Quervain's tenosynovitis due to its simplicity and low cost.
- **Integration with Imaging:** In cases of ambiguous findings, ultrasound or MRI can complement the test by providing detailed views of tendon inflammation or stenosis.
- **Enhanced Techniques:** Variations of the test, combined with imaging, have improved diagnostic accuracy and specificity.

Associated Conditions

- **Trigger Finger:** Another form of stenosing tenosynovitis, affecting the flexor tendons of the hand.
- **Radial Styloid Arthritis:** Can mimic the pain and tenderness of de Quervain's but lacks tendon involvement.
- **Intersection Syndrome:** Inflammation of the radial wrist extensor tendons proximal to the first dorsal compartment, distinguished by pain further up the forearm.

Clinical Importance

- **Early Detection:** Identifying de Quervain's tenosynovitis early prevents progression to chronic pain and dysfunction.
- **Non-Invasive:** A simple, cost-effective method for diagnosis that can be performed in any clinical setting.
- **Guides Effective Treatment:** Ensures timely intervention, reducing the need for surgical management in most cases.

References

Finkelstein H. Stenosing tendovaginitis at the radial styloid process. J Bone Joint Surg 12:509–540, 1930.

Eichhoff E. Zur Pathogenese der Tenovaginitis Stenosans. Bruns

Beitage Zur Klin Chir 139:746–755, 1927.

Elliott BG. Finkelstein's test: a descriptive error that can produce a false positive. J Hand Surg [Br] 17:481–482, 1992.

Freiberg-Köhler Syndrome

Overview

Freiberg-Köhler syndrome is a rare condition characterized by osteochondrosis of a metatarsal head, most commonly the second, and less frequently the third or fourth. It involves subchondral cancellous bone necrosis, resulting in localized pain, swelling, and restricted movement in adolescents, particularly females aged 10 to 18 years. Radiographic findings include crushing and fragmentation of the metatarsal head, and clinical symptoms may progress if untreated.

Historical Background

- The condition was first described independently by *Albert Henry Freiberg* in the United States in 1914 and *Alban Köhler* in Germany in 1908.
- Freiberg focused on the second metatarsal head, noting its vulnerability to *osteonecrosis* due to repetitive stress and vascular compromise.
- Köhler contributed to the understanding of *subchondral necrosis* in pediatric bone conditions, linking it to mechanical overloading and growth abnormalities.

Purpose

- **Diagnostic Identification:** To confirm the presence of osteonecrosis in a metatarsal head in patients presenting with localized pain and swelling in the foot.
- **Understanding Pathogenesis:** To investigate the underlying causes, such as repetitive trauma or vascular insuffi-

ciency, leading to bone necrosis.

- **Guiding Treatment:** To implement interventions aimed at pain relief, functional restoration, and prevention of deformity.

Procedure Overview

Clinical Presentation:

- **Patients typically present with:** Localized pain and tenderness over the second metatarsal head.
- Swelling, redness, and limitation of joint movement.
- Difficulty in walking or weight-bearing activities.

Radiographic Evaluation:

- **X-rays:** Show fragmentation, flattening, and sclerosis of the metatarsal head.
- **MRI or CT scans:** Provide detailed imaging to assess early changes, including bone marrow edema.
- **Differential Diagnosis:** Exclude other causes of foot pain, such as stress fractures, juvenile rheumatoid arthritis, or infection.

Treatment Plan:

- **Non-Surgical:** Rest, immobilization, and pain management with NSAIDs.
- **Surgical:** Considered in severe cases with deformity, involving metatarsal head realignment or excision.

Results and Interpretation

- **Positive Clinical Diagnosis:** Pain localized to the metatarsal head, coupled with radiological evidence of necrosis and fragmentation, confirms the diagnosis.
- **Prognosis:** Early-stage disease responds well to conservative management, while advanced cases may require surgical intervention to restore function.

Physiological Basis

- **Subchondral Necrosis:** Repetitive trauma or vascular insufficiency leads to compromised blood supply to the metatarsal head, causing osteonecrosis.
- **Mechanical Stress:** Overloading of the second metatarsal head, often due to a long or prominent second toe, exacerbates the condition.
- **Adolescent Vulnerability:** Growth plate activity and rapid skeletal development increase susceptibility in adolescent females.

Clinical Applications

- **Early Diagnosis:** Ensures timely intervention, minimizing progression to joint deformity.
- **Non-Surgical Management:** Immobilization and orthotics provide relief and prevent further stress on the affected joint.
- **Surgical Techniques:** Procedures such as joint realignment or osteotomy correct advanced deformities.

Limitations and Technical Considerations

- **Delayed Diagnosis:** Early symptoms may be mistaken for minor injuries, delaying appropriate treatment.
- **Radiological Challenges:** Subtle changes in early stages may not be apparent on standard X-rays, requiring advanced imaging like MRI.

- **Surgical Risks:** Surgical correction carries risks of joint stiffness or residual pain, necessitating careful patient selection.

Modern Relevance

- **Advanced Imaging Techniques:** MRI has improved early detection, even before significant radiographic changes appear.
- **Evolving Surgical Options:** Minimally invasive techniques and advanced implants enhance outcomes for severe cases.
- **Focus on Preventative Care:** Awareness of foot biomechanics and proper footwear can reduce the risk of repetitive stress injuries in at-risk populations.

Associated Conditions

- **Köhler Disease:** Osteonecrosis of the navicular bone, which shares similar pathophysiology.
- **Stress Fractures:** Must be differentiated from Freiberg-Köhler syndrome due to overlapping symptoms.
- **Adolescent Foot Disorders:** Includes other growth-related conditions like Sever's disease and osteochondritis dissecans.

Clinical Importance

- **Adolescent Health:** Emphasizes the need for attention to musculoskeletal complaints in adolescents to prevent long-term complications.
- **Educational Value:** Serves as a model for understanding the interplay of mechanical stress, vascular supply, and skeletal development.
- **Functional Restoration:** Early and appropriate management can restore normal gait and prevent permanent deformity, significantly improving quality of life.

References

A. H. Freiberg: Infarction of the second metatarsal bone. S. G. O., 1914, 19: 191-193. The so-called infarction of the second metatarsal bone. Journal of Bone and Joint Surgery, Boston, 1926, 8: 257-261.

A. Köhler: Ueber eine häufige, bisher anscheinend unbekannte Erkrankung einzelner kindlicher Knochen. Münchener medizinische Wochenschrift, 1908, 55: 1923-1925.

Eine typische Erkrankung des 2. Metatarsophalangealgelenkes. Münchener medizinische Wochenschrift, 1920, 67: 1289-1290.

English translation in The American Journal of Roentgenology, 1923, 10: 705-710.

Froment's Sign

Overview

Froment's sign is a clinical test used to evaluate ulnar nerve palsy, particularly focusing on the function of the adductor pollicis muscle. It is characterized by hyperflexion of the interphalangeal joint of the thumb during a key pinch motion, such as holding a piece of paper or pinching an object. This hyperflexion compensates for the weakness or paralysis of the adductor pollicis, which is innervated by the ulnar nerve, and reflects compensatory activation of the flexor pollicis longus.

Historical Background

- Named after *Jean-Jules Froment*, a French neurologist, who first described the phenomenon in the early 20th century.
- Froment's observations were pivotal in understanding *ulnar nerve dysfunction*, emphasizing the role of specific hand muscles in diagnostic testing.
- The test has since become a standard clinical tool in the evaluation of *nerve injuries* and *compression syndromes*, particularly involving the *ulnar nerve.*

Purpose

- **Assessment of Ulnar Nerve Function:** To detect dysfunction or paralysis of the adductor pollicis and other ulnar-innervated muscles.
- **Diagnosis of Ulnar Nerve Palsy:** Helps differentiate ulnar nerve involvement from other conditions affecting hand function.
- **Evaluation of Hand Strength:** Assesses compensatory mechanisms and loss of strength in thumb adduction.

Procedure Overview

- **Test Setup:** The patient is asked to hold an object, such as a piece of paper, between the thumb and index finger using a key pinch grip.
- **Observation:** The examiner attempts to pull the paper away while the patient maintains the pinch.
- **Positive Froment's Sign:** If the thumb's interphalangeal joint flexes excessively, it indicates compensatory action of the flexor pollicis longus due to weakness of the adductor pollicis.
- **Additional Features:** Jeanne's sign may accompany Froment's sign, where there is hyperextension of the metacarpophalangeal joint of the thumb, further supporting the diagnosis of ulnar nerve involvement.

Results and Interpretation

- **Positive Froment's Sign:** Indicates ulnar nerve palsy with weakness or paralysis of the adductor pollicis.
- **Compensatory Hyperflexion:** Activation of the flexor pollicis longus compensates for the inability of the adductor pollicis to provide the necessary pinch force.
- **Differentiation:** Helps distinguish ulnar nerve palsy from other neuropathies or injuries affecting hand musculature.

Physiological Basis

- **Ulnar Nerve Function:** The ulnar nerve innervates the adductor pollicis, a muscle critical for thumb adduction.
- **Compensatory Mechanism:** In ulnar nerve dysfunction, the median nerve-innervated flexor pollicis longus compensates, causing hyperflexion of the thumb's interphalangeal joint.
- **Muscle Imbalance:** Loss of adductor pollicis strength disrupts normal pinch mechanics, resulting in observable compensatory behaviors.

Clinical Applications

- **Ulnar Nerve Palsy Diagnosis:** Used to confirm and assess the severity of conditions like cubital tunnel syndrome, ulnar nerve compression, or injury.
- **Monitoring Recovery:** Useful for tracking progress in nerve repair or decompression surgeries.
- **Differentiation of Neuropathies:** Helps distinguish ulnar nerve dysfunction from injuries involving the median nerve or other hand muscles.

Limitations and Technical Considerations

- **False Positives:** Improper technique or overly forceful testing can result in false-positive results.
- **Patient Cooperation:** The test relies on the patient's ability to follow instructions and exert consistent force.
- **Incomplete Assessment:** While indicative of ulnar nerve dysfunction, Froment's sign does not assess the full extent of nerve damage or involve other ulnar-innervated muscles.

Modern Relevance

- **Standard in Neurological Exams:** Froment's sign remains a routine diagnostic tool for hand and nerve specialists.
- **Integration with Imaging:** Combined with nerve conduction studies or MRI, it provides a comprehensive evaluation of ulnar nerve conditions.
- **Surgical Planning:** The test aids in determining the need for surgical intervention in severe cases of nerve compression or injury.

Associated Conditions

- **Ulnar Nerve Compression Syndromes:** Includes cubital tunnel syndrome, Guyon's canal syndrome, and chronic compression injuries.
- **Trauma-Related Neuropathies:** Ulnar nerve injuries from fractures, lacerations, or repetitive stress.
- **Neuromuscular Disorders:** Conditions like ALS or peripheral neuropathies that involve hand muscle weakness.

Clinical Importance

- **Early Detection:** Froment's sign allows for early recognition of ulnar nerve dysfunction, enabling timely intervention.
- **Functional Assessment:** Evaluates thumb and hand strength, providing insight into the extent of muscle and nerve involvement.
- **Educational Utility:** Serves as a classic example in medical education for understanding the interplay between muscle innervation and function.

References

Froment MJ. La paralysie de l'adducteur du ponce et le signe de la prehension. Rev Neurol 28:1236–1240, 1914–15.

Froment MJ. La prehension dan les paralysies du nerf cubital et le signe du ponce. Presse Med 23:409, 1915.

Galeazzi Fracture

Overview

The Galeazzi fracture-dislocation is characterized by a fracture of the distal to middle third of the radius combined with a dislocation or disruption of the distal radioulnar joint (DRUJ). Often termed the "fracture of necessity," this injury typically requires surgical intervention to restore anatomical alignment and joint stability. The condition commonly results from a fall on an outstretched and pronated hand, leading to complex wrist and forearm injuries.

Historical Background

- **1822:** Sir Astley Paston Cooper first described the pattern of a radial fracture with DRUJ disruption and ulnar dislocation, over a century before Galeazzi's detailed report.
- **1912:** William Darrach reported a similar injury, recommending surgical excision of the distal ulna in chronic cases of DRUJ instability, now known as the Darrach procedure.
- **1922–1926:** Surgeons including Homans, Smith, Wilson, Cochrane, and Milch attempted open reductions and triangular fibrocartilage repairs, but with limited success.
- **1934:** Riccardo Galeazzi, an Italian surgeon, published his experience with 18 cases, detailing reduction techniques and immobilization methods that formed the basis of modern treatment.

Purpose

- **Restoration of Forearm Anatomy:** To realign the fractured radius and stabilize the dislocated DRUJ.
- **Functional Recovery:** To preserve pronation and supination of the forearm and prevent chronic joint instability.
- **Guidance for Surgical Repair:** To establish an evidence-based approach for open reduction and internal fixation (ORIF) with DRUJ evaluation.

Procedure Overview

- **Mechanism of Injury:** Typically caused by a fall on an outstretched pronated hand, transmitting axial force through the radius and disrupting the DRUJ.
- **Clinical Presentation:**
- Pain and swelling along the forearm and wrist.
- Visible deformity or shortening of the forearm.
- Restricted or painful supination and pronation.

Radiographic Examination:

- **AP view:** Widening of the DRUJ with possible radial shortening (>5 mm).
- **Lateral view:** Dislocation of the ulna or impaction fractures.
- Additional imaging may include CT scans for detailed joint evaluation.
- **Surgical Approach:** ORIF with plate and screw fixation for the radial fracture.
- **Intraoperative Assessment:** Evaluate DRUJ stability; repair ligaments or reconstruct the triangular fibrocartilage if required.
- **Immobilization:** Place the forearm in a position of pronation with a plaster cast postoperatively.

Results and Interpretation

- **Successful Reduction:** Proper alignment of the radius and stable reduction of the DRUJ are critical for restoring forearm function.
- **Prognostic Indicators:** Early surgical intervention improves outcomes.
- Delayed treatment can lead to nonunion, deformity, or chronic instability.

Physiological Basis

- **Axial Force Transmission:** The injury occurs as axial force transfers through the pronated forearm, leading to radial shaft fracture and DRUJ disruption.
- **Muscle Imbalance:** Forearm muscles, particularly the pronator quadratus, exacerbate DRUJ instability post-injury by pulling on the radius and ulna asymmetrically.
- **Joint Disruption:** The DRUJ, a pivotal joint for forearm rotation, becomes unstable when its ligamentous support is compromised.

Clinical Applications

- **Early Surgical Intervention:** Prevents complications like malunion, joint stiffness, and chronic pain.
- **Functional Rehabilitation:** Focuses on restoring range of motion and preventing secondary deformities.
- **Teaching and Training:** A textbook example of the importance of recogniz-

ing complex forearm injuries in trauma care.

Limitations and Technical Considerations

- **Diagnosis Challenges:** Subtle DRUJ disruptions may be missed without detailed radiographs or CT imaging.
- **Surgical Complexity:** Requires skilled orthopedic intervention to align fractures and stabilize ligaments.
- **Postoperative Issues:** Risks of stiffness, infection, and hardware complications necessitate careful follow-up.

Modern Relevance

- **Advances in Surgical Techniques:** Improved fixation devices and minimally invasive methods enhance outcomes.
- **Integration with Imaging:** CT and MRI have improved diagnostic accuracy for DRUJ and ligamentous injuries.
- **Focus on Rehabilitation:** Multidisciplinary care, including physiotherapy, ensures optimal recovery.

Associated Conditions

- **Piedmont Fracture:** An alternative term for Galeazzi fracture in some regions.
- **Reverse Monteggia Fracture:** A term highlighting the involvement of the distal radius instead of the proximal ulna.
- **Galeazzi Equivalent:** Radial shaft fractures with ulnar epiphyseal separation in children or distal ulnar fractures in adults.

Clinical Importance

- **Timely Recognition:** Early identification and intervention prevent chronic deformities and functional impairments.
- **Surgical Standard:** Demonstrates the importance of ORIF and ligament repair in managing complex forearm fractures.
- **Teaching Tool:** Widely studied in orthopedic education as a classic example of trauma management requiring multidisciplinary expertise.

References

Cooper A. A treatise on dislocations, and on fractures of the joints. London: Longman; 1824. [pp473–476] [Plate XXVIII Fig 1,2]

Darrach W. Forward dislocation at the inferior radio-ulnar joint with fractures of the lower third of the radius. Ann Surg 1912;56:801–803.

Lau FH, Chung KC. William Darrach, MD: his life and his contribution to hand surgery. J Hand Surg Am. 2006 Sep;31(7):1056-60. [PMID 16945703]

Sheehan SE, Gaviola G, Gordon R, Sacks A, Shi LL, Smith SE. Traumatic shoulder injuries: a force mechanism analysis-glenohumeral dislocation and instability. AJR Am J Roentgenol. 2013;201(2):378–93.

Homans J, Smith J. Fracture of the lower end of the radius associated with fracture or dislocation of the lower end of the ulna. Boston Med Surg J 1922;187:401–406.

Nakamura R, Horii E, Imaeda T, Tsunoda K, Nakao E. Distal radioulnar joint subluxation and dislocation diagnosed by standard roentgenography. Skeletal Radiol. 1995;24(2):91–4.

Giannoulis FS, Sotereanos DG. Galeazzi fractures and dislocations. Hand Clin. 2007;23(2):153–63. v.

Lee P, Hunter TB, Taljanovic M. Musculoskeletal colloquialisms: how did we come up with these names? Radiographics. 2004;24(4):1009–27.

Galeazzi R. Di una particolare sindrome traumatica dello scheletro dell' avambraccio. Atti e memorie della Società lombarda di chirurgia. (Of a particular traumatic syndrome of the forearm's skeleton. Acts and memories of the Lombard society of Surgery). 1934;2:663–666.

Gamekeeper's Thumb

Overview

Gamekeeper's thumb refers to the attenuation or chronic injury of the ulnar collateral ligament (UCL) at the metacarpophalangeal (MCP) joint of the thumb, leading to instability of the ulnar side of the thumb MCP joint. The condition develops due to repeated stress or chronic trauma to the UCL, often associated with occupational or repetitive activities. The term is sometimes used interchangeably with skier's thumb, which describes the acute rupture or avulsion of the UCL.

Historical Background

- **1926:** Milch first described chronic instability of the UCL at the thumb MCP joint.
- **1955:** Campbell further elaborated on the condition, associating it with Scottish gamekeepers, whose method of killing rabbits - by snapping their necks in the web space of their thumb and index finger - caused repetitive UCL injury.
- Over time, the term evolved to encompass both chronic and acute UCL injuries, reflecting the similar biomechanical etiology.

Purpose

- **Diagnosis of UCL Instability:** To identify chronic ligament attenuation or rupture in individuals with thumb instability and reduced grip strength.
- **Guidance for Treatment:** To determine whether conservative management or surgical intervention is necessary based on the degree of instability.
- **Prevent Occupational Injuries:** To highlight the importance of ergonomic techniques in preventing repetitive UCL injuries in high-risk activities.

Procedure Overview

- **Clinical Evaluation:** Patient presents with pain, weakness, and instability of the thumb MCP joint, often with a history of repetitive thumb stress or trauma.
- The thumb may exhibit a weakened pinch grip or be unable to resist valgus stress.
- **Stress Testing:** A valgus stress test is performed by applying lateral force to the thumb MCP joint.
- A positive test (excessive movement) confirms UCL instability.

Imaging:

- **X-rays:** Used to exclude avulsion fractures or bony abnormalities.
- **MRI:** Provides a detailed view of UCL integrity and evaluates for Stener lesions (interposition of the adductor aponeurosis).
- **Differentiation:** Distinguish chronic attenuation (gamekeeper's thumb) from acute rupture (skier's thumb).

Results and Interpretation

- **Positive Valgus Stress Test:** Indicates chronic UCL attenuation if there is excessive valgus angulation (>30 degrees) or laxity.
- **Imaging Findings:** MRI confirms UCL elongation or rupture and rules out associated injuries, such as Stener lesions or fractures.

- **Functional Impact:** Reduced grip strength and compromised thumb stability during precision tasks or gripping.

Physiological Basis

- **Ulnar Collateral Ligament Function:** The UCL stabilizes the MCP joint during pinching and gripping motions.
- **Chronic Stress Mechanism:** Repetitive valgus forces cause gradual elongation and weakening of the ligament, leading to instability.
- **Compensatory Changes:** Adjacent muscles and ligaments may attempt to stabilize the joint, often leading to overuse injuries.

Clinical Applications

Non-Surgical Management:

- **Mild cases with partial UCL attenuation may respond to:** Immobilization (thumb spica splint).
- Physical therapy to strengthen surrounding musculature.

Surgical Repair:

- **Complete UCL rupture or chronic instability with functional deficits typically requires:** Direct ligament repair or reconstruction.
- **Evaluation and correction of associated Stener lesions.**
- **Post-Treatment Rehabilitation:** Restores range of motion and grip strength, preventing future recurrence.

Limitations and Technical Considerations

- **Difficulty in Differentiation:** Distinguishing chronic attenuation from acute rupture can be challenging without imaging.
- **Incomplete Healing:** Chronic UCL injuries may result in persistent instability or pain even after conservative treatment.
- **False Positives:** Incorrect technique during stress testing may mimic UCL laxity.

Modern Relevance

- **Workplace Ergonomics:** Emphasizes the importance of proper hand positioning and tools to reduce repetitive thumb stress in high-risk occupations.
- **Sports Medicine Focus:** Increasing incidence among athletes, especially in sports requiring thumb gripping, such as skiing, rock climbing, or racquet sports.
- **Advances in Imaging:** High-resolution MRI improves detection of subtle UCL injuries and associated complications like Stener lesions.

Associated Conditions

- **Skier's Thumb:** Acute UCL rupture from trauma, often related to falls while holding ski poles.
- **Thumb Osteoarthritis:** Chronic UCL attenuation increases joint instability, predisposing to degenerative changes.
- **Stener Lesion:** A complication where the adductor aponeurosis interposes between the UCL and its insertion, preventing healing.

Clinical Importance

- **Functional Restoration:** Early recognition and treatment prevent long-term instability, maintaining thumb function critical for precision tasks.
- **Diagnostic Precision:** Differentiating between acute and chronic UCL injuries guides appropriate management strategies.
- **Education in Sports and Occupational Health:** Raises awareness of repetitive stress injuries, promoting preventive measures in high-risk populations.

References

Campbell CS. Gamekeeper's thumb. J Bone Joint Surg Br 71:148–149, 1955.

Milch H. Recurrent dislocation of the thumb: capsulorrhaphy. Am J Surg 6:237–239, 1929.

Garth View

Overview

The Garth view is a specialized radiographic projection designed to evaluate the glenohumeral joint, focusing on detecting dislocations, subluxations, and associated fractures or calcifications at the glenoid rim. This projection uses a unique X-ray angulation to provide a clear view of the antero-inferior and postero-superior glenoid rims, which are often obscured in standard views.

Historical Background

- Named after *William P. Garth*, who developed this projection as part of advancements in imaging techniques for evaluating *shoulder instability* and associated injuries.
- It was introduced to overcome the limitations of conventional views in detecting subtle injuries to the *glenoid* and *glenohumeral joint*, particularly in patients with recurrent dislocations or chronic instability.
- The Garth view became widely adopted for its ability to visualize both bony and soft tissue abnormalities with high accuracy.

Purpose

- **Diagnosis of Glenohumeral Instability:** To identify the direction and extent of shoulder dislocations or subluxations.
- **Detection of Glenoid Rim Injuries:** To assess for fractures, erosions, or calcifications at the glenoid rim.
- **Preoperative Evaluation:** To aid in

surgical planning for cases of recurrent dislocations or glenoid reconstruction.

Procedure Overview

- **Patient Positioning:**
- The patient is placed either seated or supine, with the arm in a neutral position or supported in a sling if injured.
- Proper alignment is critical to ensure diagnostic accuracy.
- **Cassette Placement:** The X-ray cassette is positioned posteriorly, parallel to the spine of the scapula.
- **Beam Angulation:** The X-ray beam is directed: 45 degrees caudally to the glenoid.
- 45 degrees to the plane of the thorax, ensuring optimal visualization of the joint.
- **Image Capture:** A high-quality radiograph is obtained, highlighting the glenoid rim, humeral head, and surrounding structures.
- **Interpretation:** Radiologists evaluate the alignment of the humeral head with the glenoid and any evidence of fractures, subluxations, or calcifications.

Results and Interpretation

Normal Findings:

- The humeral head aligns symmetrically with the glenoid cavity, and the glenoid rims appear intact.

Abnormal Findings:

- **Dislocations or Subluxations:** Antero-inferior or postero-superior displacement of the humeral head relative to the glenoid cavity.
- **Glenoid Rim Fractures:** Clear visualization of bony fragments or irregularities along the glenoid margins.
- **Calcifications:** Deposits near the glenoid rim indicative of chronic instability or inflammation.

Physiological Basis

- **Glenohumeral Joint Mechanics:** The shoulder joint relies on the alignment of the humeral head and glenoid cavity for stability and range of motion.
- **Injury Mechanisms:** Acute trauma or repetitive stress can lead to dislocations, subluxations, or rim fractures, compromising joint integrity.
- **Projection Utility:** The angled X-ray beam enhances visualization of critical anatomical features that are otherwise difficult to assess in standard projections.

Clinical Applications

- **Trauma Imaging:** Commonly used in acute settings to evaluate shoulder dislocations or fractures following trauma.
- **Chronic Shoulder Instability:** Helps in diagnosing recurrent dislocations and evaluating glenoid defects in patients with chronic instability.
- **Pre-Surgical Assessment:** Provides crucial information for planning surgical interventions like Bankart repair or glenoid bone grafting.

Limitations and Technical Considerations

- **Positioning Challenges:** Accurate alignment of the cassette and X-ray beam is essential; improper positioning can lead to diagnostic errors.

- **Patient Cooperation:** Pain or discomfort from acute injuries may limit the patient's ability to remain still during imaging.
- **Radiation Exposure:** While minimal, the angled beam may require careful adjustment to minimize unnecessary exposure.

Modern Relevance

- **Advancements in Imaging:** While CT and MRI are now widely used for detailed joint assessments, the Garth view remains an essential initial diagnostic tool.
- **Continued Clinical Utility:** It is a cost-effective and accessible method for evaluating glenohumeral instability in trauma and sports medicine.
- **Integration with Other Techniques:** Often used in combination with standard views to provide a comprehensive evaluation of the shoulder.

Associated Conditions

- **Anterior Shoulder Dislocation:** Frequently associated with Bankart lesions or Hill-Sachs defects.
- **Posterior Shoulder Subluxation:** Less common but detectable with the Garth view.
- **Glenoid Fractures:** Particularly fractures involving the antero-inferior and postero-superior rims.

Clinical Importance

- **Timely Diagnosis:** Ensures early detection of subtle glenoid and humeral head injuries, preventing chronic instability.
- **Enhanced Surgical Planning:** Provides critical anatomical details for reconstructive surgeries.
- **Educational Significance:** Demonstrates the importance of tailored radiographic techniques in evaluating complex joint injuries.

References

K.L. Bontrager, JP Lanpiglano. Tratado de posicionamento radiográfico e anatomia associada, 6th edition, Mosby, Elsevier, 2011: 195.

5. D J K Lee , J S Yeap,Fasir M, et al. Audit on Radiographs in Anterior Shoulder Dislocations. Med J Malaysia2005;60(1):15-20.

Glisson's disease

Overview

Glisson's disease, commonly recognized today as rickets, is a metabolic disorder of infancy and childhood caused by vitamin D deficiency. It results in inadequate calcium and phosphate deposition in developing cartilage and bone, leading to soft and deformed bones. Characteristic features include bending of the legs, pigeon chest, skull deformities, and spinal abnormalities, accompanied by systemic manifestations such as weakness, growth retardation, and joint swelling.

Historical Background

- Named after *Francis Glisson*, a 17th-century English physician, who provided the first comprehensive description of the condition in *1650* in his work "De Rachitide."
- Glisson's observations were pivotal in identifying the role of *nutrition* and *environment* in bone health, laying the groundwork for later discoveries about vitamin D metabolism.
- His detailed accounts of the clinical and anatomical manifestations of the disease remain a landmark in the history of pediatrics and metabolic disorders.

Purpose

- **Diagnosis of Bone Deformities:** To identify the characteristic skeletal abnormalities associated with vitamin D deficiency.
- **Understanding Growth Impairments:** To investigate the systemic effects of rickets on growth, muscle strength, and development.
- **Prevention and Treatment:** To guide nutritional and therapeutic strategies aimed at correcting vitamin D deficiency and preventing long-term complications.

Procedure Overview

Clinical Presentation:

- **Symptoms include:** Bowed legs or knock knees.
- Pigeon chest (protrusion of the sternum).
- Asymmetry or deformity of the skull, particularly craniotabes (softening of the skull).
- Delayed motor milestones and muscle weakness.
- Restlessness, especially at night, with potential fever.

Radiological Assessment:

- **X-rays of long bones:** Show widened growth plates, cupping and fraying at the metaphysis, and generalized osteopenia.

Laboratory Investigations:

- **Blood tests reveal:** Low serum calcium and phosphate levels.
- **Elevated alkaline phosphatase.**
- **Low 25-hydroxyvitamin D levels.**
- **Secondary hyperparathyroidism.**
- **Differential Diagnosis:** Differentiated from other causes of skeletal deformities, such as osteogenesis imperfecta or metabolic bone diseases.

Results and Interpretation

- **Positive Diagnosis:** Characteristic skeletal deformities combined with biochemical abnormalities confirm rickets.
- **Severity Assessment:** The degree of deformity and biochemical derangements correlates with the duration and extent of vitamin D deficiency.
- **Treatment Response:** Improvement in clinical symptoms and radiological findings following vitamin D and calcium supplementation confirms the diagnosis.

Physiological Basis

- **Vitamin D Deficiency:** Reduces intestinal absorption of calcium and phosphate, leading to hypocalcemia and poor mineralization of bone.
- **Skeletal Impact:** Softened and weakened bones fail to withstand normal mechanical stress, resulting in deformities and fractures.
- **Secondary Hyperparathyroidism:** Hypocalcemia stimulates parathyroid hormone (PTH) secretion, which exacerbates bone resorption and further impairs mineralization.

Clinical Applications

- **Early Detection:** Recognizing clinical signs such as bowed legs or delayed growth ensures timely intervention.
- **Nutritional Management:** Emphasizes the importance of adequate dietary intake of vitamin D, calcium, and phosphate during childhood.
- **Rehabilitation:** Physical therapy and orthotic support may be required for severe skeletal deformities.

Limitations and Technical Considerations

- **Delayed Diagnosis:** Early symptoms like irritability or mild weakness may be overlooked, leading to delayed treatment.
- **Regional Variations:** The condition is more prevalent in regions with limited sunlight exposure or poor nutritional access, complicating population-level prevention.
- **Treatment Challenges:** Severe or prolonged deficiencies may result in permanent deformities despite treatment.

Modern Relevance

- **Global Health Concerns:** Despite advances, rickets remains prevalent in developing countries and among populations with limited sun exposure or dietary deficiencies.
- **Preventive Strategies:** Public health initiatives focus on vitamin D supplementation, fortification of foods, and education about sun exposure.
- **Advances in Treatment:** Early detection through newborn screening programs and improved formulations of vitamin D have enhanced treatment outcomes.

Associated Conditions

- **Nutritional Rickets:** Often linked to inadequate dietary intake or sunlight exposure.
- **Hereditary Rickets:** Includes X-linked hypophosphatemia and vitamin D-dependent rickets caused by genetic mutations.
- **Osteomalacia:** The adult counterpart

of rickets, characterized by defective bone mineralization.

Clinical Importance

- **Pediatric Health:** Highlights the importance of balanced nutrition and sunlight exposure in skeletal development.
- **Public Health Awareness:** Draws attention to the need for global prevention strategies to combat vitamin D deficiency-related diseases.
- **Education and Research:** Glisson's disease serves as a foundation for understanding metabolic bone disorders and the role of micronutrients in health.

References

Daniel Whistler: Disputatio medica inauguralis, de morbo puerili Anglorum, quem patrio idiomate indigenae vocant The Rickets. Lugduni Batavorum, ex. off. W. C. Boxii, 1645.

Whistler's graduation thesis at Leiden. This is the first **Description** of rickets as a definite disease manifesting itself by more or less constant association of symptoms. The book attracted little attention.

Arnold Boate (Bootius, de Boot): Observationes medicae de affectibus omissis. London, T. Whittaker, 1649.

Chapter 12 contains a full first-hand account of rickets. He showed how widespread the disease was at the time. Reprinted in Opuscula Selecta Neerlandicorm, Fasc. 5, pp. 260-273. Amsterdam, 1926.

F. Glissson: De rachitide, sive morbo puerili, qui vulgo The Rickets dicitur, Tractatus opera primo ac potissimum Francisci Glissonii . . . adscitis in operis societatem Georgio Bate et Ahasvero Regemortero. London, 1650.

D. Schütte: Beobachtungen über den Nutzen des Berger Leberthrans (Oleum jecoris Aselli, von Gadus asellus L). Archiv für medizinische Erfahrung im Gebiete der praktischen Medizin, Chirurgie, Geburtshülfe und Staatsarzneikunde, 1824, 2: 79-92.

First report of the value of cod-liver oil in the treatment of rickets.

Glisson's sling

Overview

Glisson's sling is a medical device used in cervical traction to support the head and neck. It consists of a bandage strapped under the chin and the back of the head, extending over the top of the head, and is connected to an extension apparatus. This sling is frequently employed in orthopedic and neurological treatments to provide cervical stabilization, alleviate pain, and facilitate correction of deformities such as scoliosis when combined with other instruments.

Historical Background

- Named after *Francis Glisson*, a prominent 17th-century English physician known for his contributions to medical science and innovation in treatment modalities.
- The use of traction as a therapeutic measure predates modern orthopedics, but Glisson's contributions formalized the use of head-support devices for spinal conditions.
- Glisson's sling became a cornerstone in the *management of cervical spine injuries* and deformities, particularly in an era prior to advanced surgical interventions.

Purpose

- **Cervical Spine Traction:** To relieve pressure on the cervical vertebrae and spinal cord by applying gentle traction.
- **Pain Relief:** To alleviate neck pain caused by conditions like cervical spondylosis, disc herniation, or nerve com-

pression.

- **Postural Support:** To stabilize the head and neck in patients with weak musculature or postural imbalances.
- **Scoliosis Correction:** To assist in the correction of spinal deformities by aligning the cervical spine.

Procedure Overview

- **Application:** The sling is positioned with the chin cup under the jaw and straps extending to the back of the head, ensuring secure and comfortable placement.
- **Connection to Traction Apparatus:** The sling is attached to a pulley system or weights that apply controlled upward traction to the cervical spine.
- **Adjustment of Traction Force:** The tension is adjusted according to the patient's condition, typically under medical supervision to avoid overextension.
- **Duration:** Sessions typically last 20–30 minutes, depending on therapeutic goals and patient tolerance.
- **Monitoring:** Continuous observation of the patient ensures safety and minimizes the risk of complications.

Results and Interpretation

- **Positive Outcomes:** Decreased cervical pain and stiffness.
- **Improved range of motion in the neck.**
- **Enhanced alignment of the cervical vertebrae in cases of mild deformities.**
- **Suboptimal Results:** Persistent symptoms or discomfort may indicate inadequate traction force, improper sling placement, or an underlying severe condition requiring advanced interventions.

Physiological Basis

- **Spinal Decompression:** The upward traction reduces pressure on the intervertebral discs, nerve roots, and facet joints.
- **Muscle Relaxation:** Gentle tension helps relax cervical muscles, reducing spasms and improving posture.
- **Alignment Support:** Provides structural support to maintain or correct alignment of the cervical spine during recovery or therapeutic interventions.

Clinical Applications

- **Cervical Spine Disorders:** Effective in managing conditions like cervical spondylosis, radiculopathy, and whiplash injuries.
- **Post-Surgical Rehabilitation:** Used postoperatively to stabilize the cervical region and promote healing.
- **Scoliosis Management:** Integrated into multi-modal treatment plans for correcting spinal deformities, particularly in children and adolescents.
- **Neurological Disorders:** Occasionally used in conditions like cervical dystonia or muscle spasticity to improve neck posture.

Limitations and Technical Considerations

- **Patient Comfort:** Prolonged use may cause discomfort or pressure sores, particularly in sensitive individuals.

- **Traction Overload:** Excessive traction can lead to complications such as muscle strain, nerve compression, or vascular compromise.
- **Limited Effectiveness:** Severe structural abnormalities may require surgical intervention rather than conservative measures like traction.
- **Contraindications:** Not suitable for patients with severe osteoporosis, instability of the cervical spine, or vascular disorders like carotid artery stenosis.

Modern Relevance

- **Complementary Therapy:** While surgical and advanced non-invasive technologies dominate modern orthopedics, Glisson's sling remains a valuable adjunct for conservative management.
- **Portable and Accessible:** Its simplicity and cost-effectiveness make it a viable option in resource-limited settings or home-based therapy.
- **Advancements in Traction Devices:** Modern cervical traction units have incorporated the principles of Glisson's sling into more ergonomic and adjustable designs.

Associated Conditions

- **Cervical Spondylosis:** Degenerative changes in the cervical spine leading to pain and stiffness.
- **Scoliosis:** Spinal curvature disorders that may involve cervical spine alignment.
- **Whiplash Injuries:** Acute cervical spine trauma requiring stabilization and decompression.
- **Radiculopathy:** Nerve compression syndromes involving the cervical nerve roots.

Clinical Importance

- **Non-Surgical Option:** Provides a conservative approach for managing a range of cervical and spinal disorders, reducing the need for invasive procedures.
- **Ease of Use:** Its straightforward application ensures widespread utility across diverse clinical settings.
- **Teaching Tool:** Demonstrates foundational principles of traction therapy in medical education and physical therapy training.

Gorlin-Cohen Syndrome

Overview

Gorlin-Cohen syndrome is a rare congenital disorder characterized by abnormalities in the teeth, bones, connective tissue, and other systemic manifestations. Patients present with distinctive craniofacial features, orodental anomalies, and skeletal abnormalities, among other systemic complications. The syndrome is evident from birth and affects multiple organ systems, often leading to significant clinical challenges.

Historical Background

- The syndrome was first delineated in *1969* by *Robert J. Gorlin* and *Michael M. Cohen, Jr.*, along with contributions from *J. F. Holt.*
- The condition brought attention to the overlapping features of craniofacial syndromes and their systemic involvement, prompting further research into congenital syndromes involving connective tissues.
- The *unknown etiology* of this condition underscores the ongoing exploration of its genetic and developmental origins.

Purpose

- **Early Diagnosis:** To identify the condition at birth or in early infancy based on its characteristic features.
- **Treatment Planning:** To address orodental abnormalities, skeletal issues, and systemic complications in a coordinated, multidisciplinary approach.
- **Avoidance of Perinatal Complications:** To prevent complications during intubation or surgical procedures due to airway difficulties.

Procedure Overview

Clinical Examination:

- **Key findings include:** Facial asymmetry.
- Pronounced supraorbital ridge and wide nasal bridge.
- Mandibular hypoplasia with a small, pointed chin.
- Thin fingers, clinodactyly, and restricted joint mobility.

Orodental Assessment:

- **Common findings:** Malocclusion, missing permanent teeth, and retained deciduous teeth.
- Bifid uvula.

Systemic Evaluation:

- **Pulmonary and Cardiac Assessments:** Screening for primary pulmonary hypertension and bradycardia.
- **Neurological Testing:** EEG abnormalities to assess for potential neurological involvement.
- **Radiographic Imaging:** Used to identify skeletal abnormalities and assess mandibular hypoplasia.
- **Audiometry:** Evaluation for conductive deafness.

Results and Interpretation

- **Positive Diagnosis:** Based on the constellation of craniofacial, skeletal, dental, and systemic features.
- **Functional Implications:** Associated

defects like restricted mobility, deafness, and muscle wasting significantly impact daily life and require targeted therapies.

Physiological Basis

- **Connective Tissue Dysfunction:** The syndrome primarily affects connective tissues, leading to the characteristic craniofacial deformities, skeletal anomalies, and joint limitations.
- **Neurological and Cardiac Impact:** Abnormalities in systemic connective tissues may lead to pulmonary hypertension, bradycardia, and EEG abnormalities, reflecting broader systemic involvement.
- **Orodental Development:** Impaired formation and eruption of teeth result in malocclusion and retained deciduous teeth, with associated structural defects like the bifid uvula.

Clinical Applications

- **Craniofacial Surgery:** Addressing mandibular hypoplasia and facial asymmetry for functional and aesthetic improvement.
- **Orthodontic Interventions:** Correction of malocclusion and management of retained teeth.
- **Multidisciplinary Care:** Coordinated care across pediatrics, cardiology, orthopedics, and dentistry to manage systemic and local complications.
- **Pulmonary and Cardiac Monitoring:** Regular screening and management of primary pulmonary hypertension and bradycardia.

Limitations and Technical Considerations

- **Airway Management Challenges:** Mandibular hypoplasia and craniofacial abnormalities make intubation during anesthesia challenging, particularly in infants.
- **Delayed Diagnosis:** Overlapping symptoms with other craniofacial syndromes can delay an accurate diagnosis.
- **Progressive Symptoms:** Muscle wasting and joint immobility may progress, necessitating regular monitoring and therapy adjustments.

Modern Relevance

- **Advancements in Genetics:** While the syndrome's etiology remains unclear, Advances in genomic sequencing may help identify causative mutations or pathways.
- **Interdisciplinary Approaches:** Modern treatment integrates advancements in orthodontics, craniofacial surgery, and physical therapy to improve outcomes.
- **Increased Awareness:** Greater understanding of congenital craniofacial and connective tissue disorders ensures earlier detection and improved management.

Associated Conditions

- **Ehlers-Danlos Syndrome:** A connective tissue disorder with overlapping features, such as joint hypermobility and tissue fragility.
- **Pierre Robin Sequence:** Shares features like mandibular hypoplasia and airway challenges.
- **Craniofacial Syndromes:** Syndromes

such as Treacher Collins and Goldenhar Syndrome share similarities but differ in systemic involvement.

Clinical Importance

- **Comprehensive Management:** The syndrome highlights the need for coordinated, multidisciplinary care addressing systemic and craniofacial abnormalities.
- **Risk Mitigation:** Awareness of airway management challenges in these patients reduces the risk of complications during surgical interventions.
- **Educational Value:** Demonstrates the complex interplay of craniofacial, skeletal, and systemic abnormalities, serving as a case study in pediatrics and medical genetics.

References

R. J. Gorlin, M. M. Cohen, Jr: Frontometaphyseal dysplasia: A new syndrome.

American Journal of Diseases of Children, Chicago, 1969, 118: 487-494.

J. F. Holt, et al: Frontometaphyseal dysplasia. Radiologic Clinics of North America, Philadelphia, 1972, 10: 225-243.

R. J. Gorlin, R. B. Winter: Frontometaphyseal dysplasia - evidence for X-linked inheritance. American Journal of Medical Genetics, New York, 1980, 5: 81-84.

Gosselin Fracture

Overview

The Gosselin fracture is a V-shaped fracture of the distal tibia that extends into the tibial plafond, dividing it into anterior and posterior segments. It falls under the broader category of pilon fractures, which are fractures involving the weight-bearing articular surface of the tibia. These fractures commonly result from axial loading forces, often due to high-energy trauma such as falls or motor vehicle accidents.

Historical Background

- **1855:** The fracture was first mentioned by Léon Athanase Gosselin in a note published in *Mémoires de la Société de chirurgie de Paris* and *Gazette des hôpitaux*.
- **1873:** Gosselin provided a comprehensive description of the fracture, accompanied by detailed drawings, which were translated and disseminated widely by 1878.
- Gosselin's work emphasized the need for precise understanding of articular involvement and its implications on weight-bearing and joint stability.

Purpose

- **Accurate Diagnosis:** To classify fractures of the distal tibia and identify articular involvement.
- **Surgical Planning:** To evaluate fracture complexity, degree of comminution, and soft tissue involvement, guiding treatment strategies.
- **Functional Restoration:** To ensure

proper alignment and healing of the tibial plafond, which is critical for maintaining ankle joint function.

Procedure Overview

Initial Assessment:

- **Clinical examination reveals:** Swelling and tenderness around the distal tibia.
- Pain exacerbated by weight-bearing or movement.
- Deformity in severe cases.

Imaging:

- **X-rays:** Initial imaging to confirm the V-shaped fracture pattern and joint involvement.
- **CT scans:** Detailed evaluation of fracture comminution and articular congruity.
- Assists in surgical planning.

Treatment:

- **Non-Surgical:** Stable fractures with minimal displacement may be treated with immobilization in a cast or boot.

Surgical:

- **External Fixation:** Used as a temporary measure for severe fractures with soft tissue swelling.
- **Definitive Fixation:** Internal fixation with plates and screws once soft tissue swelling subsides.

Results and Interpretation

- **Positive Outcomes:** Restored alignment of the tibial plafond.
- **Maintenance of ankle joint function and reduction in post-traumatic arthritis risk.**
- **Complications:** Malunion or nonunion, particularly in highly comminuted fractures.
- Persistent articular incongruity leading to chronic pain and arthritis.

Physiological Basis

- **Axial Loading Mechanism:** High-energy trauma compresses the tibial plafond against the talus, resulting in articular and metaphyseal fractures.
- **Articular Surface Integrity:** The tibial plafond bears significant weight, and its disruption compromises joint mechanics, leading to instability and degenerative changes.
- **Soft Tissue Considerations:** Swelling and damage to the surrounding soft tissues increase the risk of complications like compartment syndrome.

Clinical Applications

- **Trauma Management:** Essential for treating high-energy injuries to the distal tibia and restoring limb functionality.
- **Post-Traumatic Arthritis Prevention:** Surgical reconstruction minimizes the risk of degenerative joint disease.
- **Orthopedic Education:** The Gosselin fracture remains a key example of articular fractures in orthopedic training and research.

Limitations and Technical Considerations

- **Soft Tissue Swelling:** Severe swelling often delays definitive surgical fixation, requiring staged procedures.
- **Articular Congruity Challenges:** Achieving perfect alignment of the tibial

plafond is difficult in comminuted fractures, increasing the risk of post-traumatic arthritis.

- **Complication Risks:** Includes infection, delayed healing, and hardware-related issues in surgically treated cases.

Modern Relevance

- **Advances in Imaging:** CT scans have enhanced the ability to assess fracture complexity and plan precise surgical interventions.
- **Improved Fixation Techniques:** Modern internal fixation methods provide better outcomes compared to historical approaches.
- **Trauma Protocols:** High-energy injuries involving Gosselin fractures are managed using comprehensive trauma care protocols, improving patient outcomes.

Associated Conditions

- **Pilon Fractures:** A broader category encompassing all fractures involving the tibial plafond.
- **Compartment Syndrome:** A common complication due to swelling in high-energy distal tibial fractures.
- **Post-Traumatic Arthritis:** A long-term sequela resulting from residual articular incongruity.

Clinical Importance

- **Functional Impact:** The tibial plafond is integral to ankle joint mechanics; proper treatment is essential to restore mobility and reduce disability.
- **Teaching Value:** The Gosselin fracture illustrates the complexity of managing intra-articular fractures and the importance of multidisciplinary care.
- **Public Health Perspective:** Highlights the need for preventive measures in high-energy trauma scenarios, such as workplace safety and road traffic regulations.

References

Gosselin LA. Les fractures en V du tibia. Bulletins et mémoires de la Société de chirurgie de Paris. 1855 p262

Gosselin LA. Leçon faite à l'hôpital Cochin sur les fractures en V du tibia. Gazette des hôpitaux. 1855. 28; p218

Gosselin LA. Clinique chirurgicale de l'hôpital de la Charité. e. 3, Paris 1879, lesson 37 p603-620. [Clinical Lectures on Surgery: Trans. Stimson LA. 1878.

Goyrand/Smith Fracture

Overview

The Goyrand/Smith fracture, commonly referred to as a Smith fracture or reverse Barton fracture, is a fracture of the distal radius characterized by volar displacement or angulation of the distal fragment. It is the opposite of a Colles fracture, which features dorsal displacement. The injury typically results from a fall on the dorsum of a flexed wrist or a direct blow to the dorsal wrist and requires careful diagnosis and management to avoid long-term complications.

Historical Background

- **1746-1814:** Jean-Gaspard-Blaise Goyrand, a French physician, first described this type of fracture in France.
- **1847:** Irish surgeon Robert William Smith provided a detailed account of the injury, naming it after himself in his publication.
- This fracture is known as the *Goyrand fracture* in French literature and remains significant in orthopedic and trauma surgery globally.

Purpose

- To achieve proper realignment and stabilization of the fractured distal radius.
- To prevent long-term complications such as malunion, carpal tunnel syndrome, or post-traumatic arthritis.
- To restore the normal range of motion and function in the wrist and hand.

Procedure Overview

Diagnosis:

- **Clinical Presentation:** Visible deformity of the distal forearm with swelling, bruising, and pain.
- Volar displacement of the distal radius fragment with the prominence of the ulna dorsally.
- **Imaging:**
- **X-rays:** Standard diagnostic tool showing fracture angulation and displacement.
- **CT scans:** Used for complex or intra-articular fractures for better visualization.

Management:

- **Non-Surgical Treatment:** Reserved for minimally displaced fractures.
- **Reduction followed by immobilization in a cast.**
- **Surgical Treatment:** Indicated for unstable, comminuted, or intra-articular fractures.
- **Open Reduction and Internal Fixation (ORIF):** Most commonly involves volar plating for stabilization.
- Other methods include external fixation or percutaneous pinning in select cases.
- **Rehabilitation:** Post-casting or surgery, patients undergo physical therapy to regain wrist mobility and strength.

Results and Interpretation

- Non-surgical treatment is effective for stable fractures with minimal displacement.

- ORIF is the preferred approach for unstable or complex fractures, providing better outcomes in terms of alignment, strength, and wrist functionality.
- Recovery time ranges from 6 weeks for simple fractures to several months for severe injuries requiring surgery.

Physiological Basis

- The distal radius plays a critical role in wrist articulation and load-bearing.
- The volar displacement seen in a Goyrand/Smith fracture disrupts the alignment of the radiocarpal joint, leading to instability and impaired wrist function if left untreated.
- Proper reduction restores biomechanical alignment and joint stability.

Clinical Applications

- Commonly treated in emergency settings following trauma, such as falls or accidents.
- Used as a diagnostic and management framework in orthopedic surgery for distal radius fractures.
- Rehabilitation focuses on restoring wrist function and preventing complications.

Limitations and Technical Considerations

- Diagnosis can be challenging in subtle cases or minimally displaced fractures; CT imaging is often necessary for accurate assessment.
- Non-surgical management may fail if the fracture remains unstable after reduction.
- Surgical complications include hardware irritation, infection, and potential for malunion or delayed union.

Modern Relevance

- **The Goyrand/Smith fracture** remains a significant injury in orthopedic trauma care, particularly with rising cases from falls in the elderly population.
- **Advances in** imaging and surgical techniques, such as volar locking plates, have improved outcomes for complex cases.

Associated Conditions

- **Carpal Tunnel Syndrome:** Median nerve compression due to fracture displacement.
- **Ulnar Styloid Fracture:** Frequently associated with Goyrand/Smith fractures.
- **Post-Traumatic Arthritis:** From untreated or improperly reduced intra-articular fractures.

Clinical Importance

- **Early Detection:** Accurate diagnosis ensures timely management and reduces long-term morbidity.
- **Specialist Involvement:** Orthopedic referral is critical for unstable or complex fractures requiring surgical intervention.
- **Patient Education:** Rehabilitation and compliance with immobilization or physical therapy are essential for optimal recovery.

The Goyrand/Smith fracture underscores the importance of precise diagnosis, appropriate management, and coordinated care to achieve the best functional outcomes. The injury's unique volar displacement makes it a distinct yet challenging fracture in orthopedic trauma.

References

Shah HM, Chung KC. Robert William Smith: his life and his contributions to medicine. J Hand Surg Am. 2008 Jul-Aug;33(6):948-51. [PMC free article] [PubMed]

Matsuura Y, Rokkaku T, Kuniyoshi K, Takahashi K, Suzuki T, Kanazuka A, Akasaka T, Hirosawa N, Iwase M, Yamazaki A, Orita S, Ohtori S. Smith's fracture generally occurs after falling on the palm of the hand. J Orthop Res. 2017 Nov;35(11):2435-2441. [PubMed]

Chung KC, Spilson SV. The frequency and epidemiology of hand and forearm fractures in the United States. J Hand Surg Am. 2001 Sep;26(5):908-15. [PubMed]

ALFFRAM PA, BAUER GC. Epidemiology of fractures of the forearm. A biomechanical investigation of bone strength. J Bone Joint Surg Am. 1962 Jan;44-A:105-14. [PubMed]

Owen RA, Melton LJ, Johnson KA, Ilstrup DM, Riggs BL. Incidence of Colles' fracture in a North American community. Am J Public Health. 1982 Jun;72(6):605-7. [PMC free article] [PubMed]

Vannabouathong C, Hussain N, Guerra-Farfan E, Bhandari M. Interventions for Distal Radius Fractures: A Network Meta-analysis of Randomized Trials. J Am Acad Orthop Surg. 2019 Jul 01;27(13):e596-e605. [PubMed]

Lawson GM, Hajducka C, McQueen MM. Sports fractures of the distal radius--epidemiology and outcome. Injury. 1995 Jan;26(1):33-6. [PubMed]

Singer BR, McLauchlan GJ, Robinson CM, Christie J. Epidemiology of fractures in 15,000 adults: the influence of age and gender. J Bone Joint Surg Br. 1998 Mar;80(2):243-8. [PubMed]

Hung LK, Wu HT, Leung PC, Qin L. Low BMD is a risk factor for low-energy Colles' fractures in women before and after menopause. Clin Orthop Relat Res. 2005 Jun;(435):219-25. [PubMed]

MILLS TJ. Smith's fracture and anterior marginal fracture of radius. Br Med J. 1957 Sep 14;2(5045):603-5.

Bonatz E, Kramer TD, Masear VR. Rupture of the extensor pollicis longus tendon. Am J Orthop (Belle Mead NJ). 1996 Feb;25(2):118-22. [PubMed]

Roth KM, Blazar PE, Earp BE, Han R, Leung A. Incidence of extensor pollicis longus tendon rupture after nondisplaced distal radius fractures. J Hand Surg Am. 2012 May;37(5):942-7. [PubMed]

Li Z, Smith BP, Tuohy C, Smith TL, Andrew Koman L. Complex regional pain syndrome after hand surgery. Hand Clin. 2010 May;26(2):281-9. [PubMed]

Christensen OM, Christiansen TG, Krasheninnikoff M, Hansen FF. Length of immobilisation after fractures of the distal radius. Int Orthop. 1995;19(1):26-9. [PubMed]

Luo P, Lou J, Yang S. Pain Management during Rehabilitation after Distal Radius Fracture Stabilized with Volar Locking Plate: A Prospective Cohort Study. Biomed Res Int. 2018;2018:5786089.

Grashey View

Overview

The Grashey view is a specialized true anteroposterior (AP) radiographic projection of the glenohumeral joint. Unlike the standard AP view, the Grashey view requires rotation of the patient to align the scapular plane parallel to the cassette. This positioning provides a tangential view of the joint, eliminating overlap between the glenoid rim and the humeral head. It is particularly useful for evaluating joint space narrowing, humeral head migration, and pathologies like Bankart lesions or osteoarthritis.

Historical Background

- Named after *Dr. Rudolph Grashey*, a pioneering radiologist known for his advancements in *roentgenology* (early X-ray imaging).
- Grashey's innovations helped refine imaging techniques to improve diagnostic accuracy, particularly for the *shoulder joint.*
- His work also contributed to *editorial leadership* in the field, succeeding *Albers-Schönberg* as editor of *Fortschritte auf dem Gebiete der Röntgenstrahlen* (Progress in the Field of X-Rays).

Purpose

- **Joint Space Evaluation:** To assess the glenohumeral joint space, crucial for diagnosing arthritis or instability.
- **Fracture and Lesion Detection:** To identify fractures of the proximal humerus, glenoid rim, or labrum (e.g., Bankart

lesions).

- **Pathology Diagnosis:** To detect conditions such as osteoporosis, osteoarthritis, and erosion of the glenoid rim.

Procedure Overview

- **Patient Positioning:** The patient stands or sits upright, with their back toward the cassette.
- Rotate the patient posteriorly by 35° to 45° to align the scapular plane parallel to the cassette.
- **Beam Alignment:** The X-ray beam is directed perpendicular to the cassette at the level of the glenohumeral joint.
- **Imaging Details:** This positioning removes overlap between the glenoid rim and the humeral head, offering a clear view of the joint space.
- **Interpretation:**
- **Radiologists assess:** Joint space narrowing (indicative of arthritis).
- Humeral head migration (suggesting instability).
- Integrity of the scapulohumeral articulation.

Results and Interpretation

- **Normal Findings:** Clear visualization of the glenohumeral joint space with no overlap of the glenoid rim and humeral head.
- No fractures or dislocations.

Abnormal Findings:

- **Joint Space Narrowing:** Indicates arthritis or degenerative joint disease.
- **Humeral Head Migration:** Suggestive of instability or rotator cuff pathology.
- **Fractures or Lesions:** Fractures of the glenoid rim, humerus, or evidence of a Bankart lesion.

Physiological Basis

- **Joint Space Visualization:** By aligning the scapular plane parallel to the cassette, the Grashey view provides a perpendicular perspective of the glenohumeral joint, accurately reflecting joint space and alignment.
- **Reduction of Overlap:** The angled positioning eliminates overlap between bony structures, ensuring precise imaging of the articular surfaces.

Clinical Applications

- **Diagnosis of Instability:** Essential for identifying subtle humeral head migration caused by ligamentous injuries or joint laxity.
- **Arthritis Assessment:** Evaluates joint space narrowing, a hallmark of degenerative changes in osteoarthritis or inflammatory arthritis.
- **Fracture Localization:** Detects proximal humerus fractures, glenoid labrum injuries, and other trauma-related changes.
- **Post-Surgical Evaluation:** Assesses the alignment and stability of the glenohumeral joint following reconstructive surgeries.

Limitations and Technical Considerations

- **Positioning Challenges:** Accurate rotation of the patient to 35°-45° is crucial, and improper alignment may compromise image quality.

- **Soft Tissue Evaluation:** Limited in detecting soft tissue abnormalities like rotator cuff tears; MRI is preferred for such evaluations.
- **Obesity or Severe Deformity:** May obscure bony landmarks, reducing diagnostic accuracy.

Modern Relevance

- **Standard of Care:** The Grashey view remains a cornerstone in shoulder radiology, providing consistent and reliable diagnostic insights.
- **Improved Techniques:** Advances in digital imaging and computerized tomography (CT) complement the Grashey view, particularly in complex cases.
- **Injury Management:** Widely used in evaluating sports injuries and degenerative conditions affecting the shoulder.

Associated Conditions

- **Bankart Lesions:** Tears or fractures of the glenoid rim associated with anterior shoulder dislocations.
- **Osteoarthritis:** Narrowing of the joint space and subchondral sclerosis seen in degenerative joint disease.
- **Proximal Humerus Fractures:** Fractures affecting the humeral head or neck, often following trauma.
- **Shoulder Instability:** Associated with ligamentous injuries or chronic dislocations.

Clinical Importance

- **Diagnostic Accuracy:** Provides a clear and unobstructed view of the glenohumeral joint, critical for early diagnosis and management.
- **Surgical Planning:** Offers detailed insights into the joint architecture, aiding in preoperative planning for reconstructive surgeries.
- **Versatility:** Useful in a wide range of conditions, from traumatic injuries to degenerative diseases, emphasizing its role in comprehensive shoulder care.

References

Pavlov H, Warren RF, Weiss CB Jr, et al. The roentgenographic evaluation of anterior shoulder instability. Clin Orthop Relat Res. 1985; (194):153-8.

Jacobson JA, Lin J, Jamadar DA et al.Aids to Successful Shoulder Arthrography Performed with a Fluoroscopically Guided Anterior Approach.Radiographics 2003; 23(2):373-378.

Grayson's Ligaments

Associated persons: Grayson J.

Overview

Grayson's ligaments are retaining ligaments found in the palmar aspect of the hand, specifically located around the neurovascular bundles. These ligaments extend from the skin to the flexor tendon sheath, providing stability and maintaining the positioning of nerves and blood vessels during finger flexion. They are most prominent around the interphalangeal (IP) joints and play a vital role in preventing bowstringing of the neurovascular bundles during finger movement.

Historical Background

- First described by *Grayson J.* in *1941*, these ligaments were identified as structural components that stabilize the *neurovascular bundles* during finger movements.
- Grayson noted their presence around the *distal interphalangeal (DIP)* and *proximal interphalangeal (PIP)* joints, describing their origin and course.
- Later, *Milford (1968)* conducted comprehensive dissections, refining the understanding of Grayson's ligaments by documenting their *fragile and membranous nature* and clarifying their functional importance and structural variations.

Purpose

- **Structural Stability:** To provide support to the digital neurovascular bundles during flexion and extension of the fingers.
- **Prevention of Bowstringing:** To maintain the anatomical alignment of nerves and vessels, preventing displacement during finger motion.
- **Surgical Navigation:** Grayson's ligaments serve as anatomical landmarks for surgeons during dissections or reconstructive surgeries involving the fingers.

Procedure Overview

Anatomical Dissection:

Grayson's ligaments are observed in pairs, with prominent positioning at the interphalangeal joints:

- **DIP Joint:** A single pair can be reliably demonstrated.
- **PIP Joint:** Two pairs are noted, with proximal and distal portions arising from the flexor sheath.
- **Microscopic Evaluation:** Detailed dissections show the ligaments to be fragile and membranous, strongest over the middle third of the phalanx and near the interphalangeal joint in the thumb.
- **Surgical Implications:** The ligaments form a tubular sheath alongside Cleland's ligaments, housing the neurovascular structures.

Results and Interpretation

- **Structural Role:** Provides a stable environment for digital vessels and nerves, crucial for normal finger function.
- **Clinical Observations:** In surgical dissection, Grayson's ligaments ensure the consistent positioning of neurovascular bundles, aiding in safe and precise operations.

Physiological Basis

- **Neurovascular Bundle Stability:** The ligaments prevent lateral displacement and bowstringing of the neurovascular bundles during finger flexion, ensuring uninterrupted function of nerves and blood flow.
- **Flexor Tendon Interaction:** By connecting the skin to the flexor sheath, they integrate the movements of superficial and deep anatomical structures, promoting coordinated finger movements.

Clinical Applications

- **Hand Surgery:** Serves as a key landmark in procedures like digital nerve repair, vascular grafting, and treatment of flexor tendon injuries.
- **Trauma Reconstruction:** Plays a role in reconstructive surgeries where the neurovascular bundle alignment must be restored.
- **Prevention of Neurological and Vascular Complications:** Protects against bowstringing and subsequent mechanical or ischemic injuries.

Limitations and Technical Considerations

- **Fragility:** As noted by Milford, Grayson's ligaments are membranous and delicate, which can complicate identification during surgery.
- **Structural Variability:** The ligament's course and strength can vary between individuals, requiring precise anatomical knowledge during dissection.
- **Surgical Challenges:** Preservation of these ligaments during surgery can be technically demanding, particularly in cases of trauma or severe scarring.

Modern Relevance

- **Advances in Hand Surgery:** Grayson's ligaments remain integral to modern reconstructive and microsurgical techniques in hand surgery.
- **Educational Significance:** Their anatomical and functional importance is emphasized in medical education for surgeons specializing in hand and reconstructive surgery.
- **Collaboration with Imaging:** Advanced imaging modalities now aid in visualizing these structures preoperatively, improving surgical outcomes.

Associated Conditions

- **Dupuytren's Contracture:** May involve fibrotic changes affecting both Grayson's and Cleland's ligaments, impacting neurovascular bundle mobility.
- **Flexor Tendon Injuries:** Disruption of these ligaments can lead to mechanical instability of the fingers.
- **Traumatic Hand Injuries:** Injuries disrupting Grayson's ligaments can compromise the positioning of neurovascular bundles, leading to functional impairments.

Clinical Importance

- **Surgical Landmark:** Aids in the identification and preservation of critical neurovascular structures during hand surgery.
- **Functional Integrity:** Plays a key role in maintaining the mechanical stability of the fingers, ensuring smooth and coordinated movements.

- **Protection Against Complications:** Prevents displacement of neurovascular bundles, reducing the risk of mechanical or ischemic injury during movement.

References

Grayson J. The cutaneous ligaments of the digits. J Anat 75:164–165, 1941.

Milford LW. Retaining ligaments of the hand. Philadelphia: WB Saunders, 1968.

Greenstick Fracture

Overview

A greenstick fracture is an incomplete fracture in which the cortex and periosteum are disrupted on only one side of the bone while remaining intact on the other. This type of fracture is most common in children due to the pliable and compliant nature of their developing bones. Greenstick fractures result from bending forces and are often associated with minor trauma, such as a fall onto an outstretched hand (FOOSH).

Historical Background

- First described in detail in the 19th century, the term "greenstick fracture" refers to the resemblance of the break to the way a green twig bends and partially breaks without snapping completely.
- Early orthopedic studies documented this unique fracture type as specific to pediatric bone anatomy due to its inherent flexibility.

Purpose

- To restore alignment and ensure proper healing of the fractured bone.
- To prevent progression to a complete fracture or displacement.
- To maintain the child's normal range of motion and avoid long-term deformity or functional impairment.

Procedure Overview

Diagnosis:

- **Clinical Signs:** Pain, tenderness, and swelling at the fracture site.

- Limited movement of the affected limb.
- **Imaging:**
- **X-ray:** Shows incomplete cortical disruption on one side of the bone.
- May involve additional imaging if complex or associated injuries are suspected.

Management:

- **Non-Surgical:** Simple greenstick fractures without significant angulation are treated with immobilization using a cast or splint.
- **Surgical:** In cases of significant angulation or instability, closed reduction may be performed under sedation or anesthesia before casting.
- **Rehabilitation:**
- Gradual reintroduction of movement and physical activity to restore function.
- Monitoring for any signs of refracture or deformity during follow-up visits.

Results and Interpretation

- Prompt and proper immobilization leads to high rates of successful healing in children.
- Reduction is typically required only in cases of significant angulation, with most children regaining full function within weeks of treatment.
- Complications, though rare, include deformity or refracture if immobilization is inadequate.

Physiological Basis

- Pediatric bones have increased elasticity and a thicker, more active periosteum compared to adults, allowing them to bend rather than break completely under stress.
- The growth plates (physes) present in children's bones contribute to their unique fracture patterns, such as greenstick and torus fractures.
- This flexibility and the remodeling capacity of pediatric bones facilitate quicker and more complete healing.

Clinical Applications

- Commonly seen in pediatric trauma cases, particularly those involving falls, sports injuries, or minor accidents.
- Used as a diagnostic and treatment framework for incomplete fractures in children.
- Orthopedic interventions focus on preventing progression to a complete fracture.

Limitations and Technical Considerations

- Diagnosing subtle greenstick fractures may be challenging with standard X-rays; additional views may be required.
- Ensuring proper alignment during immobilization is critical to avoid deformities.
- Follow-up is necessary to monitor healing and prevent complications, such as refracture.

Modern Relevance

- **Greenstick fractures** remain a common pediatric injury, with increasing relevance due to children's participation in organized sports and outdoor activities.

- **Advances in** imaging and casting techniques have improved diagnosis and outcomes for these injuries.

Associated Conditions

- **Torus Fractures:** Another pediatric-specific fracture pattern involving buckling of the cortex.
- **Growth Plate Injuries:** May occur in association with greenstick fractures and require careful monitoring for growth disturbances.
- **Refracture:** Common if activity restrictions are not followed during the healing period.

Clinical Importance

- **Early Detection:** Accurate diagnosis ensures timely intervention and minimizes long-term complications.
- **Parental Guidance:** Parents must be educated about activity restrictions and the importance of follow-up care.
- **Orthopedic Referral:** Severe or angulated fractures require prompt referral for reduction and stabilization.

Greenstick fractures highlight the unique anatomy of pediatric bones and underscore the importance of tailored approaches to pediatric trauma care. Proper management ensures rapid recovery and minimizes the risk of complications.

References

Chasm RM, Swencki SA. Pediatric orthopedic emergencies. Emerg Med Clin North Am. 2010 Nov;28(4):907-26.

Berteau JP, Gineyts E, Pithioux M, Baron C, Boivin G, Lasaygues P, Chabrand P, Follet H. Ratio between mature and immature enzymatic cross-links correlates with post-yield cortical bone behavior: An insight into greenstick fractures of the child fibula. Bone. 2015 Oct;79:190-5. [PubMed]

Cheng JC, Shen WY. Limb fracture pattern in different pediatric age groups: a study of 3,350 children. J Orthop Trauma. 1993;7(1):15-22. [PubMed]

Naranje SM, Erali RA, Warner WC, Sawyer JR, Kelly DM. Epidemiology of Pediatric Fractures Presenting to Emergency Departments in the United States. J Pediatr Orthop. 2016 Jun;36(4):e45-8. [PubMed]

Mathison DJ, Agrawal D. An update on the epidemiology of pediatric fractures. Pediatr Emerg Care. 2010 Aug;26(8):594-603; quiz 604-6. [PubMed]

Nellans KW, Kowalski E, Chung KC. The epidemiology of distal radius fractures. Hand Clin. 2012 May;28(2):113-25. [PMC free article] [PubMed]

Coban YK, Bekircan K. Greenstick Fracture of the Mandible in a Child. J Craniofac Surg. 2017 Jun;28(4):1116-1117.

Sharma S, Vashistha A, Chugh A, Kumar D, Bihani U, Trehan M, Nigam AG. Pediatric mandibular fractures: a review. Int J Clin Pediatr Dent. 2009 May;2(2):1-5. [PMC free article] [PubMed]

Chandra SR, Zemplenyi KS. Issues in Pediatric Craniofacial Trauma. Facial Plast Surg Clin North Am. 2017 Nov;25(4):581-591. [PubMed]

Noonan KJ, Price CT. Forearm and distal radius fractures in children. J Am Acad Orthop Surg. 1998 May-Jun;6(3):146-56. [PubMed]

Schmuck T, Altermatt S, Büchler P, Klima-Lange D, Krieg A, Lutz N, Muermann J, Slongo T, Sossai R, Hasler C. Greenstick fractures of the middle third of the forearm. A prospective multi-centre study. Eur J Pediatr Surg. 2010 Sep;20(5):316-20. [PubMed]

Growing Skull Fractures

Overview

Growing skull fractures (GSFs) are a rare complication of pediatric skull fractures characterized by progressive widening of a fracture line, often accompanied by brain tissue herniation. They predominantly occur in children under 3 years of age due to the unique anatomical and physiological characteristics of the developing skull. The condition is also known by other names, including leptomeningeal cyst, expanding skull fractures, and craniocerebral erosion.

Historical Background

- **1876:** The first documented case of a growing skull fracture was reported by John Halliday, who described an enlarging cranial defect resulting from a skull fracture in a child.
- Subsequent studies throughout the 20th century elucidated the role of dura mater laceration and brain pulsation in the pathogenesis of this condition, enhancing surgical and diagnostic approaches.

Purpose

- To prevent further neurological deterioration, including seizures and cognitive impairment, by surgically repairing the defect.
- To restore the integrity of the skull and protect the underlying brain tissue.
- To minimize long-term complications such as persistent cranial deformity or intracranial pressure abnormalities.

Procedure Overview

Diagnosis:

- **Clinical Features:** Persistent scalp swelling over the fracture site.
- Progressive widening of the fracture line.
- Neurological symptoms such as seizures or developmental delays.
- **Imaging:**
- **CT scans:** Visualize the fracture and associated bony defects.
- **MRI:** Evaluate the extent of brain herniation and assess the integrity of the dura mater.

Management:

- **Early Intervention:** Surgical repair is recommended to prevent worsening of the defect and associated neurological sequelae.
- **Surgical Techniques:** Craniotomy and repair of the dural tear.
- Cranioplasty using autologous or synthetic materials for bone reconstruction.

Results and Interpretation

- Successful surgical correction typically halts the progression of the fracture and alleviates neurological symptoms.
- Postoperative imaging often demonstrates closure of the fracture and normalization of intracranial structures.
- Long-term follow-up is essential to monitor for potential complications or recurrence.

Physiological Basis

- The pediatric skull is thinner and more flexible than the adult skull, with active sutures and open fontanelles that contribute to its unique fracture patterns.
- Laceration of the dura mater during the initial injury disrupts the normal healing process. The pulsatile force of the growing brain causes herniation of brain tissue through the fracture site, preventing bone repair and leading to progressive enlargement of the defect.

Clinical Applications

- Monitoring diastatic skull fractures in children under 3 years of age to identify early signs of GSF.
- Timely surgical intervention to prevent complications such as neurological deficits, infections, and cranial deformities.

Limitations and Technical Considerations

- **Challenges in Diagnosis:** Early-stage GSF may be difficult to distinguish from simple diastatic fractures.
- **MRI is critical for assessing soft tissue and dural involvement but may not always be immediately available.**
- **Surgical Risks:** Potential for postoperative infection, bleeding, or recurrence of the defect.
- Meticulous dural repair is necessary to prevent leptomeningeal cyst formation.

Modern Relevance

- **Advances in** imaging, particularly MRI, have improved early detection and surgical planning for GSFs.
- The use of synthetic materials for cranioplasty has expanded treatment options, although autologous grafts remain the preferred choice in many cases.

Associated Conditions

- **Linear and Burst Fractures:** Common precursors to GSF in infants and young children.
- **Leptomeningeal Cysts:** Often associated with dural laceration and brain herniation.
- **Seizure Disorders:** Resulting from persistent brain injury near the fracture site.

Clinical Importance

- **Early Diagnosis:** Close follow-up of diastatic skull fractures in young children is crucial to identify signs of GSF.
- **Timely Surgical Intervention:** Repairing the defect and dura mater can prevent severe neurological sequelae and cosmetic deformity.
- **Parental Education:** Parents should be informed about the importance of follow-up visits and signs of complications, such as persistent swelling or developmental delays.

Growing skull fractures emphasize the unique challenges of pediatric head trauma, requiring a multidisciplinary approach for optimal outcomes. Early detection and surgical repair remain the cornerstones of successful management.

References

Djientcheu VD, Rilliet B, Delavelle J, Argyropoulo M, Gudinchet F, de Tribolet N. Leptomeningeal cyst in newborns due to vacuum extraction: Report of two cases. Childs Nerv Syst. 1996;12:399–403. [PubMed] [Google Scholar]

Ersahin Y, Gulmen V, Palali I, Multer S. Growing skull fractures. Neurosurg Rev. 2000;23:139–44. [PubMed]

Haar FL. Complication of linear skull fracture in young children Am J Dis Child. 1975;129:1197–200. [PubMed]

Gruber FH. Posttraumatic leptomeningeal cyst. Am J Radiol. 1969;105:305–7. [PubMed] [Google Scholar]

Guilburd JN, Rakier A. Growing skull fracture: A clinical study in 15 children. Clin Neurol Neurosurg. 1997;99(1):S259.

Gupta SK, Reddy NM, Khosla VK, Mathuriya SN, Shama BS, Pathak A, et al. Growing skull fractures: A clinical study of 41 patients. Acta Neurochir (Wien) 1997;139:928–32. [PubMed] [Google Scholar]

Halliday AL, Chapman PH, Heros RC. Leptomeningeal cyst resulting from adulthood trauma. Neurosurgery. 1990;26:150–3. [PubMed] [Google Scholar]

Howship PJ. London: Longman; 1816. Practical Observations in Surgery and Morbid Anatomy; p. 494. [Google Scholar]

Kyoshima K, Gibo H, Kobayashi S, Sugita K. Cranioplasty with inner table of bone flap. Technical note. J Neurosurg. 1985;62:607–9. [PubMed] [Google Scholar]

Lende R, Erickson TC. Cranial defects developing at fracture sites in children. Trans Am Neurol Assoc. 1959;13:130–1.

Michael GM, John GP, Arnold HM. Pathogenesis and treatment of Growing Skull Fracture. Surg Neurol. 1995;43:367–73. [Google Scholar]

Miranda P, Vila M, Alvarez-Garijo JA, Perez-Nunez A. Birth trauma and development of growing fracture after coronal suture disruption. Childs Nerv Syst. 2007;23:355–8. [PubMed] [Google Scholar]

Numerow LM, Krcek JP, Wallace CJ, Tranmer BI, Auer RN, Fong TC. Growing skull fracture simulating a rounded lytic calvarial lesion. AJNR. 1991;12:783–4. [PMC free article] [PubMed] [Google Scholar]

Palaoglu S, Beskonakli E, Senel K, Taskin Y, Yaleinlar Y. Intraosseus location of posterior fossa posttraumatic leptomeningeal cyst. Neuroradiology. 1990;32:78. [PubMed] [Google Scholar]

Pezzotta S, Silvani V, Gaetani P, Spanu G, Rondini G. Growing skull fractures of childhood. Case report and review of 132 cases. J Neurosurg Sci. 1985;29:129–35. [PubMed] [Google Scholar]

Haglund Deformity, Syndrome and Disease

Overview

Haglund deformity, Haglund syndrome, and Haglund disease refer to conditions involving the posterior calcaneus. While Haglund deformity is characterized by a posterosuperior calcaneal prominence or exostosis, Haglund syndrome describes a constellation of related pathologies, including retrocalcaneal bursitis, superficial bursitis, and insertional Achilles tendinopathy. These conditions are associated with pain and inflammation due to impingement between the deformity and the Achilles tendon.

Historical Background

- *Dr. Patrik Haglund*, a Swedish orthopedic surgeon, differentiated between types of *bursitis* affecting the posterior calcaneal region and reported successful surgical treatments.
- The term *"Haglund disease"* was introduced in *1958* to describe *retrocalcaneal bursitis* related to calcaneal prominence.
- Over time, the terminology evolved, with *Haglund deformity* and *Haglund syndrome* being used to describe structural and syndromic manifestations of posterior heel pain.

Purpose

- **Haglund Deformity:** To describe the anatomical posterosuperior calcaneal prominence, which may predispose individuals to irritation and inflammation of the Achilles tendon and retrocalcaneal bursa.

- **Haglund Syndrome:** To define a broader clinical presentation involving pain, inflammation, and structural abnormalities in the posterior heel.
- **Diagnostic Classification:** To aid in differentiating between isolated bursitis, tendinopathy, and combined syndromes for targeted management.

Procedure Overview

Clinical Evaluation:

- **Examination reveals:** Posterior heel pain.
- Swelling and tenderness near the Achilles tendon insertion.
- Possible visible or palpable calcaneal prominence.

Imaging Studies:

- **X-rays:** Highlight posterosuperior calcaneal prominence.
- **Ultrasound:** Detects retrocalcaneal bursitis and Achilles tendon thickening.
- **MRI:** Assesses soft tissue involvement, including bursa inflammation and tendinopathy.
- **Surgical Options (if conservative treatment fails):**
- Removal of calcaneal exostosis.
- Bursal excision to reduce inflammation and irritation.

Results and Interpretation

- **Positive Diagnosis:** Based on imaging findings of calcaneal exostosis and evidence of bursitis or Achilles tendinopathy.
- **Surgical Success:** Pain relief and functional improvement following surgical correction of the deformity and bursal inflammation.

Physiological Basis

- **Mechanical Impingement:** The calcaneal prominence impinges the retrocalcaneal bursa and Achilles tendon, causing inflammation and pain.
- **Tendinopathy and Inflammation:** Repeated stress leads to microtrauma and chronic insertional Achilles tendinopathy.
- **Bursa Involvement:** The retrocalcaneal bursa and superficial bursa become inflamed due to friction and compression.

Clinical Applications

- **Conservative Treatment:** Rest, ice, anti-inflammatory medications, and heel lifts to reduce stress on the Achilles tendon.
- **Physical Therapy:** Stretching and strengthening exercises for the Achilles tendon and calf muscles.
- **Orthotic Devices:** Shoe modifications to reduce pressure on the posterior heel.
- **Surgical Management:** Reserved for severe cases where conservative treatment fails, addressing the deformity and associated pathologies.

Limitations and Technical Considerations

- **Overlapping Terminology:** Terms such as Haglund deformity, syndrome, and disease may lead to diagnostic confusion.

- **Surgical Risks:** Potential complications include Achilles tendon weakness and infection following surgery.
- **Incomplete Symptom Relief:** Pain may persist if all contributing factors (e.g., improper footwear, biomechanics) are not addressed.

Modern Relevance

- **Terminological Clarity:** Recent literature proposes avoiding the term "Haglund" for posterior calcaneal pathologies due to its nonspecific nature.
- **Improved Imaging:** Advances in MRI and ultrasound enhance the ability to diagnose and differentiate between various conditions affecting the posterior heel.
- **Biomechanical Interventions:** Modern orthotic designs and gait analysis address underlying biomechanical issues contributing to Haglund-related conditions.

Associated Conditions

- **Retrocalcaneal Bursitis:** Inflammation of the bursa between the Achilles tendon and calcaneus.
- **Insertional Achilles Tendinopathy:** Degeneration of the Achilles tendon at its insertion on the calcaneus.
- **Superficial Bursitis:** Inflammation of the superficial bursa overlying the Achilles tendon.

Clinical Importance

- **Early Identification:** Recognizing Haglund deformity early can prevent progression to chronic pain and tendon damage.
- **Multidisciplinary Approach:** Combines orthopedic, physical therapy, and podiatric care for optimal outcomes.
- **Educational Significance:** Highlights the importance of anatomical variations in understanding and managing musculoskeletal conditions.

References

Rössler. Zur Kenntniss der Achillodynie. Deutsch Ztschr f Chir 1895; 52: 274–91.

van Dijk CN, van Sterkenburg MN, Wiegerinck JI, Karlsson J, Maffulli N. Terminology for Achilles tendon related disorders. Knee Surg Sports Traumatol Arthrosc 2011; 19: 835–41.

Haglund P. Beitrag zur Klinik der Achillessehne. Zeitschr Orthop Chir 1928; : 49–58.

Painter CF. The classic: inflammation of the post-calcaneal bursa associated with exostosis. 1898. Clin Orthop Relat Res 2008; 466: 1521–7.

RUTHERFORD RL. Surgical correction of retrocalcaneal bursitis (Haglund's disease). J Am Podiatry Assoc 1958; 48: 538–9.

Hand-Schüller-Christian disease

Overview

Hand-Schüller-Christian disease is a rare disorder characterized by the accumulation of lipids in the body, manifesting as histiocytic granulomas primarily in bones, such as the skull, but also affecting skin and visceral organs. Common features include exophthalmos, diabetes insipidus, and osteolytic skull lesions. The disease most frequently occurs in children under six years of age and occasionally in young adults, with a slight male predominance. It is one of the clinical forms of Langerhans Cell Histiocytosis (LCH).

Historical Background

- **1865:** Sir Thomas Smith first described changes in the skull associated with the disease.
- **1891/1893:** Alfred Hand Jr. documented the condition but misdiagnosed it as tuberculosis.
- **1915:** Arthur Schüller coined the term "Landkartenschädel" (map-like skull) to describe the radiographic appearance of the affected bones.
- **1920:** Henry Asbury Christian refined the clinical understanding of the condition and highlighted the classic triad of symptoms (exophthalmos, diabetes insipidus, and skull lesions).

Purpose

- **Identification of Langerhans Cell Histiocytosis:** To classify and differentiate this form of histiocytosis from other variants like Letterer-Siwe disease.
- **Symptom Management:** To address systemic and skeletal complications such as diabetes insipidus, cranial deformities, and organ involvement.
- **Early Intervention:** To minimize progression and long-term complications.

Procedure Overview

Clinical Evaluation:

- **Symptoms include:** Unilateral or bilateral exophthalmos.
- **Polyuria and polydipsia from diabetes insipidus.**
- **Pain, swelling, and fractures due to osteolytic bone lesions.**
- **Additional Features:** hepatosplenomegaly, lymphadenopathy, and systemic weakness.

Radiographic Studies:

- **Skull X-rays:** Show characteristic map-like osteolytic lesions.
- **MRI/CT scans:** Evaluate soft tissue and CNS involvement.
- **Skeletal Survey:** Detects lesions in long bones, pelvis, ribs, and spine.
- **Biopsy:** Confirms diagnosis through histopathological examination showing Langerhans cells.
- **Laboratory Tests:** Checks for signs of endocrine dysfunction, particularly diabetes insipidus.

Results and Interpretation

- **Radiological Findings:** Characteristic skull lesions resembling a map.
- **Histological Findings:** Granulomatous inflammation with lipid-laden

macrophages and Langerhans cells.

- **Clinical Presentation:** The classic triad (exophthalmos, diabetes insipidus, skull lesions) is diagnostic but not always present.

Physiological Basis

- **Histiocytic Infiltration:** Lipid-laden macrophages accumulate in the bones, causing osteolytic lesions and deformities.
- **Endocrine Dysfunction:** Diabetes insipidus arises due to granulomatous involvement of the pituitary gland or hypothalamus.
- **Organ Involvement:** Granulomas affect the skin, liver, and spleen, leading to systemic symptoms.

Clinical Applications

- **Differential Diagnosis:** Helps distinguish Hand-Schüller-Christian disease from other histiocytosis variants and similar conditions like multiple myeloma or metastatic cancer.
- **Symptom Management:** Treats complications like diabetes insipidus and skeletal pain.
- **Monitoring:** Radiological and clinical follow-ups are essential to assess disease progression and treatment response.

Limitations and Technical Considerations

- **Diagnostic Challenges:** Early stages may lack the classic triad, making diagnosis difficult.
- **Biopsy Complications:** Invasive biopsy procedures carry risks, especially in cranial or deeply seated lesions.
- **Treatment Limitations:** While chemotherapy and corticosteroids can control symptoms, they may not cure the disease.

Modern Relevance

- **Improved Understanding:** Advances in molecular biology have linked the disease to Langerhans Cell Histiocytosis, refining its classification and treatment.
- **Targeted Therapy:** Emerging therapies targeting the MAPK pathway offer promise for more effective management.
- **Radiological Advancements:** High-resolution imaging allows earlier detection and better monitoring of disease progression.

Associated Conditions

- **Langerhans Cell Histiocytosis (LCH):** A group of disorders with similar pathophysiology.
- **Letterer-Siwe Disease:** A more aggressive and systemic variant.
- **Endocrine Disorders:** Diabetes insipidus is a hallmark feature of the condition.

Clinical Importance

- **Early Diagnosis:** Prompt identification of the disease can prevent severe deformities and systemic complications.
- **Interdisciplinary Approach:** Management often involves radiologists, endocrinologists, and oncologists for comprehensive care.
- **Educational Value:** The historical evolution of this condition highlights the importance of integrating clinical, radiological, and pathological findings.

References

T. Smith: Skull-cap showing congenital deficiency of bone.

Transactions of the Pathological Society of London, 1865, 16: 224-225.

A. Hand: Polyuria and tuberculosis.

Proceedings of the Pathological Society of Philadelphia, 1893, 16: 282-284.Archives of Pediatrics, New York, 1893: 10: 673-675. Defects of membranous bones, exophthalmos and polyuria in childhood. Is it dyspituitarism?

American Journal of the Medical Sciences, Thorofare, N.J, 1921; 162: 501.

A. Schüller: Über eigenartige Schädeldefekte im Jugendalter («Landkartenschädel»).

Fortschritte auf dem Gebiete der Röntgenstrahlen, 1915-1916; 23: 12-18. Dysostosis hypophysaria.

British Journal of Radiology, London, 1926; 31: 156-158.

H. Christian: Defects in membranous bones, exophthalmos, and diabetes insipidus; an unusual syndrome of dyspituitarism.

In: Contributions to medical and biological research, dedicated to Sir William Osler. New York, P. B. Hoeber, 1919, 1: 390-401.

Medical Clinics of North America, Philadelphia, PA., 1920; 3: 849-871.

R. S. Rowland: Xanthomatosis and the reticuloendothelial system. Correlation of an unidentified group of cases described as defects in mambraneous bones, exophthalmos and diabetes insipidus (Christian's syndrome).

Archives of Internal Medicine, Chicago, 1928, 42: 611-674.

Rowland collected 14 cases of the Hand-Schüller-Christian syndrome, and made the important generalization that it was due to xanthomatosis.

Hand-Schüller-Christian Disease

Overview

Hand-Schüller-Christian disease is a rare condition categorized under Langerhans Cell Histiocytosis (LCH), characterized by the accumulation of lipids in various tissues. It primarily manifests as histiocytic granulomas in bones (especially the skull), skin, and viscera. The disease can involve hepatosplenomegaly, lymphadenopathy, exophthalmos, and diabetes insipidus. Most commonly affecting children under six years of age, the condition presents a classic triad of exophthalmos, skull defects, and diabetes insipidus.

Historical Background

- **1865:** Sir Thomas Smith first identified the skull changes associated with this condition.
- **1891/1893:** Alfred Hand Jr. described the disease, initially misinterpreting it as tuberculosis.
- **1915:** Arthur Schüller introduced the term "Landkartenschädel" (map-like skull) for the radiographic appearance of the skull lesions.
- **1920:** Henry Asbury Christian refined the clinical picture and emphasized the classic triad of symptoms, naming it Hand-Schüller-Christian disease.

Purpose

- **Diagnostic Classification:** To differentiate Hand-Schüller-Christian disease from other forms of Langerhans Cell Histiocytosis, such as Letterer-Siwe disease.

- **Treatment Guidance:** To direct management strategies addressing systemic and skeletal complications, including hormonal and structural impairments.
- **Early Intervention:** To minimize long-term complications, including cranial deformities, hormonal imbalances, and organ dysfunction.

Procedure Overview

Clinical Evaluation:

- **Key symptoms include:** Unilateral or bilateral exophthalmos.
- Polyuria and polydipsia from diabetes insipidus.
- Pain, swelling, and fractures due to osteolytic bone lesions.
- **Additional Features:** hepatosplenomegaly, lymphadenopathy, and systemic weakness.

Radiological Imaging:

- **Skull X-rays:** Show osteolytic lesions, often described as resembling a map.
- **MRI/CT scans:** Assess soft tissue and CNS involvement.
- **Skeletal Survey:** Detects lesions in long bones, ribs, pelvis, and spine.
- **Laboratory and Histopathology:**
- Langerhans cell identification in biopsy specimens confirms diagnosis.
- Hormonal tests evaluate endocrine function, particularly pituitary involvement.
- **Biopsy:** Confirms histiocytic granulomas and lipid-laden macrophages.

Results and Interpretation

- **Radiographic Features:** Characteristic map-like lesions in membranous bones of the skull.
- **Histological Findings:** Granulomas with lipid-laden macrophages, characteristic of Langerhans cell infiltration.
- **Clinical Triad:** The combination of exophthalmos, diabetes insipidus, and skull defects confirms the diagnosis in many cases.

Physiological Basis

- **Histiocytic Granuloma Formation:** Accumulation of Langerhans cells and lipid-laden macrophages leads to granuloma formation in affected tissues.
- **Endocrine Dysfunction:** Involvement of the hypothalamus-pituitary axis causes diabetes insipidus and other hormonal disruptions.
- **Skeletal Involvement:** Granulomas erode bone, leading to osteolytic lesions, fractures, and cranial deformities.
- **Systemic Manifestations:** Hepatosplenomegaly and lymphadenopathy result from widespread tissue involvement.

Clinical Applications

- **Differential Diagnosis:** Helps distinguish Hand-Schüller-Christian disease from other histiocytosis variants like Letterer-Siwe disease.
- **Management Strategies:** Address endocrine dysfunction (e.g., with desmopressin for diabetes insipidus) and skeletal lesions.
- **Surgical Intervention:** Indicated for complications such as severe bone defor-

mities or inaccessible granulomas.

- **Radiotherapy:** Used in localized lesions affecting critical structures.

Limitations and Technical Considerations

- **Diagnostic Challenges:** The classic triad is not always present, and symptoms may overlap with other histiocytosis forms.
- **Treatment Efficacy:** Response to treatment varies; progression to systemic disease remains a risk.
- **Invasive Biopsies:** While necessary for confirmation, biopsies may be challenging in deeply seated lesions.

Modern Relevance

- **Advances in Imaging:** MRI and CT scans provide earlier detection and better monitoring of disease progression.
- **Improved Treatments:** Modern therapies target specific pathways involved in Langerhans Cell Histiocytosis, such as the MAPK pathway.
- **Genetic Research:** Recent studies investigate potential genetic causes, improving understanding of the disease's etiology.

Associated Conditions

- **Letterer-Siwe Disease:** A more severe, often fatal variant of Langerhans Cell Histiocytosis.
- **Endocrine Disorders:** Diabetes insipidus is a hallmark feature.
- **Systemic Histiocytosis:** Involvement of multiple organs, including liver, spleen, and lymph nodes.

Clinical Importance

- **Early Recognition:** Timely diagnosis can prevent severe complications such as cranial deformities and organ dysfunction.
- **Comprehensive Care:** Requires a multidisciplinary approach, involving endocrinologists, radiologists, and oncologists.
- **Educational Value:** Highlights the importance of integrating clinical, radiological, and pathological findings in rare diseases.

References

T. Smith: Skull-cap showing congenital deficiency of bone. Transactions of the Pathological Society of London, 1865, 16: 224-225.

A. Hand: Polyuria and tuberculosis. Proceedings of the Pathological Society of Philadelphia, 1893, 16: 282-284.

Archives of Pediatrics, New York, 1893: 10: 673-675. Defects of membranous bones, exophthalmos and polyuria in childhood. Is it dyspituitarism?

American Journal of the Medical Sciences, Thorofare, N.J, 1921; 162: 501.

A. Schüller: Über eigenartige Schädeldefekte im Jugendalter («Landkartenschädel»).

Fortschritte auf dem Gebiete der Röntgenstrahlen, 1915-1916; 23: 12-18. Dysostosis hypophysaria. British Journal of Radiology, London, 1926; 31: 156-158.

H. Christian: Defects in membranous bones, exophthalmos, and diabetes insipidus; an unusual syndrome of dyspituitarism.

In: Contributions to medical and biological research, dedicated to Sir William Osler. New York, P. B. Hoeber, 1919, 1: 390-401.

Medical Clinics of North America, Philadelphia, PA., 1920; 3: 849-871.

R. S. Rowland: Xanthomatosis and the reticuloendothelial system. Correlation of an unidentified group of cases described as defects in mambraneous bones, exophthalmos and diabetes insipidus (Christian's syndrome).

Archives of Internal Medicine, Chicago, 1928, 42: 611-674.

Rowland collected 14 cases of the Hand-Schüller-Christian syndrome, and made the important generalization that it was due to xanthomatosis.

Hangman's Fracture

Overview

A hangman's fracture is a traumatic injury involving bilateral fractures of the pars interarticularis of the second cervical vertebra (C2), often accompanied by anterior subluxation of C2 over CThis type of fracture is primarily caused by hyperextension and axial loading forces, commonly observed in motor vehicle accidents, diving injuries, or contact sports. Despite its name, the fracture is rarely associated with judicial hanging.

Historical Background

- **1965:** The term "hangman's fracture" was coined by Schneider et al., inspired by injuries seen during judicial hangings where hyperextension and distraction forces were applied.
- Earlier anatomical studies highlighted the vulnerability of the C2 vertebra due to its structural role and the stresses it endures during neck injuries.

Purpose

- To stabilize the cervical spine and prevent further displacement that could damage the spinal cord.
- To restore anatomical alignment and maintain cervical spine function.
- To minimize long-term complications such as chronic pain, deformity, or neurological impairment.

Procedure Overview

Diagnosis:

- **Clinical Symptoms:** Pain and tenderness in the cervical region.
- Restricted neck movement and, in severe cases, neurological deficits.

Imaging:

- **CT scans:** The gold standard for identifying fractures and displacement.
- **MRI:** Used to evaluate soft tissue injuries, including spinal cord damage and ligamentous disruptions.
- **CT Angiography:** Assesses the integrity of the vertebral arteries.

Management:

- **Non-Surgical:** Most cases, particularly Levine and Edwards Type I fractures, can be managed conservatively using a rigid cervical collar or halo orthosis for 6–12 weeks.
- **Surgical:** Indicated for unstable fractures or those with significant displacement (e.g., Type III fractures). Techniques include posterior C1–C3 fusion or anterior decompression and stabilization.

Results and Interpretation

- Proper diagnosis and timely intervention result in favorable outcomes for most patients.
- Non-surgical management with external orthosis yields excellent results for stable fractures.
- Surgical intervention effectively stabilizes complex fractures, reducing the risk of neurological complications.

Physiological Basis

- The C2 vertebra, also known as the axis, is structurally unique, supporting the skull and allowing significant cervical rotation.

- The pars interarticularis is vulnerable to hyperextension forces due to its proximity to the pedicle and transverse foramen.
- The relative stability of the fracture often prevents severe spinal cord injury due to the spacious spinal canal at this level, as described by Steele's rule of thirds.

Clinical Applications

- **Emergency Care:** Immediate immobilization with a rigid cervical collar in trauma settings.
- **Orthopedic Management:** Application of halo orthosis or surgical fixation for unstable fractures.
- **Rehabilitation:** Physical therapy to restore range of motion and strength post-recovery.

Limitations and Technical Considerations

- **Imaging Challenges:** Plain radiographs may miss subtle fractures; CT is crucial for accurate diagnosis.
- **Surgical Risks:** Surgical interventions may involve risks such as infection, hardware failure, or vascular complications.
- **Patient Compliance:** Long-term use of external orthoses requires patient adherence, particularly in non-surgical cases.

Modern Relevance

- **Advances in** imaging, including 3D CT reconstructions, have improved the diagnosis and classification of hangman's fractures.
- Surgical techniques and instrumentation, such as minimally invasive approaches, have enhanced outcomes in complex cases.

Associated Conditions

- **Vertebral Artery Injury:** Risk of vascular compromise due to proximity of the vertebral artery to the C2 pedicle.
- **Ligamentous Injury:** Frequently associated with high-energy trauma causing ligament disruption.
- **Spinal Cord Compression:** Rare due to the anatomical characteristics of the C2 region but can occur in severe cases.

Clinical Importance

- **Timely Diagnosis:** Early recognition and imaging are critical to preventing catastrophic outcomes, including paralysis or death.
- **Comprehensive Treatment:** Proper classification and tailored management strategies are essential for optimal recovery.
- **Rehabilitation:** Collaboration with physical therapists ensures restoration of function and prevention of long-term complications.

Hangman's fractures underscore the importance of interdisciplinary care and the need for precision in diagnosis and management to ensure favorable patient outcomes.

References

Spence KF, Decker S, Sell KW. Bursting atlantal fracture associated with rupture of the transverse ligament. J Bone Joint Surg Am. 1970 Apr;52(3):543-9. [PubMed]

SCHNEIDER RC, LIVINGSTON KE, CAVE AJ, HAMILTON G. "HANGMAN'S FRACTURE" OF THE CERVICAL SPINE. J Neurosurg. 1965 Feb;22:141-54. [PubMed]

Robinson AL, Olerud C, Robinson Y. Epidemiology of C2 Fractures in the 21st Century: A National Registry Cohort Study of 6,370 Patients from 1997 to 2014. Adv Orthop. 2017;2017:6516893. [PMC free article] [PubMed]

Levine AM, Edwards CC. The management of traumatic spondylolisthesis of the axis. J Bone Joint Surg Am. 1985 Feb;67(2):217-26. [PubMed]

Francis WR, Fielding JW, Hawkins RJ, Pepin J, Hensinger R. Traumatic spondylolisthesis of the axis. J Bone Joint Surg Br. 1981;63-B(3):313-8. [PubMed]

Gupta P, Kumar A, Gamangatti S. Mechanism and patterns of cervical spine fractures-dislocations in vertebral artery injury. J Craniovertebr Junction Spine. 2012 Jan;3(1):11-5. [PMC free article] [PubMed]

Pratt H, Davies E, King L. Traumatic injuries of the c1/c2 complex: computed tomographic imaging appearances. Curr Probl Diagn Radiol. 2008 Jan-Feb;37(1):26-38. [PubMed]

Tuite GF, Papadopoulos SM, Sonntag VK. Caspar plate fixation for the treatment of complex hangman's fractures. Neurosurgery. 1992 May;30(5):761-4; discussion 764-5. [PubMed]

Coric D, Wilson JA, Kelly DL. Treatment of traumatic spondylolisthesis of the axis with nonrigid immobilization: a review of 64 cases. J Neurosurg. 1996 Oct;85(4):550-4. [PubMed]

Sonntag VK, Hadley MN. Nonoperative management of cervical spine injuries. Clin Neurosurg. 1988;34:630-49. [PubMed]

Menger RP, Storey CM, Nixon MK, Haydel J, Nanda A, Sin A. Placement of C1 Pedicle Screws Using Minimal Exposure: Radiographic, Clinical, and Literature Validation. Int J Spine Surg. 2015;9:43. [PMC free article] [PubMed]

Yuan S, Wei B, Tian Y, Yan J, Xu W, Wang L, Liu X. Posterior temporary C1-2 fixation for 3-part fractures of the axis (odontoid dens and Hangman fractures). Medicine (Baltimore). 2018 Nov;97(48):e12957. [PMC free article] [PubMed]

Ryken TC, Hadley MN, Aarabi B, Dhall SS, Gelb DE, Hurlbert RJ, Rozzelle CJ, Theodore N, Walters BC. Management of isolated fractures of the axis in adults. Neurosurgery. 2013 Mar;72 Suppl 2:132-50. [PubMed]

Pehler S, Jones R, Staggers JR, Antonetti J, McGwin G, Theiss SM. Clinical Outcomes of Cervical Facet Fractures Treated Nonoperatively With Hard Collar or Halo Immobilization. Global Spine J. 2019 Feb;9(1):48-54.

Harrison's sulcus

Overview

Harrison's sulcus is a deformity of the ribs, characterized by a depression along the lower edge of the thorax at the site of diaphragmatic insertion. It is most commonly associated with conditions like rickets, severe dyspnea, and diseases causing inspiratory obstruction in infants. The characteristic appearance often results in a pear-shaped chest.

Historical Background

- *Edward Harrison*, a notable 19th-century physician, first described this thoracic deformity in relation to *rickets* and its effect on the growing rib cage.
- Over time, Harrison's name became associated with this specific rib deformity, which highlighted the relationship between *diaphragmatic tension* and *skeletal abnormalities* in infants with chronic respiratory or metabolic conditions.

Purpose

- To serve as a *clinical marker* for underlying systemic conditions such as *rickets, chronic respiratory diseases*, or *laryngeal obstruction.*
- To prompt further *diagnostic evaluation* and *intervention* in infants and children presenting with respiratory or skeletal symptoms.

Procedure Overview

- **Clinical Observation:**
- The deformity is visually identified as a depression along the lower thorax.

- Associated symptoms such as dyspnea, wheezing, or failure to thrive are evaluated.
- **Radiological Assessment:** Chest X-rays or CT scans may be used to confirm the deformity and assess associated skeletal or pulmonary abnormalities.
- **Laboratory Testing:**
- Blood tests for vitamin D, calcium, and phosphate levels to evaluate for rickets.
- Pulmonary function tests if respiratory diseases are suspected.
- **Physical Examination:** Focus on identifying related signs such as rachitic rosary, bowing of the legs, or other skeletal deformities.

Results and Interpretation

- **Positive Diagnosis:** A pronounced depression at the lower thorax with pear-shaped chest appearance.
- **Associated Findings:** Signs of rickets such as widened growth plates, bowing of the legs, and rachitic rosary.
- Pulmonary symptoms such as reduced airflow or chronic wheezing.

Physiological Basis

- **Diaphragmatic Pull:** Increased tension from the diaphragm during inspiration, especially in conditions of chronic inspiratory obstruction, causes a depression in the rib cage.
- **Weakened Rib Structure:** In diseases like rickets, reduced mineralization of bones makes the ribs more susceptible to deformation under diaphragmatic stress.
- **Increased Respiratory Effort:** Chronic respiratory conditions result in muscular tugging at the rib insertion sites, contributing to the sulcus formation.

Clinical Applications

- **Screening for Rickets:** Harrison's sulcus can be an early indicator of vitamin D deficiency or other metabolic bone diseases.
- **Respiratory Evaluation:** A marker for chronic dyspnea, prompting evaluation for conditions such as laryngeal obstruction or asthma.
- **Monitoring Progression:** Useful in assessing response to nutritional supplementation or respiratory therapies in affected children.

Limitations and Technical Considerations

- **Nonspecific Presentation:** Harrison's sulcus can result from a variety of conditions, requiring careful evaluation to identify the underlying cause.
- **Late Diagnosis:** In some cases, the sulcus may not be prominent until the disease has progressed significantly.
- **Physical Examination:** Skilled observation is required to distinguish the sulcus from other chest wall abnormalities.

Modern Relevance

- **Enhanced Diagnostic Tools:** Modern imaging techniques and biochemical testing facilitate early and accurate diagnosis of conditions associated with Harrison's sulcus.
- **Nutritional Awareness:** Increased understanding of vitamin D supplemen-

tation has reduced the prevalence of rickets but not eliminated it, particularly in high-risk populations.

- **Focus on Respiratory Health:** Advances in pediatric respiratory care help manage underlying causes of chronic dyspnea, reducing the incidence of deformities like Harrison's sulcus.

Associated Conditions

- **Rickets:** The most common cause, related to vitamin D deficiency and poor bone mineralization.
- **Chronic Dyspnea:** Conditions like laryngeal stenosis, asthma, and bronchopulmonary dysplasia.
- **Metabolic Bone Diseases:** Disorders affecting calcium and phosphate metabolism.

Clinical Importance

- **Early Indicator:** Harrison's sulcus serves as a visible and physical marker for systemic issues requiring immediate attention.
- **Comprehensive Care:** Highlights the need for an interdisciplinary approach, involving pediatrics, endocrinology, and pulmonology.
- **Preventive Medicine:** The identification of Harrison's sulcus underscores the importance of addressing nutritional deficiencies and respiratory health in early childhood.

References

E. Harrison: Remarks upon the different appearances of the back, breast and ribs in persons affected with spinal diseases.

London Medical and Physical Journal, 1820.

Herrmann-Opitz Syndrome I

Overview

Herrmann-Opitz Syndrome I is a rare genetic disorder characterized by mental retardation, acrocephalosyndactyly (a cranial and digital malformation), and peculiar facial features. These features resemble Saethre-Chotzen syndrome but include pronounced hypertelorism, brachysyndactyly of fingers and toes (with absence of the fourth finger), cryptorchidism, and other skeletal and systemic abnormalities. Movement limitations in the elbows and distinct ear morphology are additional hallmarks of this syndrome.

Historical Background

- **1969:** The syndrome was first described by Jürgen Herrmann and John Marius Opitz in a boy with no family history of the disorder.
- Herrmann and Opitz noted the unique combination of *craniofacial dysmorphisms* and *limb anomalies*, which distinguished it from other acrocephalosyndactyly syndromes.
- The syndrome's features were documented in detail, establishing it as a distinct clinical entity.

Purpose

- **Diagnostic Clarity:** To differentiate Herrmann-Opitz Syndrome I from other craniofacial syndromes, such as Saethre-Chotzen and Apert syndromes.
- **Guidance for Management:** To identify and address the specific develop-

mental, orthopedic, and systemic issues associated with the syndrome.

- **Genetic Counseling:** To provide insights into inheritance patterns and recurrence risks for affected families.

Procedure Overview

Clinical Evaluation:

- **Focus on identifying distinctive craniofacial features, including:** Hypertelorism.
- **Small chin.**
- **Deep dysmorphic ears.**
- **Assessment of limb anomalies, including:** Brachysyndactyly.
- Absence of the fourth finger.
- Cryptorchidism in males.

Radiological Imaging:

- **Cranial X-rays/CT scans:** Highlight acrocephaly and related skull deformities.
- **Skeletal surveys:** Reveal digital and limb malformations.
- **Genetic Testing:** Helps confirm diagnosis and differentiate it from similar syndromes.
- **Developmental Assessment:** Evaluates cognitive and motor delays.
- **Orthopedic Evaluation:** Examines elbow movement limitations and other skeletal deformities.

Results and Interpretation

- **Physical Findings:** Hypertelorism, brachysyndactyly, and cryptorchidism are defining features.
- **Radiological Findings:** Craniofacial anomalies consistent with acrocephaly and digital malformations.
- **Developmental Assessment:** Reveals intellectual disability of varying severity.

Physiological Basis

- **Skeletal Dysplasia:** Underlying genetic mutations affect bone and cartilage development, leading to cranial deformities and limb anomalies.
- **Neurological Involvement:** Mental retardation is associated with developmental abnormalities in brain structure and function.
- **Endocrine and Reproductive Effects:** Cryptorchidism and possible hormonal imbalances are linked to systemic developmental disruptions.

Clinical Applications

- **Early Diagnosis:** Recognizing the syndrome's distinct features aids in early intervention and management.
- **Treatment Planning:** Focuses on addressing developmental delays, orthopedic issues, and reproductive abnormalities.
- **Genetic Counseling:** Provides information for families regarding recurrence risk and potential genetic testing for relatives.

Limitations and Technical Considerations

- **Overlap with Other Syndromes:** Similarities with Saethre-Chotzen and Apert syndromes may complicate diagnosis.
- **Genetic Variability:** The underlying

genetic causes may vary, requiring advanced testing techniques.

- **Management Challenges:** Treating multiple systemic and developmental anomalies requires a multidisciplinary approach.

Modern Relevance

- **Genetic Advances:** The advent of whole-exome sequencing has improved diagnostic accuracy and understanding of the syndrome's genetic basis.
- **Early Intervention:** Enhanced developmental therapies and surgical techniques address functional and cosmetic concerns.
- **Continued Research:** Ongoing studies aim to elucidate the syndrome's pathogenesis and improve management strategies.

Associated Conditions

- **Saethre-Chotzen Syndrome:** A craniofacial dysmorphism with overlapping features but distinct genetic origins.
- **Cryptorchidism:** Common in males with this syndrome, requiring surgical correction.
- **Orthopedic Anomalies:** Limb and joint deformities may lead to lifelong functional limitations.

Clinical Importance

- **Comprehensive Care:** Herrmann-Opitz Syndrome I highlights the need for a multidisciplinary approach involving geneticists, orthopedists, endocrinologists, and developmental specialists.
- **Early Intervention:** Timely diagnosis and treatment improve quality of life and mitigate complications.
- **Educational Significance:** The syndrome's unique combination of features underscores the importance of clinical observation and detailed family histories in rare diseases.

References

J. Herrmann, J. M. Opitz: An unusual form of acrocephalosyndactyly. Birth Defects Original Article Series, New York, 1969, 5 (3): 39-42.

Herrmann-Opitz Syndrome II

Overview

Herrmann-Opitz Syndrome II is a very rare autosomal dominant genetic disorder primarily characterized by abnormalities in the skeleton and joints. Documented in only one family spanning three generations, the syndrome highlights a distinct pattern of inheritance and skeletal dysplasia.

Historical Background

- **1969:** Jürgen Herrmann and John Marius Opitz initially described Herrmann-Opitz Syndrome II in a family with consistent skeletal and joint abnormalities.
- This syndrome was differentiated from *Herrmann-Opitz Syndrome I* due to its unique clinical and genetic features, as well as its inheritance pattern.
- The observations were limited to one family, emphasizing the rarity of this condition.

Purpose

- **Genetic Understanding:** To investigate and characterize a novel genetic syndrome with a distinct autosomal dominant inheritance patter
- **Clinical Recognition:** To identify skeletal and joint abnormalities unique to this syndrome for early diagnosis and targeted interventions.
- **Research Insights:** To provide a foundation for further studies on rare genetic skeletal disorders.

Procedure Overview

- **Family History Assessment:**
- Detailed genealogical investigation to confirm autosomal dominant inheritance.
- Examination of affected members across three generations.
- **Clinical Examination:** Focus on identifying characteristic skeletal and joint abnormalities, including restricted mobility or deformities.
- **Imaging and Diagnostics:**
- Radiological studies to assess bone and joint malformations.
- Comparative imaging within the family to confirm shared phenotypic traits.
- **Genetic Testing:** Confirmation of autosomal dominant inheritance through genetic analysis.

Results and Interpretation

- **Inheritance Pattern:** Clear autosomal dominant transmission with one affected member per generation.
- **Skeletal Findings:** Abnormalities in bone formation, joint structure, and function.
- **Unique Presentation:** Consistent features observed only within the affected family, with no known cases outside this lineage.

Physiological Basis

- **Genetic Mutation:** Likely caused by a dominant mutation affecting bone and cartilage development, though the specific gene remains unidentified.

- **Skeletal Dysplasia:** Abnormal development of skeletal structures leads to deformities and joint dysfunction.
- **Joint Pathophysiology:** Structural abnormalities in joint tissues contribute to limited mobility and potential early degeneration.

Clinical Applications

- **Diagnostic Tools:** Provides a reference for clinicians encountering similar cases of autosomal dominant skeletal syndromes.
- **Family Counseling:** Assists in genetic counseling for families with rare autosomal dominant disorders.
- **Treatment Protocols:** Guides orthopedic and rehabilitation strategies to address joint and skeletal abnormalities.

Limitations and Technical Considerations

- **Limited Observations:** The syndrome's description is based on only one family, which limits the generalizability of findings.
- **Lack of Genetic Confirmation:** Absence of identified genetic mutations makes diagnosis challenging in new cases.
- **Overlap with Other Disorders:** Features may resemble other skeletal syndromes, requiring careful differential diagnosis.

Modern Relevance

- **Advances in Genetics:** Whole-genome sequencing offers potential to identify the causative mutation in this rare disorder.
- **Focus on Rare Syndromes:** Highlights the importance of documenting and studying unique familial conditions.
- **Improved Care:** Enhanced imaging and treatment options improve outcomes for individuals with similar skeletal abnormalities.

Associated Conditions

- **Herrmann-Opitz Syndrome I:** Differentiated by its features of craniofacial dysmorphism and other systemic abnormalities.
- **Other Autosomal Dominant Dysplasias:** Conditions such as Achondroplasia and Marfan Syndrome, which also affect the skeleton and joints.

Clinical Importance

- **Genetic Counseling:** The autosomal dominant inheritance pattern underscores the importance of informing affected families about recurrence risks.
- **Research Significance:** Represents a unique opportunity to study rare genetic skeletal syndromes and their underlying mechanisms.
- **Interdisciplinary Management:** Highlights the need for collaboration between geneticists, orthopedists, and rehabilitation specialists to address the multifaceted challenges of this condition.

References

J. Herrmann, J. M. Opitz: The VSR syndrome. Studies of malformation syndromes of man XXXII. Birth Defects Original Article Series, New York, 1974, X(9): 227-239.

Herrmann-Pallister Syndrome

Overview

Herrmann-Pallister Syndrome is a rare malformation and dysmorphology syndrome characterized by a triad of dwarfism, mental retardation, and skeletal anomalies. Additional symptoms include cranial synostosis, microbrachycephaly, limb abnormalities, and distinctive craniofacial features such as hypertelorism and protruding ears. The syndrome also presents with a variety of congenital musculoskeletal deformities, including aplasia of the radius and ankylosis of the knees.

Historical Background

- The syndrome was described collaboratively by *Jürgen Herrmann, John Marius Opitz, Philip D. Pallister*, and others.
- The initial description was based on *two families*, whose initials led to the earlier term *KBG syndrome*, which was later distinguished as Herrmann-Pallister syndrome.
- The unique combination of features, especially the triad of dwarfism, skeletal anomalies, and cognitive impairment, led to its identification as a distinct clinical entity.

Purpose

- **Clinical Characterization:** To identify and document the unique constellation of features distinguishing Herrmann-Pallister Syndrome from other syndromes with similar presentations.
- **Early Diagnosis:** To guide early recognition of symptoms and provide supportive care.
- **Research on Etiology:** To investigate the genetic and environmental factors contributing to the syndrome's development.

Procedure Overview

Clinical Examination:

- **Detailed physical evaluation to identify key symptoms:**
- **Craniofacial features:** hypertelorism, protruding ears, capillary hemangioma.
- **Limb abnormalities:** short ulna, valgus positioning of the hands, and missing metacarpals.
- Mental retardation and delayed development.

Radiographic Imaging:

- **Skeletal X-rays to detect abnormalities like:** Cranial synostosis.
- Dysplasia of femoral heads and aplasia of the radius.
- Ankylosis of joints, especially the knees.
- **Genetic Testing:** Advanced sequencing techniques to explore underlying mutations or confirm familial inheritance patterns.
- **Developmental Assessment:** Evaluate cognitive and motor skills for individualized therapeutic planning.
- **Orthopedic Evaluation:** Assess hip dislocation, limb deformities, and other skeletal issues for surgical and supportive interventions.

Results and Interpretation

- **Distinct Triad:** The syndrome is confirmed by the hallmark combination of dwarfism, skeletal anomalies, and cognitive impairment.
- **Radiographic Features:** Imaging reveals cranial and skeletal deformities, particularly radius aplasia and hip dysplasia.
- **Clinical Variation:** Although the syndrome presents with consistent core features, the severity of anomalies may vary among individuals.

Physiological Basis

- **Skeletal Dysplasia:** The syndrome involves disrupted bone growth and development, leading to cranial synostosis, aplasia, and limb deformities.
- **Neurological Impact:** Developmental delays and mental retardation stem from underlying neurodevelopmental anomalies.
- **Congenital Abnormalities:** The constellation of features suggests a prenatal origin, likely influenced by both genetic and environmental factors.

Clinical Applications

- **Early Interventions:** Prompt diagnosis allows for tailored therapeutic interventions, such as developmental therapies and orthopedic surgeries.
- **Genetic Counseling:** Families can receive advice on inheritance risks and recurrence probabilities in future generations.
- **Holistic Care:** Multidisciplinary management ensures comprehensive support for the diverse manifestations of the syndrome.

Limitations and Technical Considerations

- **Rare Condition:** Limited cases make it difficult to generalize findings or establish uniform treatment protocols.
- **Overlapping Features:** Similarities with other syndromes, such as Saethre-Chotzen or Apert syndromes, may lead to misdiagnosis.
- **Genetic Uncertainty:** The absence of a confirmed causative mutation complicates definitive diagnosis.

Modern Relevance

- **Improved Diagnostics:** Advances in genetic testing and imaging facilitate earlier and more accurate diagnosis.
- **Therapeutic Advances:** Innovations in orthopedic surgery and developmental interventions enhance quality of life for affected individuals.
- **Continued Research:** Ongoing studies aim to clarify the syndrome's genetic etiology and identify potential therapeutic targets.

Associated Conditions

- **Craniofacial Dysostoses:** Syndromes like Saethre-Chotzen or Apert syndromes share overlapping features.
- **Limb Anomalies:** Conditions such as radial aplasia or valgus deformities are seen in other genetic syndromes.
- **Neurodevelopmental Disorders:** Cognitive impairment aligns with other syndromes involving cranial synostosis.

Clinical Importance

- **Diagnostic Marker:** Herrmann-Pallister Syndrome highlights the importance of recognizing unique combinations of craniofacial and skeletal anomalies.
- **Multidisciplinary Management:** The syndrome underscores the need for collaboration across specialties, including pediatrics, orthopedics, and neurology.
- **Genetic Insights:** Studying the syndrome contributes to a broader understanding of rare genetic disorders and their management.

References

J. Herrmann, P. D. Palliser, J. M. Opitz: Craniosynostosis and craniosynostosis syndrome. Rocky Mountain Medical Journal, 1969, 66: 45-56.

J. Herrmann, P. D. Palliser, W. Tiddy, J. M. Opitz: The KBG syndrome - a syndrome of short stature, characteristic facies, mental retardation, macrodontia and skeletal anomalies. Birth defects Original Article Series, New York, 1975, XI (5): 7-18.

Herrmann's Syndrome

Overview

Herrmann's Syndrome is a rare familial camptodactyly syndrome, characterized by abnormalities in the fingers, wrists, and feet, including dysplasia and synostoses. It is associated with short middle phalanges, craniofacial anomalies, conductive hearing loss, strabismus, and additional systemic defects. The syndrome is inherited in an autosomal dominant manner.

Historical Background

- The syndrome was first described by *Jürgen Herrmann*, who observed a familial pattern of inherited abnormalities involving the *skeletal system* and *craniofacial structures*.
- This condition adds to the collection of syndromes attributed to Herrmann's extensive study of rare congenital disorders.

Purpose

- **Clinical Classification:** To provide a clear framework for recognizing the combination of physical and systemic features unique to this syndrome.
- **Early Diagnosis:** To ensure early identification and appropriate intervention for affected individuals.
- **Familial Understanding:** To establish inheritance patterns and guide genetic counseling for affected families.

Procedure Overview

- **Clinical Examination:**
- Evaluation of limb abnormalities such

as camptodactyly, synostoses, and short middle phalanges.

- Examination of craniofacial features and identification of associated anomalies.
- **Radiographic Imaging:** Imaging studies to confirm dysplasia, fusion of joints, and bone deformities in the hands, feet, and wrists.
- **Audiological Assessment:** Evaluation of conductive hearing loss using audiometry and tympanometry.
- **Ophthalmological Examination:** Assessment for strabismus and other ocular abnormalities.
- **Genetic Testing:** Confirmation of the autosomal dominant inheritance pattern through family pedigree analysis and genetic sequencing.
- **Developmental and Functional Testing:** Assessment of motor and developmental milestones to evaluate systemic involvement.

Results and Interpretation

- **Skeletal Abnormalities:** Dysplasia and synostoses confirmed in hands and feet, particularly involving shortened middle phalanges.
- **Craniofacial Features:** Evidence of craniofacial dysmorphisms, including unique anomalies that assist in diagnosis.
- **Audiological Findings:** Conductive hearing loss attributed to structural abnormalities in the middle ear.
- **Systemic Features:** Additional findings such as strabismus and potential motor impairments due to skeletal deformities.

Physiological Basis

- **Genetic Influence:** The syndrome's autosomal dominant inheritance pattern implicates mutations affecting skeletal development, craniofacial formation, and ear structures.
- **Skeletal Dysplasia:** Dysplastic changes in bone and joint development result in fusion (synostoses) and deformities, particularly in the digits and wrists.
- **Hearing Loss:** Structural defects in the ossicles or other components of the middle ear contribute to conductive hearing loss.
- **Craniofacial Anomalies:** Altered developmental pathways impact the symmetry and formation of facial structures.

Clinical Applications

- **Orthopedic Interventions:** Surgical correction or therapeutic management for camptodactyly, joint deformities, and mobility impairments.
- **Audiological Support:** Hearing aids or surgical interventions for conductive hearing loss.
- **Vision Therapy:** Management of strabismus through corrective lenses or surgical alignment.
- **Genetic Counseling:** Advising families about inheritance risks and recurrence probabilities in future generations.

Limitations and Technical Considerations

- **Rarity of Condition:** Limited documentation and cases make it challenging to standardize diagnostic and therapeutic approaches.

- **Overlap with Other Syndromes:** Similar skeletal and craniofacial features may be seen in other disorders, requiring careful differential diagnosis.
- **Genetic Identification:** The specific genetic mutation responsible remains unidentified, limiting confirmatory diagnostics.

Modern Relevance

- **Advances in Genetics:** Next-generation sequencing offers the potential for identifying causative mutations and improving diagnostic accuracy.
- **Innovative Therapies:** New orthopedic and audiological techniques enhance the quality of life for affected individuals.
- **Awareness of Rare Syndromes:** The syndrome underscores the need for specialized centers focusing on rare congenital disorders.

Associated Conditions

- **Camptodactyly Syndromes:** Disorders involving finger deformities, including overlapping features with Herrmann's syndrome.
- **Craniofacial Syndromes:** Conditions with craniofacial abnormalities, such as Saethre-Chotzen syndrome.
- **Hearing Loss Disorders:** Syndromes presenting with conductive hearing loss due to structural anomalies.

Clinical Importance

- **Comprehensive Management:** Herrmann's syndrome highlights the necessity for a multidisciplinary approach involving orthopedists, audiologists, geneticists, and developmental specialists.
- **Genetic Counseling:** The autosomal dominant inheritance pattern underscores the importance of educating families on reproductive planning.
- **Advancing Research:** The syndrome presents opportunities to explore the genetic basis of rare skeletal and craniofacial disorders, paving the way for targeted treatments.

References

J. Herrmann: Symphalangism and brachydactyly syndrome: Report of the WL symphalangism-brachydactyly syndrome: review of the literature and classification. Birth Defects Original Article Series, New York, 1974, 10 (5): 23-53.

S. A. Hurvitz, et al: The facio-audio-symphalangism syndrome: A report of a case and review of the literature. Clinical Genetics, Copenhagen, 1985, 28: 61-68.

Heuck-Assmann disease

Overview

Heuck-Assmann Disease is a rare condition characterized by the replacement of bone marrow with fibrous tissue, leading to compromised hematopoiesis and skeletal abnormalities. It is associated with progressive marrow fibrosis, which can result in systemic complications such as anemia, thrombocytopenia, and other hematological deficiencies.

Historical Background

- *G. Heuck* and *Herbert Assmann* were the first to describe this condition, identifying its primary feature as *fibrous transformation of bone marrow.*
- Early investigations into the disease sought to understand the underlying etiology, differentiating it from other bone marrow disorders such as aplastic anemia or myelofibrosis.

Purpose

- **Diagnostic Framework:** To establish specific clinical and pathological criteria for recognizing the disease.
- **Therapeutic Insights:** To understand the progression of marrow fibrosis and identify treatment modalities to manage hematological deficiencies.

Procedure Overview

- **Clinical Evaluation:** Symptoms include anemia, fatigue, and systemic signs of bone marrow failure.
- Patients may present with skeletal pain or deformities due to the structural changes in bones.
- **Hematological Assessment:** Complete blood counts reveal pancytopenia or specific cytopenias such as anemia and thrombocytopenia.
- **Bone Marrow Biopsy:** Biopsy confirms the replacement of marrow with fibrous tissue, which is diagnostic of Heuck-Assmann disease.
- **Radiological Imaging:** Imaging may show osteosclerosis, marrow hypoplasia, or structural bone abnormalities indicative of fibrotic transformation.
- **Molecular Testing:** To rule out genetic mutations associated with other marrow disorders, aiding in differential diagnosis.

Results and Interpretation

- **Pathological Findings:** Marrow biopsy reveals dense fibrous tissue replacing hematopoietic elements.
- **Hematological Impact:** Peripheral blood smears show features of anemia, leukopenia, and thrombocytopenia, consistent with marrow failure.
- **Skeletal Changes:** Radiological evidence of osteosclerosis and structural abnormalities, especially in long bones and the axial skeleton.

Physiological Basis

- **Bone Marrow Fibrosis:** The disease involves excessive fibroblast activity and deposition of collagen within the bone marrow, replacing normal hematopoietic cells.
- **Hematopoietic Suppression:** Fibrosis impairs the production of blood cells,

leading to systemic symptoms such as fatigue, susceptibility to infections, and bleeding tendencies.

- **Skeletal Impact:** Replacement of marrow with fibrous tissue may alter bone density and structural integrity, increasing the risk of skeletal complications.

Clinical Applications

- **Management of Anemia:** Transfusions and erythropoiesis-stimulating agents may be employed to manage symptoms of anemia.
- **Bone Marrow Support:** Hematopoietic stem cell transplantation (HSCT) may be considered in severe cases.
- **Monitoring and Supportive Care:** Regular monitoring of hematological parameters and supportive treatment for infection and bleeding risks.

Limitations and Technical Considerations

- **Diagnostic Challenges:** Overlap with other fibrotic marrow disorders, such as myelofibrosis, complicates diagnosis.
- **Limited Treatment Options:** Few targeted therapies are available, with management often focused on symptomatic relief and supportive care.
- **Progressive Nature:** The condition is typically progressive, with variable response to treatment.

Modern Relevance

- **Advances in Diagnostic Tools:** Improved imaging techniques and molecular diagnostics aid in earlier and more accurate detection of Heuck-Assmann disease.
- **Emerging Therapies:** Research into antifibrotic agents and stem cell therapies offers hope for better management.
- **Awareness of Rare Disorders:** Recognition of this rare condition highlights the importance of specialized hematological and orthopedic care.

Associated Conditions

- **Myelofibrosis:** Shares similar features of marrow fibrosis but with distinct molecular markers.
- **Osteosclerosis:** May present alongside or as a complication of Heuck-Assmann disease.
- **Anemia of Chronic Disease:** Fibrotic replacement of marrow often leads to secondary anemia.

Clinical Importance

- **Diagnostic Differentiation:** The disease serves as an important differential diagnosis in patients presenting with pancytopenia and marrow fibrosis.
- **Comprehensive Care:** Emphasizes the need for multidisciplinary management, combining hematological, orthopedic, and supportive care approaches.
- **Advancing Research:** Understanding the fibrotic mechanisms in Heuck-Assmann disease contributes to broader insights into bone marrow pathologies.

References

Heuck puublished two cases in [Virchows] Archiv für pathologische Anatomie und Physiologie und für klinische Medizin in 1879.

Hey's internal derangement

Overview

Hey's Internal Derangement, coined by William Hey, refers to the dislocation or dysfunction of the semilunar cartilages (menisci) of the knee joint. The term broadly encompasses conditions affecting the internal structures of the knee, such as meniscal injuries, ligamentous tears, and other intra-articular pathologies that impair normal joint function.

Historical Background

- The condition was first described by *William Hey*, an English surgeon in the 18th century, who introduced the term "Internal derangement of the knee" to describe injuries affecting the *semilunar cartilages*.
- Hey's work laid the foundation for understanding meniscal injuries and their impact on joint mechanics, influencing subsequent research and clinical management of knee disorders.

Purpose

- **Clinical Identification:** To diagnose and classify intra-articular knee pathologies involving the menisci or related structures.
- **Therapeutic Framework:** To guide surgical and non-surgical management strategies for knee injuries.
- **Preventive Care:** To prevent long-term complications such as osteoarthritis or chronic instability through early intervention.

Procedure Overview

- **Clinical Evaluation:**
- Symptoms include pain, locking, or clicking of the knee, often associated with limited range of motion or instability.
- Physical examinations such as the McMurray test and Apley's test are used to identify meniscal injuries.
- **Radiological Imaging:**
- MRI is the gold standard for detecting meniscal dislocations and internal knee derangements.
- X-rays may rule out bony abnormalities.
- **Arthroscopy:** Diagnostic and therapeutic arthroscopy allows direct visualization and, if necessary, repair of the injured structures.
- **Functional Assessment:** Evaluation of joint stability and mobility using specialized orthopedic tools.

Results and Interpretation

- **Imaging Findings:** MRI often reveals tears, dislocations, or degeneration of the menisci, along with any associated ligamentous injuries.
- **Arthroscopic Observations:** Confirmation of cartilage dislocation or damage, with clear identification of the affected structures.
- **Functional Impact:** Internal derangement typically results in mechanical symptoms such as knee locking, limiting the patient's ability to perform weight-bearing activities.

Physiological Basis

- **Meniscal Role:** The semilunar cartilages (menisci) serve as shock absorbers and stabilize the knee joint. Dislocation disrupts these functions, leading to joint instability and altered load distribution.
- **Pathophysiological Mechanisms:** Trauma or degeneration causes tears or dislocations, triggering inflammation, pain, and mechanical obstruction.
- **Joint Integrity:** Compromised meniscal function may accelerate cartilage wear, predisposing the joint to osteoarthritis.

Clinical Applications

- **Surgical Repair:** Arthroscopic surgery to reposition or repair dislocated menisci.
- **Rehabilitation:** Physical therapy to restore strength, mobility, and joint stability post-injury or surgery.
- **Preventive Measures:** Use of braces or modifications in activity to reduce the risk of re-injury.
- **Diagnostic Use:** Awareness of Hey's internal derangement aids clinicians in early diagnosis of meniscal pathologies.

Limitations and Technical Considerations

- **Diagnosis Challenges:** Subtle injuries or partial dislocations may be difficult to detect on imaging or physical examination.
- **Surgical Risks:** Postoperative complications, including stiffness, infection, or incomplete resolution of symptoms.
- **Progressive Nature:** Delayed treatment increases the risk of cartilage degeneration and chronic joint instability.

Modern Relevance

- **Advances in Arthroscopy:** Arthroscopic techniques have revolutionized the diagnosis and treatment of internal derangements, allowing minimally invasive interventions.
- **MRI Utilization:** High-resolution imaging provides detailed visualization of meniscal injuries, enhancing diagnostic accuracy.
- **Holistic Management:** Modern protocols emphasize a combination of surgical repair, rehabilitation, and long-term joint care to optimize outcomes.

Associated Conditions

- **Meniscal Tears:** A common component of internal derangement, often coexisting with ligament injuries.
- **Anterior Cruciate Ligament (ACL) Injuries:** Frequently associated with meniscal dislocation or dysfunction.
- **Knee Osteoarthritis:** Long-term complication of untreated or recurrent internal derangements.

Clinical Importance

- **Early Recognition:** Timely diagnosis of Hey's internal derangement prevents progression to chronic instability or degenerative joint disease.
- **Surgical Advances:** Arthroscopic repair offers an effective solution, reducing recovery time and preserving joint function.
- **Comprehensive Care:** Multidisciplinary approaches ensure that both the

structural and functional aspects of the knee are addressed.

Hilgenreiner's line

Overview

Hilgenreiner's Line is a radiographic landmark used to diagnose developmental dysplasia of the hip (DDH) in infants and young children. It is part of a system of lines on an X-ray that aids in the evaluation of hip alignment and joint congruence by providing a reference for assessing the position of the femoral head relative to the acetabulum.

Historical Background

- *Heinrich Hilgenreiner*, a German orthopedist, introduced the concept of specific radiographic lines in the early 20th century.
- The method, known in German as "Hilgenreiner's Hilfslinien" or "Hilgenreiner Beckenskiagram," was developed to improve the diagnostic accuracy of congenital hip luxation.
- Hilgenreiner's work remains foundational in pediatric orthopedics and radiology.

Purpose

- **Diagnostic Marker:** To identify developmental dysplasia of the hip (DDH) by assessing the position of the femoral head.
- **Measurement of Angles:** Serves as a baseline for measuring the acetabular index, an angle used to determine the degree of dysplasia.
- **Standardized Reference:** Provides a consistent radiographic reference for evaluating hip alignment during early childhood.

Procedure Overview

- **Patient Positioning:** The child is positioned supine during pelvic X-rays to ensure proper alignment.
- **Drawing Hilgenreiner's Line:** A horizontal line is drawn across the triradiate cartilages, which are the cartilaginous centers at the junction of the ilium, ischium, and pubis in the pelvis.
- **Additional Lines:** Perpendicular lines and other landmarks (e.g., Perkins' line) are often drawn in conjunction to assess the location of the femoral head relative to the acetabulum.
- **Angle Measurement:** The acetabular angle is measured between Hilgenreiner's line and the roof of the acetabulum to evaluate the degree of dysplasia.

Results and Interpretation

- **Normal Hip Development:** The femoral head lies within the acetabulum, and the acetabular angle falls within the normal range (≤30° at birth, reducing to ≤20° by 2 years of age).
- **Hip Dysplasia:** The femoral head is displaced superiorly or laterally, and the acetabular angle is increased, indicating a shallow or poorly developed acetabulum.

Physiological Basis

- **Development of the Hip Joint:** Proper hip joint development relies on the congruence of the femoral head and acetabulum. Displacement disrupts joint mechanics, leading to dysplasia or luxation.
- **Role of Radiographic Lines:** Hilgenreiner's line provides a horizontal reference against which deviations in femoral head alignment can be measured.

Clinical Applications

- **Diagnosis of DDH:** Used in routine screening and diagnostic imaging for infants with suspected hip dysplasia.
- **Monitoring Hip Development:** Provides a baseline for tracking changes in acetabular morphology over time.
- **Guiding Treatment:** Helps orthopedic surgeons assess the success of interventions such as Pavlik harness application or surgical reduction.

Limitations and Technical Considerations

- **Accuracy:** Variability in patient positioning may affect the accuracy of line placement and angle measurement.
- **Age-Related Changes:** Hilgenreiner's line is most useful in infants and young children, as ossification of the hip alters radiographic landmarks over time.
- **Complementary Methods:** Other radiographic markers (e.g., Perkins' line, Shenton's line) are often needed for a comprehensive evaluation.

Modern Relevance

- **Improved Imaging Techniques:** Modern radiographic and ultrasonographic methods enhance the diagnostic utility of Hilgenreiner's line by reducing variability in interpretation.
- **Standardized Screening:** Widely used in pediatric orthopedic practices and neonatal screening programs for

early detection of DDH.

- **Educational Importance:** A critical concept in teaching radiographic evaluation of the pediatric hip.

Associated Conditions

- **Developmental Dysplasia of the Hip (DDH):** Primary condition diagnosed using Hilgenreiner's line.
- **Congenital Hip Luxation:** Involves displacement of the femoral head beyond the acetabular boundary.
- **Neuromuscular Disorders:** Conditions like cerebral palsy may result in secondary hip dysplasia, detectable with this radiographic method.

Clinical Importance

- **Early Detection:** Ensures timely intervention for hip dysplasia, improving long-term outcomes and preventing complications like early-onset arthritis.
- **Guidance for Treatment:** Radiographic findings help tailor non-surgical and surgical treatment approaches.
- **Foundational Reference:** The simplicity and reliability of Hilgenreiner's line make it a cornerstone of pediatric radiology and orthopedic diagnosis.

References

H. Hilgenreiner: 10 Jahre Abduktionsschiene und Frühbehandlung der angeborenen Hüftverrenkung. Zeitschrift für orthopädische Chirurgie einschliesslich Heilgymnastik und Massage, Stuttgart, 1935, 63: 344-383.

Die angeborene Dysplasie der Hüfte. Zeitschrift für orthopädische Chirurgie einschliesslich Heilgymnastik und Massage, Stuttgart, 1935, 63: 344-383.

Hill-Sachs lesion

Overview

Hill-Sachs lesion refers to a cortical depression in the posterolateral head of the humerus, which occurs as a result of impaction against the glenoid rim during anterior shoulder dislocation. This lesion predisposes the shoulder joint to recurrent dislocations and instability, with its size and severity often correlating to the number of dislocations.

Historical Background

- **1832:** Joseph François Malgaigne noted a bony defect in the humeral head after anterior shoulder dislocation.
- **1906 & 1914:** Perthes and Schultze provided additional descriptions of this lesion.
- **1925:** Pilz demonstrated the critical importance of radiographic technique in identifying these lesions.
- **1940:** Harold Arthur Hill and Maurice David Sachs popularized the lesion through detailed radiographic studies and linked it to shoulder instability following dislocation.

Purpose

- **Diagnostic Marker:** To identify and evaluate the extent of humeral head injury following anterior shoulder dislocation.
- **Assessment of Instability:** To determine the likelihood of recurrent shoulder dislocations based on the lesion's size.
- **Preoperative Planning:** To guide

surgical intervention in cases of severe instability or recurrent dislocations.

Procedure Overview

- **Initial Imaging:** Conventional radiographs, particularly anterior-posterior (AP) views with the shoulder internally rotated, are used to identify the lesion.
- **Advanced Imaging:** Computed Tomography (CT) provides detailed visualization of the lesion's size, depth, and location.
- Associated injuries such as bony Bankart lesions can be concurrently evaluated.
- **Surgical Planning:** The imaging findings inform whether surgical techniques like remplissage or bone grafting are necessary.

Results and Interpretation

- **Radiographic Findings:** A compression fracture or groove is visible on the posterolateral humeral head.
- **Larger defects are often associated with a greater number of dislocations and increased instability.**
- **CT Findings:** Allows precise measurement of the lesion's depth and surface area.
- Reveals associated injuries such as glenoid bone loss or fractures.

Physiological Basis

- **Mechanism of Injury:** During anterior dislocation, the humeral head impacts the inferior glenoid rim, creating a cortical depression or fracture.
- **Pathophysiology:** The repetitive nature of dislocations can enlarge the defect, reducing the ability of the humeral head to maintain stability in the glenoid cavity.

Clinical Applications

- **Diagnosis of Shoulder Dislocation:** A definitive indicator of anterior shoulder dislocation, often missed without proper imaging techniques.
- **Treatment Planning:** Guides the decision between conservative management and surgical stabilization.
- **Monitoring Progression:** Identifies changes in lesion size or complications in cases of recurrent dislocations.

Limitations and Technical Considerations

- **Imaging Limitations:** Conventional radiographs may miss smaller lesions or mischaracterize their extent.
- **Surgical Challenges:** Severe lesions may require complex procedures like glenoid reconstruction or humeral head replacement.
- **Recurrent Instability:** Lesions left untreated can lead to chronic instability, pain, and functional limitations.

Modern Relevance

- **Advanced Imaging:** Modern CT and MRI techniques have enhanced the ability to detect and measure Hill-Sachs lesions accurately.
- **Surgical Innovation:** Procedures like remplissage (filling the lesion with soft tissue) are widely used to stabilize the joint.

- **Sports Medicine Focus:** Hill-Sachs lesions are a common topic in the treatment of athletes with shoulder instability.

Associated Conditions

- **Bony Bankart Lesions:** Often coexists with Hill-Sachs lesions, involving fractures or defects of the anterior glenoid rim.
- **Recurrent Shoulder Dislocations:** Strongly associated due to the loss of humeral head congruence.

Clinical Importance

- **Early Diagnosis:** Detecting Hill-Sachs lesions after the first dislocation can prevent recurrent instability.
- **Prognostic Value:** The size of the lesion correlates with the likelihood of further dislocations and helps predict surgical outcomes.
- **Interdisciplinary Management:** Involves collaboration between radiologists, orthopedic surgeons, and physical therapists for optimal outcomes.

Hill-Sachs lesion is a hallmark of anterior shoulder dislocation, significantly influencing the treatment and prognosis of recurrent instability. Early detection and intervention, guided by advanced imaging and surgical techniques, are critical in restoring joint function and preventing further injury.

References

Malgaigne JF. Chirgurue Pratique: Des Luxations scapulo-humérales. Nouveau moyens de les distinguer des fractures du col de l'humérus. Nouvelle méthode de réduction. Expériences faites à l'Hôtel-Dieu. Gazette médicale de Paris. 1832. 3:73;506-508

Berquet JE. Essai sur les luxations scapulo-humérales, accidentelles ou traumatiques: thèse présentée et publiquement soutenue à la Faculté de médecine de Montpellier. 1850 [Ref Malgaigne pp34-35]

Gyftopoulos S, Albert M, Recht MP. Osseous injuries associated with anterior shoulder instability: what the radiologist should know. AJR Am J Roentgenol. 2014;202(6):W541–50.

Harris Jr JH, Thomas P. The radiology of emergency medicine. Baltimore: Lippincott Williams and Wilkins; 2013.

Perthes G. Über Operationen bei habitueller Schulterluxation. Deutsche Ztschr. f. Chir. 1906;85:199-228

Schultze E. Die habituellen Schulterluxationen. Arch. f. kline Chir. 1914;104:138-179

Pilz W. Zur Roentgenuntersuchung der Habituellen Schulterverrenkung. Arch. f. klin. Chir 1925;135:1-22

Hill HA, Sachs MD. The grooved defect of the humeral head: a frequently unrecognized complication of dislocations of the shoulder joint. Radiology. 35: vol 6 690–700.(December 1940)

Gyftopoulos S, Albert M, Recht MP. Osseous injuries associated with anterior shoulder instability: what the radiologist should know. AJR Am J Roentgenol. 2014 Jun;202(6):W541-50. [PMID 24848847]

Somford MP, Van der Linde JA, Wiegerinck JI, Hoornenborg D, Van den Bekerom MPJ, Van Deurzen DFP. Eponymous terms in anterior shoulder stabilization surgery. Orthop Traumatol Surg Res. 2017 Dec;103(8):1257-1263. [PMID 28942024]

Calandra JJ, Baker CL, Uribe J.The incidence of Hill-Sachs lesions in initial anterior shoulder dislocations. Arthroscopy. 1989;5(4):254-7. [PMID 2590322]

Cetik O, Uslu M, Ozsar BK. The relationship between Hill-Sachs lesion and recurrent anterior shoulder dislocation. Acta Orthop Belg. 2007 Apr;73(2):175-8. [PMID 17515227]

Hoffa Fracture and Hoffa fat pad

Overview

Hoffa fracture is a rare unicondylar intra-articular fracture of the distal femur, usually involving the lateral condyle, though medial condyle fractures are also possible. The Hoffa fat pad, a fibro-fatty tissue located between the patella, femur, and tibia, plays a key role in knee joint function and movement. These conditions are significant due to their unique presentation and management challenges.

Historical Background

- *Albert Hoffa* described the unicondylar distal femur fracture that now bears his name.
- Hoffa's anatomical studies also identified the fat pad's structural and functional characteristics in the knee joint.

Purpose

- **Hoffa Fracture:** To diagnose, reduce, and stabilize intra-articular distal femur fractures to restore joint congruity and function.
- **Hoffa Fat Pad:** To understand its pathological involvement in knee pain and develop effective management strategies.

Procedure Overview

Hoffa Fracture

- **Diagnostic Imaging:** Radiographs (lateral and oblique views) and CT scans are used to confirm fracture patterns.
- **Surgical Approach:** Open reduction and internal fixation (ORIF) is performed to ensure anatomical alignment and stability.

Hoffa Fat Pad

- **Clinical Evaluation:** Anterior knee pain is assessed, often requiring MRI to evaluate for inflammation or hypertrophy.

Treatment:

- Conservative management includes RICE therapy and physical rehabilitation.
- Arthroscopic resection may be performed in chronic or refractory cases.

Results and Interpretation

- **Hoffa Fracture:** Surgical fixation restores knee joint alignment and stability, minimizing the risk of long-term complications such as arthritis or stiffness.
- **Hoffa Fat Pad:** Inflammatory changes detected on MRI are indicative of chronic irritation.
- Arthroscopic resection outcomes vary, with potential for symptom recurrence or scarring.

Physiological Basis

- **Hoffa Fracture:** Results from direct trauma, axial loading, or rotational forces, leading to shearing of the femoral condyle.
- **Requires anatomical alignment to restore joint biomechanics.**
- **Hoffa Fat Pad:** Functions as a deformable cushion to accommodate knee movements and facilitate synovial fluid distribution.
- Prone to inflammation due to vascularity

and soft tissue composition.

Clinical Applications

- **Hoffa Fracture:** Often treated in trauma cases to prevent instability and maintain weight-bearing capacity.
- **Critical for preserving functional mobility in high-demand patients.**
- **Hoffa Fat Pad:** Managed in cases of anterior knee pain, especially in athletes or active individuals.
- Integral to sports medicine and rehabilitation protocols.

Limitations and Technical Considerations

- **Hoffa Fracture:** Complex fracture patterns require advanced imaging and surgical expertise.
- **Nonunion or malunion can occur if reduction is inadequate.**
- **Hoffa Fat Pad:** Arthroscopic resection risks worsening symptoms or scar formation.
- Conservative therapies may be ineffective in chronic cases.

Modern Relevance

- **Hoffa Fracture:** Advances in surgical fixation techniques have improved outcomes.
- **Early intervention and precise management are emphasized in trauma care.**
- **Hoffa Fat Pad:** Enhanced understanding of its pathology has refined treatment, improving quality of life for affected patients.

Associated Conditions

- **Hoffa Fracture:** Frequently associated with ligament injuries, patellar dislocations, or other femoral fractures.
- **Hoffa Fat Pad:** Linked to conditions such as patella alta, impingement syndromes, and arthrofibrosis.

Clinical Importance

- **Hoffa Fracture:** Proper management ensures joint functionality and reduces the risk of debilitating complications.
- **Often observed in high-energy trauma incidents.**
- **Hoffa Fat Pad:** Early diagnosis and intervention reduce morbidity and prevent unnecessary surgical treatments.
- Significant in optimizing functional recovery in sports medicine.

References

Barbier-Brion B, Lerais J-M, Aubry S, Lepage D, Vidal C, Delabrousse E, Runge M, Kastler B (2012) Magnetic resonance imaging in patellar lateral femoral friction syndrome (PLFFS): prospective case-control study. Diagn Interv Imaging 93:e171–e182.

Calmet J, Mellado JM, Garcı´a Forcada IL, Gine´ J (2004) Open bicondylar Hoffa fracture associated with extensor mechanism injury. J Orthop Trauma 18:323–325.

Dragoo JL, Johnson C, McConnell J (2012) Evaluation and treatment of disorders of the infrapatellar fat pad. Sport Med 42:51–67.

Dua A, Shamshery PK (2010) Bicondylar Hoffa fracture: open reduction internal fixation using the swashbuckler approach. J Knee Surg 23:21–24.

Jacobson JA, Lenchik L, Ruhoy MK, Schweitzer ME, Resnick D (1997) MR imaging of the infrapatellar fat pad of Hoffa. Radiographics 17:675–691.

Larbi A, Cyteval C, Hamoui M, Dallaudiere B, Zarqane H, Viala P, Ruyer A (2014) Hoffa's disease: a report on 5 cases. Diagn Interv Imaging 95:1079–1084.

Letenneur J, Labour PE, Rogez JM, Lignon J, Bainvel JV (1997) Hoffa's fractures. Report of 20 cases (author's transl). Ann Chir 32:213–219.

Vaishya R, Singh AP, Dar IT, Singh AP, Mittal V (2009) Hoffa fracture with ipsilateral patellar dislocation resulting from household trauma. Can J Surg 52:E3–E4.

Holstein-Lewis Fracture

Overview

The Holstein-Lewis fracture is a spiral fracture of the distal third of the humerus, often resulting from blunt trauma. It is uniquely associated with radial nerve palsy due to the nerve's anatomical vulnerability at this level. Lateral displacement of the distal fragment commonly compromises nerve function, requiring careful evaluation and management.

Historical Background

- Described by *Arthur Holstein* and *Gwilym Lewis*, this fracture pattern was first recognized for its distinct association with radial nerve palsy.
- Their work underscored the clinical importance of identifying this injury to anticipate potential neurological deficits and complications.

Purpose

- To accurately diagnose the Holstein-Lewis fracture and its associated radial nerve injury.
- To provide guidance for optimal treatment strategies - whether conservative or surgical - ensuring recovery of nerve function and fracture stability.

Procedure Overview

Diagnosis:

- **Clinical Assessment:** Look for signs of radial nerve palsy, such as wrist drop or sensory loss in the dorsal hand.
- **Radiographic Imaging:** Obtain AP and lateral views to confirm the spiral fracture and displacement.
- **Neurological Evaluation:** Assess radial nerve integrity and document any deficits.

Management:

- **Conservative Treatment:** Immobilize the arm using a functional brace or coaptation splint.
- **Regular follow-up to monitor nerve recovery and fracture healing.**
- **Surgical Intervention:** Open reduction and internal fixation (ORIF) for unstable fractures or severe displacement.
- Radial nerve exploration if palsy persists or worsens.

Results and Interpretation

- Most radial nerve injuries associated with this fracture are *neuropraxias*, resolving spontaneously within weeks or months.
- Surgical intervention often leads to better anatomical alignment and functional outcomes, particularly for displaced fractures.

Physiological Basis

- The *radial nerve* travels distally along the lateral intermuscular septum at the level of the distal humerus, where it becomes vulnerable to trauma or compression by bone fragments.
- Injury leads to *motor deficits* (e.g., wrist drop) and *sensory loss* in the radial nerve's cutaneous distribution.

Clinical Applications

- Critical in *orthopedic trauma care,* as delayed recognition of radial nerve injury can lead to prolonged recovery.
- Guides decision-making in fracture management, balancing conservative versus surgical treatment.
- Plays a role in *rehabilitation protocols* for patients with nerve recovery or post-surgical stiffness.

Limitations and Technical Considerations

- **Conservative Management:** Risks delayed union or malunion, requiring secondary interventions.
- **Surgical Risks:** Radial nerve exploration can lead to scarring, infection, or failure to restore nerve function.
- **Radiographic Challenges:** Subtle displacement or overlapping of fragments may obscure the fracture pattern on plain films.

Modern Relevance

- Improvements in imaging techniques (e.g., CT scans) and surgical approaches have enhanced diagnosis and treatment precision.
- Emphasis on early neurologic evaluation ensures better functional outcomes and minimizes long-term disability.
- Multidisciplinary management, involving radiologists, orthopedic surgeons, and rehabilitation specialists, remains crucial.

Associated Conditions

- **Radial Nerve Palsy:** Present in approximately 22% of Holstein-Lewis fractures.
- **Soft Tissue Damage:** Commonly seen with high-energy trauma.
- **Vascular Injuries:** Rare but can occur in severe trauma.

Clinical Importance

- **Early Diagnosis:** Prompt identification of the Holstein-Lewis fracture and associated radial nerve injury prevents delayed treatment and complications.
- **Prognostic Value:** The degree of radial nerve dysfunction and fracture displacement determines recovery time and guides treatment decisions.
- **Interdisciplinary Management:** Collaboration between radiologists, orthopedic surgeons, and physical therapists ensures comprehensive care, from acute injury management to rehabilitation.

References

Holstein A, Lewis GM. Fractures of the humerus with radial-nerve paralysis. J Bone Joint Surg Am. 1963;45:1382–8.

Ekholm R, Ponzer S, Tornkvist H, Adami J, Tidermark J. The Holstein-Lewis humeral shaft fracture: aspects of radial nerve injury, primary treatment, and outcome. J Orthop Trauma. 2008;22(10):693–7.

Howship's lacunae

Overview

Howship's lacunae are small pits, grooves, or depressions found on the surfaces of bones. These structures are formed as a result of bone resorption by osteoclasts, which occupy these lacunae during the process of breaking down bone tissue. Typically, they are around 100 microns or more in length and are a hallmark of active bone remodeling.

Historical Background

- Named after *John Howship*, an English anatomist and surgeon, who first described these lacunae in the 19th century.
- Howship's observations contributed significantly to the understanding of bone physiology and the role of osteoclasts in bone resorption.

Purpose

- To serve as indicators of active bone remodeling.
- To provide insights into the cellular mechanisms underlying bone turnover and conditions such as osteoporosis and other metabolic bone diseases.

Procedure Overview

- **Histological Examination:** Bone samples are examined under a microscope to identify Howship's lacunae.
- **Specialized staining techniques, such as tartrate-resistant acid phosphatase (TRAP), may be used to highlight osteoclasts within the lacunae.**
- **Radiological Correlation:** In cases of significant bone resorption, imaging may indirectly reveal patterns consistent with areas of active bone turnover.

Results and Interpretation

- **Active Bone Resorption:** The presence of Howship's lacunae indicates regions where osteoclasts are breaking down bone matrix.
- **Disease Marker:** An increased number of these lacunae may suggest heightened osteoclastic activity, often seen in conditions like osteoporosis, Paget's disease, or hyperparathyroidism.

Physiological Basis

- Osteoclasts secrete acidic substances and enzymes, such as cathepsin K, to dissolve bone mineral and degrade the organic matrix.
- The lacunae represent the physical evidence of this resorptive process, reflecting the dynamic nature of bone metabolism.

Clinical Applications

- Used as a diagnostic feature in histopathological studies of bone diseases.
- Important in research for understanding mechanisms of bone loss in conditions like *osteoporosis, rheumatoid arthritis*, and *bone metastases.*
- Serves as a marker in the evaluation of the effects of anti-resorptive therapies, such as bisphosphonates.

Limitations and Technical Considerations

- **Microscopic Identification:** Requires well-preserved bone samples and skilled histopathological analysis.
- **Interpreting Lacunae:** The mere presence of lacunae is not disease-specific and must be correlated with clinical and laboratory findings.
- **Sampling Bias:** The distribution of lacunae may vary across different bone regions, potentially limiting their diagnostic reliability.

Modern Relevance

- **Advances in** imaging and molecular biology have enhanced the understanding of Howship's lacunae and their role in bone biology.
- Insights from studying these structures contribute to developing novel therapies for metabolic bone disorders.
- Plays a significant role in regenerative medicine and the study of bone healing processes.

Associated Conditions

- **Osteoporosis:** Increased numbers of Howship's lacunae due to enhanced bone resorption.
- **Hyperparathyroidism:** Overactive osteoclastic activity leading to the formation of excessive lacunae.
- **Bone Metastases:** Tumor-induced osteolysis often features pronounced Howship's lacunae.

Clinical Importance

- **Early Detection:** Identification of increased lacunae can be an early sign of metabolic bone disease.
- **Prognostic Value:** The extent of Howship's lacunae correlates with the activity of bone resorption, providing insight into disease severity.
- **Interdisciplinary Relevance:** Collaboration between pathologists, radiologists, and clinicians enhances the utility of findings related to Howship's lacunae for comprehensive disease management.

Howship's Syndrome

Overview

Howship's syndrome is characterized by pain or paresthesia radiating along the inner aspect of the thigh, often down to the knee. This pain arises due to compression or irritation of the obturator nerve, typically associated with an obturator hernia. In cases of strangulated hernia, the pain may be accompanied by abdominal discomfort. The condition is more commonly observed in elderly women and is often linked to congenital or acquired abnormalities of the obturator canal.

Historical Background

- *John Howship* was an English anatomist and surgeon who initially described the neuralgia associated with obturator nerve compression.
- *Moritz Heinrich Romberg*, a German neurologist, expanded on Howship's findings, contributing to the understanding of the nerve's involvement in hernias and associated symptomatology.

Purpose

- To identify the relationship between *obturator hernias* and *obturator nerve compression* as the cause of pain radiating to the medial thigh and knee.
- To provide a clinical framework for diagnosing and managing a rare but significant hernia type.

Procedure Overview

- **Clinical Examination:** Patients report recurrent, localized pain along the inner thigh, often exacerbated by movement or activities increasing intra-abdominal pressure.
- **Abdominal examination may reveal tenderness or signs of obstruction in cases of hernia strangulation.**
- **Imaging:** CT scans and MRI are highly effective in identifying the hernia within the obturator canal and its effect on surrounding structures.
- **Surgical Exploration:** Necessary in cases of suspected strangulated obturator hernia to confirm the diagnosis and alleviate the obstruction.

Results and Interpretation

- **Obturator Hernia:** Often a small, difficult-to-detect hernia due to its anatomical location, requiring imaging for confirmation.
- **Nerve Compression:** Confirmed by pain localization and exacerbation with movements such as thigh abduction or extension.
- **Strangulation:** Symptoms of bowel obstruction, including abdominal pain, nausea, or vomiting, may be indicative.

Physiological Basis

- The *obturator nerve* passes through the obturator canal, a narrow bony and fibrous passage in the pelvis.
- Obturator hernias compress the nerve, causing radiating pain and sensory disturbances along its distribution area.

- Strangulation of hernia contents within the canal can lead to ischemia, further exacerbating symptoms.

Clinical Applications

- **Diagnosis:** Recognition of obturator hernia as a cause of medial thigh pain aids in early intervention and reduces complications.
- **Surgical Repair:** Obturator hernias typically require surgical intervention, either open or laparoscopic, to repair the defect and relieve nerve compression.
- **Pain Management:** Addressing neuralgia with analgesics or nerve blocks can improve patient comfort preoperatively.

Limitations and Technical Considerations

- **Difficulty in Detection:** Obturator hernias are rare and challenging to diagnose without advanced imaging.
- **Nerve Damage:** Prolonged compression may cause irreversible nerve damage, emphasizing the importance of early intervention.
- **Recurrent Hernias:** Despite surgical repair, there is a risk of recurrence, necessitating careful follow-up.

Modern Relevance

- **Advances in Imaging:** Improved diagnostic capabilities with CT and MRI have increased the detection rate of obturator hernias.
- **Minimally Invasive Surgery:** Laparoscopic techniques allow for precise hernia repair with reduced recovery times and improved outcomes.
- **Geriatric Focus:** Awareness of Howship's syndrome is particularly relevant in aging populations with higher prevalence of hernias.

Associated Conditions

- **Bowel Obstruction:** Strangulated obturator hernia can lead to small bowel obstruction, a surgical emergency.
- **Neuropathy:** Chronic compression of the obturator nerve can result in persistent pain or paresthesia.
- **Pelvic Trauma:** Trauma or prior surgeries involving the pelvis may predispose patients to obturator hernias.

Clinical Importance

- **Early Diagnosis:** Prompt identification of Howship's syndrome can prevent complications such as bowel strangulation.
- **Prognostic Value:** The severity of nerve compression and the extent of hernia strangulation guide surgical urgency and outcomes.
- **Interdisciplinary Management:** Effective management requires collaboration between general surgeons, radiologists, and neurologists.

References

J. Howship: Practical Remarks on the Discrimination and Appearance of Surgical Disease. London, Churchill, 1840.

M. H. von Romberg: Pathologie und Therapie der Senisbilitäts- und Motilitätsneurosen. 1857. 3rd edition (unfinished) of Romberg's Lehrbuch der Nervenkrankheiten des Menschen, page 89.

Hutchinson/Chauffer's Fractures

Overview

The Hutchinson fracture, also referred to as the Chauffeur's fracture, is an intra-articular fracture of the distal radius involving the radial styloid. This type of fracture typically results from axial loading or a direct blow, often in conjunction with wrist dorsiflexion and abduction. While historically associated with occupational injuries among early automobile chauffeurs, this fracture is now predominantly seen in modern settings due to falls on outstretched hands (FOOSH) or high-impact trauma.

Historical Background

- **1866:** First described by Jonathan Hutchinson, a British surgeon, as a radial styloid fracture resulting from direct trauma.
- **Early 20th Century:** The term "Chauffeur's fracture" emerged, credited to Just Lucas-Championnière, referencing injuries sustained by chauffeurs starting cars with hand cranks. This mechanism became obsolete with Advances in automotive technology.
- **1904:** The French surgeon highlighted the occupational origins of the fracture, solidifying the eponym in medical literature.

Purpose

- To accurately identify and manage fractures involving the radial styloid and associated ligamentous injuries.
- To restore the functional anatomy of the wrist, ensuring joint stability and preventing complications such as arthritis or chronic pain.

Procedure Overview

Diagnosis:

- **Clinical Presentation:** Pain localized to the wrist, particularly near the radial styloid.
- Swelling and limited wrist mobility.
- Tenderness over the radial styloid on palpation.
- **Imaging:**
- **X-rays:** Initial imaging modality showing the fracture and displacement.
- **CT scans:** Useful in complex cases to assess intra-articular extension and associated ligamentous injuries.
- **MRI:** Occasionally used for soft tissue and ligament evaluation.

Management:

- **Non-Surgical:** Indicated for minimally displaced fractures.
- **Immobilization using a cast or splint for 4–6 weeks.**
- **Surgical:** Required for significantly displaced or unstable fractures.
- Techniques include open reduction and internal fixation (ORIF) with plates or screws, and, in some cases, arthroscopic-assisted reduction.

Results and Interpretation

- With appropriate treatment, most patients achieve near-normal wrist function and mobility.

- Non-operative treatments are effective for stable fractures, but surgical intervention provides superior outcomes for displaced fractures.
- Early diagnosis and appropriate intervention reduce the risk of long-term complications like joint stiffness or osteoarthritis.

Physiological Basis

- The radial styloid plays a key role in wrist stability and articulation with the scaphoid.
- Disruption of the radioscaphocapitate ligament, often associated with Chauffeur's fractures, can lead to instability and joint misalignment if untreated.
- The mechanism of injury involves compression forces transmitted through the scaphoid to the radial styloid, resulting in an avulsion or fracture.

Clinical Applications

- **Emergency Medicine:** Immediate immobilization and pain management in acute settings.
- **Orthopedic Surgery:** Repair of displaced fractures to restore anatomical alignment and prevent joint instability.
- **Rehabilitation:** Physical therapy to restore range of motion and strength post-treatment.

Limitations and Technical Considerations

- **Imaging Challenges:** Complex intra-articular fractures may require advanced imaging modalities for accurate diagnosis.
- **Surgical Risks:** Potential complications include infection, hardware failure, or residual stiffness.
- **Healing Considerations:** Delayed union or nonunion may occur, particularly in comminuted fractures.

Modern Relevance

- Improved imaging and surgical techniques have enhanced the management of Chauffeur's fractures.
- The transition from occupational injuries to trauma-related cases reflects changes in societal and technological trends.
- Awareness of associated ligamentous injuries has improved functional outcomes.

Associated Conditions

- **Scapholunate Ligament Injury:** Often accompanies radial styloid fractures, necessitating thorough evaluation.
- **Lunate Dislocation:** A potential complication of untreated ligamentous disruptions.
- **Triangular Fibrocartilage Complex (TFCC) Injury:** Common in high-impact injuries affecting wrist articulation.

Clinical Importance

- **Early Diagnosis:** Crucial for preventing long-term complications such as arthritis or chronic wrist pain.
- **Interdisciplinary Management:** Collaboration among emergency physicians, radiologists, and orthopedic surgeons ensures optimal patient outcomes.
- **Rehabilitation:** Essential for restoring wrist functionality and preventing stiff-

ness post-treatment.

The Hutchinson/Chauffeur's fracture underscores the importance of understanding wrist biomechanics and emphasizes advancements in diagnostic and surgical techniques for achieving favorable patient outcomes.

References

Lee P, Hunter TB, Taljanovic M. Musculoskeletal colloquialisms: how did we come up with these names? Radiographics. 24 (4): 1009-27.

SPRINGER B. Emergency Radiology, Imaging and Intervention. (2010)

Goldfarb CA, Yin Y, Gilula LA et-al. Wrist fractures: what the clinician wants to know. Radiology. 2001;219 (1): 11-28.

Saffar P, Cooney WP. Fractures of the Distal Radius. Informa HealthCare. (1995)

Yochum TR, Rowe LJ. Essentials of Skeletal Radiology. Philadelphia, Pa. : Lippincott Williams & Wilkins, c2005.

Schatzker J, Tile M. The Rationale of Operative Fracture Care. Springer Verlag. (2005)

Robinson P. Essential Radiology for Sports Medicine. Springer Verlag. (2010) ISBN:1441959726.

Caldwell RA, Shorten PL, Morrell NT. Common Upper Extremity Fracture Eponyms: A Look Into What They Really Mean. J Hand Surg Am. 2019 Apr;44(4):331-334. [PubMed]

Meena S, Sharma P, Sambharia AK, Dawar A. Fractures of distal radius: an overview. J Family Med Prim Care. 2014 Oct-Dec;3(4):325-32. [PMC free article] [PubMed]

Karl JW, Olson PR, Rosenwasser MP. The Epidemiology of Upper Extremity Fractures in the United States, 2009. J Orthop Trauma. 2015 Aug;29(8):e242-4. [PubMed]

Hotchkiss Terrible Triad

Overview

The Hotchkiss Terrible Triad (TTE) of the elbow is a complex and severe orthopedic injury involving three components: an elbow dislocation, a radial head fracture, and a coronoid process fracture. This triad disrupts the bony and ligamentous stabilizers of the elbow, often resulting in instability and a high potential for complications such as chronic pain, stiffness, and arthritis.

Historical Background

- **1996:** The terrible triad of the elbow was first described by Hotchkiss. He identified the combination of elbow dislocation, radial head fracture, and coronoid process fracture as a serious and challenging condition requiring meticulous management.

- Elbow dislocations and their complications have been documented for centuries, but the comprehensive understanding and association of the three injuries were formally defined by Hotchkiss.

Purpose

- To restore joint congruence, stability, and functionality in a highly unstable elbow.

- To reduce the risk of secondary complications, such as recurrent instability, arthrosis, and contractures.

- To allow for early postoperative mobilization and limit stiffness.

Procedure Overview

Diagnosis:

- **Clinical Examination:** Visible deformity, swelling, and restricted motion of the elbow.
- Pain and instability on palpation or attempted motion.
- **Imaging:** X-rays: Initial imaging to confirm dislocation and associated fractures.
- **CT Scan:** Essential post-reduction to identify and classify fractures and to plan surgical intervention.

Treatment:

- **Non-Surgical:** Rarely indicated due to the high instability associated with TTE.
- **Reserved for very minor fractures with stable elbow reduction.**
- **Surgical:** Focus on restoring bony and ligamentous stabilizers.
- **Key steps:**
- **Radial Head:** Fixation or replacement, depending on the extent of comminution.
- **Coronoid Process:** Osteosynthesis using plates, screws, or anchors if significant.
- **Lateral Collateral Ligament (LCL):** Repair or reconstruction to restore elbow stability.
- **Medial Collateral Ligament (MCL):** Debate exists, but systematic repair is not always required.
- Postoperative management emphasizes early mobilization to prevent stiffness.

Results and Interpretation

- Successful surgical treatment often results in restored elbow stability and good functional outcomes.
- Early motion can prevent flexion-extension contractures and chronic stiffness, critical for patient satisfaction and long-term elbow function.
- Long-term outcomes hinge on the quality of anatomical reduction and repair.

Physiological Basis

- The *coronoid process* is the key to anteroposterior stability in the humero-ulnar joint, with at least 50% of its height required for stability.
- The *radial head* plays a vital role in resisting valgus and rotational forces.
- The *lateral collateral ligament complex* is critical for posterolateral stability, and its disruption can lead to recurrent dislocation or subluxation.
- The elbow joint's intricate combination of bony and soft tissue structures makes it highly vulnerable to instability following the terrible triad injury.

Clinical Applications

- **Orthopedic Surgery:** A precise and systematic surgical approach is essential for optimal outcomes.
- **Physical Therapy:** Postoperative rehabilitation focuses on regaining range of motion while avoiding overstressing repaired structures.
- **Trauma Management:** Emergency reduction and stabilization to prevent neurovascular compromise and further joint damage.

Limitations and Technical Considerations

- **Injury Complexity:** The multiplicity of injuries requires a comprehensive surgical plan, often involving multiple approaches.
- **Postoperative Stiffness:** Early motion is crucial, but it must be balanced against the risk of disrupting the surgical repair.
- **Associated Injuries:** Neurovascular damage and collateral ligament involvement may complicate treatment.

Modern Relevance

- **Advances in** imaging and surgical techniques have significantly improved the management and prognosis of TTE.
- The development of prosthetic implants for the radial head and refined ligament reconstruction techniques has enhanced outcomes.
- Increased understanding of biomechanics and injury patterns allows for individualized treatment plans.

Associated Conditions

- **Posterolateral Rotatory Instability:** Common due to lateral ligament complex disruption.
- **Elbow Arthrosis:** Long-term complication of untreated or inadequately treated TTE.
- **Chronic Stiffness:** Can develop despite surgical intervention if mobilization is delayed.

Clinical Importance

- TTE is a *high-stakes injury* requiring meticulous evaluation and management.
- The restoration of stability and mobility is critical to avoid permanent disability.
- A multidisciplinary approach, including orthopedic surgeons, radiologists, and physical therapists, ensures comprehensive care.
- Early recognition and intervention can prevent complications and improve long-term functional outcomes.
- The *Hotchkiss Terrible Triad* emphasizes the delicate interplay between bone and ligament structures in the elbow, underscoring the importance of a systematic and multidisciplinary approach to achieve successful outcomes.

References

Hotchkiss R.N. In: fourth ed. Rockwood C.A., Green D.P. Jr., Bucholz R.W., Heckman J.D., editors. vol. 1. Lippincott-Raven; Philadelphia: 1996. Fractures and dislocations of the elbow; pp. 929–1024. (Rockwood and Green's Fractures in Adults). [Google Scholar]

O'Driscoll S.W., Jupiter J.B., King G.J.W., Hotchkiss R.N., Morrey B.F. The unstable elbow. J. Bone Jt. Surg. Am. 2000;82:724–738. [Google Scholar]

Amstrong A.D. The terrible triad injury of the elbow. Curr. Opin. Orthop. 2005;16:267–270. [Google Scholar]

Agha R.A., Sohrabi C., Mathew G., Franchi T., Kerwan A., O'Neill N for the PROCESS Group The PROCESS 2020 guideline: updating Consensus preferred reporting of CasE series in surgery (PROCESS) guidelines. Int. J. Surg. 2020;84:231–235. [PubMed] [Google Scholar]

Van Riet R.P., Morrey B.F. Documentation of associated injuries occurring with radial head fracture. Clin. Orthop. 2008;466:130–134. [PMC free article] [PubMed] [Google Scholar]

McKee M.D., Pugh D.M.W., Wild L.M., Schemitsch E.H., King G.J.W. Standard surgical protocol to treat elbow dislocations with radial head and coronoid fractures. Surgical technique. J. Bone Jt. Surg. Am. 2005;87:22–32. [PubMed]

Pugh D.M.W., Wild L.M., Schemitsch E.H., King G.J.W., McKee M.D. Standard surgical protocol to treat elbow dislocations with radial head and coronoid fractures. J. Bone Jt. Surg. Am. 2004;86:1122–1130.

Chemama B., Bonnevialle N., Peter O., Mansat P., Bonnevialle P. Terrible triade du coude : description et prise en charge. Rev.

Chir. Orthopédique Traumatol. 2010;96:191–198. [Google Scholar]

Jéro^me P., Thierry B., Pierre M. Terrible triad of the elbow: treatment protocol and outcome in a series of eighteen cases. Injury Int. J. Care Injured. 2015;46:8–12. [PubMed] [Google Scholar]

Jaffe-Lichtenstein Syndrome

Overview

Jaffe-Lichtenstein syndrome is a monostotic form of fibrous dysplasia characterized by excessive proliferation of single or multiple fibrous lesions within the bones. These lesions predominantly affect the long bones and can lead to painful deformities, pathological fractures, scoliosis, chest deformities, and other skeletal abnormalities. Irregular macular dermal pigmentation may also be present. The syndrome typically manifests during the first two decades of life and is considered benign but constitutional. Familial cases, though rare, have been reported.

Historical Background

- The syndrome was first described in *1942* by *Henry Lewis Jaffe* and *Louis Lichtenstein*, who reported 15 cases of monostotic fibrous dysplasia.
- Additional cases were later documented by Schlumberger, who expanded the understanding of the condition.
- The syndrome is distinct from the similar *McCune-Albright syndrome*, described by Fuller Albright and characterized by skin pigmentation and endocrinopathies.

Purpose

- To understand the pathophysiology and clinical presentation of monostotic fibrous dysplasia and distinguish it from other forms of fibrous dysplasia, including McCune-Albright syndrome.
- To provide a framework for the diagnosis and management of this rare condition.

Procedure Overview

- **Clinical Evaluation:** Symptoms often include localized bone pain, deformity, and limping.
- **A thorough history and physical examination are crucial to identifying features such as skin pigmentation or skeletal asymmetry.**
- **Imaging:** X-rays reveal characteristic lesions with ground-glass appearance, thinning of the cortex, and expanded bone with irregular trabecular patterns.
- **Advanced imaging such as CT or MRI may be used for detailed evaluation of bone integrity and deformity.**
- **Biopsy:** Histological confirmation involves identifying fibrous connective tissue with irregular bone trabeculae, which is diagnostic for fibrous dysplasia.

Results and Interpretation

- **Lesions:** Monostotic lesions tend to be localized to one bone, while polyostotic forms may involve multiple skeletal sites.
- **Radiographic Findings:** Lesions show characteristic radiolucent areas with sclerotic margins.
- **Progression:** The disorder progresses gradually, with skeletal changes becoming more prominent during childhood or adolescence.

Physiological Basis

- Fibrous dysplasia results from a somatic mutation in the *GNAS1* gene, which affects osteoblastic differentiation and leads to the replacement of normal bone with fibrous tissue.
- This abnormal bone remodeling predisposes affected areas to fractures and deformities.

Clinical Applications

- **Diagnosis:** Early diagnosis allows for monitoring of bone lesions to prevent fractures and deformity.
- **Surgical Intervention:** Corrective surgery may be required for severe deformities or pathological fractures.
- **Pain Management:** Analgesics and bisphosphonates may be used to reduce bone pain and stabilize lesions.

Limitations and Technical Considerations

- **Radiographic Challenges:** Early lesions may be subtle and difficult to detect without advanced imaging techniques.
- **Differential Diagnosis:** The syndrome must be differentiated from similar conditions such as McCune-Albright syndrome or osteogenesis imperfecta.
- **Surgical Risks:** Surgery may lead to complications, including recurrent fractures or delayed healing.

Modern Relevance

- **Genetic Insights:** Advances in molecular biology have improved the understanding of GNAS1 mutations in fibrous dysplasia.
- **Minimally Invasive Treatments:** Emerging therapies, such as targeted bisphosphonate treatment, offer hope for better management of bone lesions.
- **Multidisciplinary Care:** Collaboration among orthopedic surgeons, endo-

crinologists, and geneticists is vital for optimal outcomes.

Associated Conditions

- **McCune-Albright Syndrome:** Distinguished by endocrinopathies and café-au-lait spots in addition to fibrous dysplasia.
- **Pathological Fractures:** Increased risk due to weakened structural integrity of bones.
- **Scoliosis and Deformities:** Frequently observed in cases with extensive skeletal involvement.

Clinical Importance

- **Early Diagnosis:** Identifying lesions early allows for timely intervention to prevent severe deformities and fractures.
- **Prognostic Value:** The extent and location of lesions guide management strategies and predict functional outcomes.
- **Interdisciplinary Management:** Effective treatment requires coordination between orthopedic surgeons, radiologists, and genetic counselors.

References

H. L. Jaffe: "Osteoid-osteoma,", benign osteoblastic tumor composed of osteoid atypical bone. Archives of Surgery, Chicago, 1935, 31: 709-728.

F. Albright, A. M. Butler, A. O. Hampton, P. Smith: Syndrome characterized by osteitis fibrosa disseminata, areas of pigmentation and endocrine dysfunction, with precocious puberty in females: report of five cases. New England Journal of Medicine, Boston, 1937, 216: 727-746.

H. L. Jaffe, L. Lichtenstein: Fibrous dysplasia of bone. A condition affecting one, several or many bones, the graver cases of which may present with abnormal pigmentation of skin, premature sexual development, hyperthyroidism or still other extraskeletal abnormalities. Archives of Pathology, Chicago, 1942, 33: 777-816. This review was based upon clinical, radiological and histological studies of 23 cases.

D. J. McCune, H. Bruch: Osteodystrophia fibrosa: report of a case in which the condition was combined with precocious puberty, pathologic pigmentation of the skin and hyperthyroidism, with a review of the literature. American Journal of Diseases of Children, Chicago, 1937, 54: 806-848.

Jaffe-Lichtenstein-Sutro Syndrome

Overview

Jaffe-Lichtenstein-Sutro syndrome is a condition characterized by localized pain in one or more large joints, commonly the knee, accompanied by functional limitation in joint articulation. Systemic symptoms are notably absent, and the condition is primarily limited to the affected joint. The syndrome is associated with mild to moderate movement restriction and is not associated with systemic inflammatory markers or disease.

Historical Background

- The syndrome was described and delineated by *Henry Lewis Jaffe*, *Louis Lichtenstein*, and *C. J. Sutro*, who collectively studied joint pain syndromes without systemic involvement.
- Early investigations emphasized the absence of systemic symptoms and focused on the localized joint manifestations, distinguishing this syndrome from other arthropathies.

Purpose

- To identify the specific features of joint pain that lack systemic involvement and differentiate this syndrome from other inflammatory or degenerative joint diseases.
- To improve the understanding and management of localized joint pain with functional limitations.

Procedure Overview

- **Clinical Assessment:** Focused on localized joint pain and its impact on movement.
- **History-taking includes the duration, nature, and extent of joint pain.**
- **Physical Examination:** Evaluates range of motion, tenderness, swelling, and stiffness in the affected joint.
- **Imaging:** X-rays or MRI may be used to rule out degenerative or structural abnormalities in the joint.
- **Exclusion of Systemic Conditions:** Laboratory tests are conducted to ensure the absence of systemic inflammatory markers (e.g., CRP, ESR) or autoimmune indicators.

Results and Interpretation

- **Localized Findings:** Pain and functional limitation confined to the affected joint.
- **Imaging:** May show minor structural changes, but no systemic or inflammatory signs.
- **Clinical Differentiation:** Absence of systemic symptoms and markers confirms diagnosis and distinguishes it from other joint diseases.

Physiological Basis

- The underlying pathophysiology remains unknown, but the syndrome appears to involve localized joint dysfunction without systemic involvement.
- It may represent a unique response to stress or injury within the joint capsule or surrounding tissues.

Clinical Applications

- **Diagnosis:** Provides a framework for identifying patients with localized joint pain lacking systemic symptoms.
- **Management:** Focused on pain relief and maintaining joint function through physical therapy and conservative measures.

Limitations and Technical Considerations

- **Diagnosis of Exclusion:** Requires careful differentiation from systemic inflammatory conditions such as rheumatoid arthritis or osteoarthritis.
- **Subjectivity of Pain:** The reliance on subjective pain reports may complicate diagnosis.

Modern Relevance

- **Growing Recognition:** Increasing awareness of joint-specific pain syndromes has enhanced early diagnosis and management.
- **Emphasis on Joint Preservation:** Modern approaches focus on preserving joint function and preventing long-term complications.

Associated Conditions

- **Localized Joint Disorders:** May coexist with or mimic early osteoarthritis or mechanical joint dysfunction.

Clinical Importance

- **Early Diagnosis:** Enables targeted management to prevent progression and improve quality of life.
- **Symptom Relief:** Focuses on alleviating pain and restoring joint mobility through conservative measures.
- **Differentiation from Systemic Conditions:** Accurate identification avoids unnecessary systemic treatments and interventions.

References

H. L. Jaffe, L. Lichtenstein, C. J. Sutro: Pigmented villonodular synovitis, and bursitis, tenosynovitis. A discussion of the synovial and bursal equivalents of the tenosynovial lesion commonly denoted as xanthoma, xanthogranuloma, giant-cell tumor, or myeloplaxoms of the tendon sheath, with some consideration of this tendon sheath lesion itself. Archives of Pathology, Chicago, 1941, 31: 731-765.

Jefferson Fracture

Overview

The Jefferson fracture is a burst fracture of the atlas (C1), which typically occurs due to an axial load applied to the spine, such as a direct blow to the vertex of the head. This mechanism compresses the atlas between the occipital condyles and the axis (C2), resulting in lateral displacement of the C1 articular masses and fractures of its anterior and posterior arches. While these fractures are often stable due to the anatomical configuration of the atlas, associated injuries, including ligament damage and spinal cord involvement, can complicate the clinical picture.

Historical Background

- First described by *Sir Geoffrey Jefferson*, an eminent British neurosurgeon, in 1920. Jefferson highlighted the unique pattern of this fracture and its distinct mechanism involving axial loading of the cervical spine.
- His work contributed significantly to the understanding of cervical spine injuries, and the fracture was subsequently named in his honor.

Purpose

- To understand and diagnose cervical spine injuries, particularly those resulting from high-energy axial loading forces.
- To guide treatment strategies aimed at stabilizing the spine and preventing neurological complications.

Procedure Overview

- **Clinical Assessment:**
- Symptoms include neck pain, limited mobility, and, in some cases, neurological deficits.
- Neurological evaluation is critical to rule out spinal cord injury.
- **Imaging Studies:**
- **X-ray:** Open-mouth (odontoid) and lateral views to assess the C1-C2 alignment and fractures.
- **CT Scan:** Gold standard for visualizing the fracture pattern and evaluating lateral displacement.
- **MRI:** Used to assess ligamentous injury and spinal cord involvement.

Results and Interpretation

- **Imaging Findings:**
- Bilateral fractures of the anterior and posterior arches of the atlas.
- Lateral displacement of the C1 lateral masses.
- Occasionally, evidence of ligamentous injury or instability on MRI.
- **Neurological Assessment:**
- In many cases, the spinal cord remains unharmed due to the spacious nature of the spinal canal at the C1 level.
- Neurological deficits, when present, may indicate severe ligament damage or other associated injuries.

Physiological Basis

- The atlas (C1) acts as a transitional structure between the skull and the cervical spine, designed to bear axial loads.
- Axial compression forces from trauma result in a burst fracture, where the anterior and posterior arches fail under pressure.
- The lateral spread of the C1 articular masses accommodates the impact, often sparing the spinal cord from injury.

Clinical Applications

- **Stabilization:** Non-operative methods, such as external immobilization with a cervical collar or halo vest, are often sufficient for stable fractures.
- Surgical stabilization may be required in cases of significant instability or ligament damage.
- **Rehabilitation:** Early mobilization with careful supervision helps prevent complications such as muscle atrophy or stiffness.

Limitations and Technical Considerations

- **Imaging Challenges:**
- Open-mouth X-rays require precise positioning, which can be difficult in patients with pain or limited mobility.
- CT scans provide clearer imaging but may not detect subtle ligamentous injuries.
- **Risk of Missed Diagnosis:** Delays in diagnosis may occur if imaging studies are not carefully reviewed, especially in patients with concurrent injuries.

Modern Relevance

- Improved imaging modalities, such as high-resolution CT and MRI, have enhanced the accuracy of diagnosing Jefferson fractures.
- Advanced surgical techniques and instrumentation now offer better outcomes in unstable cases.
- Awareness of the fracture's mechanism has led to improved safety protocols in high-risk activities, such as sports and industrial work.

Associated Conditions

- **Occipital Condyle Injuries:** Concurrent injuries to the occiput may accompany a Jefferson fracture.
- **Transverse Ligament Disruption:** Instability due to transverse ligament injury is a significant concern.

Clinical Importance

- **Early Diagnosis:** Accurate and prompt identification of the fracture prevents long-term complications such as chronic instability.
- **Risk Stratification:** Differentiating between stable and unstable fractures guides appropriate management strategies.
- **Prevention of Neurological Injury:** Ensuring proper alignment and stabilization minimizes the risk of spinal cord damage.
- **Comprehensive Management:** Requires a multidisciplinary approach involving radiologists, orthopedic surgeons, and physical therapists for optimal outcomes.

References

Jefferson G. Fracture of the atlas vertebra: report of four cases, and a review of those previously recorded. Br J Surg. 1920;7(27):407–22.

Jersey Finger

Overview

Jersey Finger, also known as rugby or sweater finger, refers to the avulsion of the flexor digitorum profundus (FDP) tendon from its insertion on the volar base of the distal phalanx. This injury typically occurs when a flexed finger is forcibly hyperextended, as often seen in sports when an athlete grabs an opponent's jersey. The fourth digit (ring finger) is most commonly affected due to its unique anatomical susceptibility.

Historical Background

- The term "Jersey Finger" emerged in the context of sports medicine to describe injuries encountered in high-speed contact sports such as rugby and American football.
- Though the specific year of its first recognition is unclear, it became a well-recognized injury with the increasing popularity of contact sports in the mid-20th century, particularly in athletes attempting tackles.

Purpose

- **Early Diagnosis:** Prevent long-term functional impairment of the affected digit.
- **Restore Functionality:** Surgical or non-surgical treatment aims to reestablish active flexion at the distal interphalangeal joint (DIP).
- **Prevent Complications:** Early intervention avoids tendon retraction, stiffness, or chronic weakness.

Procedure Overview

- **Clinical Presentation:**
- The affected digit appears extended at the DIP joint.
- Inability to flex the DIP joint actively while passive motion remains intact.
- Commonly associated with tenderness and swelling at the distal phalanx.
- **Imaging:**
- **X-rays:** Rule out avulsion fractures and assess bony fragments.
- **Ultrasound:** Evaluate tendon anatomy, especially in non-fracture cases.
- **MRI:** Occasionally required for chronic or complex injuries.

Treatment:

- **Non-Surgical:** Rarely indicated, limited to minor injuries without retraction.
- **Surgical:** Tendon repair using pull-out sutures or anchor-based fixation.
- For chronic cases, tendon grafting or reconstruction may be required.
- Timing is critical; surgery is ideally performed within two weeks of injury.
- **Postoperative Care:** Immobilization followed by a structured physical therapy program for optimal recovery.

Results and Interpretation

- Early surgical intervention offers the best prognosis, with functional recovery in most cases.
- Delayed diagnosis or improper management often results in chronic stiffness, weakness, or tendon adhesions.

Physiological Basis

- **The FDP tendon enables flexion at the DIP joint by anchoring at the distal phalanx.**
- **Forced hyperextension against active contraction results in avulsion at its weakest point:** the insertion on the distal phalanx.
- The fourth digit is predisposed due to its unique role in grip mechanics and its comparatively weaker anatomical structure.

Clinical Applications

- **Sports Medicine:** Commonly encountered in athletes; rapid diagnosis and treatment prevent long-term disability.
- **Orthopedic Surgery:** Complex cases require expertise in tendon repair or reconstruction techniques.
- **Rehabilitation:** Essential to restore mobility, grip strength, and prevent re-injury.

Limitations and Technical Considerations

- **Delayed Diagnosis:** Leads to tendon retraction, complicating surgical repair.
- **Chronic cases require advanced techniques, such as tendon grafting.**
- **Surgical Challenges:** Proper tensioning of the tendon is critical to avoid complications like quadriga (inability to flex adjacent digits).
- **Risk of infection, adhesion forma-**

tion, and repair failure.**

- **Postoperative Recovery:** Requires strict compliance with immobilization and physical therapy protocols.

Modern Relevance

- Increased participation in high-speed sports has led to a rise in the incidence of jersey finger injuries.
- Advancements in imaging and surgical techniques have improved outcomes significantly.
- Emphasis on early detection and interprofessional management ensures better long-term results.

Associated Conditions

- **Quadriga Syndrome:** Over-tensioning during tendon repair affects adjacent digits.
- **Avulsion Fractures:** Commonly associated with FDP avulsion.
- **Tendon Adhesions:** Scar tissue formation limits motion, requiring aggressive physical therapy.

Clinical Importance

- Jersey Finger represents a *functional emergency* in sports medicine, as delays in treatment can lead to permanent loss of finger flexion and grip strength.
- Accurate diagnosis, timely surgical repair, and structured rehabilitation are essential for optimal recovery.
- Collaboration between sports physicians, orthopedic surgeons, radiologists, and rehabilitation specialists is critical to achieving favorable outcomes.
- By addressing the unique challenges of jersey finger, modern orthopedic and sports medicine can ensure athletes return to full functionality with minimal complications.

References

Lunn PG, Lamb DW. "Rugby finger"--avulsion of profundus of ring finger. J Hand Surg Br. 1984 Feb;9(1):69-71.

Folmar RC, Nelson CL, Phalen GS. Ruptures of the flexor tendons in hands of non-rheumatoid patients. J Bone Joint Surg Am. 1972 Apr;54(3):579-84. [PubMed]

Bachoura A, Ferikes AJ, Lubahn JD. A review of mallet finger and jersey finger injuries in the athlete. Curr Rev Musculoskelet Med. 2017 Mar;10(1):1-9. [PMC free article] [PubMed]

Yeh PC, Shin SS. Tendon ruptures: mallet, flexor digitorum profundus. Hand Clin. 2012 Aug;28(3):425-30, xi.

Ootes D, Lambers KT, Ring DC. The epidemiology of upper extremity injuries presenting to the emergency department in the United States. Hand (N Y). 2012 Mar;7(1):18-22. [PMC free article] [PubMed]

de Jong JP, Nguyen JT, Sonnema AJ, Nguyen EC, Amadio PC, Moran SL. The incidence of acute traumatic tendon injuries in the hand and wrist: a 10-year population-based study. Clin Orthop Surg. 2014 Jun;6(2):196-202.

BOYES JH, WILSON JN, SMITH JW. Flexor-tendon ruptures in the forearm and hand. J Bone Joint Surg Am. 1960 Jun;42-A:637-46. [PubMed]

Manske PR, Lesker PA. Avulsion of the ring finger flexor digitorum profundus tendon: an experimental study. Hand. 1978 Feb;10(1):52-5. [PubMed]

Leddy JP, Packer JW. Avulsion of the profundus tendon insertion in athletes. J Hand Surg Am. 1977 Jan;2(1):66-9.

Klauser A, Frauscher F, Bodner G, Halpern EJ, Schocke MF, Springer P, Gabl M, Judmaier W, zur Nedden D. Finger pulley injuries in extreme rock climbers: depiction with dynamic US. Radiology. 2002 Mar;222(3):755-61. [PubMed]

Zemirline A, Asmar G, Liverneaux PA. Conservative treatment in Jersey finger: a case report. J Plast Reconstr Aesthet Surg. 2013 Nov;66(11):1616-8. [PubMed]

Pappas N, Gay AN, Major N, Bozentka D. Case report: pseudotendon formation after a type III flexor digitorum profundus avulsion. Clin Orthop Relat Res. 2011 Aug;469(8):2385-8. [PMC free article] [PubMed]

Polfer EM, Sabino JM, Katz RD. Zone I Flexor Digitorum Profundus Repair: A Surgical Technique. J Hand Surg Am. 2019 Feb;44(2):164.e1-164.e5. [PubMed]

Halát G, Negrin LL, Unger E, Koch T, Streicher J, Erhart J, Platzer P, Hajdu S. Introduction of a new repair technique in bony avulsion of the FDP tendon: A biomechanical study. Sci Rep. 2018 Jul 02;8(1):9906. [PMC free article] [PubMed]

Tuttle HG, Olvey SP, Stern PJ. Tendon avulsion injuries of the distal phalanx. Clin Orthop Relat Res. 2006 Apr;445:157-68. [PubMed]

Becker H. Primary repair of flexor tendons in the hand without immobilisation-preliminary report. Hand. 1978 Feb;10(1):37-47. [PubMed]

Becker H, Orak F, Duponselle E. Early active motion following a beveled technique of flexor tendon repair: report on fifty cases. J Hand Surg Am. 1979 Sep;4(5):454-60. [PubMed]

Gillig JD, Smith MD, Hutton WC, Jarrett CD. The effect of flexor digitorum profundus tendon shortening on jersey finger surgical repair: a cadaveric biomechanical study. J Hand Surg Eur Vol. 2015 Sep;40(7):729-34. [PubMed]

Jones Fracture

Overview

The Jones fracture refers to a fracture of the proximal diaphysis of the 5th metatarsal, distal to the tuberosity, and typically without joint involvement. It is caused by foot inversion, twisting, or repetitive stress, and is distinct from avulsion fractures at the base of the metatarsal. The term is sometimes inconsistently applied, leading to classification using the Zone I, II, III system, which more accurately identifies the fracture's location and assists in determining appropriate treatment and management.

Historical Background

- Named after *Sir Robert Jones*, a pioneering general surgeon and orthopedist.
- In *1902*, Jones reported a personal case of a fracture sustained while dancing, describing the injury as resulting from "indirect violence." This led to its association with the name "Jones fracture."
- In *1960*, Stewart differentiated avulsion fractures of the tuberosity from fractures at the proximal diaphysis, reserving the term "Jones fracture" for the latter.
- Later classifications by *Torg et al. (1984)* and *Lawrence and Botte (1993)* further refined the understanding and terminology for these fractures.

Purpose

- To identify and treat fractures of the *5th metatarsal* that are prone to delayed healing or nonunion due to their anatomical and vascular characteristics.

- To classify these fractures for better prognosis and treatment planning, distinguishing them from avulsion injuries and stress fractures.

Procedure Overview

- **Clinical Examination:**
- Patients typically present with localized pain, swelling, and tenderness over the base of the 5th metatarsal.
- Pain is exacerbated by weight-bearing activities or inversion of the foot.
- **Imaging Studies:**
- **X-ray:** Standard AP, lateral, and oblique views of the foot reveal the fracture location and extent.
- **MRI or CT:** Used for further evaluation of stress fractures or chronic injuries.

Results and Interpretation

- **Zone Classification:**
- **Zone 1:** Tuberosity avulsion fractures, sometimes involving the tarsometatarsal joint.
- **Zone 2:** Jones fracture at the metaphyseal-diaphyseal junction, often extending into the fourth-fifth intermetatarsal facet.
- **Zone 3:** Diaphyseal stress fractures, distal to the fourth and fifth metatarsal articulation.
- **Radiographic Findings:**
- Clear fracture line in the affected zone.
- Delayed healing or signs of nonunion may be evident in chronic cases.

Physiological Basis

- The 5th metatarsal's proximal diaphysis has a *watershed area* with limited blood supply, making fractures in this region more prone to delayed union or nonunion.
- Stress fractures and acute injuries are influenced by repetitive loading or inversion forces that place undue strain on the lateral aspect of the foot.

Clinical Applications

- **Non-Operative Management:**
- Indicated for stable fractures or avulsion injuries (Zone 1).
- Immobilization using a cast or boot with non-weight-bearing activity for 6-8 weeks.
- **Surgical Management:**
- Recommended for displaced fractures, Zone 2 (Jones fractures), or Zone 3 stress fractures.
- Open reduction and internal fixation (ORIF) with screws or plates may be required.
- **Rehabilitation:**
- Progressive weight-bearing after healing is confirmed radiographically.
- Physical therapy to restore range of motion and strength.

Limitations and Technical Considerations

- **Delayed Healing:** Zone 2 fractures are particularly prone to nonunion due to poor vascular supply.

- **Misclassification:** Differentiating between Zone 1 and Zone 2 fractures can be challenging without advanced imaging.
- **Surgical Risks:** Risks include infection, hardware failure, or further injury during the recovery phase.

Modern Relevance

- The Zone classification system has improved treatment outcomes by enabling tailored management strategies for specific fracture types.
- **Advances in** imaging and surgical techniques now allow better outcomes even in complex cases.
- Recognition of the importance of biomechanics and repetitive stress in sports medicine has helped in the prevention and early diagnosis of Jones fractures.

Associated Conditions

- **Stress Fractures:** Chronic repetitive loading in Zone 3 can mimic or coexist with Jones fractures.
- **Avulsion Fractures:** Zone 1 fractures caused by peroneus brevis or plantar fascia forces are often confused with Jones fractures.
- **Ligament Injuries:** Concurrent sprains of the lateral ankle ligaments may accompany the fracture.

Clinical Importance

- **Early Diagnosis:** Timely identification prevents complications like delayed union or nonunion, particularly in Zone 2 fractures.
- **Prognostic Value:** Zone classification guides treatment and helps predict healing time and outcomes.
- **Interdisciplinary Management:** Collaboration between radiologists, orthopedic surgeons, and physical therapists ensures comprehensive care.
- **Athletic Considerations:** Common in athletes due to repetitive stress; requires tailored management to expedite return to play.

References

Stewart IM. Jones's fracture: fracture of base of fifth metatarsal. Clin Orthop. 1960;16:190-8. [PMID 13834594]

Torg JS, Balduini FC, Zelko RR, Pavlov H, Peff TC, Das M. Fractures of the base of the fifth metatarsal distal to the tuberosity. Classification and guidelines for non-surgical and surgical management. J Bone Joint Surg Am. 1984 Feb;66(2):209-14. [PMID 6693447]

Lawrence SJ, Botte MJ. Jones' fractures and related fractures of the proximal fifth metatarsal. Foot Ankle. 1993 Jul-Aug;14(6):358-65. [PMID 8406253]

Torg JS. Fractures of the base of the fifth metatarsal distal to the tuberosity. Orthopedics. 1990;13(7):731–7. [PMID 2197611].

Torg JS, Balduini FC, Zelko RR, Pavlov H, Peff TC, Das M. Fractures of the base of the fifth metatarsal distal to the tuberosity. Classification and guidelines for non-surgical and surgical management. J Bone Joint Surg Am. 1984;66(2):209–14 [PMID 6693447]

Petrisor BA, Ekrol I, Court-Brown C. The epidemiology of metatarsal fractures. Foot Ankle Int. 2006 Mar;27(3):172-4. [PMID 16539897]

Zwitser EW, Breederveld RS. Fractures of the fifth metatarsal; diagnosis and treatment. Injury. 2010 Jun;41(6):555-62. [PMID 19570536]

Polzer H, Polzer S, Mutschler W, Prall WC. Acute fractures to the proximal fifth metatarsal bone: development of classification and treatment recommendations based on the current evidence. Injury. 2012 Oct;43(10):1626-32. [PMID 22465516]

Jumper's Fracture

Overview

Jumper's Fracture, also known as suicidal jumper's fracture, refers to sacral fractures typically sustained from high-energy trauma such as falls from heights or vehicular accidents. These fractures are serious injuries often associated with pelvic instability, neurological deficits, and complex management requirements. A thorough neurological examination is critical to diagnosis and treatment planning.

Historical Background

- The term "jumper's fracture" emerged as these injuries were frequently observed in individuals who suffered falls from significant heights.
- **Advances in** imaging modalities like CT scans, beginning in the late 20th century, have significantly improved the diagnosis of sacral fractures, including jumper's fractures.

Purpose

- **Neurological Preservation:** Early identification and decompression of nerves to prevent permanent neurological deficits.
- **Stability Restoration:** Ensure structural stability of the sacral region and pelvic ring for effective rehabilitation.
- **Pain and Function Recovery:** Enable mobility and minimize chronic pain through appropriate intervention.

Procedure Overview

- **Clinical Presentation:**
- Symptoms include lower back pain, buttock pain, bruising, swelling, or laceration over the sacral area.
- Neurological signs include perineal or genital sensory changes, loss of sphincter tone, and lower extremity motor deficits.
- High suspicion is necessary for patients with high-energy trauma or persistent low back pain in athletes without clear injury.

Imaging:

- **X-rays:** Often insufficient due to the complexity of sacral anatomy.
- **CT scans:** Gold standard for identifying fracture patterns and associated pelvic injuries.
- **MRI:** Used to evaluate neurological structures and soft tissue involvement.

Management:

- **Non-Surgical:** Appropriate for stable fractures or stress fractures; involves immobilization and gradual rehabilitation.
- **Surgical:** Techniques like nerve decompression, fragment reduction, and lumbopelvic fixation are employed for unstable fractures.
- Minimally invasive approaches, such as sacroplasty, are gaining popularity to reduce complications.

Results and Interpretation

- Successful management often results in the resolution of pain and restoration of neurological function.

- Complications like malunion, infection, and hardware failure can impact long-term outcomes.

Physiological Basis

- The sacrum connects the spine to the pelvis, transferring forces from the upper body to the lower extremities. Fractures disrupt this critical load-bearing structure.
- High-energy impacts can cause both transverse and vertical fracture patterns, often associated with ligamentous injuries to the pelvic ring.

Clinical Applications

- **Trauma Management:** Critical in addressing injuries sustained in high-energy events such as falls and vehicular accidents.
- **Orthopedic Surgery:** Advanced fixation techniques for complex fracture patterns.
- **Rehabilitation:** Multidisciplinary care to restore function and prevent long-term disability.

Limitations and Technical Considerations

- **Complex Diagnosis:** High rates of missed or delayed diagnoses due to the subtle clinical presentation.
- **Overlapping symptoms with lumbar spinal conditions can mislead evaluation.**
- **Surgical Challenges:** High risk of perioperative complications, including neural injuries and excessive blood loss.
- **Postoperative complications like infection and hardware failure require vigilant follow-up.**
- **Patient Factors:** Osteoporotic fractures in elderly patients necessitate careful management to avoid further injury.

Modern Relevance

- Improved imaging modalities have enhanced early diagnosis, particularly in subtle or stress-related sacral fractures.
- Minimally invasive techniques, such as lumbopelvic fixation, offer promising results with fewer complications.
- Increased awareness among clinicians is crucial to prevent missed diagnoses and optimize treatment outcomes.

Associated Conditions

- **Pelvic Ring Injuries:** Often coexist with sacral fractures, necessitating integrated management.
- **Neurological Deficits:** Compression of sacral nerve roots leading to lower limb or sphincter dysfunction.
- **Osteoporosis:** Predisposes elderly patients to low-energy sacral fractures.

Clinical Importance

- Early and accurate diagnosis of jumper's fractures is critical to prevent long-term neurological complications and pelvic instability.
- Multidisciplinary management involving trauma surgeons, orthopedic specialists, and rehabilitation experts ensures comprehensive care.
- **Advances in** surgical techniques and minimally invasive approaches have significantly improved patient outcomes in complex sacral fractures.

- By addressing the diagnostic and treatment challenges of jumper's fractures, healthcare professionals can ensure optimal recovery and reduce the risk of chronic disability.

References

M van Berkel D, Ong T, Drummond A, et al. ASSERT (Acute Sacral inSufficiEncy fractuRe augmenTation) randomised controlled, feasibility in older people trial: a study protocol. BMJ Open 2019;9:e032111. [PMC free article] [PubMed]

Bydon M, De la, Garza-Ramos R, Macki M, Desai A, Gokaslan AK, Bydon A. Incidence of sacral fractures and in-hospital postoperative complications in the United States: an analysis of 2002–2011 data. Spine (Phila Pa 1976) 2014;39:E1103–E1109. [PubMed] [Google Scholar]

Lyders EM, Whitlow CT, Baker MD, Morris PP. Imaging and treatment of sacral insufficiency fractures. AJNR Am J Neuroradiol 2010;31:201–210. [PMC free article] [PubMed] [Google Scholar]

Tamaki Y, Nagamachi A, Inoue K, et al. Incidence and clinical features of sacral insufficiency fracture in the emergency department. Am J Emerg Med 2017;35:1314–1316. [PubMed] [Google Scholar]

Rommens PM, Arand C, Hofmann A, Wagner D. When and how to operate fragility fractures of the pelvis? Indian J Orthop 2019;53:128–137. [PMC free article] [PubMed] [Google Scholar]

Bydon M, Fredrickson V, De la, Garza-Ramos R, et al. Sacral fractures. Neurosurg Focus 2014;37:E12. [PubMed]

Beckmann NM, Chinapuvvula NR. Sacral fractures: classification and management. Emerg Radiol 2017;24:605–617.

Schroeder GD, Kurd MF, Kepler CK, et al. The development of a universally accepted sacral fracture classification: a survey of AOSpine and AOTrauma members. Global Spine J 2016;6:686–694.

Sakaguchi M, Maebayashi T, Aizawa T, Ishibashi N. Risk factors for sacral insufficiency fractures in cervical cancer after whole pelvic radiation therapy. Anticancer Res 2019;39:361–367. [PubMed] [Google Scholar]

Vajapey S, Matic G, Hartz C, Miller TL. Sacral stress fractures: a rare but curable cause of back pain in athletes. Sports Health 2019;11:446–452. [PMC free article] [PubMed] [Google Scholar]

Beckmann N, Cai C. CT characteristics of traumatic sacral fractures in association with pelvic ring injuries: correlation using the Young-Burgess classification system. Emerg Radiol 2017;24:255–262. [PubMed] [Google Scholar]

Park YS, Baek SW, Kim HS, Park KC. Management of sacral fractures associated with spinal or pelvic ring injury. J Trauma Acute Care Surg 2012;73:239–242. [PubMed] [Google Scholar]

Meinberg EG, Agel J, Roberts CS, Karam MD, Kellam JF. Fracture and dislocation classification compendium-2018. J Orthop Trauma 2018;32:S1–S170. [PubMed] [Google Scholar]

Burgess AR, Eastridge BJ, Young JW, et al. Pelvic ring disruptions: effective classification system and treatment protocols. J Trauma 1990;30:848–856. [PubMed] [Google Scholar]

Rommens PM, Hofmann A. Comprehensive classification of fragility fractures of the pelvic ring: recommendations for surgical treatment. Injury 2013;44:1733–1744. [PubMed] [Google Scholar]

Jüngling's disease

Overview

Jüngling's disease, also known as Perthes-Jüngling disease, is a specific osteitic manifestation of Boeck's sarcoidosis, presenting as a slowly progressive polycystic osteitis. It predominantly affects the bones of the fingers, toes, and nasal bone, and may involve surrounding soft tissues. It is thought to be associated with an infection by Mycobacterium tuberculosis strains. The disease is marked by cystic bone lesions and soft tissue involvement.

Historical Background

- First described by *Adolph Otto Jüngling* and later expanded by *Georg Clemens Perthes*, Jüngling's disease gained recognition for its unique polycystic osteitis presentation within the broader context of sarcoidosis.
- The linkage between sarcoidosis and tuberculosis-like infections remains a point of historical and ongoing debate, as this association was originally theorized when sarcoidosis was poorly understood.

Purpose

- To identify and characterize the *skeletal manifestations of sarcoidosis*, particularly in its polycystic osteitis form.
- To aid in distinguishing Jüngling's disease from other cystic bone conditions such as *osteomyelitis, enchondromas, and bone metastases.*

Procedure Overview

- **Clinical Examination:** Patients may present with localized swelling, pain, and restricted movement in affected areas (e.g., fingers, toes, or nasal bone).
- **Imaging Studies:**
- **X-ray:** Reveals cystic lesions in the bones, typically polycystic, with a lytic appearance.
- **MRI and CT:** Further delineate the extent of bony and soft tissue involvement.
- **Laboratory Tests:**
- Elevated serum angiotensin-converting enzyme (ACE) levels are often associated with sarcoidosis.
- Tests for latent or active Mycobacterium tuberculosis infection, such as tuberculin skin test or interferon-gamma release assays.

Results and Interpretation

- **Radiographic Findings:**
- Cystic bone lesions with distinct polycystic patterns.
- Involvement of surrounding soft tissues, often with granulomatous inflammation.
- **Histological Analysis:** Granulomas without caseation, characteristic of sarcoidosis, are typically found in affected tissues.
- **Differential Diagnosis:** Differentiates from other conditions such as enchondromas, metastatic bone disease, or osteomyelitis, which can mimic similar radiographic appearances.

Physiological Basis

- Sarcoidosis, a multisystem granulomatous disorder, leads to the formation of *non-caseating granulomas* in multiple organs, including the bones.
- In Jüngling's disease, the granulomas induce osteitic changes, resulting in cystic lesions and local tissue destruction.
- Possible involvement of *Mycobacterium tuberculosis* complicates the disease process by introducing infectious or immune-mediated mechanisms.

Clinical Applications

- **Diagnosis of Sarcoidosis:** Jüngling's disease may serve as a skeletal marker of systemic sarcoidosis, prompting further systemic evaluation.
- **Treatment of Osteitis:** Addresses bone-specific symptoms with corticosteroids or immunosuppressive therapies targeting the underlying sarcoid process.
- **Differentiation of Cystic Bone Diseases:** Helps in distinguishing sarcoid-related osteitis from malignant or infectious processes.

Limitations and Technical Considerations

- **Invasive Procedures:** Biopsy is often required for definitive diagnosis, adding potential risks of infection or complications.
- **Overlap in Imaging Findings:** Radiological appearance can mimic other cystic bone diseases, requiring correlation with clinical and laboratory findings.

- **Incomplete Understanding:** The role of Mycobacterium tuberculosis in the disease process remains speculative and may complicate treatment strategies.

Modern Relevance

- **Advances in** imaging modalities, such as *high-resolution MRI and PET scans*, allow for earlier detection and characterization of polycystic lesions.
- Improved understanding of the immunopathology of sarcoidosis has led to more targeted therapies for conditions like Jüngling's disease.
- Studies continue to explore the relationship between sarcoidosis and *latent tuberculosis infections*, especially in endemic regions.

Associated Conditions

- **Sarcoidosis:** Multisystem granulomatous disease affecting the lungs, lymph nodes, skin, and other organs.
- **Tuberculosis:** Coexistent or mimicking conditions may confuse the diagnostic process.
- **Bone Metastases and Osteomyelitis:** Must be ruled out during the evaluation of similar bone lesions.

Clinical Importance

- **Early Detection:** Recognizing Jüngling's disease as a manifestation of sarcoidosis aids in early diagnosis and systemic management.
- **Differential Diagnosis:** Essential to distinguish this condition from infectious or neoplastic bone diseases to guide appropriate therapy.
- **Systemic Monitoring:** Skeletal involvement in sarcoidosis often signals systemic disease, necessitating comprehensive evaluation.
- **Therapeutic Implications:** Proper diagnosis allows for effective use of corticosteroids and immunosuppressive agents, preventing disease progression and complications.

References

O. Jüngling: Ostitis tuberculosa multiplex cystica (eine eigenartige Form der Knochentuberkulose). Fortschritte auf dem Gebiete der Röntgenstrahlen, Hamburg, 1919-1921, 27: 375-383.

G. C. Perthes, in: Münchener medizinische Wochenschrift, 1922, 69: 99.

Kager Triangle/Fat Pad

Overview

The Kager Triangle, also known as the Kager Fat Pad or pre-Achilles fat pad, is an anatomical triangular structure composed of lipomatous (fat) tissue. It is bordered by:

- The *flexor hallucis longus muscle and tendon* anteriorly.
- The *superior cortex of the calcaneus* inferiorly.
- The *Achilles tendon* posteriorly.

The triangle plays a significant role in evaluating the integrity of the Achilles tendon and adjacent structures, particularly in conditions like Achilles tendon rupture.

Historical Background

- The term *Kager triangle* originates from *Dr. Hans Kager*, who first described this anatomical feature in his publication.
- The specific term "Kager triangle" was formally cited in a *1977 German publication*, although its clinical importance was recognized much earlier.

Purpose

- **Diagnostic Imaging:** The Kager triangle is an essential radiological landmark for assessing the Achilles tendon and detecting abnormalities such as ruptures, calcifications, or inflammation.
- **Surgical Guidance:** Identifies anatomical boundaries during procedures involving the posterior ankle, such as Achilles tendon repairs or retrocalcaneal bursectomies.

Procedure Overview

Radiographic Assessment:

- **Lateral ankle X-ray:** Used to visualize the triangle and identify deformities caused by Achilles tendon injuries.
- **Ultrasound and MRI:** Advanced modalities are used for detailed evaluation, especially in cases of suspected soft tissue injury.
- **Physical Examination:** While the triangle itself is not directly palpable, related conditions like tendon ruptures or bursitis may produce tenderness in the region.

Results and Interpretation

- **Normal Appearance:** A well-defined triangular space with clear borders, indicating an intact Achilles tendon and no abnormal fluid or masses in the retrocalcaneal bursa.
- **Pathological Findings:**
- Deformity or obliteration of the triangle on radiographs is a hallmark sign of an Achilles tendon rupture.
- Fluid or swelling in the region may indicate retrocalcaneal bursitis or adjacent soft tissue inflammation.

Physiological Basis

- The Kager triangle functions as a *protective cushion* for the Achilles tendon and adjacent structures, absorbing stress during movement.
- Its lipomatous composition helps reduce friction between the tendon, calcaneus, and surrounding tissues, ensuring

smooth ankle function.

Clinical Applications

- **Achilles Tendon Evaluation:** Critical in diagnosing tendon ruptures, particularly partial tears or complete disruptions.
- **Postoperative Monitoring:** Ensures proper healing and alignment following Achilles tendon repair surgery.
- **Differential Diagnosis:** Helps distinguish between Achilles tendon rupture, retrocalcaneal bursitis, and other posterior ankle pathologies.

Limitations and Technical Considerations

- **Imaging Challenges:** Conventional radiographs may not detect subtle abnormalities; advanced imaging like MRI may be necessary.
- **Non-specific Findings:** Changes in the triangle can result from multiple conditions, necessitating a comprehensive clinical evaluation.
- **Radiographic Quality:** Proper positioning is essential for accurate visualization; poor technique can obscure important details.

Modern Relevance

- **Advances in Imaging:** MRI and high-resolution ultrasound provide superior detail, making the Kager triangle a key feature in modern diagnostic protocols for Achilles tendon injuries.
- **Sports Medicine:** Increasing awareness of Achilles injuries in athletes has emphasized the importance of this anatomical landmark.

Associated Conditions

- **Achilles Tendon Rupture:** The most common condition associated with deformation of the Kager triangle.
- **Retrocalcaneal Bursitis:** Swelling in the retrocalcaneal bursa may alter the triangle's appearance.
- **Calcaneal Fractures:**
- **Can disrupt the inferior border of the triangle.**
- **Haglund Deformity:** Prominent calcaneal exostosis may compress the retrocalcaneal bursa and distort the triangle.

Clinical Importance

- **Early Detection:** Changes in the Kager triangle on imaging are often the first indication of Achilles tendon rupture, facilitating prompt diagnosis and treatment.
- **Prognostic Value:** Helps monitor healing and predict recovery outcomes following surgical or conservative treatment of Achilles injuries.
- **Surgical Relevance:** Serves as a key anatomical landmark during posterior ankle surgeries, ensuring precise and safe procedures.
- **Interdisciplinary Management:** Involves collaboration among radiologists, orthopedic surgeons, and physical therapists to optimize patient outcomes.

References

Ly JQ, Bui-Mansfield LT. Anatomy of and abnormalities associated with Kager's fat Pad. AJR Am J Roentgenol 2004; 182: 147–54.

RUTHERFORD RL. Surgical correction of retrocalcaneal bursitis (Haglund's disease). J Am Podiatry Assoc 1958; 48: 538–9.

Kaplan's Dislocation

Overview

Kaplan's Dislocation refers to a complex dislocation of the metacarpophalangeal (MCP) joint, most commonly affecting the index finger. It involves the metacarpal head buttonholing into the palm, making closed reduction challenging and often necessitating surgical intervention. The injury disrupts surrounding joint ligaments, significantly impairing joint function.

Historical Background

- In *1876*, Farabeuf et al. first described complex MCP dislocations involving the thumb.
- *Kaplan in 1957* described the specific anatomy and pathophysiology of the MCP dislocation of the index finger, highlighting the challenges in closed reduction due to buttonholing of the metacarpal head into the palm.

Purpose

- **Restoration of Joint Function:** Ensures proper joint alignment and mobility.
- **Prevention of Long-term Complications:** Mitigates risks like osteonecrosis, arthritis, or chronic stiffness.
- **Anatomical Repair:** Addresses ligament and volar plate injuries to restore joint stability.

Procedure Overview

- **Clinical Presentation:**
- Pain, swelling, and visible deformity at the MCP joint.
- Puckering of the palmar skin over the metacarpal head, indicative of a complex dislocation.
- Limited or absent joint mobility.
- **Imaging:**
- **X-rays:** Confirm dislocation and classify as simple or complex.
- **MRI/CT (if necessary):** Evaluate associated ligamentous or osteochondral injuries.

Reduction Techniques:

- **Simple Dislocations:** Managed with closed reduction by hyperextending the MCP joint and pushing the proximal phalanx over the metacarpal head.
- **Avoid longitudinal traction, as it risks converting a simple dislocation into a complex one.**
- **Complex Dislocations:** Require open reduction, usually via a dorsal approach.
- Ensures safe manipulation of displaced structures and repair of ligamentous injuries.
- **Post-procedure Care:** Immobilization for a short duration followed by guided rehabilitation to restore range of motion.

Results and Interpretation

- Prompt and appropriate management typically results in good functional outcomes.
- Delay in treatment or inadequate reduction can lead to chronic stiffness, joint instability, or degenerative changes.

Physiological Basis

- The MCP joint consists of the metacarpal head articulating with the base of the proximal phalanx, surrounded by a capsule and stabilized by collateral ligaments and the volar plate.
- In complex dislocations, the metacarpal head buttonholes through the volar plate and ligaments, disrupting the joint's structural integrity and hindering reduction.

Clinical Applications

- **Orthopedic Surgery:** Open reduction techniques for complex dislocations.
- **Emergency Medicine:** Initial diagnosis and closed reduction attempts for simple dislocations.
- **Rehabilitation:** Post-reduction physiotherapy to regain mobility and strength.

Limitations and Technical Considerations

- **Closed Reduction:** Limited to simple dislocations.
- **Risk of converting to complex dislocation if traction is applied.**
- **Open Reduction:** Requires precise surgical technique to avoid neurovascular injury.
- The dorsal approach is preferred for its safety and effective visualization.

Modern Relevance

- **Advances in** imaging and surgical techniques have improved outcomes in managing Kaplan's dislocations.
- Enhanced understanding of pathophysiology ensures timely identification and appropriate categorization of dislocations, guiding optimal treatment.

Associated Conditions

- **Ligamentous Injuries:** Frequently accompany MCP dislocations.
- **Osteochondral Fractures:** May complicate the reduction process.
- **Arthritis:** A long-term complication of inadequately treated dislocations.

Clinical Importance

- **Emergency Intervention:** Immediate management prevents complications like joint stiffness and chronic pain.
- **Functional Preservation:** Early surgical repair restores joint congruity and mobility.
- **Education and Awareness:** Training healthcare providers on recognizing Kaplan's dislocation ensures timely and effective care.

Kaplan's dislocation, while rare, poses significant challenges that require a clear understanding of anatomy, appropriate diagnostic tools, and skilled intervention to optimize outcomes.

References

Kozmaryn LM. The collateral ligament of the digits of the hand:Anatomy, physiology, biomechanics, injury, and treatment. J Hand Surg. 2017;42:904–15. [PubMed] [Google Scholar]

Dinh P, Franklin A, Hutchinson B, Schnall SB, Fassola I. Metacarpophalangeal joint dislocation. J Am Acad Orthop Surg. 2009;17:318–24. [PubMed] [Google Scholar]

Barry K, McGee H, Curtin J. Complex dislocation of the metacarpophalangeal joint of the index finger:A comparison of the surgical approaches. J Hand Surg Br. 1988;13:466–8. [PubMed] [Google Scholar]

Calfee RP, Sommerkamp TG. Fracture-dislocation about the finger joints. J Hand Surg Am. 2009;34:1140–7. [PubMed]

Kaplan EB. Dorsal dislocation of the metacarpophalangeal joint of the index finger. J Bone Joint Surg Am. 1957;39:1081–6. [PubMed] [Google Scholar]

Rubin G, Orbach H, Rinott M, Rozen N. Complex dorsal metacarpophalangeal dislocation:Long-term follow-up. J Hand Surg. 2016;41:e229–33. [PubMed] [Google Scholar]

Vigneswaran V, Bhardwaj P. Dorsal dislocation of the metacarpophalangeal joint of the index finger. J Bone Joint Surg Am. 1957;39-A:1081–6. [PubMed] [Google Scholar]

Patterson RW, Maschke SD, Evans PJ, Lawton JN. Dorsal approach for open reduction of complex metacarpophalangeal joint dislocations. Orthopedics. 2008;31:1099. [PubMed] [Google Scholar]

Light TR, Ogden JA. Complex dislocation of the index metacarpophalangeal joint in children. J Pediatr Orthop. 1988;8:300–5. [PubMed] [Google Scholar]

Meurer WJ, Kronick SL, Lowell MJ, Desmond JS, Mudgal CS. Complex metacarpophalangeal dislocation. Int J Emerg Med. 2008;1:227–8.

Kienbock Disease

Overview

Kienböck Disease, also known as lunatomalacia, refers to avascular necrosis (AVN) of the lunate bone, one of the carpal bones in the wrist. It leads to the progressive collapse of the lunate, causing chronic pain, limited motion, and, if untreated, arthritis. It most commonly affects males aged 20 to 40 years and is the second most common AVN of the carpal bones.

Historical Background

- **1910:** Austrian radiologist Robert Kienböck first described the condition, linking it to AVN of the lunate.
- Since then, the disease has been studied extensively, with a focus on its multifactorial etiology and progression.

Purpose

- **Preserve Joint Function:** Prevent progressive degeneration of the wrist by maintaining motion and grip strength.
- **Alleviate Pain:** Manage chronic discomfort associated with lunate collapse.
- **Prevent Arthritis:** Minimize secondary degenerative changes in the wrist.

Procedure Overview

Diagnosis:

- Patients present with wrist pain, stiffness, and weakness, often without a history of significant trauma.
- Physical examination reveals tenderness

over the lunate, reduced grip strength, and decreased range of motion.

Imaging:

- **X-rays:** Reveal sclerosis and collapse of the lunate in advanced stages.
- **MRI:** Best modality to detect early-stage avascular necrosis.
- **CT scans:** Useful for assessing bone morphology and joint alignment.

Staging (Lichtman Classification):

- **Stage I:** Normal radiographs; changes visible on MRI.
- **Stage II:** Sclerosis of the lunate without collapse.
- **Stage IIIA:** Collapse of the lunate without scapholunate dissociation.
- **Stage IIIB:** Collapse with scapholunate dissociation.
- **Stage IV:** Advanced arthritis.

Treatment Options:

- **Non-Surgical:** Activity modification, splinting, NSAIDs.
- **Surgical:** Revascularization: Enhances blood supply to the lunate.
- **Joint-leveling procedures:** Radial shortening or ulnar lengthening to address ulnar negative variance.
- **Partial or total wrist fusion:** For advanced disease with arthritis.

Results and Interpretation

- Early diagnosis and intervention improve outcomes.
- Surgical procedures aim to slow disease progression, alleviate pain, and maintain wrist function. In late stages, joint fusion provides pain relief at the expense of motion.

Physiological Basis

- The lunate relies on a sparse vascular supply, primarily from dorsal and volar branches of the radiocarpal and intercarpal arches. Poor collateral circulation makes it prone to ischemia.
- Overload due to *ulnar negative variance*, abnormal lunate morphology, or repetitive microtrauma exacerbates vascular compromise, leading to AVN.

Clinical Applications

- Early-stage interventions include *revascularization techniques* and unloading procedures to preserve wrist motion.
- Advanced-stage management often requires *fusion procedures* to restore joint stability and mitigate pain.

Limitations and Technical Considerations

Late-stage diagnosis limits the success of motion-preserving interventions.

- **Surgical outcomes depend on:** Precise identification of the stage.
- Addressing the underlying anatomical or mechanical contributors.
- *Complications* of surgery include infection, stiffness, and hardware failure.

Modern Relevance

- **Advances in** imaging, such as MRI, allow earlier detection of Kienböck disease.
- Surgical innovations, including

vascularized bone grafts and arthroscopy, have improved treatment outcomes and reduced complications.

Associated Conditions

- **Ulnar Negative Variance:** Shortened ulna relative to the radius is a significant predisposing factor.
- **Trauma:** Though not always present, repetitive microtrauma increases the risk.
- **Arthritis:** A common sequela of untreated Kienböck disease.

Clinical Importance

- **Progressive Nature:** Left untreated, Kienböck disease leads to severe wrist arthritis and significant functional impairment.
- **Early Intervention:** Prevents lunate collapse and secondary joint degeneration.
- **Holistic Management:** Requires a multidisciplinary approach involving orthopedic surgeons, physical therapists, and radiologists to optimize outcomes.

Kienböck disease highlights the importance of understanding carpal anatomy, biomechanics, and vascular supply in diagnosing and managing wrist pathologies effectively.

References

Murphey MD, Foreman KL, Klassen-Fischer MK, Fox MG, Chung EM, Kransdorf MJ. From the radiologic pathology archives imaging of osteonecrosis: radiologic-pathologic correlation. Radiographics. 2014 Jul-Aug;34(4):1003-28.

Arnaiz J, Piedra T, Cerezal L, Ward J, Thompson A, Vidal JA, Canga A. Imaging of Kienböck disease. AJR Am J Roentgenol. 2014 Jul;203(1):131-9.

Rhee PC, Jones DB, Moran SL, Shin AY. The effect of lunate morphology in Kienböck disease. J Hand Surg Am. 2015 Apr;40(4):738-44.

Thienpont E, Mulier T, Rega F, De Smet L. Radiographic analysis of anatomical risk factors for Kienböck's disease. Acta Orthop Belg. 2004 Oct;70(5):406-9.

Lutsky K, Beredjiklian PK. Kienböck disease. J Hand Surg Am. 2012 Sep;37(9):1942-52.

Quenzer DE, Linscheid RL, Vidal MA, Dobyns JH, Beckenbaugh RD, Cooney WP. Trispiral tomographic staging of Kienböck's disease. J Hand Surg Am. 1997 May;22(3):396-403.

Goldfarb CA, Hsu J, Gelberman RH, Boyer MI. The Lichtman classification for Kienböck's disease: an assessment of reliability. J Hand Surg Am. 2003 Jan;28(1):74-80.

Schmitt R, Heinze A, Fellner F, Obletter N, Strühn R, Bautz W. Imaging and staging of avascular osteonecroses at the wrist and hand. Eur J Radiol. 1997 Sep;25(2):92-103.

van Leeuwen WF, Tarabochia MA, Schuurman AH, Chen N, Ring D. Risk Factors of Lunate Collapse in Kienböck Disease. J Hand Surg Am. 2017 Nov;42(11):883-888.e1.

Wagner JP, Chung KC. A historical report on Robert Kienböck (1871-1953) and Kienböck's Disease. J Hand Surg Am. 2005 Nov;30(6):1117-21. [PubMed]

Viegas SF, Patterson RM, Todd PD, McCarty P. Load mechanics of the midcarpal joint. J Hand Surg Am. 1993 Jan;18(1):14-8. [PubMed]

Schuind F, Cooney WP, Linscheid RL, An KN, Chao EY. Force and pressure transmission through the normal wrist. A theoretical two-dimensional study in the posteroanterior plane. J Biomech. 1995 May;28(5):587-601. [PubMed]

van Leeuwen WF, Oflazoglu K, Menendez ME, Ring D. Negative Ulnar Variance and Kienböck Disease. J Hand Surg Am. 2016 Feb;41(2):214-8. [PubMed]

Murphey MD, Foreman KL, Klassen-Fischer MK, Fox MG, Chung EM, Kransdorf MJ. From the radiologic pathology archives imaging of osteonecrosis: radiologic-pathologic correlation. Radiographics. 2014 Jul-Aug;34(4):1003-28.

Klippel's deformity

Overview

Klippel's Deformity, also known as Sprengel's deformity, is a congenital condition characterized by the elevation and malposition of the scapula. It is frequently associated with other skeletal anomalies, including vertebral and rib abnormalities, and often results in cosmetic concerns, limited shoulder movement, and asymmetry of the neck and shoulders.

Historical Background

- The deformity is named after *Maurice Klippel*, a French neurologist, who first described the condition in association with other skeletal anomalies.
- The condition has also been studied in-depth by other clinicians and radiologists, leading to its synonymous designation as *Sprengel's deformity.*

Purpose

- **Functional Evaluation:** Assessment focuses on shoulder mobility and the impact of the deformity on daily activities.
- **Aesthetic Consideration:** Evaluation of asymmetry for potential surgical or non-surgical interventions.
- **Diagnosis of Associated Conditions:** Identify related anomalies, such as Klippel-Feil syndrome, cervical ribs, or spinal malformations.

Procedure Overview

- **Clinical Examination:**
- Observing for elevated scapula, shoulder asymmetry, and restricted shoulder abduction.
- Assessing associated anomalies like rib or vertebral deformities.
- **Radiographic Imaging:**
- **X-rays:** Detect the high scapular position and related skeletal anomalies.
- **MRI and CT scans:** Used for detailed visualization of musculoskeletal abnormalities and planning corrective surgery.

Results and Interpretation

- **Clinical Findings:**
- Elevated scapula, often with inferior rotation and medial displacement.
- Restricted shoulder movement, particularly abduction.
- **Radiographic Findings:**
- Evidence of hypoplastic or dysplastic scapula.
- Associated vertebral anomalies, such as cervical fusion or rib anomalies.

Physiological Basis

- The deformity arises due to *failure of the scapula to descend* to its normal position during embryonic development.
- The abnormal scapular position affects the biomechanics of the shoulder girdle, limiting the range of motion and causing asymmetry.

Clinical Applications

- **Orthopedic Assessment:** Evaluates shoulder function and potential for improving mobility through physical therapy or surgery.

- **Cosmetic Surgery:** Addressing aesthetic concerns through procedures like scapular repositioning.
- **Diagnosis of Syndromes:** Identifying Klippel's deformity as a part of syndromic conditions such as Klippel-Feil syndrome or other congenital abnormalities.

Limitations and Technical Considerations

- **Radiographic Limitations:** X-rays may not fully visualize soft tissue anomalies; MRI or CT may be required for comprehensive evaluation.
- **Surgical Challenges:** Corrective surgery is complex and may involve risks such as nerve damage or incomplete functional recovery.
- **Delayed Diagnosis:** Mild cases may be overlooked in childhood, leading to delayed management of functional limitations or cosmetic concerns.

Modern Relevance

- **Pediatric Orthopedics:** Enhanced imaging techniques allow earlier diagnosis and intervention in affected children.
- **Reconstructive Surgery Advances:** Improvements in surgical techniques have increased the success rate of scapular repositioning and functional restoration.
- **Public Awareness:** Increased focus on early detection through routine pediatric evaluations.

Associated Conditions

- **Klippel-Feil Syndrome:** Fusion of cervical vertebrae, often co-occurring with Klippel's deformity.
- **Cervical Ribs:** Extra ribs arising from cervical vertebrae.
- **Scoliosis:** Spinal curvature commonly seen in affected individuals.
- **Congenital Muscular Torticollis:** Neck muscle tightness causing head tilt, sometimes associated with this deformity.

Clinical Importance

- **Early Diagnosis:** Early recognition allows for timely interventions, including physical therapy or surgical correction.
- **Improved Quality of Life:** Addressing functional limitations through targeted therapies helps enhance daily living activities.
- **Aesthetic and Psychological Support:** Corrective measures can address cosmetic concerns, boosting self-esteem in affected individuals.
- **Interdisciplinary Care:**Collaboration between pediatricians, orthopedic surgeons, and physical therapists ensures comprehensive management.

Klippel-Feil deformity

Overview

Klippel-Feil deformity is a rare congenital anomaly characterized by a reduced number of cervical vertebrae or multiple hemivertebrae fused into a single osseous mass, resulting in a short, wide neck with restricted motion. Additional hallmark features include a low hairline, facial asymmetry, and limited cervical mobility. The condition often has a wide range of associated abnormalities affecting the skeletal, muscular, and neurological systems. It is more prevalent in females (65%) and can vary greatly in severity.

Historical Background

- **1743:** Victor Albrecht von Haller (1708–1777) documented anatomical features suggestive of this condition.
- **1746:** Giovanni Battista Morgagni (1682–1771) described a similar condition in his anatomical studies.
- **1893:** Sir Jonathan Hutchinson (1828–1913) is believed to have provided the first clinical description of Klippel-Feil syndrome.
- **1912:** Maurice Klippel and André Feil offered a comprehensive interpretation of the deformity, leading to its eponymous designation.
- *Nielsen's syndrome*, a combination of Klippel-Feil syndrome and *Bonnevie-Ullrich syndrome (pterygium colli)*, was later defined.

Purpose

- **Early Diagnosis:** Facilitates timely identification of associated anomalies such as scoliosis, torticollis, or neurological deficits.
- **Functional Assessment:** Evaluates the extent of neck mobility and its impact on daily activities.
- **Preventive Management:** Addresses complications such as spinal instability or neurological impairment.

Procedure Overview

- **Clinical Examination:** Observation for hallmark features like a short neck, low hairline, and restricted cervical mobility.
- Assessment of associated anomalies such as facial asymmetry, scoliosis, or torticollis.
- **Radiographic Imaging:**
- **X-rays:** Detect reduced cervical vertebrae and bony fusions.
- **MRI and CT scans:** Evaluate soft tissue involvement, spinal cord abnormalities, and nerve compression.
- **Genetic Testing:** Performed in familial cases to confirm suspected inheritance patterns.

Results and Interpretation

- **Clinical Findings:**
- Hallmark features include a short, wide neck, low posterior hairline, and restricted cervical motion.
- Neurological symptoms such as nystagmus, ataxia, or spastic quadriplegia may be present in severe cases.

- **Radiographic Features:**
  - Fusion of two or more cervical vertebrae, hemivertebrae, or anomalies in the thoracic or lumbar spine.
  - Possible evidence of scoliosis, kyphosis, or thoracic outlet syndrome.

Physiological Basis

- The deformity arises due to a *failure of normal segmentation* of the cervical vertebrae during embryonic development, leading to fused vertebral segments and associated anomalies.
- The resulting structural abnormalities often lead to *neurological compression*, *skeletal deformities*, and limitations in neck movement.

Clinical Applications

- **Orthopedic Surgery:** For correction of severe scoliosis, kyphosis, or spinal instability.
- **Neurological Interventions:** Addressing nerve compression or associated neurological deficits.
- **Physical Therapy:** Improving range of motion and preventing muscle atrophy.
- **Multidisciplinary Care:** Managing associated symptoms such as respiratory or swallowing difficulties.

Limitations and Technical Considerations

- **Variable Severity:** The wide spectrum of presentation necessitates individualized treatment plans.
- **Surgical Risks:** Neurological structures are at risk during corrective surgeries, requiring meticulous planning and execution.
- **Delayed Diagnosis:** Mild cases may be overlooked, delaying appropriate intervention.
- **Genetic Counseling:** Important in familial cases, but genetic testing may not always pinpoint causative mutations.

Modern Relevance

- **Advanced Imaging:** MRI and CT scans provide detailed insights into spinal cord and skeletal anomalies, improving diagnostic accuracy.
- **Improved Surgical Techniques:** Allow for safer correction of severe deformities and associated conditions like scoliosis or thoracic outlet syndrome.
- **Enhanced Genetic Understanding:** Helps in identifying inheritance patterns and potential gene mutations.

Associated Conditions

- **Bonnevie-Ullrich Syndrome (Pterygium Colli):** When combined with Klippel-Feil syndrome, it is termed Nielsen's syndrome.
- **Scoliosis and Kyphosis:** Common skeletal deformities associated with the condition.
- **Torticollis:** Neck muscle abnormalities leading to head tilt.
- **Neurological Impairments:** Spastic quadriplegia, synkinesis, or sensory deficits may occur due to spinal cord involvement.

Clinical Importance

- **Early Diagnosis:** Enables prompt intervention to prevent complications such as progressive scoliosis or neurological deficits.
- **Holistic Management:** Multidisciplinary approach addressing orthopedic, neurological, and respiratory aspects of the condition.
- **Improved Quality of Life:**
- Through physical therapy, surgical correction, and supportive care.
- **Genetic Counseling:** Essential for families with hereditary cases to understand risks and recurrence probabilities.

References

A. von Haller: Icones anatomicae quibus praecipuae aliquae partes corporis humani delineatae proponutur et arterianum potissimum historia continuatr.

8 parts, Gottingae, A. Vandenhoeck, 1743-1756.

M. Klippel, A. Feil:

Un cas d'absence des vertèbres cervicales avec cage thoracique remontant jusqu' à la base du crâne (cage thoracique cervicale).

Nouvelle iconographie de la Salpêtrière, Paris, 1912; 25: 223-250.

English translation in Bick, Classics of Orthopaedics, 511-516.

Köhler's disease I

Overview

Köhler's disease I is a rare condition involving avascular necrosis of the tarsal navicular bone, primarily affecting children between the ages of 3 to 8 years. This condition occurs due to repetitive compressive forces disrupting the blood supply to the navicular bone, which is not fully ossified at this developmental stage. Clinical presentations include medial foot pain, tenderness on palpation, and sometimes a slight limp. The condition is more prevalent in males and is usually unilateral.

Historical Background

- **1908:** The disease was first described by Alban Köhler, a German radiologist, who noted its radiographic features and associated symptoms.
- **1910:** Albert Mouchet and Hans Jessen Panner contributed additional descriptions and case studies, establishing the pathological basis of the condition.
- The disorder's discovery marked a significant advancement in understanding pediatric avascular necrosis and skeletal development.

Purpose

- **Early Detection:** Identifying avascular necrosis in its initial stages to prevent long-term deformities.
- **Management of Symptoms:** Addressing pain, swelling, and gait abnormalities in affected children.

- **Preserving Bone Integrity:** Preventing further fragmentation or collapse of the navicular bone through timely intervention.

Procedure Overview

- **Clinical Examination:**
- Observation for localized pain, tenderness, and swelling over the medial side of the foot.
- Assessment of limping or gait abnormalities.
- **Radiographic Imaging:** X-rays are the primary diagnostic tool, showing sclerosis, fragmentation, and flattening of the navicular bone.
- **Advanced Imaging:** MRI or CT scans may be utilized in ambiguous cases to assess the extent of necrosis and soft tissue involvement.

Results and Interpretation

- **Radiographic Features:**
- The navicular bone appears flattened, fragmented, and sclerotic.
- As the condition progresses, signs of reossification may become evident, indicating healing.
- **Clinical Findings:**
- Pain and swelling localized to the medial side of the foot.
- Affected children may exhibit a slight limp or difficulty bearing weight on the affected side.

Physiological Basis

- **Pathogenesis:**
- Köhler's disease I is caused by ischemia and necrosis of the tarsal navicular bone due to repetitive compressive forces that impair its blood supply.
- The condition occurs during a critical period of skeletal development when the navicular bone is highly susceptible to vascular disruption.

Clinical Applications

- **Non-Surgical Management:** Rest, activity modification, and the use of orthopedic devices like arch supports or casts to offload pressure on the navicular bone.
- **Physical Therapy:** To restore normal gait patterns and strengthen supporting muscles once acute symptoms subside.
- **Follow-Up Imaging:** Monitoring reossification and recovery of the navicular bone to ensure proper healing.

Limitations and Technical Considerations

- **Delayed Diagnosis:** Symptoms can be mild or asymptomatic, leading to delayed presentation and diagnosis.
- **Radiographic Limitations:** Early stages of the disease may not be apparent on X-rays, necessitating advanced imaging techniques.
- **Recurrence or Persistence:** Rare cases may progress to long-term deformities if untreated or if the vascular supply does not recover adequately.

Modern Relevance

- **Improved Imaging Techniques:** MRI and CT scans enable earlier and more accurate diagnosis, especially in ambiguous cases.

- **Enhanced Treatment Protocols:** Modern orthopedic interventions, such as custom orthotics, improve outcomes and reduce recovery time.
- **Increased Awareness:** Greater recognition of Köhler's disease I among pediatricians and orthopedic surgeons ensures timely intervention.

Associated Conditions

- **Panner's Disease:** A similar avascular necrosis condition affecting the capitellum of the humerus, which also shares a link to repetitive stress.
- **Sever's Disease:** Involves the calcaneal apophysis and presents with heel pain, commonly observed in active children.

Clinical Importance

- **Early Diagnosis:** Timely identification prevents the progression of necrosis and deformity.
- **Prognosis:** Early intervention leads to complete recovery in most cases, with minimal long-term effects.
- **Multidisciplinary Approach:** Collaboration between pediatricians, orthopedic specialists, and physical therapists ensures optimal patient outcomes.
- **Parental Guidance:** Educating caregivers about the benign nature of the disease and the importance of adherence to treatment plans promotes faster recovery.

References

A. Köhler: Über eine häufige, bisher anscheinend unbekannte Erkrankung einzelner kindlicher Knochen. Münchener medizinische Wochenschrift. 1908, 55: 1923-1925.

König's Syndrome I

Overview

König's Syndrome I is a condition involving osteochondritis dissecans, a joint disorder affecting the subchondral bone and articular cartilage. This disorder leads to inflammatory processes and necrosis within the subchondral bone, with the eventual formation of loose fragments in the joint cavity. It typically affects tubular bones, particularly weight-bearing joints like the knee, elbow, or ankle. While asymptomatic for extended periods, patients may experience sharp pain in the affected joint, exacerbated by activity or pressure, and occasional joint locking.

Historical Background

- **1888:** The condition was first described by Franz König, a German surgeon, who identified the formation of loose bodies in joint cavities due to subchondral inflammation and necrosis.
- **1870:** Prior to König's description, Sir James Paget had observed similar findings, particularly noting loose bodies as part of joint pathologies.
- König's work clarified the role of *osteochondritis* in the progression of the disease and the subsequent detachment of necrotic fragments.

Purpose

- **Identifying Early Symptoms:** Recognize joint inflammation and early necrosis to prevent progression to chronic joint dysfunction.
- **Managing Joint Stability:** Reduce the likelihood of joint locking and improve

functionality.

- **Preventing Chronic Complications:** Minimize the risk of degenerative arthritis associated with prolonged untreated osteochondritis.

Procedure Overview

- **Clinical Evaluation:**
- Assessment of joint pain, swelling, and range of motion.
- Identification of transitory joint locking episodes.
- **Imaging Techniques:**
- **X-rays:** To detect subchondral bone necrosis and loose bodies in the joint cavity.
- **MRI:** Provides detailed visualization of cartilage integrity and early subchondral changes.
- **CT scans:** Used for precise mapping of bony fragments and joint architecture.
- **Arthroscopy:** Utilized for direct visualization and, if necessary, removal of loose bodies.

Results and Interpretation

- **Imaging Findings:**
- Presence of loose bodies within the joint cavity.
- Subchondral necrosis and cartilage defects seen on **MRI or** X-rays.
- **Clinical Presentation:**
- Sharp, localized joint pain with intermittent locking episodes.
- Swelling and tenderness over the affected joint.

Physiological Basis

- **Pathogenesis:**
- König's Syndrome I originates with ischemic necrosis in the subchondral bone, leading to fragmentation of the cartilage and detachment into the joint cavity.
- The inflammatory response contributes to further joint degradation and the formation of loose bodies.

Clinical Applications

- **Non-Surgical Management:**
- Rest, physiotherapy, and anti-inflammatory medications for mild cases.
- Immobilization to allow natural healing of subchondral bone.
- **Surgical Interventions:**
- **Arthroscopic Removal:** Extraction of loose bodies to alleviate symptoms.
- **Microfracture Technique:** Stimulates cartilage repair by creating small bone perforations.
- **Osteochondral Grafting:** For advanced cases requiring cartilage restoration.

Limitations and Technical Considerations

- **Delayed Diagnosis:** Early stages may be asymptomatic, delaying treatment and increasing the risk of complications.
- **Treatment Variability:** Outcomes depend on the location and severity of the necrotic lesion.
- **Post-Treatment Arthritis:** In some cases, residual joint degeneration may persist despite treatment.

Modern Relevance

- **Advances in Imaging:** MRI provides earlier detection of subchondral necrosis, improving treatment timelines.
- **Minimally Invasive Surgery:** Arthroscopic techniques have reduced recovery times and improved outcomes.
- **Preventive Strategies:** Improved understanding of biomechanical stress on joints has influenced preventive care in athletes and at-risk populations.

Associated Conditions

- **Osteochondritis Dissecans:** Related condition involving similar processes in joints like the knee or elbow.
- **Avascular Necrosis:** Overlapping pathology seen in other joints due to disrupted blood supply.

Clinical Importance

- **Early Diagnosis:** Identifying the condition during its asymptomatic phase prevents progression to chronic dysfunction.
- **Prognostic Indicator:** The size and location of necrotic lesions influence long-term outcomes and recovery potential.
- **Interdisciplinary Approach:** Collaboration between radiologists, orthopedic surgeons, and physiotherapists optimizes treatment and rehabilitation.
- **Patient Education:** Counseling patients on activity modifications and compliance with treatment plans aids in recovery and reduces recurrence.

References

F. König: Über freie Körper in den Gelenken. Deutsche Zeitschrift für Chirurgie, Leipzig, 1887/1888, 27: 90-109.

Lehrbuch der allgemeinen Chirurgie für Aerzte und Studierende. Berlin, 1889, page 751.

Koslowski's Syndrome

Overview

Koslowski's Syndrome is a rare dwarfing skeletal dysplasia characterized by disproportionate short stature, primarily affecting the trunk. Key features include waddling gait, limited joint mobility, kyphoscoliosis, pectus carinatum, bowed legs, and irregular metaphyses. The condition also presents with occasional hyperopia and genua valga, with affected adults typically reaching a height of 130–165 cm. Radiographic findings include platyspondyly and broad, short basilar parts of the iliac bones. It is inherited in an autosomal dominant manner.

Historical Background

- **1960s:** First detailed description provided by Kazimierz S. Koslowski, a Polish radiologist, who identified the skeletal anomalies characteristic of the syndrome.
- **1970s:** Further expanded upon by Pierre Maroteaux and Jürgen W. Spranger, who detailed the clinical and radiographic features, particularly in relation to other skeletal dysplasias.

Purpose

- **Identify Key Skeletal Dysplasias:** Differentiate Koslowski's syndrome from other forms of skeletal dysplasia through clinical and radiographic markers.
- **Monitor Growth and Mobility:** Assess growth patterns and address limitations in mobility to improve quality of life.
- **Guide Genetic Counseling:** Provide families with information regarding inheritance patterns and recurrence risks.

Procedure Overview

- **Clinical Examination:**
- Evaluate growth patterns, joint mobility, and spinal curvature.
- Identify hallmark features such as pectus carinatum and bowed legs.
- **Radiographic Imaging:**
- **X-rays:** Document platyspondyly, broad iliac bones, and irregular metaphyses.
- **MRI/CT scans:** Evaluate joint and spinal abnormalities in greater detail.
- **Genetic Testing:** Confirm autosomal dominant inheritance and rule out differential diagnoses.

Results and Interpretation

- **Radiographic Findings:**
- Presence of platyspondyly and shortened basilar parts of the iliac bones.
- Irregular metaphyses and bowed legs observed in affected individuals.
- **Clinical Presentation:** Truncal shortening with waddling gait, limited joint mobility, and postural abnormalities like kyphoscoliosis.

Physiological Basis

- **Skeletal Dysplasia Pathogenesis:** Abnormal cartilage and bone growth lead to disproportionate skeletal development, particularly affecting the spine, pelvis, and long bones.
- **Genetic Component:** Autosomal

dominant mutations impair growth factor pathways, causing short stature and skeletal deformities.

Clinical Applications

- **Orthopedic Interventions:** Address kyphoscoliosis, bowed legs, and pectus carinatum through corrective surgeries and bracing.
- **Physical Therapy:** Improve joint mobility and reduce discomfort associated with gait abnormalities.
- **Vision Correction:** Manage associated hyperopia with ophthalmologic interventions.

Limitations and Technical Considerations

- **Differential Diagnosis:** Overlap with other skeletal dysplasias may complicate diagnosis; genetic testing can confirm Koslowski's syndrome.
- **Surgical Challenges:** Skeletal deformities may increase risks associated with orthopedic surgeries.
- **Progressive Features:** Conditions like kyphoscoliosis may worsen over time, requiring continuous monitoring.

Modern Relevance

- **Advances in Imaging:** High-resolution imaging modalities provide earlier and more accurate detection of skeletal abnormalities.
- **Genetic Insights:** Identification of specific gene mutations aids in prenatal diagnosis and genetic counseling.
- **Improved Therapies:** Development of targeted therapies and surgical techniques enhances patient outcomes.

Associated Conditions

- **Hyperopia:** Refractive error commonly seen in affected individuals.
- **Kyphoscoliosis:** Progressive spinal curvature leading to postural and functional limitations.
- **Pectus Carinatum:** Abnormal protrusion of the chest wall.

Clinical Importance

- **Early Diagnosis:** Recognition of skeletal abnormalities and joint limitations in early childhood enables timely interventions.
- **Prognostic Value:** Identifying the severity of kyphoscoliosis and joint deformities helps predict mobility outcomes.
- **Holistic Management:** Collaboration among orthopedic surgeons, geneticists, and physical therapists ensures comprehensive care.
- **Genetic Counseling:** Educating families on inheritance patterns helps manage expectations and future planning.

References

K. Koslowski, P. Maroteaux, J. Spranger: La dysostose spondylométaphysaire. La presse médicale, Paris, 1967, 75: 2769-2774.

K. Koslowski, F. A. Beemer, G. Bens, et al: Spondylometaphyseal dysplasia: report of 7 cases and assay of classification. In C. J. Papadatos, C. S. Bartsocas (editors): Skeletal Dysplasias. New York, Alan R. Liss, 1982.

Lauge-Hansen Classification

Overview

The Lauge-Hansen Classification is a detailed system for classifying ankle fractures based on the stability of the ankle mortise and the mechanism of injury. It incorporates two descriptive terms: the initial position of the foot at the time of injury and the direction of the injuring force through the talus. This classification identifies five main mechanisms:

- *Supination-Adduction*
- *Supination-Eversion*
- *Pronation-Eversion*
- *Pronation-Abduction*
- *Pronation-Dorsiflexion*

Despite its comprehensive nature, its complexity often limits its routine clinical use.

Historical Background

- **1950:** Niels Lauge-Hansen, a Danish surgeon, introduced the classification in his seminal work, which provided a biomechanical understanding of ankle injuries and their resulting fracture patterns.
- The classification was based on experimental studies where Lauge-Hansen recreated injury mechanisms to correlate trauma forces with specific fracture types.

Purpose

- **Guide Fracture Diagnosis:** Link the mechanism of injury to predictable fracture patterns and joint instability.
- **Assist in Treatment Planning:** Provide a framework for understanding injury severity and necessary surgical or nonsurgical interventions.
- **Standardized Communication:** Create a uniform system for clinicians to describe and document ankle injuries.

Procedure Overview

- **Initial Examination:**
- Gather patient history, including mechanism of injury and foot position during trauma.
- Perform clinical assessment for tenderness, deformities, and joint stability.
- **Radiographic Imaging:**
- Use AP, lateral, and mortise views to identify fracture lines and dislocations.
- Correlate findings with specific injury patterns described by the classification.
- **Classification Assignment:** Categorize the injury based on foot position (supination/pronation) and direction of the force (adduction/eversion/abduction/dorsiflexion).

Results and Interpretation

- **Supination-Adduction (SA):** Involves vertical fractures of the medial malleolus and transverse fractures of the distal fibula.
- **Supination-Eversion (SE):** Results in transverse fractures of the medial malleolus or deltoid ligament rupture

and spiral fibular fractures.

- **Pronation-Eversion (PE):** Typically leads to medial ligament rupture, fibular fractures, and posterior malleolar fractures.
- **Pronation-Abduction (PA):** Produces transverse medial malleolar fractures and compression fractures of the fibula.
- **Pronation-Dorsiflexion (PD):** Associated with anterior tibial margin fractures and posterior malleolar fractures.

Physiological Basis

- **Biomechanics of Trauma:** Injury forces through the talus disrupt the stability of the ankle mortise, creating predictable fracture patterns.
- **Ankle Mortise Stability:** Damage to the ligaments or bony structures compromises the mortise, affecting ankle joint function.

Clinical Applications

- **Treatment Guidance:** Helps determine the need for closed reduction, open reduction, or internal fixation.
- **Surgical Planning:** Guides surgical approaches, particularly for complex injury patterns.
- **Rehabilitation Strategies:** Tailors postoperative rehabilitation based on injury severity and involved structures.

Limitations and Technical Considerations

- **Complexity of the System:** The detailed classification can be difficult to apply in busy clinical settings.
- **Variability in Practice:** Not universally adopted, even in its origin location, due to its intricacy.
- **Subjectivity in Diagnosis:** Determining the exact mechanism of injury retrospectively may be challenging.

Modern Relevance

- **Enhanced Imaging Techniques:** Modern modalities like CT and MRI complement the classification by providing detailed visualizations of fractures and soft tissue injuries.
- **Educational Tool:** Still valuable for teaching ankle biomechanics and injury patterns to orthopedic trainees.
- **Research Applications:** Continues to inform studies on ankle injury mechanisms and outcomes.

Associated Conditions

- **Ligamentous Injuries:** Medial or lateral ligament tears often accompany ankle fractures.
- **Chronic Ankle Instability:** Repeated injuries can lead to long-term joint instability.
- **Post-Traumatic Arthritis:** Improper healing of ankle fractures increases the risk of arthritis.

Clinical Importance

- **Early Diagnosis:** Identifying injury mechanisms early helps prevent misdiagnosis and improper management.
- **Prognostic Value:** The classification predicts the severity of fractures and the likelihood of complications like

malunion or arthritis.

- **Standardized Treatment:** Facilitates structured approaches to ankle injury management across different healthcare settings.
- **Interdisciplinary Collaboration:** Promotes coordination among radiologists, orthopedic surgeons, and physical therapists for optimal outcomes.

References

LAUGE-HANSEN N. Fractures of the ankle. V. Pronation-dorsiflexion fracture. AMA Arch Surg 1953; 67: 813–20.

LAUGE-HANSEN N. Fractures of the ankle. IV. Clinical use of genetic roentgen diagnosis and genetic reduction. AMA Arch Surg 1952; 64: 488–500.

LAUGE-HANSEN N. Fractures of the ankle. III. Genetic roentgenologic diagnosis of fractures of the ankle. Am J Roentgenol Radium Ther Nucl Med 1954; 71: 456–71.

Le Fort facial Fractures

Overview

Le Fort facial fractures refer to a classification system for midfacial fractures involving the separation of the maxilla from the skull base along three specific planes of injury. These fractures are divided into Le Fort I, II, and III, with increasing severity and anatomical complexity. They may occur as unilateral or bilateral injuries and often result from high-energy trauma such as motor vehicle accidents or blunt facial injuries.

Historical Background

- **1866:** Alphonse Guérin demonstrated that fractures of the maxilla could be diagnosed by clinical evaluation, even when displacement was minimal or absent.
- **1900-1901:** René Le Fort, a French surgeon, conducted experimental studies by dropping bricks on cadaver heads to study fracture patterns.
- He identified predictable fracture patterns based on the magnitude and direction of blunt force trauma.
- These experiments culminated in the development of the Le Fort classification system in 1901.
- Le Fort credited Guérin for his earlier observations and emphasized that accurate diagnosis allows for better treatment of maxillary fractures.

Purpose

- **Fracture Classification:** Standardize the description of midfacial fractures into predictable patterns (Le Fort I, II,

III).

- **Guide Treatment:** Enable appropriate surgical or nonsurgical management based on fracture complexity and location.
- **Facilitate Diagnosis:** Assist clinicians in identifying fractures through physical examination and imaging.

Procedure Overview

- **Imaging Studies:** CT scans are the gold standard for diagnosing and classifying Le Fort fractures, providing detailed visualization of fracture lines.
- **Physical Examination:**
- Check for mobility of facial bones, bruising, swelling, or misalignment.
- Assess for associated injuries such as airway obstruction, dental trauma, or visual impairment.
- **Classification:**
- **Le Fort I:** Fracture across the piriform aperture and maxillary sinus walls.
- **Le Fort II:** Fracture involving the orbital rim, floor, and medial orbital wall.
- **Le Fort III:** Fracture extending through the nasal bridge, orbital walls, and zygomatic arch.

Results and Interpretation

- **Le Fort I:** Known as a "floating palate," the fracture separates the maxilla at the level of the nasal cavity.
- **Le Fort II:** Known as a "pyramidal fracture," with the nasal bridge, maxilla, and orbital floor affected.
- **Le Fort III:** Known as a "craniofacial disjunction," resulting in complete separation of the midface from the skull base.

Physiological Basis

- **Impact Force Distribution:**
- The maxilla's structural anatomy dictates how forces are absorbed and distributed during trauma.
- The buttress system of the midface directs forces along predictable planes, resulting in the characteristic fracture patterns described by Le Fort.
- **Loss of Structural Integrity:** Fractures compromise the maxilla's support for critical structures, including the orbit, nasal cavity, and airway.

Clinical Applications

- **Surgical Planning:** Accurate classification aids in determining the surgical approach, such as open reduction and internal fixation.
- **Airway Management:** Patients with Le Fort II and III fractures often require airway stabilization.
- **Rehabilitation:** Guides postoperative care, including management of dental, nasal, or orbital complications.

Limitations and Technical Considerations

- **Complex Fracture Patterns:** Some fractures do not fit neatly into the Le Fort categories, making diagnosis and treatment challenging.
- **Imaging Limitations:** Severe soft tissue swelling can obscure fractures on X-rays, emphasizing the importance of CT imaging.

- **Associated Injuries:** High-energy trauma often results in concurrent cranial or cervical spine injuries, complicating management.

Modern Relevance

- **Advanced Imaging:** Modern CT and 3D reconstructions improve diagnostic accuracy and surgical planning.
- **Trauma Protocols:** The Le Fort classification remains integral to trauma guidelines for managing maxillofacial injuries.
- **Interdisciplinary Collaboration:** Collaboration among surgeons, radiologists, and emergency physicians is critical for optimal outcomes.

Associated Conditions

- **Airway Obstruction:** Fractures may result in swelling or hematomas that compromise breathing.
- **Dental and Ocular Injuries:** Often associated with Le Fort II and III fractures.
- **Neurological Impairments:** Le Fort III fractures can involve cranial nerves, leading to visual or sensory deficits.

Clinical Importance

- **Early Diagnosis:** Recognizing fracture patterns early prevents complications such as airway obstruction or infection.
- **Prognostic Value:** Le Fort III fractures indicate severe trauma and carry a higher risk of complications.
- **Treatment Planning:** Ensures that surgical intervention is tailored to fracture type and associated injuries.
- **Interdisciplinary Management:** Involves teamwork across multiple specialties, including maxillofacial surgery, anesthesiology, and neurology, to achieve the best outcomes.

References

Guerin AFM. Des fractures des maxillaires supérieurs. Nouveau moyen de les reconnaitre dans les cas fréquents ou elles ne s'accompagnent pas de déplacement [Fractures of the upper jawbones. New means of recognizing them in frequent cases or they are not accompanied by displacement] In: Archives générales de médecine, 1866,Vol.2, pp5-13

Le Fort R. Étude expérimentale sur les fractures de la machoire supérieure. Revue chir de Paris 1901; 23:208-27; 360-79; 479-507

Tessier P. The classic reprint: experimental study of fractures of the upper jaw. I and II. René Le Fort, M.D., Lille, France. Plast Reconstr Surg. 1972 Dec;50(6):497–506. [PMID 4563382]

Tessier P. The classic reprint: experimental study of fractures of the upper jaw. III. René Le Fort, M.D., Lille, France. Plast Reconstr Surg. 1972 Dec;50(6):600-7. [PMID 4564611]

Dyer PV. Experimental study of fractures of the upper jaw: a critique of the original papers published by René Le Fort. Trauma 1999; 1:81-84.

Lequesne View

Overview

The Lequesne View is a radiographic technique designed to evaluate the articular space in the anterior and posterior compartments of the hip joint. This imaging method is particularly useful in assessing cartilage loss and joint space narrowing in conditions such as osteoarthritis. It provides a standardized projection of the hip to ensure precise evaluation of joint anatomy and alignment.

Historical Background

- **1952:** The technique was first described by Dr. Michel Lequesne, a prominent researcher in the field of radiology and musculoskeletal disorders. Lequesne aimed to develop a standardized imaging view to address inconsistencies in diagnosing joint space abnormalities.
- The Lequesne view was initially introduced as part of a broader study on the progression of hip osteoarthritis, providing a more accurate assessment of joint space narrowing.

Purpose

- **Assess Joint Space Narrowing:** The technique allows for accurate measurement of the articular space in the hip joint, particularly in the anterior and posterior compartments.
- **Diagnose Osteoarthritis:** By identifying changes in joint space and alignment, the Lequesne view aids in diagnosing osteoarthritis and other degenerative joint diseases.
- **Monitor Disease Progression:**
- Useful in evaluating the progression of conditions such as hip dysplasia, impingement syndromes, and post-traumatic arthritis.

Procedure Overview

- **Patient Positioning:**
- The patient is placed in orthostasis (standing upright), with the hip of interest positioned along the X-ray chassis.
- The shoulders are angled at 65°, while the foot on the side to be studied is aligned parallel to the chassis.
- **Radiographic Beam:**
- The X-ray beam is directed through the hip joint.
- Proper alignment is verified by ensuring a visible distance between the femoral heads on the radiograph.
- **Imaging Objective:** Capture a clear view of the anterior and posterior articular compartments to assess joint integrity.

Results and Interpretation

- **Normal Findings:**
- Uniform joint space across anterior and posterior compartments.
- No visible osteophytes, subchondral sclerosis, or deformities.
- **Abnormal Findings:**
- Narrowing of joint space indicative of cartilage loss.
- Presence of bony growths or irregularities associated with degenerative chang-

es.

Physiological Basis

- **Joint Space Narrowing:** Cartilage degeneration leads to reduced articular space, which is visible on radiographs as a key sign of osteoarthritis.
- **Anterior-Posterior Discrepancies:** The Lequesne view highlights variations in joint space that may not be apparent on conventional radiographs.

Clinical Applications

- **Osteoarthritis Evaluation:** Detects early signs of hip osteoarthritis, including joint space narrowing and osteophyte formation.
- **Pre-Surgical Assessment:** Provides critical information for planning procedures such as total hip arthroplasty or hip resurfacing.
- **Monitoring Disease Progression:** Tracks changes in joint space over time to evaluate treatment efficacy or disease progression.

Limitations and Technical Considerations

- **Patient Positioning:** Accurate positioning is essential to avoid artifacts or distorted measurements.
- **Limited Soft Tissue Visualization:** While effective for bone and joint evaluation, the technique provides limited information about surrounding soft tissues.
- **Radiation Exposure:** Requires careful consideration, particularly in younger patients or those requiring frequent imaging.

Modern Relevance

- **Enhanced Diagnostic Precision:** Advances in digital radiography and 3D imaging have improved the accuracy and reproducibility of the Lequesne view.
- **Integration with Advanced Modalities:** Often combined with CT or MRI for comprehensive hip evaluations.
- **Research Applications:** Used in clinical trials to assess the efficacy of new treatments for osteoarthritis and related conditions.

Associated Conditions

- **Hip Osteoarthritis:** The most common condition evaluated using the Lequesne view.
- **Femoroacetabular Impingement (FAI):** Detects subtle structural changes contributing to impingement syndromes.
- **Post-Traumatic Arthritis:** Identifies degenerative changes following hip injuries.

Clinical Importance

- **Early Diagnosis:** Enables detection of joint space narrowing before advanced degenerative changes occur.
- **Prognostic Value:** Measurement of joint space narrowing provides insight into the severity and progression of osteoarthritis.
- **Pre-Surgical Planning:** Ensures accurate assessment of joint morphology and alignment before surgical intervention.
- **Standardized Imaging:** Provides a consistent and reproducible method for evaluating hip joint integrity, enhancing

diagnostic confidence.

References

Musculoskeletal Radiographic Views and Eponyms; 10.1594/essr2013/P-0158.

Léri-Joanny Syndrome

Overview

Léri-Joanny syndrome, also known as melorheostosis or "candle bone disease," is a rare disorder of bone characterized by irregular linear areas of increased density along the shafts of long bones. This condition arises from ostal or periostal osteosclerosis, yet it occurs in the setting of normal mineral metabolism. It manifests in two forms: monostotic, affecting a single bone, and polystotic, involving multiple bones. Early onset of the disease can lead to complications such as premature closure of the epiphysis, resulting in dwarfism. Restricted limb motion may also occur due to ankylosis, muscle involvement, or both.

Historical Background

- **1922:** First described by French physician André Léri and his colleague Joanny in their study of sclerotic bone conditions.
- **Etymology:** The term "melorheostosis" derives from the Greek words "melos" (limb), "rheo" (flow), and "ostosis" (bone), reflecting the radiographic appearance resembling melted wax.
- Their observations laid the foundation for understanding the unique radiographic and clinical features of the condition.

Purpose

- **Characterize Bone Lesions:** To distinguish melorheostosis from other sclerotic bone disorders, such as osteopoikilosis or osteopathia striata.
- **Guide Symptom Management:** To

identify affected areas and provide relief from pain, functional impairment, and stiffness.

- **Monitor Disease Progression:** To assess whether the condition is worsening, particularly in cases involving ankylosis or soft tissue calcification.

Procedure Overview

- **Radiographic Imaging:** X-rays are the primary diagnostic tool, showing irregular linear densities that resemble melted wax running along the bone's surface.
- Advanced imaging, such as CT and MRI, may help evaluate soft tissue involvement and periosteal excrescences.
- **Clinical Evaluation:** Comprehensive assessment of limb motion, pain, and any associated skeletal deformities.

Results and Interpretation

- **Characteristic Radiographic Findings:**
- Linear sclerotic streaks along the shafts of long bones.
- Densities resembling melted wax on the surface of affected bones.
- Potential premature closure of the epiphysis in early-onset cases.
- **Functional Impact:**
- Restricted joint mobility and possible ankylosis.
- Pain and stiffness in the affected limbs.

Physiological Basis

- **Pathophysiology:** Melorheostosis is believed to result from a postzygotic somatic mutation in the MAP2K1 gene, leading to abnormal osteoblast activity.
- **Impact on Bone:** The abnormal periosteal and endosteal bone growth creates the characteristic sclerotic streaks and may disrupt normal bone and joint function.

Clinical Applications

- **Differential Diagnosis:** Differentiates melorheostosis from other skeletal dysplasias and conditions, such as Paget's disease or osteopetrosis.
- **Pain Management:** Guides intervention strategies for reducing pain and discomfort caused by sclerosis or soft tissue involvement.
- **Surgical Planning:** Provides insights for surgical correction of deformities or ankylosis to improve limb function.

Limitations and Technical Considerations

- **Radiographic Limitations:** X-rays may not reveal the full extent of soft tissue involvement or subtle lesions, requiring supplemental imaging techniques like CT or MRI.
- **Variable Presentation:** The condition's presentation can vary widely, making diagnosis challenging, particularly in its early stages.
- **Rare Occurrence:** The rarity of the condition can lead to delayed diagnosis or misdiagnosis in clinical practice.

Modern Relevance

- **Genetic Insights:** Advances in understanding genetic mutations, such as MAP2K1, provide deeper insights into disease mechanisms and potential targeted therapies.
- **Advanced Imaging Techniques:** Improved imaging modalities enable more precise diagnosis and monitoring of disease progression.
- **Novel Treatment Approaches:** Ongoing research explores the use of targeted therapies and regenerative techniques to manage skeletal deformities.

Associated Conditions

- **Ankylosis:** Joint stiffness and fusion due to abnormal bone growth.
- **Dwarfism:** Premature epiphyseal closure in early-onset cases.
- **Soft Tissue Calcification:** Involvement of surrounding tissues, further impairing mobility.

Clinical Importance

- **Early Diagnosis:** Identifying the condition early allows for better management of symptoms and prevention of severe deformities.
- **Prognostic Value:** Imaging findings provide insights into disease severity and potential functional impairment.
- **Interdisciplinary Management:** Collaboration among radiologists, orthopedic surgeons, and physical therapists ensures optimal outcomes.
- **Surgical Interventions:** Required in cases with significant joint immobility or skeletal deformity to restore function and alleviate pain.

References

A. Leri, J. P. Joanny:Une affection non décriete des os: Hyperostose «en coulée» sur toute la longueur d'un membre ou "mélorhéostose".

Bulletins et memoires de la Société medicale des hôpitaux de Paris, 1922, 46: 1141-1145.

Lisfranc Fracture

Overview

The Lisfranc fracture, associated with Jacques Lisfranc de Saint-Martin, refers to injuries involving the tarsometatarsal (TMT) joint complex, where the forefoot meets the midfoot. These fractures often result from direct trauma or axial loading on a plantarflexed foot, leading to disruption of the Lisfranc ligament, which stabilizes the joint. The condition can involve fractures, dislocations, or a combination of both and often requires surgical intervention to restore joint alignment and function.

Historical Background

- **1799:** William Hey described forefoot amputation at the junction of the metatarsals and cuneiforms, a precursor to Lisfranc's work.
- **1815:** Jacques Lisfranc de Saint-Martin described a simple and rapid method for forefoot amputation through the TMT joint, which could be performed in under a minute.
- **1823:** Lisfranc clarified that he had not invented the procedure but had refined the surgical anatomy of the TMT joint, enabling efficient operations.
- Lisfranc's detailed descriptions and refinement of the disarticulation at the TMT joint led to the joint, ligament, and injury being eponymously attributed to him.

Purpose

- **Stabilize the TMT Joint:** Ensure anatomical alignment of the forefoot and midfoot following injury.
- **Prevent Chronic Instability:** Address ligamentous disruption and fractures to avoid post-traumatic arthritis or deformity.
- **Restore Functionality:** Enable normal gait and weight-bearing after injury.

Procedure Overview

- **Diagnosis:**
- **Clinical Exam:** Swelling, bruising (often on the plantar midfoot), and pain on dorsiflexion or rotation of the forefoot.
- **Imaging:**
- X-rays reveal the "fleck sign," a bony fragment indicating ligamentous avulsion. **CT or** MRI may be required for subtle injuries.
- **Management:**
- **Non-Surgical:** For non-displaced injuries, immobilization with a cast and non-weight-bearing status for 6–8 weeks.
- **Surgical:** Open reduction and internal fixation (ORIF) or primary arthrodesis for displaced fractures or severe ligament injuries.

Results and Interpretation

- **Post-Treatment Outcomes:** Successful anatomical reduction often restores stability and prevents arthritis.
- Poor outcomes may result from delayed treatment or improper reduction.

- **Complications:** Persistent pain, limited mobility, and secondary arthritis are possible without proper alignment.

Physiological Basis

- The *Lisfranc ligament* plays a critical role in stabilizing the medial cuneiform and the second metatarsal.
- Disruption of this ligament destabilizes the TMT joint complex, leading to deformity and altered weight-bearing mechanics.
- Associated fractures exacerbate instability and increase the risk of long-term complications, such as arthritis.

Clinical Applications

- **Trauma Management:** Treats injuries resulting from high-impact forces, such as car accidents or sports injuries.
- **Rehabilitation Planning:** Guides physiotherapy protocols post-surgery to restore gait and strength.
- **Preventing Chronic Issues:** Timely intervention minimizes risks of arthritis or deformities.

Limitations and Technical Considerations

- **Diagnosis Challenges:** Subtle injuries may be missed on plain radiographs; advanced imaging is often necessary.
- **Surgical Complexity:** ORIF requires precise alignment of small bones, and complications like hardware failure can occur.
- **Delayed Recovery:** Weight-bearing restrictions and prolonged immobilization may affect recovery time.

Modern Relevance

- **Advanced Imaging:** MRI and CT have improved the detection of subtle injuries, enabling early diagnosis.
- **Improved Techniques:** Innovations in surgical fixation and arthrodesis have enhanced outcomes.
- **Sports Medicine Focus:** Greater awareness of Lisfranc injuries in athletes has improved treatment protocols and performance outcomes.

Associated Conditions

- **Post-Traumatic Arthritis:** Chronic pain and joint degeneration from untreated or poorly managed injuries.
- **Plantar Arch Collapse:** Deformity resulting from loss of midfoot stability.
- **Neuropathy or Vascular Injury:** Rare complications from severe trauma.

Clinical Importance

- **Early Diagnosis:** Detecting Lisfranc injuries promptly prevents chronic instability and deformity.
- **Prognostic Value:** Proper anatomical reduction is critical for functional outcomes and long-term joint health.
- **Interdisciplinary Management:** Collaboration among orthopedic surgeons, radiologists, and physical therapists ensures optimal recovery.
- **Functional Rehabilitation:** Post-treatment therapy is essential for restoring mobility and strength in the affected foot.

References

Hey W. Excision of the metatarsal bones. In: Practical observations in surgery. 1803 p530-537

Averill C. A short treatise on operative surgery, describing the principal operations as they are practised in England and France; designed for the use of students in operating on the dead body. London: Jackson, Borough. 1825

Cassebaum WH. Lisfranc fracture-dislocations. Clin Orthop Relat Res. 1963;30:116-29. [PMID 5888997]

Foster SC, Foster RR. Lisfranc's tarsometatarsal fracture-dislocation. Radiology. 1976 Jul;120(1):79-83. [PMID 935468]

Gupta RT, Wadhwa RP, Learch TJ, Herwick SM. Lisfranc injury: imaging findings for this important but often-missed diagnosis. Curr Probl Diagn Radiol. 2008 May-Jun;37(3):115-26. [PMID 18436111]

Kalia V, Fishman EK, Carrino JA, Fayad LM. Epidemiology, imaging, and treatment of Lisfranc fracture-dislocations revisited. Skeletal Radiol. 2012 Feb;41(2):129-36. [PMID 21431438]

Castro M, Melão L, Canella C, Weber M, Negrão P, Trudell D, Resnick D. Lisfranc joint ligamentous complex: MRI with anatomic correlation in cadavers. AJR Am J Roentgenol. 2010 Dec;195(6):W447-55. [PMID 21098178]

Johnson A, Hill K, Ward J, Ficke J Anatomy of the Lisfranc ligament. Foot Ankle Spec. 2008 Feb;1(1):19-23. [PMID 19825687]

Myerson MS, Fisher RT, Burgess AR, Kenzora JE. Fracture dislocations of the tarsometatarsal joints: end results correlated with pathology and treatment. Foot Ankle. 1986 Apr;6(5):225-42. [PMID 3710321]

Hatem SF. Imaging of lisfranc injury and midfoot sprain. Radiol Clin North Am. 2008 Nov;46(6):1045-60, vi. [PMID 19038612]

Lover's Fracture

Overview

Lover's Fracture, also known as Don Juan fracture or Casanova fracture, refers to a type of calcaneal (heel bone) fracture. It primarily involves the calcaneal body and can be either intra-articular (involving the joint) or extra-articular (not involving the joint). This injury often results from a high-energy axial load, such as jumping or falling from a significant height, and is frequently associated with concurrent spinal injuries like lumbar burst fractures.

Historical Background

- The term "Lover's Fracture" originates from the image of a suitor jumping from a great height, such as a balcony, to escape an angry lover's spouse. While the exact year of its coinage is unclear, its association with dramatic escapes has made it a memorable and descriptive eponym in orthopedic literature.
- This condition's connection with lumbar burst fractures was recognized due to the similar axial loading mechanism involved in high-impact injuries.

Purpose

- **Diagnosis:** Identify the fracture pattern and any associated injuries, especially spinal fractures.
- **Treatment Goals:** Restore the anatomical alignment of the calcaneus.
- Preserve joint function and prevent arthritic complications.
- Ensure early mobilization and weight-bearing capabilities.

Procedure Overview

- **Diagnosis:**
- **Clinical Presentation:** Patients typically present with pain, swelling, and bruising over the heel following a high-impact event. They may also exhibit difficulty or inability to bear weight.
- **Imaging:** X-rays: Initial imaging modality to evaluate the calcaneus and associated fractures.
- **CT scans:** Provide detailed views of fracture patterns and joint involvement.
- **MRI:** Used for soft tissue assessment if needed.

Classification:

- **Essex-Lopresti Classification:** Tongue-type fractures: Extends from the posterior facet to the Achilles tendon insertion.
- **Joint depression fractures:** More complex intra-articular fractures.
- **Sanders Classification:** Based on CT scans to guide surgical decision-making.

Treatment:

- **Non-Surgical:** For extra-articular fractures or intra-articular fractures with minimal displacement. Involves immobilization in a cast or splint and non-weight bearing for several weeks.
- **Surgical:** Open reduction and internal fixation (ORIF) for displaced intra-articular fractures.
- Minimally invasive techniques, such as percutaneous fixation, for certain fracture patterns.

Results and Interpretation

- Properly treated Lover's Fractures generally have favorable outcomes, but delays in diagnosis or improper management can lead to chronic pain, reduced function, and post-traumatic arthritis.
- Surgical intervention offers better restoration of joint congruency and long-term functionality compared to non-surgical approaches in complex cases.

Physiological Basis

- The calcaneus serves as the primary weight-bearing bone in the heel and absorbs significant forces during activities like walking and running.
- High-energy axial loads, such as falls from heights, cause compression of the calcaneus, leading to fractures that may propagate into the subtalar joint and disrupt normal foot biomechanics.

Clinical Applications

- Early identification and classification of the fracture guide treatment decisions.
- Surgical reconstruction techniques focus on restoring the calcaneal shape and joint surface to optimize long-term outcomes.

Limitations and Technical Considerations

- **Challenges in Diagnosis:** These fractures are often missed initially, especially when associated spinal injuries divert attention.
- **Surgical Risks:** Include infection, wound healing complications, and implant failure.

- **Post-Treatment Morbidity:** Even with optimal treatment, patients may experience stiffness, reduced mobility, and subtalar arthritis.

Modern Relevance

- **Advances in** imaging and surgical techniques have improved the diagnosis and management of calcaneal fractures.

- Minimally invasive approaches and biologics for bone healing are being explored to reduce complications and enhance recovery.

Associated Conditions

- **Lumbar Burst Fractures:** Resulting from similar axial loading mechanisms.

- **Tibial Plateau Fractures:** May occur in concurrent high-energy trauma.

- **Soft Tissue Injuries:** Include damage to the Achilles tendon or surrounding ligaments.

Clinical Importance

- **Comprehensive Assessment:** Given the high-energy nature of the trauma, associated injuries, particularly spinal fractures, must be ruled out.

- **Long-Term Outcomes:** Failure to restore the anatomy of the calcaneus can lead to chronic pain, deformity, and arthritis, emphasizing the importance of accurate diagnosis and appropriate treatment.

- **Multidisciplinary Management:** Coordination among orthopedic surgeons, radiologists, and rehabilitation specialists is crucial for optimal outcomes.

References

Daftary A, Haims AH, Baumgaertner MR. Fractures of the calcaneus: a review with emphasis on CT. Radiographics. 25 (5): 1215-26. doi:10.1148/rg.255045713 - Pubmed citation

Lee P, Hunter TB, Taljanovic M. Musculoskeletal colloquialisms: how did we come up with these names?. Radiographics. 2004;24 (4): 1009-27.

Reichel R, Monstein HJ, Jansen HW, Philipson L, Benecke BJ (May 1982). "Small nuclear RNAs are encoded in the nontranscribed region of ribosomal spacer DNA". Proc. Natl. Acad. Sci. U.S.A. 79 (10): 3106–10. doi:10.1073/pnas.79.10.3106. PMID 6179077.

Tomasini M, Meciani L, Sartorelli E (December 1965). "[Observations on the subject of digitalis therapy of chronic pulmonary heart disease]". Minerva Med. (in Italian). 56 (101): 4470–82. PMID 5862705.

Lee P, Hunter TB, Taljanovic M (2004). "Musculoskeletal colloquialisms: how did we come up with these names?". Radiographics. 24 (4): 1009–27. doi:10.1148/rg.244045015. PMID 15256625.

Fikhman BA, Sirotiuk LV, Petukhov VG (April 1966). "[Photometric analysis of bacterial suspensions. IV. On the possibility of using the osmotic effect to determine the relationship between live and dead cells in suspensions of tularemia bacteria]". Zh. Mikrobiol. Epidemiol. Immunobiol. (in Russian). 43 (4): 130–4. PMID 6004727.

Ventrucci M, Gullo L, Daniele C, Bartolucci C, Priori P, Platé L, Bonora G, Labò G (1983). "Comparative study of serum pancreatic isoamylase, lipase, and trypsin-like immunoreactivity in pancreatic disease". Digestion. 28 (2): 114–21. doi:10.1159/000198973. PMID 6197334.

Belmonte M, Scardovi C, Tabacchi G (April 1966). "[Rheographic control cerebral hemodynamic effects induced by roentgen irradiation on the cervical sympathetic system in subjects with tapeto-retinal degenerations]". Ann Ottalmol Clin Ocul (in Italian). 92 (4): 235–46. PMID 5961258.

Masztalerz A, Bujwidowa B, Jagielska I, Masztalerzowa Z, Potoczek J, Szczepańska H, Warych B (September 1983). "[Social class and dental and occlusal conditions]". Czas Stomatol (in Polish). 36 (9): 691–5. PMID 6584293.

Saito Y (December 1973). "[Comparison of ACTH and insulin actions on sugar transport in their target organs]". Nihon Naibunpi Gakkai Zasshi (in Japanese). 49 (12): 1436–46. doi:10.1507/endocrine1927.49.12_1436. PMID 4359527.

Wilesmith JW, Bode R, Pritchard DG, Stuart FA, Sayers PE (August 1986). "Tuberculosis in East Sussex. I. Outbreaks of tuberculosis in cattle herds (1964-1984)". J Hyg (Lond). 97 (1): 1–10. doi:10.1017/s0022172400064305. PMID 3734437.

Hopkins NF, Spinks TJ, Rhodes CG, Ranicar AS, Jamieson CW (January 1983). "Positron emission tomography in venous ulceration and liposclerosis: study of regional tissue function". Br Med J (Clin Res Ed). 286 (6362): 333–6. doi:10.1136/bmj.286.6362.333. PMID 6402087.

Awachie JB (November 1965). "The ecology of Echinorhynchus truttae Schrank, 1788 (Acanthocephala) in a trout stream in North Wales". Parasitology. 55 (4): 747–62.

Luschka's joints

Overview

Luschka's joints, also known as uncovertebral joints, are small synovial articulations located in the cervical spine (C2 to C7). These joints are formed between the lateral edges of the vertebral bodies below (with upward-projecting lips) and the vertebral bodies above (with downward-projecting lips). They provide stability while allowing for specific movements in the cervical spine, such as flexion and extension, while limiting lateral flexion.

Historical Background

- **1858:** Hubert von Luschka, a German anatomist, first described these unique articulations in his work on the anatomy of the human spine.
- His detailed anatomical studies expanded the understanding of cervical spine mechanics and pathology, giving the joints their eponymous name.

Purpose

- **Structural Stability:** Stabilizes the cervical spine during movement by preventing excessive lateral flexion.
- **Facilitation of Movement:** Allows for smooth flexion and extension in the cervical spine.
- **Reduction of Friction:** Minimizes wear and tear between adjacent vertebral bodies.

Procedure Overview

- **Imaging for Diagnosis:** Plain X-rays, CT, and MRI are used to evaluate Luschka's joints. These modalities detect degenerative changes such as osteophyte formation or joint hypertrophy.
- **Clinical Examination:** Palpation and range-of-motion tests may indicate pain or restricted movement linked to uncovertebral joint pathology.
- **Management:**
- **Conservative:** Physical therapy, anti-inflammatory medications, and ergonomic modifications.
- **Surgical:** In severe cases, decompression or discectomy may address nerve impingement due to joint hypertrophy.

Results and Interpretation

- **Normal Function:** In healthy spines, these joints facilitate smooth, stable motion without pain or restriction.
- **Pathological Findings:** Degeneration or hypertrophy can lead to nerve root impingement, causing cervical radiculopathy, pain, or stiffness.

Physiological Basis

- **Structural Design:** The unique upward and downward projections of adjacent vertebrae form a joint space that is lined with synovium and supported by cartilage.
- **Mechanical Role:** These joints guide and limit motion, ensuring that cervical spine movements are efficient and within safe ranges.

Clinical Applications

- **Cervical Spine Disorders:** Diagnosing and managing conditions like cervical radiculopathy and degenerative joint disease.
- **Guidance for Surgery:** Understanding Luschka's joints is critical for planning cervical spine surgeries, especially in procedures involving decompression or fusion.
- **Postural Ergonomics:** Rehabilitation programs often consider these joints when addressing neck pain and improving posture.

Limitations and Technical Considerations

- **Complexity of Diagnosis:** Pathologies may overlap with other cervical spine conditions, requiring advanced imaging for accurate identification.
- **Surgical Challenges:** Due to their proximity to critical neural structures, surgical interventions around Luschka's joints demand precision.
- **Natural Degeneration:** These joints undergo age-related changes, complicating differentiation between normal and pathological findings.

Modern Relevance

- **Advanced Imaging Techniques:** High-resolution CT and MRI have enhanced the ability to evaluate Luschka's joints for subtle degenerative or pathological changes.
- **Minimally Invasive Procedures:** Innovations in minimally invasive spine surgery have improved outcomes for conditions involving these joints.
- **Ergonomic Awareness:** Growing attention to cervical spine health in the context of technology use highlights the relevance of Luschka's joints in maintaining mobility and preventing pain.

Associated Conditions

- **Cervical Radiculopathy:** Hypertrophy or osteophyte formation at Luschka's joints may compress adjacent nerve roots.
- **Cervical Spondylosis:** Degeneration of these joints contributes to stiffness, pain, and decreased range of motion.
- **Facet Joint Syndrome:** Can coexist with uncovertebral joint degeneration, exacerbating symptoms.

Clinical Importance

- **Early Diagnosis:** Identifying uncovertebral joint degeneration can prevent the progression of cervical radiculopathy.
- **Guidance for Treatment:** Detailed knowledge of Luschka's joints aids in tailoring conservative or surgical interventions.
- **Prognostic Value:** Assessing the degree of joint degeneration provides insight into the expected outcomes of treatment.
- **Interdisciplinary Approach:** Collaboration among radiologists, orthopedic surgeons, and physical therapists ensures comprehensive care.

Luxatio Erecta

Overview

Luxatio erecta, or inferior glenohumeral dislocation, is a rare form of shoulder dislocation, accounting for about 0.5% of all shoulder dislocations. It typically results from trauma involving forced hyperabduction of the upper limb. The characteristic clinical presentation includes the arm held in an abducted position, flexed elbow, and pronated forearm. Complications such as fractures, rotator cuff tears, and neurological injuries are common, occurring in up to 80% of cases, emphasizing the need for early diagnosis and prompt treatment.

Historical Background

- The condition was first described by *Middeldorpf and Scharm in 1859*, marking its recognition in medical literature.
- *Murrad, in 1920*, documented the first case of bilateral luxatio erecta, an extremely rare presentation with fewer than 30 cases reported to date.
- A recent meta-analysis by *Nambiar et al.* highlights a 15% prevalence of bilateral cases among 199 patients with this condition.

Purpose

- **Immediate Objective:** Reduce the dislocated joint to restore anatomical alignment and relieve pain.
- **Long-Term Objective:** Prevent complications such as recurrent dislocations, neurological deficits, and adhesive capsulitis while preserving joint function.

Procedure Overview

Diagnosis:

- **Clinical Presentation:** The arm is abducted overhead, with the elbow flexed and the forearm pronated. The patient is unable to lower the arm actively.
- **Imaging:** X-rays (anteroposterior and axillary lateral views): Confirm diagnosis and evaluate for associated fractures.
- **CT scans:** Used for further characterization of fractures or joint damage.
- **MRI:** Essential for assessing rotator cuff tears and soft tissue injuries.
- **Reduction Techniques:** Traction-Contre-Traction Method: Involves applying traction to the abducted arm while counter-traction stabilizes the torso.
- **Smooth Rotation Technique:** Includes anterior translocation of the humeral head, followed by gentle traction and rotation to reposition it into the glenoid fossa.
- Adequate anesthesia and muscle relaxation are critical to ensure a successful and painless reduction.
- **Post-Reduction Care:**
- Immobilization of the arm in adduction and internal rotation for 2–3 weeks.
- Physical therapy to restore range of motion and strength.
- **Surgical Intervention:**
- Reserved for cases with irreducible dislocations, severe fractures, or significant neurological injury.

- Open reduction is performed to restore the joint's anatomical alignment and address associated injuries.

Results and Interpretation

- **Successful Reduction:** Immediate relief from pain and restoration of shoulder alignment. Post-reduction imaging confirms the absence of residual displacement.
- **Complications:** Despite reduction, patients may develop chronic issues like adhesive capsulitis, recurrent instability, or neurological deficits.

Physiological Basis

- The *glenohumeral joint* has the greatest range of motion among all joints, making it highly susceptible to dislocations.
- Forced hyperabduction causes the humeral neck to act as a lever against the acromion, displacing the humeral head inferiorly. This mechanism leads to soft tissue injuries, including damage to the rotator cuff and neurovascular structures.

Clinical Applications

- Knowledge of luxatio erecta is crucial for emergency care providers, orthopedic surgeons, and physical therapists to ensure timely diagnosis and effective management.
- Early intervention reduces the risk of complications and optimizes functional recovery.

Limitations and Technical

Considerations

- **Challenges in Reduction:** Requires skill and experience to avoid causing additional soft tissue or neurovascular damage.
- **Imaging Challenges:** Subtle fractures or soft tissue injuries may be missed without advanced imaging modalities like CT or MRI.
- **Prolonged Immobilization:** Can lead to joint stiffness and delayed recovery.

Modern Relevance

- Advanced imaging techniques like CT and MRI have improved diagnostic accuracy, enabling detailed evaluation of complex injuries.
- Minimally invasive surgical techniques and enhanced physical therapy protocols have significantly improved outcomes in patients with luxatio erecta.

Associated Conditions

- **Fractures:** Commonly involve the glenoid, greater tuberosity, or humeral head.
- **Rotator Cuff Tears:** Observed in up to 80% of cases.
- **Neurovascular Injuries:** Neurological deficits are seen in 60% of cases, often involving the axillary or radial nerve.
- **Adhesive Capsulitis:** A long-term complication affecting joint mobility.

Clinical Importance

- **Prompt Diagnosis:** Clinicians should be aware of the characteristic clinical presentation and confirm the diagnosis using imaging.

- **Early Reduction:** Immediate reduction of the dislocation prevents secondary damage to the joint and surrounding structures.
- **Rehabilitation:** Early initiation of physical therapy minimizes the risk of chronic complications like stiffness and instability.
- **Comprehensive Care:** A multidisciplinary approach involving radiologists, orthopedic surgeons, and rehabilitation specialists ensures optimal outcomes for patients with luxatio erecta.

References

H Acosta CAX, Da Silva Resch E, Rodrigues R. Luxatio erecta bilateral: um relato de caso. Rev Bras Ortop. 2012;47(1):130–2.

Lippert J, Desai B. Bilateral luxatio erecta: a case report. Case Reports Clin Med. 2018;7:608–12.

Tsuchida T, Yang K, Kimura Y, Taniwaki M, Ishigaki S, Itoi E. Luxatio erecta of bilateral shoulders. J Shoulder Elb Surg. 2001;10(6):595–7.

Camarda L, Martorana U, D'Arienzo M. A case of bilateral luxatio erecta. J Orthop Traumatol. 2009;10:97–9.

Petty K, Price J, Kharasch M, Novack J. Bilateral luxatio erecta: a case report. J Emerg Med. 2014;46(2):176–9.

Karaoglu S, Guney A, Ozturk M, Kekec Z. Bilateral luxatio erecta humerI. Arch Orthop Trauma Surg. 2003;123:308–10.

Mesa M, Carpintero P, Carpintero J. Bilateral luxatio erecta humeri. Acta Orthop Belg. 1996;62(2):116–9.

Kumar KS, O'Rourke S, Pillay JG. Hands up: a case of bilateral inferior shoulder dislocation. Emerg Med J. 2001;18(5):404–5.

Musmeci E, Gaspari D, Sandri A, Regis D, Bartolozzi P. Bilateral luxatio erecta humeri associated with a unilateral brachial plexus and bilateral rotator cuff injuries. J Orthop Trauma. 2008;22(7):498–500.

Nambiar M, Owen D, Moore P, Carr A, Thomas M. Traumatic inferior shoulder dislocation: a review of management and outcome. Eur J Trauma Emerg Surg. 2018;44(1):45–51.

Garcia R, Ponsky T, Brody F, Long J. Bilateral luxatio erecta complicated by venous thrombosis. J Trauma. 2006;60(5):1132–4.

Freundlich BD. Luxatio erecta. J Trauma. 1983;23(5):434–6.

Nho SJ, Dodson CC, Bardzik KF, Brophy RH, Domb BG, MacGillivray JD. The two-step maneuver for closed reduction of inferior glenohumeral dislocation (luxatio erecta to anterior dislocation to reduction). J Orthop Trauma. 2006;20(5):354–7.

Reddy SV, Jaiswal A, Kanwar CS. A rare case of bilateral luxatio erecta with bilateral greater tuberosity fracture following a fall due to seizure. J Clin Orthop Trauma. 2019;10(3):503–6.

Mackenzie's operation

Overview

Mackenzie's operation is a surgical modification of Syme's amputation performed at the ankle joint. In Mackenzie's version, the skin flap for closure is derived specifically from the inner side, offering a distinct variation that may be beneficial in certain clinical scenarios. This approach prioritizes flap viability and weight-bearing function.

Historical Background

- **1843:** James Syme introduced his method of ankle disarticulation, Syme's amputation, emphasizing functionality and durable weight-bearing stumps.
- **Late 19th Century:** Richard James Mackenzie modified Syme's procedure by advocating for the creation of a skin flap from the inner side of the ankle to improve the closure and weight-bearing capabilities.

Purpose

- **Improved Weight-Bearing Stump:** Enhances the function of the residual limb for prosthetic use.
- **Optimized Flap Viability:** Utilizes robust skin from the inner side for a durable, well-vascularized closure.
- **Prevention of Complications:** Reduces risks of ischemia and breakdown by utilizing the medial skin flap.

Procedure Overview

- **Patient Preparation:** Standard preoperative steps, including vascular assessment and anesthesia, are followed.
- **Incision and Flap Creation:** A skin incision is made, emphasizing the inner side to preserve sufficient soft tissue for flap formation.
- **Joint Disarticulation:** The ankle joint is disarticulated, similar to Syme's original procedure.
- **Flap Closure:** The medial skin flap is folded over the stump and securely sutured to create a durable and functional end-bearing residual limb.

Results and Interpretation

- **Successful Outcomes:** Many patients achieve functional, weight-bearing stumps that adapt well to prosthetics.
- **Potential Complications:** Flap ischemia, poor healing, or stump discomfort may occur if technical execution or patient factors are suboptimal.

Physiological Basis

- **Preservation of Weight-Bearing:** The operation maintains the heel pad as a natural cushion for weight-bearing, minimizing discomfort.
- **Enhanced Circulation:** By using the medial skin flap, the procedure leverages better vascular supply compared to alternative flaps.

Clinical Applications

- **Amputation Indications:** Severe trauma, infections, tumors, or peripheral vascular disease requiring limb salvage through ankle disarticulation.
- **Prosthetic Compatibility:** Mackenzie's operation produces a residual limb well-suited for modern prosthetic designs.
- **Pediatric Cases:** May be particularly useful in children due to the durability and growth potential of the flap.

Limitations and Technical Considerations

- **Surgical Expertise:** Requires precision in flap creation and closure to ensure a functional stump.
- **Patient Factors:** Not all patients are candidates, especially those with compromised medial skin integrity.
- **Prosthetic Challenges:** Stump shape and size may require custom prosthetic adjustments.

Modern Relevance

- **Enhanced Prosthetics:** Advances in prosthetic technology have renewed interest in amputation techniques that prioritize durable, weight-bearing stumps.
- **Tailored Applications:** Mackenzie's operation is now considered a valuable option for specific cases requiring ankle disarticulation.

Associated Conditions

- **Peripheral Vascular Disease:** Used in cases where limb ischemia necessitates amputation.
- **Severe Trauma:** Suitable for patients with non-salvageable injuries below the knee.

- **Oncological Surgery:** May be employed when tumors involve the foot or lower ankle region.

Clinical Importance

- **Early Intervention:** Provides a surgical solution for severe lower-limb pathologies requiring amputation.
- **Functional Outcomes:** Delivers a durable, weight-bearing stump that adapts well to prosthetics.
- **Prosthetic Compatibility:** Tailors the stump for efficient prosthetic fitting and patient rehabilitation.
- **Customization:** Allows for variations in technique based on patient-specific anatomy and vascular supply.

References

R. J. Mackenzie: On amputation at the ankle-joint by internal lateral flap. Monthly Journal of Medical Science, Edinburgh, 1849, 9: 951-954.

Mafucci's Syndrome

Overview

Maffucci's syndrome is a rare congenital disorder characterized by the presence of multiple enchondromas (benign cartilage tumors) and cavernous hemangiomas (vascular anomalies). The syndrome typically manifests during childhood, leading to bone deformities, pathological fractures, and an increased risk of developing malignancies such as chondrosarcoma and angiosarcoma. The lesions are asymmetrical, affecting both skin and bones, and often remain asymptomatic.

Historical Background

- **1881:** Angelo Maffucci first described the syndrome in a patient with multiple enchondromas and hemangiomas.
- **1889:** Alfred Kast and Friedrich Daniel von Recklinghausen independently reported cases of the same disorder, though they were possibly unaware of Maffucci's earlier work.
- The term "Kast-Maffucci syndrome" was initially used but later simplified to Maffucci's syndrome, reflecting Maffucci's primary contributions.
- **1981:** The centenary of Maffucci's original work was commemorated by Tilsley and Burden, reaffirming the syndrome's clinical and historical importance.

Purpose

- **Diagnosis and Classification:** Identifies the presence of enchondromas and hemangiomas to differentiate

Maffucci's syndrome from other similar conditions, such as Ollier's disease.

- **Early Risk Assessment:** Facilitates the monitoring of potential complications, including malignant transformation into chondrosarcoma or angiosarcoma.

Procedure Overview

- **Imaging Studies:**
- X-rays, CT scans, and MRIs to evaluate enchondromas and bone deformities.
- Doppler ultrasound and angiography to assess vascular lesions.
- **Biopsy:**
- Performed on suspicious lesions to confirm malignancy.
- **Genetic Testing:** Occasionally used to identify potential familial cases or underlying genetic mutations.

Results and Interpretation

- **Imaging Findings:** Radiographs typically show multiple, irregularly distributed enchondromas within the metaphyses and diaphyses of long bones.
- Soft tissue masses corresponding to hemangiomas may be evident.
- **Clinical Presentation:** Progressive skeletal deformities and occasional pigmentation abnormalities, but typically no pain unless complicated by fractures or malignancy.

Physiological Basis

- **Enchondromas:** Represent benign cartilage growths within bones, disrupting normal ossification and leading to deformities.
- **Cavernous Hemangiomas:** Vascular malformations that affect skin and soft tissues, often exacerbating the disfigurement caused by enchondromas.

Clinical Applications

- **Differential Diagnosis:** Distinguishes Maffucci's syndrome from similar disorders, such as Ollier's disease, by identifying hemangiomas and the asymmetrical distribution of lesions.
- **Management of Complications:** Guides the treatment of fractures, deformities, and malignant transformations.
- **Monitoring Malignancy Risk:** Regular follow-ups to detect and address sarcomas early.

Limitations and Technical Considerations

- **Complex Diagnosis:** Early signs may be subtle, requiring detailed imaging and clinical evaluation to avoid misdiagnosis.
- **Surgical Challenges:** Operative management of deformities and tumors may be complicated by extensive vascular lesions.
- **Genetic Insights:** Limited understanding of the genetic basis hampers familial risk prediction.

Modern Relevance

- **Improved Imaging Techniques:** Advanced modalities like MRI provide better visualization of lesions, aiding in early diagnosis.
- **Enhanced Surgical Interventions:** Minimally invasive procedures and prosthetic technologies improve patient outcomes.

- **Oncology Collaboration:** Cross-disciplinary management between orthopedics and oncology ensures comprehensive care.

Associated Conditions

- **Ollier's Disease:** Enchondromatosis without vascular lesions, often mistaken for Maffucci's syndrome.
- **Chondrosarcoma:** Malignant transformation of enchondromas, commonly seen in Maffucci's syndrome.
- **Angiosarcoma:** Malignant transformation of vascular lesions, though less common than chondrosarcoma.

Clinical Importance

- **Early Detection:** Facilitates prompt intervention to manage deformities and prevent fractures.
- **Risk Monitoring:** Regular assessments minimize delays in identifying malignancies.
- **Multidisciplinary Approach:** Involves orthopedists, oncologists, and geneticists for optimal management.
- **Prosthetic Adaptation:** Supports functional recovery following surgical interventions.

References

A. Maffucci: Di un caso encondroma ed angioma multiplo. Contribuzione alla genesi embrionale dei tumori. Movimento medico-chirurgico, Napoli,1881,3:399-412 & 565-575.

Alfred Kast, F. D. von Recklinghausen: Ein Fall von Enchondrom mit ungewöhnlicher Multiplikation. Virchows Archiv für pathologische Anatomie und Physiologie und für klinische Medicin, Berlin, 1889, 118: 1-18.

F. Anderson: Maffucci's syndrome. Report of a case with a review of the literature. South African Medical Journal, Cape Town, 1965, 39: 1066-1070.

D. A. Tilsley, P. W. Burden: A case of Maffucci's syndrome. British Journal of Dermatology, Oxford, 1981, 105: 331-336.

Maisonneuve Fracture

Overview

The Maisonneuve fracture is a spiral fracture of the proximal third of the fibula caused by an external rotation injury to the ankle. It is typically associated with disruption of the distal tibiofibular syndesmosis and the interosseous membrane. Additionally, the injury often includes a fracture of the medial malleolus or a rupture of the deep deltoid ligament. Radiographs reveal widening of the ankle mortise and may show avulsion fractures of the medial or posterior malleoli.

Historical Background

- **1840:** Jacques Gilles Maisonneuve described this fracture mechanism through cadaveric studies. He demonstrated how an external rotational force applied to the foot could propagate through the interosseous membrane to cause a proximal fibula fracture.
- Since its initial description, this fracture pattern has become a classic example of how rotational forces affect the lower extremity and has influenced orthopedic diagnostic and treatment strategies.

Purpose

- **Accurate Diagnosis:** Identifying proximal fibula fractures in association with ankle injuries to ensure the integrity of the distal tibiofibular syndesmosis is assessed.
- **Comprehensive Evaluation:** Helps guide appropriate treatment strategies by evaluating the extent of syndesmotic and ligamentous injuries.

Procedure Overview

- **Clinical Examination:**
- Look for tenderness along the fibula and signs of ankle instability.
- Assess for pain and swelling in the proximal fibula area even if the primary complaint is at the ankle.
- **Imaging:**
- Radiographs of the ankle show mortise widening or medial malleolar fractures.
- Full-length tibiofibular radiographs identify the proximal fibula fracture.
- Stress radiographs assess syndesmotic stability.
- **MRI or** CT may be required to confirm ligamentous and interosseous membrane involvement.

Results and Interpretation

- **Radiographic Findings:**
- Spiral fracture of the proximal fibula.
- Widening of the ankle mortise, indicative of syndesmotic instability.
- Possible avulsion fractures of the medial or posterior malleoli.
- **Clinical Presentation:**
- Pain and swelling at the ankle and proximal fibula.
- Tenderness along the interosseous membrane.

Physiological Basis

- **Force Transmission:**
- External rotation force applied to the foot transmits through the ankle, rupturing the deltoid ligament or fracturing the medial malleolus.
- The force then propagates proximally through the interosseous membrane, resulting in a spiral fracture of the fibula.
- **Instability Mechanism:**
- Disruption of the distal tibiofibular syndesmosis compromises the stability of the ankle joint.

Clinical Applications

- **Orthopedic Surgery:** Essential for determining whether surgical stabilization of the syndesmosis and fixation of associated fractures are required.
- **Rehabilitation:** Post-treatment, patients require physical therapy to regain ankle and lower limb function.

Limitations and Technical Considerations

- **Diagnostic Challenges:** The proximal fibula fracture may be overlooked if radiographs are limited to the ankle region.
- **Incomplete Imaging:** Stress radiographs or advanced imaging may be necessary for subtle injuries to the syndesmosis or interosseous membrane.
- **Delayed Diagnosis:** Missed proximal fibula fractures can result in chronic instability or nonunion.

Modern Relevance

- **Enhanced Imaging:** Modern imaging techniques such as MRI have improved the diagnosis of ligamentous injuries associated with Maisonneuve fractures.

- **Surgical Advances:** Improved surgical techniques for syndesmotic fixation have enhanced outcomes for these injuries.
- **Awareness:** Recognition of this fracture pattern ensures comprehensive management, even when the proximal fibula fracture is not immediately apparent.

Associated Conditions

- **Deltoid Ligament Rupture:** Often accompanies medial malleolar fractures or occurs as an isolated injury in Maisonneuve fractures.
- **Posterior Malleolus Fracture:** May occur in association with Maisonneuve fractures, necessitating specific management.

Clinical Importance

- **Early Diagnosis:** Prompt identification of the Maisonneuve fracture prevents missed proximal fibula injuries and ensures timely management.
- **Comprehensive Management:** Involves stabilizing the syndesmosis, treating fractures, and addressing associated soft tissue injuries.
- **Prognostic Significance:** Proper treatment minimizes long-term complications, such as chronic instability or post-traumatic arthritis.
- **Interdisciplinary Care:** Collaboration between orthopedic surgeons, radiologists, and rehabilitation specialists is crucial for optimal outcomes.

References

Maisonneuve JG. Recherches sur la fracture du péroné. Archives générales de médecine 1840;7:165-187 and 433-473

Pankovich AM. Maisonneuve fracture of the fibula. J Bone Joint Surg Am. 1976 Apr;58(3):337-42. [PMID 816799]

Israeli A, Horoszowski H, Chechick A, Farine I. Beware the "simple" fibular fracture (a clue for severe unstable ankle injury. Br J Sports Med. 1981 Dec; 15(4): 269–271. [PMC1858905]

Hanson JA, Fotoohi M, Wilson AJ. Maisonneuve fracture of the fibula: implications for imaging ankle injury. American Journal of Roentgenology. 1999;173: 702-702.

Kalyani BS, Roberts CS, Giannoudis PV. The Maisonneuve injury: a comprehensive review. Orthopedics. 2010 Mar;33(3):190-5. [PMID 20205369]

Millen JC, Lindberg D. Maisonneuve fracture. J Emerg Med. 2011 Jul;41(1):77-8. [PMID 19157747]

Stufkens SA, van den Bekerom MP, Doornberg JN, van Dijk CN, Kloen P. Evidence-based treatment of Maisonneuve fractures. J Foot Ankle Surg. 2011 Jan-Feb;50(1):62-7 [PMID 21172642]

Taweel NR, Raikin SM, Karanjia HN, Ahmad J. The proximal fibula should be examined in all patients with ankle injury: a case series of missed maisonneuve fractures. J Emerg Med. 2013 Feb;44(2):e251-5. [PMID 23079149]

Malgaigne Fracture

Overview

Malgaigne fracture is a type of unstable pelvic fracture caused by vertical shear forces that result in two ipsilateral pelvic ring fractures. These fractures typically include one anterior and one posterior to the acetabulum, most often involving the superior and inferior pubic rami and the sacroiliac joint or sacral wing. The injury is severe, often associated with instability, high-energy trauma, and a significant risk of complications.

Historical Background

- **1847:** Described by Joseph François Malgaigne, a French surgeon and anatomist, in his seminal work on fractures and dislocations. Malgaigne provided detailed descriptions of pelvic ring injuries, emphasizing the instability and potential complications associated with this type of fracture. His name became associated with the fracture pattern due to his pioneering analysis of pelvic ring injuries.

Purpose

- **Stabilizing Diagnosis:** The classification and identification of Malgaigne fractures aid in understanding the severity and instability of the pelvic injury.
- **Guiding Treatment:** Diagnosis directs the choice of intervention, whether surgical or conservative, based on fracture stability and associated injuries.

Procedure Overview

- **Clinical Assessment:** Patients present with severe pelvic pain, instability, and an inability to bear weight.
- Check for associated injuries, including vascular or visceral trauma.
- **Radiographic Evaluation:** Initial radiographs (AP pelvis) reveal ipsilateral fractures of the pelvic ring.
- CT scans provide detailed images of the sacroiliac joint and sacral fractures, confirming vertical instability.

Results and Interpretation

- **Radiological Findings:**
- Ipsilateral vertical fractures through the superior and inferior pubic rami.
- Fractures involving the sacroiliac joint or sacral wing.
- Widening or displacement indicating vertical instability.
- **Clinical Presentation:** Severe pelvic pain, deformity, and potential signs of shock or neurovascular compromise.

Physiological Basis

- **Force Mechanism:** A high-energy vertical shear force, such as a fall from a height or vehicular collision, transmits through the pelvic ring, disrupting its structural integrity.
- **Instability:** Disruption of the pelvic ring results in significant biomechanical instability, leading to compromised weight-bearing capacity and potential damage to surrounding soft tissues, blood vessels, and nerves.

Clinical Applications

- **Surgical Fixation:** Often necessary to stabilize the pelvic ring, restore weight-bearing function, and prevent chronic instability.
- **Rehabilitation:** Focused on regaining mobility, strength, and functional independence following fracture stabilization.

Limitations and Technical Considerations

- **Complex Diagnosis:** Vertical instability can be subtle and may require advanced imaging techniques for accurate assessment.
- **Risk of Complications:** Associated vascular injuries, nerve damage, and organ involvement may complicate treatment and recovery.
- **Surgical Challenges:** Proper alignment and fixation can be technically demanding due to the complex anatomy of the pelvis.

Modern Relevance

- **Improved Imaging:** Advances in CT and MRI allow for better visualization of fracture patterns and associated injuries.
- **Enhanced Surgical Techniques:** Innovations in surgical hardware and minimally invasive procedures have improved outcomes for unstable pelvic fractures.

Associated Conditions

- **Vascular Injuries:** Disruption of pelvic vessels can lead to significant bleeding and hemodynamic instability.
- **Neurological Damage:** Involvement of the lumbosacral plexus may cause sensory or motor deficits.
- **Visceral Complications:** Injuries to pelvic organs, such as the bladder or urethra, are common in high-energy pelvic trauma.

Clinical Importance

- **Early Diagnosis:** Timely identification of Malgaigne fractures is crucial for preventing complications and initiating stabilization.
- **Surgical Precision:** Precise surgical intervention ensures the restoration of pelvic stability and prevents long-term disability.
- **Holistic Management:** Effective treatment requires a multidisciplinary approach, including orthopedic surgeons, trauma specialists, and rehabilitation experts.
- **Prognostic Implications:** Successful management significantly improves quality of life, though recovery may be prolonged depending on the severity of the injury and associated complications.

References

Malgaigne JF. Double vertical fractures of the pelvis. In: A Treatise on Fractures, Vol 1 (fractures) Philadelphia: Lippincott, 1859. pp523-527

Bucholz RW. The pathological anatomy of Malgaigne fracture-dislocations of the pelvis. J Bone Joint Surg Am. 1981 Mar;63(3):400-4. [PMID 7204439]

Mallet Finger

Overview

Mallet finger, also referred to as baseball finger, is a deformity caused by disruption of the extensor tendon at the distal interphalangeal joint (DIPJ). This condition results in an inability to actively extend the distal phalanx, which droops into a flexed position. It commonly occurs due to trauma or minor injuries, often during sports or household activities. Mallet finger can lead to functional impairment if untreated, but non-surgical management is effective in most cases.

Historical Background

- The term "Mallet finger" has origins in the 19th century, coined to describe the hammer-like deformity caused by sports-related injuries.
- Alternative names such as *baseball finger* arose from its prevalence in athletes, especially those involved in high-velocity or contact sports.
- The evolution of treatment modalities over decades reflects a deeper understanding of tendon injury mechanisms and outcomes.

Purpose

- **Immediate Objective:** Restore proper alignment of the extensor tendon and preserve DIPJ functionality.
- **Long-Term Objective:** Prevent deformities such as swan neck deformity and avoid complications like chronic pain or impaired joint mobility.

Procedure Overview

Diagnosis:

- **Clinical Presentation:** Drooping of the distal phalanx with an inability to extend actively.

Imaging:

- X-rays (AP, lateral, and oblique) are essential to differentiate between bony and tendinous injuries.
- Ultrasound may aid in assessing soft tissue involvement if required.

Treatment:

- **Nonoperative Management:** Splinting of the DIPJ in full extension or slight hyperextension for 6-8 weeks.
- **Splints such as stack splints or custom-fabricated splints are commonly used.**
- **Operative Management:** Reserved for cases with large avulsion fractures, subluxation of the DIPJ, or failed conservative treatment.
- Techniques include pin fixation, tendon reconstruction, or direct repair of bony fragments.
- **Follow-Up:**
- Regular evaluations to ensure proper alignment and healing.
- Physical therapy to restore strength and range of motion after splint removal.

Results and Interpretation

- **Successful Nonoperative Treatment:** Restoration of full or near-full extension of the DIPJ with minimal lag (<10°).
- **Operative Outcomes:** Generally

favorable, but complications like infection, tendon rupture, or joint incongruity may occur.

Physiological Basis

- The *extensor tendon* facilitates straightening of the DIPJ. Mallet finger occurs when this tendon is disrupted, leaving the *flexor digitorum profundus* unopposed, causing the distal phalanx to remain in a flexed position.
- If untreated, chronic flexion may lead to joint instability, deformities like swan neck deformity, and impaired hand functionality.

Clinical Applications

- Applicable in primary care, sports medicine, and orthopedic surgery for managing trauma-induced or chronic extensor tendon injuries.
- Early diagnosis and splinting are critical in preventing long-term complications.

Limitations and Technical Considerations

- **Challenges in Nonoperative Management:** Skin complications like maceration and ulceration due to prolonged splint use.
- **Patient compliance is critical, as interruptions in splinting can lead to recurrent deformities.**
- **Surgical Risks:** Infection, secondary displacement, and extensor tendon rupture.
- Potential for joint stiffness or avascular necrosis in severe cases.

Modern Relevance

- **Advances in** splint design and surgical techniques have improved outcomes for mallet finger injuries.
- Minimally invasive approaches and early rehabilitation protocols enhance recovery and minimize complications.

Associated Conditions

- **Swan Neck Deformity:** Hyperextension at the proximal interphalangeal joint due to imbalance between extensor and flexor forces.
- **Chronic Extensor Lag:** Residual inability to fully extend the DIPJ despite treatment.
- **Nail Deformities:** Resulting from improper splinting or secondary complications.

Clinical Importance

- **Prompt Management:** Early diagnosis and splinting are crucial to avoid chronic deformities and functional impairments.
- **Multidisciplinary Care:** Collaboration among primary care providers, orthopedic specialists, and physical therapists ensures comprehensive care.
- **Patient Education:** Emphasizing compliance with splinting protocols and follow-up visits is key to successful outcomes. Rehabilitation post-treatment is vital to restore joint function and strength.

Mallet finger, though often perceived as minor, demands systematic evaluation and care to prevent long-term morbidity and optimize hand function.

References

Kootstra TJM, Keizer J, van Heijl M, Ferree S, Houwert M, van der Velde D. Delayed Extension Block Pinning in 27 Patients With Mallet Fracture. Hand (N Y). 2021 Jan;16(1):61-66. [PMC free article] [PubMed]

Kralj R, Barcot Z, Vlahovic T, Kurtanjek M, Petracic I. The patterns of phalangeal fractures in children and adolescents: a review of 512 cases. Handchir Mikrochir Plast Chir. 2019 Feb;51(1):49-53. [PubMed]

Reddy M, Ho CA. Comparison of Percutaneous Reduction and Pin Fixation in Acute and Chronic Pediatric Mallet Fractures. J Pediatr Orthop. 2019 Mar;39(3):146-152. [PubMed]

Lin JS, Samora JB. Outcomes of Splinting in Pediatric Mallet Finger. J Hand Surg Am. 2018 Nov;43(11):1041.e1-1041.e9. [PubMed]

Rosinsky P, Sarig O, David Y, Oron A. [MALLET FINGER - DIAGNOSIS, CLASSIFICATION AND TREATMENT]. Harefuah. 2018 Feb;157(2):104-107. [PubMed]

Lin JS, Samora JB. Surgical and Nonsurgical Management of Mallet Finger: A Systematic Review. J Hand Surg Am. 2018 Feb;43(2):146-163.e2. [PubMed]

Yee J, Waseem M. StatPearls [Internet]. StatPearls Publishing; Treasure Island (FL): Aug 8, 2022. Mallet Finger Injuries. [PubMed]

Lamaris GA, Matthew MK. The Diagnosis and Management of Mallet Finger Injuries. Hand (N Y). 2017 May;12(3):223-228. [PMC free article] [PubMed]

Bachoura A, Ferikes AJ, Lubahn JD. A review of mallet finger and jersey finger injuries in the athlete. Curr Rev Musculoskelet Med. 2017 Mar;10(1):1-9. [PMC free article] [PubMed]

Jabłecki J, Syrko M. Zone 1 extensor tendon lesions: current treatment methods and a review of literature. Ortop Traumatol Rehabil. 2007 Jan-Feb;9(1):52-62. [PubMed]

Niechajev IA. Conservative and operative treatment of mallet finger. Plast Reconstr Surg. 1985 Oct;76(4):580-5. [PubMed]

Valdes K, Naughton N, Algar L. ICF components of outcome measures for mallet finger: A systematic review. J Hand Ther. 2016 Oct-Dec;29(4):388-395. [PubMed]

Kinninmonth AW, Holburn F. A comparative controlled trial of a new perforated splint and a traditional splint in the treatment of mallet finger. J Hand Surg Br. 1986 Jun;11(2):261-2. [PubMed]

Katzman BM, Klein DM, Mesa J, Geller J, Caligiuri DA. Immobilization of the mallet finger. Effects on the extensor tendon. J Hand Surg Br. 1999 Feb;24(1):80-4. [PubMed]

Fritz D, Lutz M, Arora R, Gabl M, Wambacher M, Pechlaner S. Delayed single Kirschner wire compression technique for mallet fracture. J Hand Surg Br. 2005 May;30(2):180-4.

March Fracture

Overview

March fractures, also known as metatarsal stress fractures, are overuse injuries that typically affect the second or third metatarsal bones. These fractures are caused by repetitive stress rather than a single traumatic event, making them common in athletes, military recruits, and individuals engaging in prolonged weight-bearing activities. These injuries are associated with pain and swelling in the forefoot and are typically managed conservatively, although complications like nonunion may necessitate surgical intervention.

Historical Background

- The term "March fracture" was first described in *1855*, referencing the foot pain and swelling observed in *Prussian soldiers* during long marches.
- The fracture has since been recognized in other populations, particularly those engaged in high-impact activities like athletics and military training.

Purpose

- **Primary Objective:** Relieve symptoms such as pain and swelling and promote bone healing.
- **Long-Term Objective:** Restore functionality, prevent recurrence, and reduce complications such as nonunion.

Procedure Overview

Diagnosis:

- **Clinical Features:** Gradual onset of forefoot pain, aggravated by activity.

- Swelling and tenderness localized to the affected metatarsal.
- **Imaging:** Initial X-rays may appear normal; stress fractures are often detectable only after 2-3 weeks when callus formation becomes evident.
- **MRI or** bone scans can detect fractures earlier and differentiate from other conditions like soft tissue injuries.

Management:

- **Nonoperative Treatment:** Activity modification: Rest and avoidance of weight-bearing activities.
- **Immobilization:** Use of a stiff-soled shoe or walking boot for pain relief and to prevent further stress.
- **Physical therapy:** Strengthening exercises and gradual return to activity.
- **Surgical Treatment:** Reserved for cases of nonunion or persistent pain.
- Options include intramedullary nailing or open reduction and internal fixation (ORIF).

Results and Interpretation

- **Nonoperative Outcomes:** Most cases resolve with rest and immobilization, achieving full recovery within 6-8 weeks.
- **Surgical Outcomes:** Effective in cases of nonunion, though recovery may be prolonged, sometimes requiring months for full healing.

Physiological Basis

- **Stress fractures result from a mismatch between bone remodeling processes:** Osteoclastic Activity: Bone resorption increases during periods of increased mechanical stress.
- **Osteoblastic Activity:** Bone formation lags behind, leading to microfractures that eventually consolidate into stress fractures.
- The second metatarsal is particularly vulnerable due to its length, rigidity, and high torsional forces during gait.

Clinical Applications

- Common in sports medicine and orthopedics for managing overuse injuries in active populations.
- Preventive measures, including footwear modifications and training adjustments, are crucial in high-risk groups like military recruits and athletes.

Limitations and Technical Considerations

- **Challenges in Diagnosis:** Early stress fractures may not be visible on initial X-rays, requiring advanced imaging modalities.
- **Treatment Challenges:** Noncompliance with activity modification can delay healing.
- Nonunion and chronic pain may necessitate surgical intervention, which involves risks like infection or hardware failure.

Modern Relevance

- With increasing participation in recreational sports and military activities, march fractures remain a prevalent concern.
- **Advances in** imaging and minimally invasive surgical techniques have improved diagnosis and outcomes.
- Emphasis on preventive strategies has grown, focusing on footwear, training

regimens, and early detection.

Associated Conditions

- **Bone Insufficiency:** Stress fractures in individuals with osteoporosis or other bone-weakening conditions.
- **Nutritional Deficiencies:** Conditions like vitamin D or calcium deficiency can predispose individuals to stress fractures.
- **Chronic Pain Syndromes:** Resulting from untreated or inadequately treated fractures.

Clinical Importance

- **Prevention:** Education on stretching, proper footwear, and gradual training progression is key.
- **Multidisciplinary Management:** Collaboration among physicians, physical therapists, and nurses ensures comprehensive care.
- **Prognosis:** Most fractures heal well with conservative management.
- Early detection and adherence to treatment protocols are critical in preventing complications such as nonunion and recurrent fractures.
- March fractures are a significant yet manageable condition in active populations. Early intervention and preventive measures can optimize outcomes and reduce the risk of long-term disability.

References

Jacobs JM, Cameron KL, Bojescul JA. Lower extremity stress fractures in the military. Clin Sports Med. 2014 Oct;33(4):591-613. [PubMed]

Sanderlin BW, Raspa RF. Common stress fractures. Am Fam Physician. 2003 Oct 15;68(8):1527-32. [PubMed]

Pegrum J, Dixit V, Padhiar N, Nugent I. The pathophysiology, diagnosis, and management of foot stress fractures. Phys Sportsmed. 2014 Nov;42(4):87-99. [PubMed]

Patel DS, Roth M, Kapil N. Stress fractures: diagnosis, treatment, and prevention. Am Fam Physician. 2011 Jan 01;83(1):39-46. [PubMed]

Miller TL, Jamieson M, Everson S, Siegel C. Expected Time to Return to Athletic Participation After Stress Fracture in Division I Collegiate Athletes. Sports Health. 2018 Jul-Aug;10(4):340-344. [PMC free article] [PubMed]

Saunier J, Chapurlat R. Stress fracture in athletes. Joint Bone Spine. 2018 May;85(3):307-310. [PubMed]

Bolin D, Kemper A, Brolinson PG. Current concepts in the evaluation and management of stress fractures. Curr Sports Med Rep. 2005 Dec;4(6):295-300. [PubMed]

Patel DR. Stress fractures: diagnosis and management in the primary care setting. Pediatr Clin North Am. 2010 Jun;57(3):819-27.

Marfan's hypermobility Syndrome

Overview

Marfan's hypermobility syndrome is a condition characterized by a marfanoid habitus, marked joint hypermobility, and significant skin hyperextensibility. Unlike classic Marfan syndrome, it lacks the hallmark features of aortic involvement or lens displacement. However, some cases have been associated with valvular heart disease. The etiology remains unknown, and it is considered distinct from other connective tissue disorders.

Historical Background

- **1896:** Antoine Bernard-Jean Marfan first described Marfan syndrome, characterized by long limbs, arachnodactyly, and other connective tissue anomalies.
- The differentiation of *Marfan's hypermobility syndrome* as a distinct entity emerged later, emphasizing the absence of aortic and lens abnormalities typical of Marfan syndrome.

Purpose

- **Differentiating Marfan Subtypes:** The syndrome helps clinicians distinguish between Marfan syndrome and other marfanoid presentations with joint and skin hypermobility.
- **Targeted Management:** Understanding the absence of aortic or ocular involvement aids in focusing management on musculoskeletal and dermatological manifestations.

Procedure Overview

- **Clinical Examination:**
- Assessment of marfanoid features, including long limbs, tall stature, and joint hypermobility using the Beighton score.
- Evaluation of skin hyperextensibility and other connective tissue anomalies.
- **Imaging and Testing:**
- Echocardiography to rule out aortic and valvular heart abnormalities.
- Ophthalmologic evaluation to confirm the absence of lens dislocation.

Results and Interpretation

- **Typical Findings:**
- Hypermobile joints with a Beighton score indicative of significant laxity.
- Hyperextensible skin that far exceeds the typical range in classic Marfan syndrome.
- Absence of aortic root dilation or ectopia lentis.
- **Potential Variability:** Some cases may show valvular heart abnormalities, necessitating regular monitoring.

Physiological Basis

- **Connective Tissue Abnormality:** The syndrome is thought to result from an underlying defect in connective tissue, affecting joint capsules, skin elasticity, and potentially heart valves.
- **Distinction from Marfan Syndrome:** Unlike Marfan syndrome, there is no involvement of fibrillin-1 mutations or associated aortic and ocular pathology.

Clinical Applications

- **Symptom Management:** Focused on treating joint hypermobility-related issues such as pain, dislocations, and reduced mobility.
- **Surveillance for Heart Disease:** Regular cardiac evaluations in cases with valvular involvement.

Limitations and Technical Considerations

- **Complex Diagnosis:** Differentiating Marfan's hypermobility syndrome from similar conditions such as Ehlers-Danlos syndrome or hypermobility spectrum disorders may be challenging.
- **Variable Presentation:** The absence of major systemic complications like aortic involvement makes the diagnosis more reliant on subtle musculoskeletal and dermatological signs.

Modern Relevance

- **Growing Awareness:** Increased recognition of hypermobility-related disorders highlights the importance of identifying Marfan's hypermobility syndrome as a distinct clinical entity.
- **Personalized Treatment Approaches:** Advances in understanding connective tissue disorders contribute to better management strategies tailored to individual presentations.

Associated Conditions

- **Valvular Heart Disease:** Mitral valve prolapse and other valvular abnormalities have been reported in some cases.
- **Musculoskeletal Issues:** Recurrent joint dislocations, chronic pain, and early-onset osteoarthritis may occur.

Clinical Importance

- **Early Diagnosis:** Timely identification helps in addressing joint and skin symptoms while avoiding unnecessary screening for aortic or ocular involvement.
- **Improved Quality of Life:** Managing hypermobility-related complications can significantly enhance mobility and reduce pain.
- **Differentiating Similar Syndromes:** Clear distinction from other marfanoid and connective tissue disorders ensures appropriate clinical focus and avoids overdiagnosis.

References

C. Roederer: Syndrome d'Ehlers-Danlos atypique coincidant avec une dolichostenomélie. Archives francaises de pédiatrie, Paris, 1951, 8: 192-195.

B. A. Walker, et al: The marfanoid hypermobility syndrome. Annals of Internal Medicine, Philadelphia, 1969, 71: 349-352.

Marfan's symptom

Overview

Marfan's symptom is a clinical manifestation characterized by rachitic epiphyseal swelling of the medial malleolus (malleolus medialis) of the lower leg. This swelling, commonly referred to as a "double knuckle," is evident as a step-like deformity on palpation and is associated with rachitic conditions affecting bone growth and development.

Historical Background

- **1896:** Antoine Bernard-Jean Marfan, a French pediatrician, first described the systemic condition now known as Marfan syndrome.
- The specific symptom of rachitic epiphyseal swelling of the medial malleolus was later identified and included under the descriptive spectrum of Marfan-related signs.

Purpose

- **Diagnostic Aid:** Marfan's symptom serves as a physical clue to underlying metabolic or developmental bone disorders, especially in cases of suspected rickets or other systemic skeletal abnormalities.
- **Early Recognition of Rachitic Conditions:** The symptom highlights the presence of bone deformities that may benefit from early medical intervention.

Procedure Overview

- **Clinical Examination:** The medial malleolus is palpated for evidence of swelling and step-like deformities.
- Assessment for other signs of rickets, such as bowing of the legs or skeletal abnormalities, is performed.
- **Radiographic Imaging:** X-rays are often used to confirm the presence of rachitic changes at the epiphyseal plates and surrounding structures.

Results and Interpretation

- **Typical Findings:**
- A visible and palpable "double knuckle" deformity at the medial malleolus.
- Radiographs reveal widening and irregularity at the epiphyseal plate, indicative of rickets or similar disorders.
- **Variable Presentation:** The severity of the symptom may vary depending on the underlying condition and the age of the patient.

Physiological Basis

- **Epiphyseal Changes:** The swelling and step-like deformity are caused by defective mineralization and cartilage ossification at the epiphyseal plates, often due to vitamin D deficiency or metabolic bone disease.
- **Rachitic Influence:** Rickets causes softening and weakening of bones, leading to characteristic deformities like those observed in Marfan's symptom.

Clinical Applications

- **Screening Tool:** Marfan's symptom can aid in the early detection of rickets and other bone growth disorders in pediatric patients.
- **Guiding Treatment:** Identification of this symptom helps in directing investigations toward the underlying metabolic or nutritional deficiencies.

Limitations and Technical Considerations

- **Non-Specific Symptom:** While indicative of rachitic or metabolic conditions, Marfan's symptom alone is not diagnostic and requires further clinical and radiological correlation.
- **Age Dependency:** The manifestation is more pronounced in growing children and may be less noticeable in adults.

Modern Relevance

- **Awareness in Pediatric Practice:** The recognition of Marfan's symptom remains relevant in identifying early bone deformities and addressing systemic conditions like rickets.
- **Advances in Imaging:** Modern radiographic techniques have improved the precision of diagnosing epiphyseal abnormalities.

Associated Conditions

- **Rickets:** The most common underlying condition, characterized by vitamin D deficiency and defective bone mineralization.
- **Metabolic Bone Diseases:** Other systemic conditions causing abnormal epiphyseal growth or ossification may also present with Marfan's symptom.

Clinical Importance

- **Early Diagnosis:** Recognition of Marfan's symptom facilitates timely identification and treatment of underlying rachitic or metabolic disorders.
- **Guiding Nutritional Interventions:** Prompts correction of vitamin D deficiency or other nutritional deficiencies to prevent further skeletal complications.
- **Highlighting Systemic Impact:** The symptom underscores the systemic nature of rachitic and metabolic bone conditions, emphasizing the need for comprehensive management.

References

J. B. A. Marfan: Quatre leçons sur le rachitisme. Nourisson, 1922, 10.

Maladies des os. Paris, 1912.

Marfan's syndrome I

Overview

Marfan's syndrome I is a genetic connective tissue disorder primarily affecting the musculoskeletal, cardiovascular, and ocular systems. Patients exhibit a characteristic asthenic build with tall stature, long limbs, arachnodactyly (spider-like fingers), joint laxity, and skeletal deformities such as scoliosis and chest wall abnormalities. Cardiovascular complications, especially aortic aneurysm or rupture, are the leading causes of mortality. The condition is autosomal dominant in 75% of cases, with variable expression, and sporadic mutations account for the remaining 25%.

Historical Background

- **1896:** Antoine Bernard-Jean Marfan, a French pediatrician, first described the syndrome in a five-year-old girl presenting with characteristic skeletal abnormalities, including long, thin fingers (arachnodactyly).
- Further studies throughout the 20th century detailed the condition's systemic involvement, particularly the cardiovascular and ocular complications.
- The genetic basis was identified as mutations in the *FBN1 gene* encoding fibrillin-1, a protein crucial for connective tissue structure.

Purpose

- **Clinical Identification:** To enable early diagnosis and management of life-threatening complications, particularly cardiovascular abnormalities.
- **Genetic Counseling:** To inform affected individuals and their families about inheritance patterns, risks, and preventive measures.

Procedure Overview

- **Clinical Examination:** Height, arm span-to-height ratio, joint laxity, and skeletal abnormalities (e.g., scoliosis, pectus excavatum).
- Ocular examination for lens dislocation and retinal detachment.
- Cardiovascular evaluation using echocardiography to assess aortic dilation and valvular dysfunction.
- **Genetic Testing:** Identification of mutations in the FBN1 gene confirms the diagnosis.
- **Diagnostic Criteria:** Ghent Nosology combines clinical findings and family history for diagnostic accuracy.

Results and Interpretation

- **Key Findings:**
- Disproportionately long limbs and fingers (arachnodactyly).
- Lens subluxation (ectopia lentis) seen in ocular imaging.
- Echocardiographic evidence of aortic root dilation or aneurysm.
- Positive genetic test for FBN1 mutation confirms diagnosis.

Physiological Basis

- **Connective Tissue Dysfunction:** The FBN1 gene mutation affects fibrillin-1, a glycoprotein essential for the structural integrity of connective tissue and regulation of growth factors.

- **Cardiovascular Impact:** Weakening of the aortic wall predisposes to aneurysms and rupture, often the leading cause of death.
- **Skeletal Abnormalities:** Overgrowth of bones due to disrupted signaling pathways involving connective tissue components.

Clinical Applications

- **Preventive Cardiovascular Management:** Beta-blockers and angiotensin receptor blockers (e.g., losartan) to reduce stress on the aortic wall.
- Regular echocardiographic monitoring for aortic root dilation.
- **Orthopedic Interventions:** Surgical correction of scoliosis or severe chest wall deformities.
- **Ophthalmologic Care:** Lens replacement surgery for ectopia lentis and management of glaucoma or retinal detachment.

Limitations and Technical Considerations

- **Variable Expression:** Wide phenotypic variability complicates diagnosis, particularly in mild cases.
- **Overlap with Other Syndromes:** Differential diagnosis is necessary to distinguish from other marfanoid syndromes such as Loeys-Dietz syndrome.
- **Incomplete Genetic Testing:** Not all cases show detectable FBN1 mutations, requiring reliance on clinical findings.

Modern Relevance

- **Improved Survival:** Advances in cardiovascular management, including prophylactic aortic surgery, have significantly increased life expectancy.
- **Enhanced Diagnosis:** Use of genetic testing and updated diagnostic criteria (Ghent Nosology) ensures earlier and more accurate diagnosis.

Associated Conditions

- **Loeys-Dietz Syndrome:** Similar features but associated with craniofacial abnormalities and higher vascular rupture risk.
- **Ehlers-Danlos Syndrome:** Joint hypermobility and skin extensibility overlap but lack Marfan's skeletal and ocular findings.
- **Achard Syndrome:** Similar skeletal features but without eye or heart involvement.

Clinical Importance

- **Early Diagnosis:** Critical for preventing life-threatening aortic complications through surveillance and timely interventions.
- **Prognostic Value:** Severity of cardiovascular manifestations determines life expectancy and quality of life.
- **Interdisciplinary Management:** Coordination among cardiologists, geneticists, orthopedic surgeons, and ophthalmologists is essential for comprehensive care.
- **Genetic Counseling:** Empowers families with knowledge of inheritance patterns and options for prenatal or

preimplantation genetic diagnosis.

References

A. B. Marfan: Un cas de déformation congénitale des quatre membres, plus prononcée aux extrémités, caracterisée par l'allongement des os avec un certain degré d'aminicissement. Bulletins et memoires de la Société medicale des hôpitaux de Paris, 1896, 13: 220-226.

La dolichosténomélie (dolichomélie, arachnodactylie). Ann Méd, 1938, 44:5-29.

H. J. M. Weve: Ueber Arachnodaktylie (Dystrophia mesodermalis congenita, Typus Marfan). Archiv für Augenheilkunde, Wiesbaden, 1931, 104: 1-46.

Maroeteaux-Lamy Syndrome I

Overview

Maroteaux-Lamy Syndrome I is a rare lysosomal storage disorder caused by a deficiency in the enzyme arylsulfatase B, leading to impaired degradation of dermatan sulfate and chondroitin sulfate. The condition is characterized by progressive skeletal deformities, dwarfism, hearing loss, and multi-organ involvement, including cardiac valve disease and hepatosplenomegaly. Onset and severity vary, with two distinct forms: a severe type presenting in early childhood and a milder type with later onset.

Historical Background

- **1963:** Pierre Maroteaux and Maurice Emile Joseph Lamy described the syndrome, distinguishing it from other mucopolysaccharidoses by its unique clinical and biochemical features.
- Prior to their work, the condition was often confused with *Hurler syndrome* due to overlapping clinical presentations.
- **Advances in** enzymatic and genetic analysis in the later 20th century confirmed the deficiency of *arylsulfatase B* as the underlying cause.

Purpose

- **Clinical Diagnosis:** To distinguish Maroteaux-Lamy Syndrome from other mucopolysaccharidoses through clinical features and enzymatic assays.
- **Therapeutic Intervention:** Early identification allows for enzyme

replacement therapy and supportive care to improve quality of life.

Procedure Overview

- **Clinical Examination:** Assessment of growth parameters, skeletal deformities (e.g., kyphosis, genu valgum), and corneal clouding.
- **Laboratory Testing:** Measurement of arylsulfatase B activity in leukocytes or fibroblasts.
- Elevated levels of dermatan sulfate and chondroitin sulfate in urine.
- **Imaging:** Radiographic evidence of dysostosis multiplex, including thickened ribs, shortened long bones, and pelvic deformities.
- **Genetic Testing:** Identification of mutations in the ARSB gene.

Results and Interpretation

- **Key Findings:**
- Reduced or absent arylsulfatase B enzyme activity confirms the diagnosis.
- Radiological findings consistent with dysostosis multiplex.
- Normal intelligence differentiates Maroteaux-Lamy Syndrome from other forms of mucopolysaccharidosis with cognitive impairment.

Physiological Basis

- **Enzyme Deficiency:** Mutation in the ARSB gene leads to reduced arylsulfatase B activity, causing accumulation of dermatan sulfate and chondroitin sulfate in lysosomes.
- **Connective Tissue Impact:** Excess mucopolysaccharides disrupt connective tissue function, leading to skeletal abnormalities, joint stiffness, and cardiac valve defects.

Clinical Applications

- **Enzyme Replacement Therapy (ERT):** Use of recombinant human arylsulfatase B (e.g., Galsulfase) to slow disease progression and reduce non-skeletal complications.
- **Surgical Interventions:** Correction of severe skeletal deformities, including kyphosis and genu valgum.
- Valve replacement for cardiac involvement.
- **Symptom Management:** Physical therapy for joint mobility.
- Supportive care for hearing loss and vision issues.

Limitations and Technical Considerations

- **Variable Severity:** Mild cases may remain undiagnosed until later in life due to delayed onset of symptoms.
- **Incomplete Response to ERT:** Skeletal abnormalities are less responsive to enzyme replacement compared to other systemic symptoms.
- **Diagnostic Challenges:** Overlapping features with other mucopolysaccharidoses require careful differentiation through biochemical and genetic testing.

Modern Relevance

- **Advances in Treatment:** Enzyme replacement therapy has transformed the management of Maroteaux-Lamy Syndrome, improving life expectancy and reducing systemic complications.

- **Early Diagnosis:** Newborn screening programs may enable earlier detection and intervention.

Associated Conditions

- **Hurler Syndrome:** Similar skeletal deformities but with cognitive impairment.
- **Morquio Syndrome:** Skeletal dysplasia with significant spine and joint involvement but without hepatosplenomegaly.

Clinical Importance

- **Early Diagnosis:** Crucial for initiating enzyme replacement therapy and preventing irreversible complications.
- **Prognostic Value:** Severity of skeletal and systemic involvement determines the patient's quality of life and longevity.
- **Interdisciplinary Management:** Requires collaboration among geneticists, orthopedists, cardiologists, and physical therapists to address multisystem involvement.
- **Genetic Counseling:** Educates families on inheritance patterns and risks for future offspring.

References

P. Maroteaux, B. Levêque, J. Marie, M. Lamy. Une nouvelle dysostose avec élimination urinaire de chondroitine-sulfat B. La presse médicale, Paris, 1963, 71: 1949-1851.

P. Maroteaux, M. Lamy: Hurler's disease, Morquio's disease, and related mucopolysaccharidoses. Jurnal of Pediatrics, St. Louis, 1965, 67: 312-323.

Maroteaux-Lamy Syndrome II

Overview

Maroteaux-Lamy Syndrome II, a rare familial form of idiopathic osteolysis, is characterized by progressive bone resorption, primarily affecting the phalanges of the hands and feet. The condition typically presents between the ages of 8 and 22, leading to ulcers, bone sequestra, and eventual loss of digits upon healing. Although it shares some features with other skeletal dysplasias, Maroteaux-Lamy Syndrome II is distinguished by its familial nature and autosomal dominant inheritance.

Historical Background

- **1965:** Maroteaux and Lamy, pioneers in the study of connective tissue and lysosomal disorders, described this syndrome, building on their previous work on Maroteaux-Lamy Syndrome I.
- **Recognition of osteolysis as a primary feature helped differentiate this condition from other forms of skeletal dysplasia.**
- **1970s:** Reports emerged linking a similar clinical presentation to vinyl chloride exposure, highlighting potential environmental factors mimicking the syndrome.

Purpose

- **Clinical Differentiation:** To distinguish Maroteaux-Lamy Syndrome II from other osteolytic conditions, including those caused by environmental exposures or systemic diseases.

- **Therapeutic Planning:** Early identification allows for symptomatic management and preventive care to reduce complications such as ulceration and digit loss.

Procedure Overview

- **Clinical Examination:** Inspection for ulcers on digits, shortened phalanges, and evidence of progressive bone loss.
- **Radiological Imaging:** X-rays to identify progressive osteolysis of the phalanges and other affected bones.
- **Genetic Testing:** Confirmation of autosomal dominant inheritance through family history and genetic studies.
- **Environmental Assessment:** Evaluation for exposure to potential toxins like vinyl chloride that may mimic the syndrome.

Results and Interpretation

- **Radiographic Findings:**
- Progressive resorption of the bones in the phalanges, with eventual loss of visible bone structures.
- Evidence of healed ulcers without active infection or significant inflammation.
- **Genetic Confirmation:** Identification of a hereditary pattern supports a diagnosis of Maroteaux-Lamy Syndrome II.

Physiological Basis

- **Bone Resorption:** Pathological activation of osteoclasts or suppression of osteoblast activity leads to progressive bone loss.
- **Ulcer Formation:** Reduced structural integrity and vascular compromise predispose to ulceration, particularly on pressure-bearing areas.
- **Idiopathic Nature:** Unlike other forms of osteolysis, no specific enzyme deficiency or metabolic abnormality has been identified.

Clinical Applications

- **Symptomatic Management:** Treatment of ulcers to prevent secondary infections and promote healing.
- **Prosthetic Fitting:** For individuals with significant digit loss, prosthetics may restore some functionality.
- **Preventive Measures:** Avoidance of environmental exposures, such as vinyl chloride, which may exacerbate symptoms.

Limitations and Technical Considerations

- **Diagnostic Challenges:** Overlap with other idiopathic osteolytic disorders or environmental exposures can complicate diagnosis.
- **Progressive Nature:** Lack of curative treatment necessitates ongoing monitoring and management of complications.
- **Variable Presentation:** Age of onset and severity vary widely, even within families.

Modern Relevance

- **Advances in Genetic Studies:** Emerging genetic tools may help identify specific mutations associated with this condition, improving diagnostic accuracy.

- **Toxicology Awareness:** Awareness of chemical exposures mimicking the syndrome informs public health and workplace safety initiatives.

Associated Conditions

- **Vinyl Chloride-Induced Osteolysis:** Environmental exposure presenting with similar clinical and radiographic features.
- **Other Forms of Idiopathic Osteolysis:** Gorham-Stout disease and Winchester syndrome share overlapping characteristics but differ in systemic manifestations.

Clinical Importance

- **Early Diagnosis:** Identification of the syndrome facilitates preventive care and symptomatic management to reduce complications.
- **Prognostic Insights:** Recognizing the autosomal dominant inheritance pattern provides critical information for genetic counseling.
- **Environmental Considerations:** Distinguishing familial cases from toxin-induced conditions informs both treatment and prevention strategies.
- **Multidisciplinary Management:** Collaboration among geneticists, orthopedic specialists, and dermatologists optimizes outcomes for affected individuals.

References

P. Maroteaux, M. Lamy: Acro-ostéolyse dominante. Archives francaises de pédiatrie, Paris, 1961, 18: 693-702.

D. K. Harris, W. G. Adams: Acro-osteolysis occurring in men engaged in the polymerization of vinyl chloride. British Medical Journal, London, 1967, 3: 712-714.

Maroteaux-Lamy Syndrome III

Overview

Maroteaux-Lamy Syndrome III, also referred to as pycnodysostosis, is a rare congenital bone disorder manifesting early in infancy. It is characterized by short-limbed dwarfism, craniofacial abnormalities, and increased bone fragility, leading to frequent fractures, particularly in the lower extremities. Distinctive craniofacial features include a large skull with persistent fontanelle, frontal and occipital bossing, parrot-like nose, and dental anomalies. Skeletal deformities such as genu valgum, kyphosis, and scoliosis are common. The syndrome is autosomal recessive, and parental consanguinity has been documented in some cases.

Historical Background

- **1957:** Pierre Maroteaux and Maurice Lamy first described the syndrome in the context of their research into mucopolysaccharidosis disorders.
- *Henri de Toulouse-Lautrec (1864–1901)*, the famous French painter, is often retrospectively considered a classic case of Maroteaux-Lamy Syndrome III, leading to its association with the term *Toulouse-Lautrec syndrome.*
- Subsequent studies in the late *20th century* further elaborated on its genetic basis and clinical features, establishing the syndrome as a distinct skeletal dysplasia.

Purpose

- **Diagnostic Clarity:** To differentiate Maroteaux-Lamy Syndrome III from other forms of short-limbed dwarfism, such as Maroteaux-Lamy Syndrome I or osteogenesis imperfecta.
- **Genetic Counseling:** Early recognition aids in providing genetic advice to families with a history of autosomal recessive disorders.

Procedure Overview

- **Clinical Examination:** Identification of hallmark craniofacial and skeletal abnormalities such as a large skull, short limbs, and genu valgum.
- **Radiographic Imaging:** X-rays showing generalized osteosclerosis, shortened long bones, and persistent fontanelles.
- **Genetic Testing:** Confirmation of autosomal recessive inheritance via molecular analysis of relevant genes.
- **Family History Analysis:** Documentation of consanguinity and recurrence in siblings provides diagnostic clues.

Results and Interpretation

- **Radiographic Findings:** Shortened and thickened long bones with widened metaphyses.
- Persistent fontanelles and delayed cranial suture closure.
- Evidence of frequent pathological fractures, especially in the lower extremities.
- **Genetic Findings:** Confirmation of autosomal recessive inheritance in families with documented consanguinity.

Physiological Basis

- **Bone Fragility:** Reduced bone remodeling activity due to impaired osteoclastic function leads to increased fragility and susceptibility to fractures.
- **Craniofacial Deformities:** Dysregulation of bone growth results in disproportionately large calvarium, frontal bossing, and parrot-like nose.
- **Skeletal Deformities:** Disrupted bone and cartilage development contributes to kyphosis, genu valgum, and scoliosis.

Clinical Applications

- **Orthopedic Management:** Corrective surgeries for genu valgum and scoliosis to improve mobility and reduce complications.
- **Fracture Prevention and Treatment:** Use of low-impact activity regimens and bone-strengthening therapies to mitigate fractures.
- **Dental Care:** Management of dental anomalies through specialized orthodontic interventions.

Limitations and Technical Considerations

- **Diagnostic Complexity:** Overlap with other syndromes like osteogenesis imperfecta can complicate early diagnosis.
- **Variable Expression:** Severity and presentation vary widely, even among individuals with similar genetic profiles.
- **Management Challenges:** Progressive deformities and frequent fractures necessitate ongoing multidisciplinary care.

Modern Relevance

- **Advances in Genetic Research:** Improvements in molecular diagnostics have enhanced early detection and understanding of the genetic mechanisms underlying the syndrome.
- **Orthopedic Innovations:** Progress in surgical techniques and prosthetics has improved the quality of life for affected individuals.

Associated Conditions

- **Other Skeletal Dysplasias:** Similar features may appear in Maroteaux-Lamy Syndrome I, cleidocranial dysplasia, or osteogenesis imperfecta.
- **Toulouse-Lautrec Syndrome:** Retrospective association with the French painter highlights the cultural and historical significance of the condition.

Clinical Importance

- **Early Diagnosis:** Timely identification prevents complications such as severe fractures and progressive deformities.
- **Prognostic Clarity:** Understanding the syndrome's natural history aids in planning long-term care and intervention.
- **Genetic Counseling:** Identification of autosomal recessive inheritance supports family planning and risk assessment.
- **Multidisciplinary Approach:** Involves collaboration between orthopedic surgeons, geneticists, and pediatricians for optimal outcomes.

References

U. Montanari: Acondroplasia e distosi cleidocranica digitale. Chirurgia degli organi di movimento, Bologna, 1923, 7: 379-391.

F. Collado-Otero: Una forma mas de distrofia osea. Acta pediatrica española, Madrid, 1956, 14: 1-27.

P. Maroteaux, M. Lamy: La pycnodysostose. La presse médicale, Paris, 1962, 70: 999-1002.

P. Maroteaux, M. Lamy: The malady of Toulouse-Lautrec. Journal of the American Medical Association, Chicago, 1965, 191: 715-717.

Maroteaux-Lamy Syndrome IV

Overview

Maroteaux-Lamy Syndrome IV is a familial bone dysplasia characterized by short-trunk dwarfism, back and hip pain, and limited joint movement, often accompanied by a variety of skeletal and systemic anomalies. The disorder typically manifests between the ages of 5 and 10 years. It follows an X-linked recessive inheritance pattern, primarily affecting males, though carrier females may show mild symptoms.

Historical Background

- **1963:** Pierre Maroteaux and Maurice Lamy first identified and documented this subtype in their broader work on mucopolysaccharidosis-related syndromes.
- **1970s:** Advances in genetic research further delineated the X-linked recessive nature of this subtype, differentiating it from other forms of Maroteaux-Lamy syndromes.
- **Recent Years:** Genetic studies have identified specific mutations associated with this syndrome, further clarifying its molecular basis.

Purpose

- **Clinical Identification:** To distinguish Maroteaux-Lamy Syndrome IV from other forms of mucopolysaccharidosis and short-trunk dwarfism.
- **Family Counseling:** To provide genetic counseling for families with a history of X-linked recessive disorders.

Procedure Overview

- **Clinical Assessment:** Examination for hallmark features such as short trunk, joint stiffness, and progressive skeletal deformities.
- **Radiological Evaluation:** X-rays showing shortened vertebral bodies, hip dysplasia, and other bone abnormalities.
- **Genetic Testing:** Identification of specific X-linked mutations responsible for the syndrome.

Results and Interpretation

- **Radiographic Features:** Evidence of shortened vertebral height, pelvic deformities, and hip joint abnormalities.
- **Clinical Findings:** Limited joint movement, particularly in the hips and spine, and characteristic short-trunk stature.
- **Genetic Confirmation:** Detection of mutations on the X chromosome confirms the diagnosis.

Physiological Basis

- **Skeletal Abnormalities:** Defective cartilage and bone formation result in short-trunk dwarfism and joint stiffness.
- **Pain and Mobility Issues:** Structural deformities in the spine and hips lead to chronic pain and reduced joint mobility.

Clinical Applications

- **Orthopedic Interventions:** Surgical correction for severe skeletal deformities, such as spinal curvature or hip dysplasia.
- **Physical Therapy:** Programs designed to maintain joint mobility and reduce

pain.

- **Pain Management:** Use of medications and supportive devices to manage chronic back and hip pain.

Limitations and Technical Considerations

- **Diagnostic Challenges:** Overlap with other forms of Maroteaux-Lamy syndrome and related skeletal dysplasias can complicate diagnosis.
- **Genetic Variability:** Variability in phenotypic expression may lead to underdiagnosis in mild cases.
- **Management Difficulties:** Progressive nature of the disorder requires lifelong multidisciplinary care.

Modern Relevance

- **Genetic Advances:** Progress in molecular diagnostics has enabled early identification and carrier detection.
- **Improved Management:** Advances in orthopedic and rehabilitative care have improved quality of life for affected individuals.

Associated Conditions

- **Skeletal Dysplasias:** Overlap with other forms of dwarfism and cartilage disorders.
- **Joint Disorders:** High prevalence of hip dysplasia, kyphosis, and scoliosis.

Clinical Importance

- **Early Detection:** Early recognition allows for timely intervention to prevent complications such as severe deformities.
- **Genetic Counseling:** Identification of X-linked inheritance enables better family planning and risk assessment.
- **Interdisciplinary Care:** Involves collaboration among orthopedic surgeons, geneticists, and physiotherapists for optimal outcomes.

References

A. W. Jacobsen: Hereditary osteochondrodystrophia deformans. A family with twenty members affected in 5 generations. Journal of the American Medical Association, Chicago, 1939, 113: 121-124.

P. Maroteaux, M. Lamy, J. Bernard: La dysplasie spondylo-epiphysaire tardive. La presse médicale, Paris, 1957, 65: 1205-1208.

Maroteaux's MEDTS Syndrome

Overview

Maroteaux's MEDTS Syndrome is a rare skeletal dysplasia characterized by moderate dwarfism predominantly affecting the trunk, with relatively normal length of the extremities. It is frequently associated with early-onset arthrosis of the hips. The syndrome is inherited in an autosomal recessive pattern and affects both sexes equally.

Historical Background

- **1960s:** The syndrome was first documented by Pierre Maroteaux, a prominent French geneticist and pediatrician specializing in skeletal dysplasias.
- **1966:** Maroteaux provided a detailed clinical and radiological description of MEDTS (Moderate Dwarfism with Trunk Shortening) syndrome in his foundational work on hereditary skeletal disorders.

Purpose

- **Diagnostic Clarification:** To differentiate Maroteaux's MEDTS Syndrome from other forms of skeletal dysplasia, such as achondroplasia or Marfan syndrome.
- **Genetic Counseling:** To assist families in understanding inheritance patterns and potential risks to offspring.

Procedure Overview

- **Clinical Assessment:** Detailed examination to identify disproportionate truncal dwarfism, normal limb proportions, and associated hip arthrosis.
- **Radiological Studies:** X-rays to evaluate vertebral abnormalities, hip arthrosis, and potential joint deformities.
- **Genetic Testing:** Confirmatory testing to identify mutations associated with autosomal recessive inheritance of the condition.

Results and Interpretation

- **Clinical Findings:** Moderate truncal dwarfism with normal limb proportions.
- Early-onset hip pain and limited mobility due to arthrosis.
- **Radiographic Features:** Evidence of shortened vertebral bodies, early degenerative changes in the hip joints, and preserved limb bone morphology.
- **Genetic Confirmation:** Identification of specific autosomal recessive mutations confirms the diagnosis.

Physiological Basis

- **Skeletal Abnormalities:** Impaired growth and development of the vertebral column lead to truncal shortening.
- **Hip Degeneration:** Early-onset arthrosis results from abnormal cartilage and joint structure, leading to limited mobility and pain.

Clinical Applications

- **Orthopedic Management:** Surgical interventions, such as hip replacements, may be necessary for severe arthrosis.
- **Physical Therapy:** Tailored exercises to maintain joint mobility and reduce pain.
- **Genetic Counseling:** Provides valuable information for affected families regarding recurrence risks in subsequent generations.

Limitations and Technical Considerations

- **Diagnostic Overlap:** Similarities with other forms of dwarfism can delay accurate diagnosis.
- **Management Challenges:** Progressive hip arthrosis and joint degeneration may require ongoing orthopedic interventions.
- **Genetic Variability:** Phenotypic variability may make it challenging to recognize mild cases.

Modern Relevance

- **Advances in Imaging:** High-resolution imaging modalities allow for earlier detection of vertebral and hip abnormalities.
- **Genetic Research:** Improved understanding of the genetic basis of MEDTS syndrome has enhanced diagnostic accuracy and family counseling.

Associated Conditions

- **Skeletal Dysplasias:** Often compared to or confused with other forms of dwarfism.
- **Arthrosis:** Predominantly affects the hip joints, leading to pain and functional impairment.

Clinical Importance

- **Early Detection:** Timely diagnosis helps mitigate complications such as severe arthrosis and functional limitations.
- **Personalized Management:** Interdisciplinary care ensures optimal outcomes for physical and functional well-being.
- **Family Counseling:** Genetic insights allow families to make informed decisions about reproductive options.

References

P. Maroteaux: Spondyloepiphyseal dysplasias and metatropic dwarfism. Birth Defects Original Article Series, New York, 1969, 5: 35-41.

Maroteaux's Syndrome I

Overview

Maroteaux's Syndrome I is a rare pediatric condition primarily observed during the winter months, characterized by swelling, redness, heat, and minimal pain in the fingers and, occasionally, the toes. The condition predominantly affects infants and children and tends to resolve with time or environmental changes.

Historical Background

- **1960s:** The syndrome was first described by Pierre Maroteaux, a French pediatrician and geneticist, in his studies on rare pediatric disorders.
- **1965:** Maroteaux detailed the seasonal nature and benign course of the syndrome, emphasizing its occurrence during cold weather in children.

Purpose

- **Clinical Recognition:** To distinguish Maroteaux's Syndrome I from other inflammatory or rheumatologic conditions that involve swelling and redness of the digits.
- **Preventative Measures:** To identify environmental or behavioral modifications that might prevent episodes.

Procedure Overview

- **Clinical Observation:** Diagnosis is based on visual signs (swelling, redness, and heat in the fingers or toes) and a history of seasonal onset.
- **Exclusion of Other Conditions:** Rule out more serious conditions like chilblains, frostbite, or inflammatory arthritis through detailed history and clinical examination.

Results and Interpretation

- **Findings:** Localized swelling and redness in affected digits.
- Minimal pain, despite notable physical changes.
- **Diagnostic Clarity:** Symptoms align with a benign course and spontaneous resolution as the primary indicators of Maroteaux's Syndrome I.

Physiological Basis

- **Seasonal Influence:** Cold weather appears to trigger a localized inflammatory response in the digits.
- **Peripheral Circulation:** Changes in blood flow to the fingers and toes in response to cold may contribute to swelling and redness.

Clinical Applications

- **Pediatric Management:** Educating caregivers about the benign and self-limiting nature of the syndrome.
- **Environmental Adjustments:** Advising warm clothing and hand protection during winter months to minimize episodes.

Limitations and Technical Considerations

- **Exclusion Challenges:** Similarity to conditions like chilblains or other vascular disorders may complicate diagnosis.

- **Minimal Intervention:** As the syndrome is self-limiting, medical intervention is rarely needed, making long-term study difficult.

Modern Relevance

- **Increased Awareness:** The syndrome is now recognized more readily in pediatric practices, reducing unnecessary interventions.
- **Preventative Focus:** Highlighting the importance of environmental factors and simple protective measures.

Associated Conditions

- **Chilblains (Pernio):** Differentiated by more severe pain and potential ulceration.
- **Rheumatologic Conditions:** Rarely misdiagnosed as inflammatory arthritis due to overlapping symptoms.

Clinical Importance

- **Early Recognition:** Prevents unnecessary diagnostic workups or treatments for a benign and self-resolving condition.
- **Parental Reassurance:** Educates caregivers about the non-threatening nature of the syndrome.
- **Environmental Adaptation:** Simple interventions, such as keeping extremities warm, can significantly reduce episodes.

References

P. Maroteaux: Cinq observations d'une affection microgeodique des phalanges du nourrison d'etiologie inconnue. Annales de radiologie, Paris, 1970, 13: 229-236.

Maroteaux's Syndrome II

Overview

Maroteaux's Syndrome II is a rare skeletal dysplasia characterized by metaphyseal dysostosis that is limited to the knees. The condition is congenital and presents at birth. It follows an autosomal recessive inheritance pattern, making it a genetic disorder that typically manifests in children born to consanguineous parents.

Historical Background

- **1960s:** Pierre Maroteaux, a prominent French pediatrician and geneticist, identified and described the syndrome during his extensive research into rare skeletal dysplasias.
- **1965:** Maroteaux's formal description established the condition as a distinct entity with localized metaphyseal involvement, distinguishing it from other forms of dysostosis.

Purpose

- **Diagnostic Clarity:** To identify and diagnose cases of metaphyseal dysostosis localized to the knees and differentiate it from other generalized skeletal dysplasias.
- **Genetic Counseling:** To provide families with an understanding of the autosomal recessive inheritance and the associated risks for offspring.

Procedure Overview

- **Clinical Evaluation:** Diagnosis begins with observation of skeletal deformities localized to the knee region and radiological imaging for confirmation.

- **Radiographic Analysis:** X-rays reveal irregular metaphyseal changes in the bones forming the knee joint, with no other skeletal abnormalities.
- **Genetic Testing:** In suspected familial cases, genetic testing can confirm the autosomal recessive inheritance pattern.

Results and Interpretation

- **Radiographic Findings:** X-rays show abnormal metaphyseal widening and irregularities at the distal femur and proximal tibia.
- **Clinical Signs:** Patients may exhibit short stature, restricted knee movement, or mild angular deformities of the legs.
- **Genetic Confirmation:** Autosomal recessive inheritance patterns confirmed in familial cases.

Physiological Basis

- **Genetic Mutation:** Likely involves mutations affecting the genes responsible for normal endochondral ossification and bone remodeling at the metaphysis of the knee.
- **Localized Effect:** The dysplasia uniquely impacts the knee region without affecting other skeletal sites, a hallmark of this syndrome.

Clinical Applications

- **Orthopedic Management:** Early intervention for knee deformities or misalignment to improve mobility and prevent complications.
- **Genetic Counseling:** Families with affected children benefit from understanding the genetic basis and recurrence risks.

Limitations and Technical Considerations

- **Diagnostic Challenges:** Rarity and localized nature may lead to underdiagnosis or misclassification.
- **Treatment Limitations:** The genetic basis limits curative options, leaving management primarily supportive or corrective.

Modern Relevance

- **Improved Diagnostics:** Advances in genetic testing and imaging techniques have made early diagnosis more accurate.
- **Therapeutic Advances:** Orthopedic interventions for associated deformities have evolved, improving patient quality of life.

Associated Conditions

- **Other Metaphyseal Dysplasias:** Conditions like Schmid metaphyseal chondrodysplasia may share radiographic similarities but differ in systemic involvement.
- **Skeletal Dysplasia Syndromes:** Differentiated from generalized skeletal dysplasias through its unique localization.

Clinical Importance

- **Early Identification:** Facilitates timely orthopedic intervention to prevent progressive deformities.
- **Genetic Counseling:** Supports families in understanding inheritance risks and planning for future pregnancies.

- **Localized Management:** Allows for targeted interventions, minimizing systemic impacts on the patient.

References

P. Maroteaux, P. Savart, J. Lefebvre, et al: Les formes partielles de la dysostose metaphysaire. La presse médicale, Paris, 1963, 71: 1523-1526.

Maroteaux-Spranger-Wiedemann Syndrome

Overview

Maroteaux-Spranger-Wiedemann Syndrome is a rare congenital skeletal disorder that manifests as disproportionate dwarfism with a long trunk and short limbs, alongside other skeletal abnormalities. The condition presents at birth and progresses during infancy, leading to significant disability in adolescence. Survival into adulthood is rare, and both autosomal recessive and autosomal dominant inheritance patterns have been reported.

Historical Background

- **1960s-1970s:** The syndrome was first described collaboratively by Pierre Maroteaux, Jürgen W. Spranger, and Hans-Rudolf Wiedemann, who identified its unique skeletal and developmental features.
- Their work contributed to the understanding of rare skeletal dysplasias and differentiated this syndrome from other forms of dwarfism.

Purpose

- **Diagnostic Characterization:** To define and diagnose this syndrome based on clinical and radiographic findings, allowing for early intervention.
- **Genetic Understanding:** To study the transmission patterns and identify potential genetic markers for the condition.

Procedure Overview

- **Clinical Examination:** Observing physical features such as short limbs, long trunk, narrow chest, and prominent joints.
- **Radiographic Imaging:** X-rays to identify skeletal abnormalities, including narrow thoracic cavity and joint malformations.
- **Genetic Analysis:** Testing to determine inheritance patterns and differentiate autosomal dominant from recessive cases.

Results and Interpretation

- **Physical Features:** Infants present with dwarfism, narrow chest, and limited joint movement. A linear fold resembling a tail may be observed.
- **Radiographic Findings:** Radiographs show shortened limb bones, narrow thoracic cavity, and progressive skeletal deformities.
- **Progression:** Symptoms worsen during childhood and adolescence, with progressive disability and limited survival into adulthood.

Physiological Basis

- **Skeletal Dysplasia:** Caused by abnormal endochondral ossification, leading to shortened limb bones and disproportionate body growth.
- **Joint Abnormalities:** Prominent and limited joint movement results from malformed cartilage and connective tissue.

Clinical Applications

- **Orthopedic Management:** Early interventions, such as bracing or surgery, to address joint and spinal deformities.
- **Physical Therapy:** To maintain mobility and manage progressive disability.
- **Genetic Counseling:** Advising families about inheritance risks and recurrence probabilities.

Limitations and Technical Considerations

- **Diagnostic Challenges:** Early diagnosis is difficult due to overlapping features with other skeletal dysplasias.
- **Treatment Limitations:** No curative treatment exists; management focuses on symptom relief and functional support.

Modern Relevance

- **Advances in Genetic Testing:** Improved understanding of the genetic basis of the syndrome may lead to more accurate diagnoses and targeted therapies.
- **Supportive Care Developments:** Better orthopedic and rehabilitative interventions are improving quality of life for affected individuals.

Associated Conditions

- **Other Skeletal Dysplasias:** Conditions such as achondroplasia and metaphyseal dysplasias share features but are distinct in progression and inheritance.
- **Respiratory Complications:** Narrow

thoracic cavity can result in respiratory issues, especially in infancy.

Clinical Importance

- **Early Recognition:** Timely diagnosis can improve outcomes by initiating early interventions to address deformities and disabilities.
- **Genetic Counseling:** Families benefit from understanding inheritance patterns and the likelihood of recurrence in future pregnancies.
- **Supportive Care Focus:** Enhances quality of life through multidisciplinary management, including orthopedic, respiratory, and physical therapy specialists.

References

P. Maroteaux, J. Spranger, H. R. Wiedemann: Der metatrophische Zwergwuchs. Archiv für Kinderheilkunde, 1966, 173: 211-226.

Melnick-Needles Syndrome

Overview

Melnick-Needles Syndrome is an extremely rare genetic disorder classified as a type of generalized bone dysplasia. It is characterized by distinct craniofacial features, including micrognathia, exophthalmos, and hypertelorism, alongside skeletal abnormalities such as bowing of the limbs, cubitus valgus, and genu valgum. Affected individuals often present with stunted growth, abnormal gait, and susceptibility to respiratory and ear infections. The syndrome has a significant female predominance with a male-to-female ratio of 1:7, as inheritance is primarily X-linked dominant, lethal in males, and survivable in females.

Historical Background

- **1954:** John Melnick and Carl F. Needles first described this syndrome in their study of patients with unique craniofacial and skeletal abnormalities.
- Their work highlighted the distinct inheritance pattern and its predominance in females, attributing the condition to an *X-linked dominant genetic mutation.*

Purpose

- **Diagnostic Clarity:** To establish clear diagnostic criteria for recognizing craniofacial and skeletal abnormalities associated with this syndrome.
- **Genetic Insights:** To understand the genetic basis and inheritance patterns, especially the condition's lethality in

males.

- **Management Protocols:** To develop supportive care and preventive strategies for recurrent infections and skeletal deformities.

Procedure Overview

- **Clinical Assessment:** Comprehensive evaluation of craniofacial features and skeletal deformities, noting abnormalities such as bowed limbs and cubitus valgus.
- **Imaging Studies:** X-rays to identify bone dysplasia, including bowing of long bones and shortening of distal phalanges.
- **Genetic Testing:** Confirmation of mutations in the FLNA gene, which is implicated in this syndrome.

Results and Interpretation

- **Craniofacial Features:** Patients exhibit micrognathia, hypertelorism, full cheeks, and large ears.
- **Skeletal Findings:** Radiographs reveal bowing of the upper arms and legs, cubitus valgus, and genu valgum, along with shortened distal phalanges.
- **Clinical Presentation:** Stunted growth, abnormal gait, and frequent infections are hallmark symptoms.
- **Inheritance Patterns:** The condition follows an X-linked dominant pattern, affecting predominantly females.

Physiological Basis

- **Genetic Mutation:** The syndrome is caused by mutations in the FLNA gene, which encodes filamin A, a protein involved in cytoskeletal structure and cell signaling.
- **Skeletal Dysplasia:** Abnormal bone development leads to the characteristic craniofacial and skeletal deformities.
- **Infectious Susceptibility:** Structural abnormalities in the respiratory tract and ears contribute to recurrent infections.

Clinical Applications

- **Orthopedic Management:** Braces or corrective surgeries for bowed limbs and joint deformities.
- **Infection Control:** Preventive measures and early treatment for respiratory and ear infections.
- **Supportive Care:** Multidisciplinary approach involving genetics, orthopedics, and pediatrics to improve quality of life.

Limitations and Technical Considerations

- **Diagnostic Challenges:** Overlap of features with other skeletal dysplasias may complicate diagnosis.
- **Limited Treatment Options:** Management is largely symptomatic, as no curative treatment exists.
- **Male Lethality:** The high lethality in males limits the understanding of the condition's full spectrum.

Modern Relevance

- **Advances in Genetic Testing:** Increased availability of genetic testing has improved early diagnosis and risk assessment.
- **Targeted Therapies:** Research into

FLNA-related pathways holds promise for future therapeutic interventions.

- **Improved Supportive Care:** Advances in orthopedic techniques and infection management enhance patient outcomes.

Associated Conditions

- **Other FLNA-Related Disorders:** Conditions such as periventricular nodular heterotopia may share genetic underpinnings.
- **Skeletal Dysplasias:** Disorders with overlapping features include osteogenesis imperfecta and Marfan's syndrome.

Clinical Importance

- **Early Diagnosis:** Recognizing the craniofacial and skeletal features allows for timely interventions to manage deformities and infections.
- **Prognostic Value:** Understanding the inheritance pattern and malc lethality informs genetic counseling for affected families.
- **Multidisciplinary Care:** Collaboration among specialists ensures comprehensive management of the syndrome's complex features.

References

J. Melnick, C. F. Needles: An undiagnosed bone dysplasia. A 2 family study of 4 generations and 3 generations. American Journal of Roentgenology, 1966, 97: 39-48.

Jürgen W. Spranger, Leonard O. Langer, Jr., Hans-Rudolf Wiedemann: Bone dysplasias. An Atlas of Constitutional Disorders of Skeletal Development. Stuttgart and Philadelphia: G. Fischer and W. B. saunders, 1974.

B. Leiber, G. Olbrich, N. Moelter et al: Melnick-Needles-Syndrom. Monatsschrift für Kinderheilkunde, Berlin, 1975, 123: 178.

J. P. Fryns, R. Maertens, H. van den Bergh: Osteodysplastia – a rare skeletal dysplasia. Acta paediatrica Belgica, Bruxelles, 1979, 32: 65.

F. Majewski et al: Serpentine fibula – polycystic kidney syndrome and Melnick-Needles syndrome are different disorders. European Journal of Pediatrics, Berlin, 1993, 152: 916-921.

Monteggia Fracture

Overview

Monteggia fracture-dislocation is a significant orthopedic injury characterized by a fracture of the proximal ulna coupled with dislocation of the radial head at the proximal radioulnar and radiocapitellar joints. It often results from direct trauma to the forearm or a fall on an outstretched hand, making it a high-impact injury. Left untreated, it can cause chronic instability, nonunion, or nerve complications, especially involving the posterior interosseous nerve.

Historical Background

- **1812:** Giovanni Battista Monteggia, a Milanese surgeon, first described the injury as a proximal ulna fracture associated with radial head dislocation in his seminal work, *Istituzioni chirurgiche – Volume V*.
- **1967:** José Luis Bado, an Uruguayan orthopedic surgeon, expanded upon Monteggia's initial work, categorizing the injury into four distinct types based on the direction of dislocation and the mechanism of injury.

Purpose

- **Clinical Classification:** To provide a systematic classification of Monteggia fractures, aiding in diagnosis and treatment.
- **Effective Treatment:** To establish optimal strategies for surgical and nonsurgical management of these injuries.
- **Prevent Chronic Complications:** To identify and address potential long-term issues such as joint instability or nerve damage.

Procedure Overview

Initial Diagnosis: Obtain anteroposterior (AP) and lateral X-rays of the forearm, elbow, and wrist to assess the fracture and radial head dislocation.

Classification: Classify the injury using Bado's Types:

- **Type I:** Anterior radial head dislocation (most common).
- **Type II:** Posterior radial head dislocation.
- **Type III:** Lateral radial head dislocation.
- **Type IV:** Fracture of both bones of the forearm with radial head dislocation.
- **Surgical Intervention:**
- Perform open reduction and internal fixation (ORIF) of the ulna to stabilize the fracture.
- Simultaneously reduce the radial head dislocation.
- **Postoperative Management:** Immobilization with a long arm cast, followed by physical therapy for joint mobility restoration.

Results and Interpretation

- **Radiographic Findings:** Clear visualization of the ulna fracture and misalignment of the radial head in relation to the capitellum confirms the diagnosis.
- **Clinical Outcome:** Successful treatment results in restored forearm

stability, range of motion, and nerve function.

- Delayed or improper treatment may lead to malunion, nonunion, or chronic instability.

Physiological Basis

- **Biomechanics:** The proximal ulna and radial head form a critical component of the elbow joint and the forearm rotation mechanism. Disruption of this alignment impacts pronation, supination, and elbow flexion/extension.
- **Neurological Concerns:** The posterior interosseous nerve is at risk due to proximity to the radial head. Injuries may result in motor deficits without sensory loss.

Clinical Applications

- **Orthopedic Surgery:** Surgical intervention is the primary approach for reducing fractures and dislocations in Monteggia injuries.
- **Rehabilitation Programs:** Postoperative care focuses on mobility exercises and strength training to restore function.
- **Pediatric Considerations:** In children, Monteggia fractures may be managed conservatively if promptly identified.

Limitations and Technical Considerations

- **Delayed Diagnosis:** Unrecognized injuries may lead to chronic instability and necessitate complex reconstructive surgeries.
- **Surgical Risks:** Potential complications include infection, nonunion, and nerve damage.
- **Technical Expertise:** Precise reduction and fixation require skilled orthopedic surgeons to ensure joint congruency and stability.

Modern Relevance

- **Advanced Imaging:** CT scans and MRIs provide enhanced visualization of the injury, aiding in preoperative planning.
- **Improved Fixation Techniques:** Modern surgical hardware, including locking plates and intramedullary nails, improves outcomes in Monteggia injuries.
- **Early Recognition Protocols:** Educational initiatives for emergency physicians aim to reduce delayed diagnoses.

Associated Conditions

- **Posterior Interosseous Nerve Palsy:** Often associated with radial head dislocation in Type I fractures.
- **Elbow Instability:** Chronic instability can occur if the radial head is not properly reduced.

Clinical Importance

- **Early Diagnosis:** Prompt recognition and treatment prevent long-term complications, including nerve injuries and joint instability.
- **Functional Recovery:** Timely surgical intervention ensures restoration of elbow and forearm functionality.
- **Prognostic Value:** Classification into Bado's types guides treatment plans and predicts surgical outcomes.

- **Comprehensive Care:** Multidisciplinary management, including physical therapy and periodic monitoring, optimizes patient recovery.

References

Monteggia GB. Lussazioni delle ossa delle estremita superiori. In: Monteggia GB. Instituzioni Chirurgiches. Vol. 5. Maspero; Milan, Italy: 1814. p131-133.

Andjelković S et al Giovanni Battista Monteggia (1762-1815). Srp Arh Celok Lek. 2015 Jan-Feb;143(1-2):105-7. [PMID 25845262] [Free Full text]

Rehim SA et al. Monteggia fracture-dislocations: A Historical Review. J Hand Surg Am. 2014 Jul; 39(7): 1384–1394. [PMC4266382]

Conforti M. Monteggia GB. Dizionario Biografico degli Italiani, Volume 76; 2012

Acerbi FE. Della vita di Giambatista Monteggia, professore di chirurgia. 1816 [Archive text]

McGarvey WC, Clanton TO. Peroneal Tendon Dislocations. Foot and Ankle Clinics. Vol 1, 2: 1996 [Free Full Text]

Bado JL. The Monteggia lesion. Clin Orthop Relat Res. 1967 Jan-Feb;50:71-86. [PMID 6029027]

Rehim SA, Maynard MA, Sebastin SJ, Chung KC. Monteggia fracture dislocations: a historical review. J Hand Surg [Am]. 2014;39(7):1384–94.

Eathiraju S, Mudgal CS, Jupiter JB. Monteggia fracture-dislocations. Hand Clin. 2007;23(2):165–77. v.

Müller-Ribbing-Clément Syndrome

Overview

Müller-Ribbing-Clément syndrome is a rare bone disturbance characterized by moderate dwarfism, obliteration of hollow bones, and premature degenerative arthropathy, particularly affecting the hip joints. Despite these abnormalities, the body proportions remain normal. Clinical features often include prominent and painful joints, limited mobility, and a waddling gait. Symptoms generally manifest between 5 and 10 years of age, with early signs of dysplasia appearing as young as 2 to 3 years.

Historical Background

- **1925:** Harold Arthur Thomas Fairbank, a British orthopedic surgeon, first described this syndrome in his pioneering work on skeletal dysplasia.
- **1945:** Walther Müller and Seved Ribbing further elaborated on the condition, delineating its distinct characteristics and variations.- 1960s: Robert Clément contributed additional observations, leading to the combined eponym Müller-Ribbing-Clément syndrome.
- The correct eponym is debated, with *Fairbank's disease* often considered appropriate due to Fairbank's initial description.

Purpose

- **Diagnostic Clarity:** To differentiate this condition from other forms of skeletal dysplasia and degenerative joint diseases.

- **Management of Symptoms:** To guide interventions that minimize joint damage and improve mobility.
- **Recognition of Variants:** To identify and classify the Ribbing and Fairbank forms for targeted management.

Procedure Overview

- **Diagnostic Imaging:** X-rays reveal obliteration of hollow bones, irregular epiphyses, and changes in the carpal bones and phalanges.
- **Clinical Evaluation:** Assess joint mobility, gait abnormalities, and early signs of coxa vara and genu valgum.
- **Differentiation of Variants:**
- **Ribbing Form:** Mild involvement of hand bones, flat epiphyses.
- **Fairbank Form:** Small epiphyses, delayed ossification, and notable changes in metacarpal bones and phalanges.

Results and Interpretation

- **Radiographic Findings:** Flattened epiphyses, irregular ossification patterns, and degenerative changes in major joints, especially the hips.
- **Clinical Presentation:** Moderate dwarfism with an average height of 152 cm, thoracic kyphosis, and back pain are key indicators.
- **Functional Outcomes:** Mobility is often compromised, but the condition rarely causes significant disability.

Physiological Basis

- **Bone Dysplasia:** The syndrome involves abnormal ossification, leading to flattened epiphyses and degenerative changes.
- **Joint Degeneration:** Premature arthropathy results from mechanical stress and altered bone architecture.
- **Growth Disturbance:** Stunted stature arises from delayed and irregular ossification of long bones.

Clinical Applications

- **Orthopedic Management:** Surgical correction may be required for severe coxa vara or genu valgum.
- **Physical Therapy:** Strengthening exercises and gait training can improve mobility and reduce pain.
- **Pediatric Monitoring:** Early recognition and intervention during growth years help prevent severe deformities.

Limitations and Technical Considerations

- **Diagnostic Challenges:** The syndrome may be misdiagnosed as another form of skeletal dysplasia, leading to delayed treatment.
- **Surgical Risks:** Joint surgeries, particularly in the hips, carry risks of complications due to bone fragility.
- **Lack of Genetic Understanding:** The exact genetic basis remains unknown, complicating counseling and prediction of inheritance patterns.

Modern Relevance

- **Advances in Imaging:** MRI and CT scans now provide better visualization of joint structures and early bone changes.
- **Improved Therapies:** Joint preservation techniques and customized prosthetics enhance mobility and quality of life.
- **Genetic Studies:** Ongoing research may uncover the molecular basis of the condition, leading to targeted therapies.

Associated Conditions

- **Coxa Vara and Genu Valgum:** Common deformities leading to gait disturbances.
- **Early-Onset Osteoarthritis:** Accelerated joint degeneration, particularly in the hips.
- **Thoracic Kyphosis:** Contributes to back pain and posture abnormalities.

Clinical Importance

- **Early Diagnosis:** Early recognition of dysplasia and skeletal abnormalities allows for timely intervention.
- **Functional Outcomes:** Proper management can maintain mobility and minimize complications like severe arthropathy.
- **Prognostic Insights:** Differentiating between the Ribbing and Fairbank forms provides insights into disease progression and therapy options.
- **Interdisciplinary Care:** Collaboration among pediatricians, orthopedic surgeons, and physical therapists is essential for comprehensive management.

References

H. A. T. Fairbank: Generalized disease of the skeleton.

Proceedings of the Royal Society of Medicine, 1935, 28: 1611-1619. An Atlas of General Affections of the Skeleton.

Edinburgh, E. S. Livingstone, 1951, pp. 91-105. Dysplasia epiphysialis multiplex.

British Journal of Surgery, London, 1947, 34: 225-232.

S. Ribbing: Studien über hereditäre multiple epiphysenstörungen.

Acta Radiologica. Supplement, 1937, 34: 1-105. Hereditary multiple diaphyseal sclerosis.

Acta Radiologica, Stockholm, 1949, 31: 522-536.

W. Müller: Das Bild der multiplen erblichen Störungen der Epiphysenverknoecherung.

Zeitschrift für Orthopädie und ihre Grenzgebiete, Stuttgart, 1939, 69: 257.

J. Spranger, L. O. Langer, H.-R. Wiedemann: Bone Dysplasias. Fischer-Saunder, Stuttgart. Philadelphia, 1974. Pp. 10-15.

Müller-Weiss Syndrome

Overview

Müller-Weiss syndrome is a bilateral, symmetrical osteochondrosis of the navicular bone in the foot, primarily affecting adults. It is often marked by pain in the midfoot, which is exacerbated by walking or other weight-bearing activities. However, some cases may remain asymptomatic. The syndrome is distinguished from Köhler's disease by its later age of onset and its typical occurrence in adults rather than children.

Historical Background

- **1927:** Walther Müller and Konrad Weiss first described the condition, providing a detailed explanation of its osteochondrotic nature and emphasizing its distinction from Köhler's disease.
- The syndrome was named after these two pioneers in *radiology and orthopedic pathology*, who were instrumental in recognizing the unique features of adult navicular osteonecrosis.

Purpose

- **Diagnostic Classification:** To distinguish Müller-Weiss syndrome from similar conditions like Köhler's disease and other causes of midfoot pain.
- **Guidance for Treatment:** To develop management strategies that address pain, mobility, and progression of the condition.

Procedure Overview

- **Clinical Examination:** Evaluate for midfoot pain, tenderness over the navicular bone, and reduced mobility in the foot.
- **Radiographic Assessment:**
- X-rays typically show fragmentation, collapse, or lateral displacement of the navicular bone.
- Advanced imaging, such as **MRI or** CT scans, may reveal osteonecrosis, sclerosis, and joint incongruity.
- **Functional Evaluation:** Assess the impact on ambulation and daily activities to tailor treatment.

Results and Interpretation

- **Radiographic Findings:** Flattened, fragmented navicular bone with sclerosis and possible lateral displacement.
- **Clinical Presentation:** Symptoms range from chronic midfoot pain to asymptomatic cases detected incidentally.
- **Functional Outcomes:** Pain and reduced mobility can significantly impair quality of life, particularly in severe cases.

Physiological Basis

- **Osteonecrosis:** Reduced blood supply to the navicular bone leads to necrosis and subsequent collapse.
- **Weight-Bearing Stress:** The navicular bone, a key component of the medial arch, is particularly vulnerable to chronic loading and repetitive trauma, exacerbating the condition.

- **Symmetrical Manifestation:** The bilateral nature of the disease reflects its systemic or biomechanical predisposition.

Clinical Applications

- **Non-Surgical Management:** Use of orthotics, pain management with NSAIDs, and physical therapy to improve mobility.
- **Surgical Options:** In severe cases, surgical interventions such as navicular excision, arthrodesis, or osteotomy may be required to restore function.
- **Preventive Measures:** Identifying high-risk individuals, particularly those with foot deformities or repetitive stress injuries, can help prevent progression.

Limitations and Technical Considerations

- **Diagnostic Challenges:** Overlap with other midfoot conditions, such as arthritis or Köhler's disease, can delay diagnosis.
- **Surgical Risks:** Procedures to stabilize or reconstruct the navicular bone carry risks of complications, including arthritic changes or limited range of motion.
- **Limited Awareness:** The condition is underrecognized, leading to misdiagnosis or inappropriate treatment.

Modern Relevance

- **Advances in Imaging:** Modern imaging techniques, such as MRI, have improved early detection and assessment of osteonecrosis.
- **Customized Orthotics:** Innovations in orthotic design provide better support for patients with navicular dysfunction.
- **Minimally Invasive Surgery:** New surgical techniques aim to reduce recovery time and improve outcomes.

Associated Conditions

- **Flatfoot Deformity:** Patients with preexisting flatfoot are more prone to developing Müller-Weiss syndrome.
- **Osteoarthritis:** Chronic joint stress may lead to secondary arthritis in the midfoot.
- **Post-Traumatic Changes:** A history of foot trauma or repetitive stress increases susceptibility.

Clinical Importance

- **Early Diagnosis:** Timely recognition of the condition can prevent progression to severe deformity and chronic pain.
- **Functional Preservation:** Management strategies aim to maintain ambulation and prevent joint deterioration.
- **Improved Quality of Life:** Effective pain relief and mobility restoration can significantly enhance daily living activities.
- **Interdisciplinary Approach:** Collaboration between radiologists, orthopedic surgeons, and physical therapists is essential for comprehensive care.

References

W. Müller: Über eine eigenartige doppelseitige Veränderung des Os naviculare pedis beim Erwachsenen. Deutsche Zeitschrift für Chirurgie, Leipzig, 1927; 201: 84-87.

K. Weiss: Über die "Malazie" des Os naviculare pedis. Fortschritte auf dem Gebiete der Röntgenstrahlen, 1927, 45: 63-67.

Mumenthaller Sign

Overview

Mumenthaler Sign is a clinical diagnostic maneuver used to assess ulnar nerve integrity by observing the absence of skin dimpling in the hypothenar eminence during specific hand movements. The sign involves testing the contraction of the palmaris brevis (PB) muscle, an ulnar-innervated muscle responsible for hypothenar skin wrinkling. Absence of this finding may indicate ulnar nerve compromise.

Historical Background

- **1960s:** The sign was described by M. Mumenthaler, a neurologist who focused on peripheral nerve injuries. He identified this clinical observation as a subtle indicator of ulnar nerve dysfunction, particularly in cases involving hypothenar muscle compromise.

Purpose

- **Diagnostic Indicator:** To detect ulnar nerve compromise by assessing the functional status of the palmaris brevis muscle.
- **Localization of Lesion:** Provides clues about whether the ulnar nerve lesion is located at the superficial branch, deep branch, or proximal level.

Procedure Overview

- **Patient Position:** The patient is seated with their hand resting on a stable surface, palm up.
- **Test Maneuver:** The examiner asks the patient to abduct the small finger against resistance.
- **Observation:** During this maneuver, the examiner observes for the presence of skin dimpling or wrinkling in the proximal hypothenar eminence.
- **Findings:** Positive Mumenthaler Sign: Absence of dimpling suggests compromised innervation of the palmaris brevis muscle.

Results and Interpretation

- **Positive Finding:** Absence of dimpling in the hypothenar region suggests ulnar nerve dysfunction, potentially at the level of the wrist or above.
- **Negative Finding:** Presence of hypothenar dimpling indicates intact palmaris brevis function and suggests an absence of significant ulnar nerve compromise.

Physiological Basis

- **Palmaris Brevis Function:** The palmaris brevis muscle, innervated by the ulnar nerve, plays a role in wrinkling the skin of the hypothenar eminence.
- **Nerve Innervation Variability:** While typically innervated by the superficial branch of the ulnar nerve, the muscle may receive innervation from the deep branch or mixed branches, which can complicate the interpretation of findings.

Clinical Applications

- **Peripheral Neuropathy:** Useful in diagnosing ulnar neuropathy caused by entrapment, trauma, or systemic conditions like diabetes.

- **Localizing Lesions:** Helps differentiate between proximal and distal lesions of the ulnar nerve.

- **Post-Surgical Assessment:** Used to monitor recovery following ulnar nerve surgeries, such as cubital tunnel release.

Limitations and Technical Considerations

- **Variable Innervation:** Variability in the innervation of the palmaris brevis muscle may lead to inconsistent findings.

- **Non-Specificity:** Absence of dimpling may also occur due to unrelated factors, such as muscle atrophy or other nerve injuries.

- **Patient Cooperation:** The accuracy of the test depends on the patient's ability to perform the maneuver and the examiner's observation skills.

Modern Relevance

- **Peripheral Nerve Diagnostics:** Remains a valuable, non-invasive method to identify early signs of ulnar nerve injury.

- **Complementary Use:** Used alongside nerve conduction studies (NCS) and imaging for comprehensive diagnosis.

Associated Conditions

- **Ulnar Neuropathy:** Entrapment at the Guyon's canal or cubital tunnel syndrome.

- **Traumatic Injuries:** Fractures or lacerations affecting the ulnar nerve pathway.

- **Systemic Neuropathies:** Diabetic neuropathy or entrapment syndromes exacerbated by systemic diseases.

Clinical Importance

- **Early Diagnosis:** Enables the detection of subtle ulnar nerve dysfunction before significant motor or sensory loss develops.

- **Prognostic Indicator:** The presence or absence of hypothenar dimpling helps predict the severity and potential recovery of ulnar nerve lesions.

- **Interdisciplinary Management:** Facilitates collaboration between neurologists, orthopedic surgeons, and physiotherapists for comprehensive patient care.

References

Mannerfelt L. Studies on the hand in ulnar nerve paralysis: a clinicalexperimental investigation in the normal and anomalous innervation. Acta Orthop Scand Suppl 87:17–34, 91, 1966.

Mumenthaler M. Die Ulnarisparesen. Stuttgart: G Thieme, 1961.

Nélaton's Syndrome

Overview

Nélaton's Syndrome is a rare hereditary disorder characterized by sensory abnormalities in the lower extremities, often leading to ulceration, destruction of bones and joints, and other skeletal deformities. It typically manifests between the ages of 15 and 35 years, often during puberty. The syndrome has a wide array of features, including acroosteolysis, Charcot arthropathy, vasomotor dysfunction, and occasionally systemic involvement, such as deafness and optic atrophy.

Historical Background

- **1855:** Auguste Nélaton, a French surgeon, first described associated sensory and ulcerative changes in the lower extremities.
- **1940s-1950s:** Further contributions were made by Derek Ernst Denny-Brown and Eric Perrin Hicks, who expanded on the neurological and sensory pathology underlying the condition.
- **1957:** André Thévenard documented cases involving optic atrophy, adding a broader understanding of systemic manifestations.
- The eponym reflects contributions from these figures and others, including *E. M. Smith*, in recognizing the full spectrum of clinical features.

Purpose

- **Diagnostic Identification:** To identify patients with sensory neuropathy and associated osseous and vascular complications.
- **Management Planning:** To guide the treatment of ulcerative lesions, skeletal deformities, and neuropathic complications effectively.

Procedure Overview

- **Clinical Assessment:** Evaluate for ulcerative lesions, Charcot foot deformities, and sensory deficits in the lower extremities.
- Conduct a thorough neurological examination for shooting pain and loss of deep tendon reflexes.
- **Radiographic Imaging:** Assess for acroosteolysis, osteoporosis, and Charcot joint deformities.
- **Additional Tests:**
- Perform audiological testing for progressive deafness.
- Optical assessments for signs of optic atrophy.

Results and Interpretation

- **Key Findings:**
- Sensory neuropathy with loss of pain sensation leading to ulceration.
- Radiographic signs include metatarsophalangeal joint destruction, osteoporosis, and Charcot arthropathy.
- Systemic involvement in some cases, including optic and cochlear atrophy.

Physiological Basis

- **Neurological Component:** Primary degeneration of the posterior root ganglia leads to sensory deficits, which predispose to ulceration and skeletal deformities.

- **Vascular and Skeletal Changes:** Chronic pressure-point ulceration leads to osteolysis, fractures, and deformities.
- Vasomotor dysfunction may exacerbate local tissue damage and lead to peripheral complications, such as elephant foot.

Clinical Applications

- **Neurological Disorders:** Diagnosis and management of hereditary sensory neuropathies.
- **Orthopedic Management:** Surgical and non-surgical management of Charcot arthropathy, fractures, and skeletal deformities.
- **Preventive Care:** Strategies to prevent ulcerative lesions in patients with sensory deficits.

Limitations and Technical Considerations

- **Diagnostic Complexity:** Overlap with other hereditary sensory neuropathies may complicate diagnosis.
- **Progression Variability:** Wide variability in age of onset and symptom severity requires individualized care.
- **Genetic Uncertainty:** Sporadic and recessive cases may obscure family history.

Modern Relevance

- **Peripheral Neuropathy Research:** Advances in understanding genetic and molecular mechanisms of posterior root ganglia degeneration have expanded diagnostic and therapeutic options.
- **Surgical Advances:** Enhanced surgical techniques for managing Charcot deformities and ulcerative complications.
- **Interdisciplinary Care:** Collaboration between neurologists, orthopedists, and vascular specialists has improved patient outcomes.

Associated Conditions

- **Charcot Arthropathy:** Neuropathic joint disease leading to severe deformities in weight-bearing joints.
- **Elephant Foot:** Severe vasomotor dysfunction causing hypertrophy and swelling in the lower extremities.
- **Sensory Neuropathies:** Overlap with other hereditary sensory neuropathies.

Clinical Importance

- **Early Detection:** Early recognition can prevent progressive skeletal deformities and chronic ulceration.
- **Comprehensive Management:** Requires a combination of orthopedic intervention, neurological care, and vascular support for optimal outcomes.
- **Genetic Counseling:** Vital for families with a history of autosomal dominant or recessive inheritance.

References

A. Nélaton: Affection singulière des os du pied. Gazette des hôpitaux, Paris, 1852, 4: 13.

D. E. Denny Brown: Hereditary sensory radicular neuropathy. Journal of Neurology, Neurosurgery and Psychiatry, London, 1951, 14: 237-252.

E. P. Hicks: Hereditary perforating ulcer of the foot. The Lancet, London,1922,1:319-321.

E. M. Smith: Familial neurotrophic osseous atrophy: A familial neurotrophic condition of the feet with anesthesia and loss of bone. Journal of the American Medical Association, Chicago, 1934, 102: 593-595.

A. Thévenard: L'acropathie ulcéro-mutilante familiale. Revue neurologique, Paris, 1942, 74: 193-212.

Nélaton's tumour

Overview

Nélaton's Tumour refers to a central bone tumor, often presenting as a lesion within the bone's medullary cavity. While its clinical presentation and behavior may vary, these tumors typically disrupt normal bone structure and may result in pain, swelling, and functional impairment depending on the extent of the lesion. The term is largely of historical interest but serves as an important reference in orthopedic and oncological studies of bone neoplasms.

Historical Background

- **1835-1836:** Baron Guillaume Dupuytren contributed significantly to early descriptions of bone pathology, including central lesions of the bone.
- **1851:** Auguste Nélaton, a French surgeon, described the tumor in greater detail, associating it with central lesions of the bone, which later bore his name.
- The naming of *Nélaton's Tumour* highlights the early collaborative efforts in understanding skeletal neoplasms and emphasizes their recognition as distinct pathological entities.

Purpose

- **Diagnosis and Classification:** To identify and differentiate central bone tumors from other bone lesions or systemic conditions.
- **Guidance for Treatment:** To direct surgical or non-surgical interventions based on the tumor's characteristics, such as size, location, and histological type.

Procedure Overview

- **Clinical Examination:** Assessment of localized pain, swelling, or restricted motion in the affected bone region.
- **Imaging Techniques:**
- **X-rays:** To identify medullary involvement and assess the extent of cortical thinning or disruption.
- **MRI/CT:** To evaluate soft tissue extension, vascular involvement, and precise anatomical localization.
- **Histopathological Examination:** Biopsy to confirm the tumor's type, grade, and malignancy potential.

Results and Interpretation

- **Imaging Findings:** Lesions localized in the medullary cavity with evidence of cortical expansion or thinning.
- **Histological Features:** Identification of cellular patterns that distinguish benign from malignant lesions.
- **Clinical Course:** Slow or rapid progression depending on the tumor type and aggressiveness.

Physiological Basis

- **Tumor Pathogenesis:** Arises from the central medullary cavity due to abnormal proliferation of bone-forming cells or secondary invasion by metastatic cells.
- **Bone Remodeling Disruption:** Tumors interfere with the balance between osteoblastic and osteoclastic activity, leading to structural instability and potential fractures.

Clinical Applications

- **Orthopedic Oncology:** Critical for diagnosing and managing central bone tumors such as enchondromas, osteosarcomas, or metastatic lesions.
- **Surgical Planning:** Guides resection margins and reconstructive strategies, especially in long bones.
- **Prognostic Evaluation:** Determines the likelihood of recurrence or metastatic spread based on tumor characteristics.

Limitations and Technical Considerations

- **Diagnostic Challenges:** Differentiating between benign and malignant central tumors may require extensive imaging and histopathological studies.
- **Risk of Mismanagement:** Delay in diagnosis or incomplete resection may lead to tumor progression or recurrence.
- **Surgical Risks:** Interventions involving the medullary cavity pose risks of infection, nerve injury, or fracture complications.

Modern Relevance

- **Advancements in Imaging:** Use of advanced techniques such as positron emission tomography (PET) for early and precise tumor detection.
- **Targeted Therapies:** Development of chemotherapy and radiotherapy protocols tailored to specific tumor types.
- **Minimally Invasive Techniques:** Introduction of endoscopic surgeries and percutaneous interventions for selected cases.

Associated Conditions

- **Enchondroma:** A benign tumor arising from cartilage cells within the medullary cavity.
- **Osteosarcoma:** A malignant central bone tumor characterized by aggressive growth and metastasis potential.
- **Metastatic Lesions:** Secondary tumors arising from cancers of other organs, such as the breast or lung.

Clinical Importance

- **Early Diagnosis:** Early detection through imaging and biopsy is critical to prevent complications like fractures or metastasis.
- **Comprehensive Management:** Requires interdisciplinary collaboration among orthopedic surgeons, radiologists, and oncologists.
- **Patient-Centered Care:** Focuses on preserving function and minimizing morbidity through timely and appropriate treatment.

References

A. Nélaton: Élements de pathologie chriurgicale. 'Paris, 1847-1848, volume 2, p 46.

G. Dupuytren: Des kystes qui se dévelop dans l'épaisser des os, et de leurs différentes espéces. In his: Leçons orales de clinique chirurgicale faites à l'Hôtel-Dieu de Paris. 1839, pp 129-148.

Nievergelt's Syndrome

Overview

Nievergelt's Syndrome is a rare hereditary bone disease marked by symmetrical dysplasia of the radius, ulna, tibia, and fibula. It is characterized by skeletal deformities such as radioulnar synostosis, luxation of ulna or radial heads, brachydactyly, and deformities of the lower legs and feet. The condition has variable expression and typically manifests from birth. Inheritance is autosomal dominant, with a higher prevalence in males.

Historical Background

- **1874:** Wilhelm Heinrich Erb contributed foundational knowledge to neuromuscular and skeletal diseases, creating a context for understanding skeletal dysplasias.
- **1944:** Kurt Nievergelt provided a detailed description of this syndrome, identifying it in a father and three sons with distinct skeletal deformities, linking the features to autosomal dominant inheritance.
- Later, *Hubert S. Pearlman* and other researchers expanded the clinical understanding of its manifestations and genetic implications.

Purpose

- **Diagnosis and Genetic Understanding:** To identify and classify skeletal deformities and determine the hereditary pattern of the syndrome.
- **Guidance for Treatment:** To provide therapeutic options aimed at preserving function and minimizing disability.
- **Parental Identification in Legal Cases:** Due to its high penetrance, the condition has been cited as proof of parentage in disputed instances.

Procedure Overview

- **Clinical Evaluation:** Physical examination focusing on deformities of the upper and lower extremities.
- **Imaging Techniques:**
- **X-rays:** To evaluate bony dysplasias such as radioulnar synostosis, brachydactyly, and rhomboid-shaped tibia and fibula.
- **CT/MRI:** For a detailed assessment of joint abnormalities and synostoses.
- **Genetic Testing:** Screening for mutations linked to autosomal dominant inheritance patterns.

Results and Interpretation

- **Radiographic Findings:** Symmetric dysplasia of the radius and ulna, with evidence of radioulnar synostosis and luxation of the radial head.
- Characteristic rhomboid-shaped tibia and fibula.
- **Clinical Manifestations:** Dysplastic elbows, genu valgum, clubfoot, and deformities of the great toes.
- Flexion contractures in fingers and short digits (brachydactyly).
- **Inheritance Pattern:** Autosomal dominant with variable penetrance, explaining differing severities among affected individuals.

Physiological Basis

- **Bone Dysplasia:** Disruption in normal bone growth and joint development leads to deformities and synostoses.
- **Connective Tissue Abnormalities:** Abnormal connective tissue development contributes to joint luxations and restricted mobility.

Clinical Applications

- **Orthopedic Management:** Surgical interventions to correct genu valgum, clubfoot, or severe dysplasias.
- Prosthetics or orthotics to improve mobility in severe deformities.
- **Genetic Counseling:** Important for families with a history of the syndrome to predict and manage inheritance risks.
- **Forensic Applications:** The syndrome's strong genetic penetrance has been used in legal contexts for parentage verification.

Limitations and Technical Considerations

- **Diagnostic Complexity:** Variable expression and overlap with other skeletal syndromes may complicate diagnosis.
- **Surgical Challenges:** Operations on dysplastic bones and malformed joints carry higher risks of complications.
- **Genetic Testing:** Identifying causative mutations remains challenging in some cases due to genetic heterogeneity.

Modern Relevance

- **Advancements in Imaging:** Use of high-resolution imaging for detailed skeletal analysis.
- **Molecular Genetics:** Progress in genetic testing offers better diagnostic and predictive capabilities.
- **Personalized Medicine:** Tailored treatment plans based on the severity of deformities and genetic background.

Associated Conditions

- **Radioulnar Synostosis:** Fusion of the radius and ulna limiting forearm rotation.
- **Clubfoot (Talipes Equinovarus):** Congenital deformity affecting the alignment of the foot.
- **Brachydactyly:** Shortened digits associated with restricted joint movement.

Clinical Importance

- **Early Detection:** Identifying skeletal dysplasia at birth allows for timely intervention to reduce long-term disability.
- **Functional Preservation:** Orthopedic and physical therapy interventions are crucial to maintain mobility and limb function.
- **Genetic Counseling:** Helps families understand inheritance patterns and plan for future pregnancies.
- **Research Potential:** Offers insights into the genetic and developmental pathways underlying bone dysplasias.

Nievergelt's Syndrome, with its distinctive

skeletal features and inheritance pattern, serves as an important model for understanding genetic bone dysplasias. **Advances in** *diagnostics and treatment continue to improve outcomes for affected individuals.*

References

K. Nievergelt: Positiver Vaterschaftsnachweis auf Grund erblicher Fehlbildungen der Extremitäten. Archiv der Julius Klaus Stiftung für Vererbungsforschung, Sozialanthropologie und Rassenhygiene, Zürich, 1944, 157-194.

H. S. Pearlman, et al: Familial tarsal and carpal synostosis with radial-head subluxation (Nievergelt's syndrome). Journal of Bone and Joint Surgery, Boston, 1964, 46-A: 585-592.

K. A. Solonen, M. Sulamaa: Nievergelt syndrome and its treatment: a case report. Annales chirurgicae et gynaecologiae fenniae, Helsinki, 1958, 47: 142-147.

Nightstick Fracture

Overview

A nightstick fracture is an isolated fracture of the ulnar shaft, often caused by direct trauma to the medial forearm. It derives its name from the mechanism of injury associated with defending oneself against a blow, such as from a police baton or "nightstick." These fractures typically present with localized pain, tenderness, and dysfunction of the affected arm. While traditionally managed non-operatively, current approaches emphasize a balance between surgical and conservative treatments based on the injury's severity and associated complications.

Historical Background

- The term "nightstick fracture" originated from injuries sustained when individuals defended against blows to the forearm with a police baton. Although no specific year is attributed to its nomenclature, the concept has been recognized for decades in clinical practice.

- **Advances in** imaging and surgical techniques have since refined the understanding and management of this injury.

Purpose

- **Primary Objective:** Ensure proper alignment and healing of the ulna to restore forearm function.

- **Secondary Objective:** Prevent complications such as nonunion, deformity, and compromised range of motion.

Procedure Overview

Diagnosis:

- **Clinical Evaluation:** Pain, swelling, and tenderness over the ulnar shaft.
- Rule out open fractures and associated injuries (e.g., Monteggia fractures or wrist instability).
- **Imaging:**
- X-rays of the forearm, elbow, and wrist in multiple views.
- A "perfect" lateral elbow view to assess radial head alignment with the capitellum.

Treatment:

- **Nonoperative Management:** Preferred for minimally displaced fractures (<50% displacement, <10° angulation).
- Immobilization with a functional brace or cast for 4-6 weeks.
- Gradual return to activity with physical therapy.
- **Surgical Management:** Indicated for displaced fractures, instability, or polytrauma.
- **Techniques include:**
- **Plate fixation:** Gold standard with low nonunion rates.
- **Intramedullary fixation:** Minimally invasive but slightly higher risk of nonunion.

Results and Interpretation

- **Nonoperative Outcomes:** Most isolated ulnar shaft fractures heal with proper immobilization, with union achieved in 6-8 weeks.
- **Surgical Outcomes:** Plate fixation provides robust stability and high rates of union, with patients typically regaining full range of motion and strength.

Physiological Basis

- The *ulna* is a long bone in the forearm that provides structural support and serves as an attachment point for muscles. Direct trauma or excessive rotational forces can disrupt its integrity, leading to isolated fractures.
- Proper alignment during healing ensures that rotational movements of the forearm, facilitated by the radius, remain functional.

Clinical Applications

- Management of isolated ulnar fractures is common in emergency and orthopedic settings.
- Understanding the associated injuries (e.g., Monteggia fractures) is critical to avoid delayed diagnoses and complications.

Limitations and Technical Considerations

- **Diagnostic Challenges:** Subtle fractures may be missed without thorough radiographic evaluation.
- **Differentiating between simple and complex fracture patterns requires experience.**
- **Treatment Challenges:** Nonunion, though rare, can occur in conservatively managed fractures.
- Surgical complications include infection, hardware failure, and soft tissue irritation.

Modern Relevance

- Improved imaging techniques and surgical advancements have enhanced the accuracy of diagnosis and outcomes.
- Awareness of this injury among emergency department clinicians ensures timely referrals and reduces complications.

Associated Conditions

- **Monteggia Fracture-Dislocation:** Concurrent fracture of the ulna with radial head dislocation.
- **Wrist Injuries:** Instabilities or fractures involving the distal radioulnar joint (DRUJ).

Clinical Importance

- **Prevention:** Appropriate protective measures and fall prevention strategies can reduce the incidence.
- **Multidisciplinary Care:** Coordination between emergency clinicians, radiologists, and orthopedic surgeons ensures optimal outcomes.
- **Prognosis:** Most patients achieve full recovery with appropriate treatment, though compliance with immobilization and follow-up care is crucial.

Nightstick fractures remain a common injury, particularly in trauma settings. With proper diagnosis and management, the prognosis is excellent, underscoring the importance of timely and accurate intervention.

References

Hooper G. Isolated fractures of the shaft of the ulna. Injury. 1974 Nov;6(2):180-4. [PubMed]

Cai XZ, Yan SG, Giddins G. A systematic review of the non-operative treatment of nightstick fractures of the ulna. Bone Joint J. 2013 Jul;95-B(7):952-9. [PubMed]

Ali M, Clark DI, Tambe A. Nightstick Fractures, Outcomes of Operative and Non-Operative Treatment. Acta Medica (Hradec Kralove). 2019;62(1):19-23. [PubMed]

Du Toit FP, Gräbe RP. Isolated fractures of the shaft of the ulna. S Afr Med J. 1979 Jul 07;56(1):21-5. [PubMed]

Dymond IW. The treatment of isolated fractures of the distal ulna. J Bone Joint Surg Br. 1984 May;66(3):408-10.

Ekelund AL, Nilsson OS. Early mobilization of isolated ulnar-shaft fractures.Acta Orthop Scand.1989 Jun;60(3):261-2.

de Jong T, de Jong PC. Ulnar-shaft fracture needs no treatment. A pilot study of 10 cases. Acta Orthop Scand. 1989 Jun;60(3):263-4. [PubMed]

Zych GA, Latta LL, Zagorski JB. Treatment of isolated ulnar shaft fractures with prefabricated functional fracture braces. Clin Orthop Relat Res. 1987 Jun;(219):194-200. [PubMed]

Sarmiento A, Kinman PB, Murphy RB, Phillips JG. Treatment of ulnar fractures by functional bracing. J Bone Joint Surg Am. 1976 Dec;58(8):1104-7. [PubMed]

Gupta RP, Danielsson LG. Dorsally angulated solitary metaphyseal greenstick fractures in the distal radius: results after immobilization in pronated, neutral, and supinated position. J Pediatr Orthop. 1990 Jan-Feb;10(1):90-2. [PubMed]

Altner PC, Hartmann JT. Isolated fractures of the ulnar shaft in the adult. Surg Clin North Am. 1972 Feb;52(1):155-70. [PubMed]

Riska EB, von Bonsdorff H, Hakkinen S, Jaroma H, Kiviluoto O, Paavilainen T. Primary operative fixation of long bone fractures in patients with multiple injuries. J Trauma. 1977 Feb;17(2):111-21. [PubMed]

Mackay D, Wood L, Rangan A. The treatment of isolated ulnar fractures in adults: a systematic review. Injury. 2000 Oct;31(8):565-70.

Nursemaid's Elbow

Overview

Nursemaid's elbow, also known as radial head subluxation, is a common orthopedic injury in young children where the radial head slips from under the annular ligament. This results in pain and restricted motion, particularly in the forearm's supination. Diagnosis is typically clinical and based on history, and treatment involves a simple reduction maneuver that restores normal arm function immediately.

Historical Background

- The term "nursemaid's elbow" originates from the early 20th century when the condition was observed in children cared for by nursemaids who inadvertently caused the injury by pulling the child's arm.
- First systematically described in medical literature in the early 1900s, its mechanism and treatment have since been well-documented.

Purpose

- **Primary Objective:** To relieve pain and restore normal arm function by repositioning the radial head.
- **Secondary Objective:** To educate caregivers on preventing recurrence by avoiding traction on the child's arm.

Procedure Overview

Diagnosis:

- Based on history and physical examination, with a clear account of axial traction on an extended and pronated forearm.
- Symptoms include pain, refusal to move the arm, and holding the arm in a pronated position.
- Imaging is rarely necessary unless the mechanism or symptoms suggest a fracture or other pathology.

Treatment:

- **Reduction Techniques:** Supination-Flexion Method: The forearm is supinated while the elbow is flexed.
- **Hyperpronation Method:** The forearm is hyperpronated without flexing the elbow.
- Both methods aim to reposition the radial head under the annular ligament.

Results and Interpretation

- Reduction is often confirmed by a palpable or audible click during the maneuver.
- Pain relief and immediate return of arm function within minutes indicate successful treatment.
- No further immobilization is required if the reduction is successful.

Physiological Basis

- The *annular ligament* encircles the radial head and stabilizes it against the ulna.
- Axial traction on a pronated and extended forearm stretches the annular ligament, allowing the radial head to slip out, resulting in subluxation.
- Reduction maneuvers reposition the radial head under the ligament and restore normal joint mechanics.

Clinical Applications

- Commonly seen in children under five due to their ligamentous laxity and smaller radial heads.
- Routine in pediatric emergency and primary care settings.

Limitations and Technical Considerations

- **Challenges in Diagnosis:** Atypical presentations or unclear history can complicate diagnosis.
- **Imaging is warranted if other injuries are suspected.**
- **Reduction Considerations:** Some children may require repeated attempts or sedation if the reduction is unsuccessful initially.

Modern Relevance

- Nursemaid's elbow remains a frequent presentation in pediatric care, often associated with play activities or accidents.
- The simplicity of the reduction and the immediate resolution of symptoms make it a satisfying condition to treat for both healthcare providers and caregivers.

Associated Conditions

- **Recurrent Subluxation:** Due to ligamentous laxity, some children experience repeated episodes.
- **Misdiagnosed Fractures:** Rare cases where fractures mimic the presentation of nursemaid's elbow.

Clinical Importance

- **Prevention:** Educating caregivers to avoid lifting or pulling a child by their arms significantly reduces recurrence.
- **Prognosis:** Excellent if treated promptly; untreated cases may lead to persistent pain and dysfunction.
- **Caregiver Reassurance:** Addressing caregiver concerns and explaining the benign nature of the injury and its simple treatment is essential.

References

Mohd Miswan MF, Othman MS, Muhamad Effendi F, Ibrahim MI, Rozali KN. Pulled/nursemaid's elbow. Malays Fam Physician. 2017;12(1):26-28. [PMC free article] [PubMed]

Wong K, Troncoso AB, Calello DP, Salo D, Fiesseler F. Radial Head Subluxation: Factors Associated with Its Recurrence and Radiographic Evaluation in a Tertiary Pediatric Emergency Department. J Emerg Med. 2016 Dec;51(6):621-627. [PubMed]

Mak S, Beltran LS, Bencardino J, Orr J, Jazrawi L, Cerezal L, Beltran J. MRI of the annular ligament of the elbow: review of anatomic considerations and pathologic findings in patients with posterolateral elbow instability. AJR Am J Roentgenol. 2014 Dec;203(6):1272-9. [PubMed]

Karasick D. Nursemaid elbow revisited and a review of congenital radioulnar synostosis. Radiographics. 2004 Nov-Dec;24(6):1608-10; author reply 1608-10. [PubMed]

Chen H, Shao Y, Li S. Replacement or repair of terrible triad of the elbow: A systematic review and meta-analysis. Medicine (Baltimore). 2019 Feb;98(6):e13054. [PMC free article] [PubMed]

Wang Q, Du MM, Pei XJ, Luo JZ, Li YZ, Liu YC, Wang X, Cao JC, Han JH. External Fixator-assisted Ulnar Osteotomy: A Novel Technique to Treat Missed Monteggia Fracture in Children. Orthop Surg. 2019 Feb;11(1):102-108. [PMC free article] [PubMed]

Cope B, Tracy M. Not just another nursemaid's: an enigmatic paediatric humeral fracture. BMJ Case Rep. 2018 Oct 02;2018 [PMC free article] [PubMed]

Pawelec B, Waśko MK, Pomianowski S. Neglected Iatrogenic Elbow Joint Dislocation. Didactic Case Report. Ortop Traumatol Rehabil. 2018 Feb 27;20(1):57-63. [PubMed]

Galbiatti JA, Cardoso FL, Ferro JAS, Godoy RCG, Belluci SOB, Palacio EP. Terrible triad of the elbow: evaluation of surgical treatment. Rev Bras Ortop. 2018 Jul-Aug;53(4):460-466. [PMC free article] [PubMed]

Hill CE, Cooke S. Common Paediatric Elbow Injuries. Open Orthop J. 2017;11:1380-1393.

Ollier's disease

Overview

Ollier's Disease is a rare disorder of bone development characterized by the presence of multiple nonossified cartilaginous masses, known as enchondromas, within the metaphyses of bones. These lesions predominantly affect the growing ends of long bones, leading to asymmetrical skeletal deformities, including limb shortening and angular deformities. While the condition often stabilizes after adolescence, complications such as fractures and malignant transformation can occur. The condition is typically sporadic, with rare familial cases.

Historical Background

- **1876:** The disease was first described by Louis Xavier Édouard Léopold Ollier, a French surgeon who extensively studied bone pathology and named the condition enchondromatosis in cases of multiple enchondromas.
- **1881:** Angelo Maffucci, an Italian pathologist, later identified the association of enchondromas with vascular abnormalities such as hemangiomas and phleboliths, which now constitute Maffucci Syndrome.
- Over the years, Ollier's work has remained foundational in understanding skeletal dysplasias and benign cartilaginous tumors.

Purpose

- **Clinical Identification:** To diagnose and differentiate Ollier's disease from other skeletal dysplasias and syndromes.
- **Management of Complications:** To monitor for malignant transformation of enchondromas into chondrosarcomas, a potential complication.
- **Research in Bone Pathology:** Provides insights into abnormal cartilage development and skeletal growth.

Procedure Overview

- **Clinical Examination:** Evaluate limb deformities, asymmetry, and potential limb shortening.
- **Radiographic Analysis:** X-rays reveal multiple lytic lesions with a cartilaginous matrix, often localized in the metaphyseal regions of long bones.
- **Advanced Imaging:** MRI and CT scans assess lesion size, distribution, and any indications of malignant transformation.
- **Histological Examination:** Biopsy may be performed to rule out malignancy, particularly in symptomatic or enlarging lesions.

Results and Interpretation

- **Radiographic Findings:** Presence of multiple cartilaginous masses in the metaphyseal regions, often causing bony deformities and asymmetrical limb lengths.
- Bone lesions typically appear as well-demarcated, radiolucent areas with calcifications.
- **Clinical Manifestations:**
- Asymmetric limb shortening, angular deformities, and occasional fractures.
- Lesions are typically evident by 1 to 4 years of age, with minimal progression

after puberty.

- **Histology:** Benign cartilaginous tissue is found within the lesions unless malignant transformation occurs.

Physiological Basis

- **Cartilaginous Abnormality:** Enchondromas result from an abnormal proliferation of cartilage at the growth plate, disrupting normal endochondral ossification.
- **Skeletal Growth Defect:** The accumulation of cartilaginous tissue impairs bone growth, leading to asymmetry and deformity.

Clinical Applications

- **Orthopedic Interventions:** Corrective surgeries to manage limb length discrepancies or angular deformities.
- Internal fixation or bone grafting for fractures.
- **Oncological Monitoring:** Regular follow-ups to detect early signs of malignant transformation, such as pain, rapid lesion growth, or destruction of the bone cortex.
- **Pediatric Management:** Early diagnosis allows for timely intervention to minimize long-term skeletal complications.

Limitations and Technical Considerations

- **Diagnostic Challenges:** Differentiating Ollier's disease from other syndromes, such as Maffucci Syndrome, and detecting early signs of malignancy can be difficult.
- **Surgical Risks:** Procedures for limb correction or tumor excision carry risks of infection, recurrence, and complications in skeletal growth.
- **Prognostic Uncertainty:** Variable progression and outcomes, including the risk of chondrosarcoma, make prognosis challenging.

Modern Relevance

- **Advances in Imaging:** Improved imaging modalities, such as MRI, allow for better visualization and monitoring of lesions.
- **Genetic Insights:** Ongoing research into the genetic basis of enchondromatosis could lead to targeted therapies in the future.
- **Interdisciplinary Care:** Collaboration among orthopedic surgeons, oncologists, and geneticists is critical for managing complex cases.

Associated Conditions

- **Maffucci Syndrome:** Characterized by enchondromatosis along with vascular anomalies such as hemangiomas and phleboliths.
- **Chondrosarcoma:** Malignant transformation of enchondromas occurs in approximately 25–30% of cases of Ollier's disease.

Clinical Importance

- **Early Diagnosis:** Timely identification of enchondromas and skeletal abnormalities enables early intervention, reducing functional impairment.
- **Surveillance for Malignancy:** Regular monitoring is essential to detect

chondrosarcoma, a life-threatening complication, at an early stage.

- **Functional Preservation:** Surgical and non-surgical interventions aim to improve mobility, correct deformities, and enhance quality of life.
- **Pediatric Considerations:** Focused care during the growing years minimizes the progression of skeletal deformities.

Ollier's disease, though rare, requires a multidisciplinary approach for effective management. **Advances in** *imaging, genetics, and surgical techniques continue to improve the prognosis and quality of life for affected individuals.*

References

L. X. E. L. Ollier: Dyschondroplasie. Lyon médical 1898, 88: 484-492.

Exostoses multiples. Mémoires et comptes rendus de la Société des sciences médicales de Lyon, (1889), 1890; 29, 2: 12.

Ollier's layer

Overview

Ollier's Layer refers to the inner layer of the periosteum, the dense connective tissue membrane covering the outer surface of bones. This layer is rich in osteoblasts, the cells responsible for bone formation and remodeling. It plays a critical role in bone growth, repair, and regeneration.

Historical Background

- **1876:** The term and concept were associated with the works of Louis Xavier Édouard Léopold Ollier, a French surgeon renowned for his pioneering research in bone pathology and periosteal functions.
- Ollier extensively studied the *periosteum*, elucidating its vital role in *bone growth and healing*. His foundational research emphasized the periosteum's osteogenic potential, particularly the function of its inner layer.

Purpose

- **Bone Growth and Development:** To support longitudinal and appositional bone growth during childhood and adolescence.
- **Bone Healing:** To facilitate fracture repair through osteoblast-mediated bone regeneration.
- **Bone Remodeling:**
- To maintain bone strength and adapt to mechanical stresses by forming new bone tissue.

Procedure Overview

- **Structure Examination:** The periosteum is dissected and microscopically examined to study the Ollier's layer.
- **Histological Analysis:** The osteoblast density, activity, and alignment within Ollier's layer are analyzed.
- **Bone Regeneration Studies:** Experimentally, the osteogenic capacity of the periosteum, particularly Ollier's layer, is assessed in bone grafting and fracture healing models.

Results and Interpretation

- **Cellular Composition:** Ollier's layer is rich in osteoblasts, which are cuboidal cells involved in the synthesis of bone matrix.
- **Bone Regeneration:** The layer demonstrates a high capacity for forming new bone tissue, especially in response to injury or mechanical stimulation.
- **Histological Features:** Microscopic examination reveals active osteoblasts aligned along the inner periosteal surface, with robust extracellular matrix deposition.

Physiological Basis

- **Bone Formation:** Osteoblasts in Ollier's layer produce collagen and other proteins that form the osteoid matrix, which is subsequently mineralized to become bone.
- **Healing Response:** During fractures, this layer is activated, contributing significantly to the periosteal callus, a critical structure for stabilizing and repairing broken bones.

Clinical Applications

- **Orthopedic Surgeries:** Leveraging the osteogenic potential of Ollier's layer in bone grafting and defect repair.
- **Fracture Healing:** Understanding the role of Ollier's layer enhances strategies for promoting bone regeneration in non-union fractures.
- **Biomaterials Development:** Inspired by the regenerative properties of Ollier's layer, advanced materials mimic its osteogenic function in scaffold designs.

Limitations and Technical Considerations

- **Age-Dependent Activity:** The osteoblast activity in Ollier's layer diminishes with age, reducing its regenerative potential in older individuals.
- **Injury Susceptibility:** Damage to the periosteum, including Ollier's layer, can impair bone healing and remodeling.
- **Histological Analysis Challenges:** Precise identification of Ollier's layer and quantifying its osteogenic activity require advanced imaging and staining techniques.

Modern Relevance

- **Tissue Engineering:** Studies of Ollier's layer guide the development of osteogenic scaffolds for bone tissue engineering.
- **Regenerative Medicine:** Insights into periosteal layers have fostered advancements in cell-based therapies for bone defects.
- **Biomechanical Research:** Understanding Ollier's layer's role in

adapting bone to mechanical stresses informs rehabilitation strategies for orthopedic injuries.

Associated Conditions

- **Periosteal Injury:** Damage to Ollier's layer impairs fracture healing and bone growth.
- **Osteoporosis:** Reduced osteoblast function in Ollier's layer contributes to the imbalance between bone formation and resorption.

Clinical Importance

- **Bone Regeneration Potential:** Harnessing the osteogenic capacity of Ollier's layer is critical in orthopedic interventions.
- **Fracture Healing:** Activation of Ollier's layer during injury underlines its importance in the natural healing process.
- **Target for Therapies:** Stimulating osteoblasts in Ollier's layer could enhance bone repair and counteract age-related bone loss.
- **Insights for Research:** The cellular and molecular dynamics of Ollier's layer continue to be a focal point for understanding bone biology and pathology.

Ollier's layer remains a cornerstone in understanding the periosteum's osteogenic potential, with broad implications for orthopedic research, clinical practice, and regenerative medicine.

References

L. X. E. L. Ollier: Des moyens chirurgicaux de favoriser la reproduction des os après les résections, etc. Gazette hebdomadaire de médecine et de chirurgie, Paris, 1858, 5: 572-577, 651-653, 733-736, 769-770, 853-857, 890, 899-905.

Ollier-Thiersch graft

Overview

The Ollier-Thiersch graft is a split-thickness skin graft characterized by its thin nature, consisting of the epidermis and a portion of the dermis. This grafting technique, originally devised by Louis Xavier Édouard Léopold Ollier and later refined by Karl Thiersch, is utilized to promote wound healing and restore skin coverage in cases of burns, ulcers, or large tissue defects.

Historical Background

- **1872:** Louis Xavier Édouard Léopold Ollier, a French surgeon, introduced a novel method of skin grafting to aid in wound healing and tissue repair.
- Later in the same century, *Karl Thiersch*, a German surgeon, refined and popularized the technique by adjusting the method of harvesting the graft and its thickness.
- The combined contributions of Ollier and Thiersch led to the term *Ollier-Thiersch graft*, though it is more commonly referred to as the *Thiersch graft* in modern medical practice.

Purpose

- **Wound Coverage:** To provide a protective covering for open wounds, preventing infection and fluid loss.
- **Aesthetic and Functional Recovery:** To promote regeneration of damaged skin, minimizing scarring and restoring function.
- **Burn Treatment:** Used in managing second- and third-degree burns

to accelerate healing and reduce complications.

Procedure Overview

- **Preparation:** The wound bed is debrided to ensure a clean surface for graft adherence.
- Hemostasis is achieved to prevent interference with graft survival.
- **Graft Harvesting:** A thin layer of skin, including the epidermis and part of the dermis, is removed using a dermatome or razor blade from a donor site, such as the thigh or buttock.
- **Application:** The harvested graft is placed over the prepared wound bed and secured with sutures, staples, or adhesive strips.
- **Postoperative Care:** The area is dressed with non-adherent gauze to prevent dislodgment, and the graft is monitored for adherence and signs of infection.

Results and Interpretation

- **Initial Healing:** The graft adheres to the wound bed, with capillary ingrowth ensuring its survival.
- **Regeneration:** Epithelialization begins at the edges and progresses centrally, restoring skin coverage.
- **Outcome:** Successful grafting results in durable skin coverage with minimal scarring and restoration of function, though pigmentation and texture differences may persist.

Physiological Basis

- **Partial Thickness:** The inclusion of dermal components allows for improved graft survival and integration into the recipient site.
- **Angiogenesis:** Capillary ingrowth from the wound bed ensures the graft receives nutrients and oxygen for survival.
- **Regeneration:** The remaining dermal structures in the donor site promote rapid healing and epithelial regeneration.

Clinical Applications

- **Burn Management:** Effective for covering large burns where autologous grafting is preferred.
- **Chronic Wounds:** Useful in treating ulcers, including venous and diabetic ulcers.
- **Trauma Repair:** Provides skin coverage for extensive traumatic injuries.
- **Reconstructive Surgery:** Employed in procedures requiring restoration of skin integrity and aesthetics.

Limitations and Technical Considerations

- **Graft Fragility:** Thin grafts are more prone to tearing and require careful handling during application.
- **Pigmentation Variance:** Donor and recipient site color differences may result in cosmetic irregularities.
- **Donor Site Morbidity:** Harvesting can lead to pain, scarring, or delayed healing at the donor site.
- **Infection Risk:** Both donor and

recipient sites are susceptible to infection if not properly managed.

Modern Relevance

- **Tissue Engineering:** Advances in artificial skin substitutes and regenerative techniques are inspired by the principles of split-thickness grafting.
- **Burn Centers:** The Ollier-Thiersch graft remains a cornerstone technique in specialized burn units.
- **Global Adoption:** The technique's simplicity and effectiveness ensure its widespread use, particularly in resource-limited settings.

Associated Conditions

- **Severe Burns:** Especially in cases requiring extensive skin coverage.
- **Chronic Ulcers:** Including diabetic, venous, and pressure ulcers.
- **Post-Trauma Defects:** Large wounds resulting from accidents or surgical excisions.

Clinical Importance

- **Early Intervention:** Immediate grafting reduces infection risks and promotes rapid wound closure.
- **Reduced Morbidity:** Effective for covering wounds with minimal donor site complications.
- **Wound Healing Efficacy:** Accelerates healing while maintaining the integrity and function of the affected area.
- **Versatile Application:** Used across a range of surgical and traumatic wound scenarios.

The Ollier-Thiersch graft is a foundational method in reconstructive surgery, with enduring relevance due to its simplicity, effectiveness, and adaptability to various clinical scenarios.

References

L. X. E. L. Ollier: Greffes cutanées ou autoplastiques. Bulletin de l'Académie de médecine, Paris, 1872, 2 sér., 1: 243-250.

Open Book Fracture

Overview

Open book fracture is a severe and rare type of pelvic fracture caused by high-energy trauma. It involves disruption of the pubic symphysis and often includes ligamentous and posterior pelvic ring injuries, leading to a widening of the pelvic ring resembling an "open book." These fractures are associated with high morbidity and mortality due to complications like hemorrhage, vascular injuries, and damage to internal organs, necessitating a multidisciplinary approach for optimal management.

Historical Background

- The term "open book fracture" originates from the resemblance of the separated pelvic bones to an opened book.
- This type of fracture gained recognition in trauma literature as motor vehicle accidents and high-energy injuries became more prevalent in the 20th century, especially with the rise of automobile use.

Purpose

- **Primary Objective:** To stabilize the pelvic ring and control hemorrhage to reduce morbidity and mortality.
- **Secondary Objective:** To restore pelvic anatomy and function and minimize long-term complications.

Procedure Overview

- **Initial Evaluation:**
- Follows Advanced Trauma Life Support (ATLS) guidelines focusing on airway, breathing, and circulation.
- Identification of pelvic instability via clinical exam and imaging.
- Immediate control of hemorrhage using pelvic binders or external fixators.
- **Imaging Studies:**
- **X-rays:** AP pelvis radiographs to identify pubic diastasis and sacroiliac joint widening.
- **CT Scan:** For detailed assessment of fractures and associated organ injuries.
- **Definitive Treatment:**
- **Non-Surgical Management:** Pelvic binders or sheets for stable fractures with minimal displacement.
- **Surgical Intervention:** Required for unstable fractures involving open reduction and internal fixation (ORIF) or external fixation for severe instability.
- **Supportive Care:**
- Angiographic embolization or pre-peritoneal packing to control hemorrhage.
- Multidisciplinary management for associated injuries, including vascular, genitourinary, and gastrointestinal complications.

Results and Interpretation

- **Immediate Outcome:** Stabilization of the pelvis and cessation of hemorrhage lead to increased survival rates.
- **Long-Term Outcome:** With appropriate surgical reconstruction and rehabilitation, patients can achieve functional recovery, though some may develop chronic pelvic pain or gait disturbances.

Physiological Basis

- The pelvis serves as a *load-bearing structure* and provides protection for critical vascular and organ systems.
- High-energy trauma leads to ligamentous rupture (e.g., sacrospinous and sacrotuberous ligaments) and/or fractures in the anterior and posterior pelvic ring, compromising stability.
- Hemorrhage occurs due to injury to major pelvic vessels or venous plexuses, necessitating immediate intervention to prevent hypovolemic shock.

Clinical Applications

- **Trauma Settings:** Managing life-threatening hemorrhage and pelvic instability.
- **Surgical Reconstruction:** Restoring pelvic anatomy and alignment to enable mobility.
- **Rehabilitation:** Post-operative physical therapy to regain strength and functionality.

Limitations and Technical Considerations

- **Challenges in Diagnosis:** Occult injuries may be missed without advanced imaging like CT scans.
- **Associated injuries to internal organs can complicate diagnosis and management.**
- **Surgical Considerations:** Delayed surgical intervention increases the risk of infection, malunion, or nonunion.
- Pre-existing conditions like osteoporosis can complicate fixation.

Modern Relevance

- Increased use of *pelvic binders* and advanced imaging modalities has improved early diagnosis and stabilization.
- Trauma systems now emphasize the multidisciplinary approach for managing open book fractures, including emergency care, surgery, and post-operative rehabilitation.

Associated Conditions

- **Vascular Injuries:** Damage to the iliac arteries or veins leading to hemorrhagic shock.
- **Organ Injuries:** Bladder rupture, urethral injury, and rectal tears.
- **Spinal Injuries:** Frequently associated with high-energy trauma.

Clinical Importance

- **Early Intervention:** Rapid identification and hemorrhage control are critical for survival.
- **Use of pelvic binders can significantly reduce mortality.**
- **Multidisciplinary Care:** Requires coordination between trauma surgeons, orthopedic specialists, vascular surgeons, and rehabilitation therapists.
- **Prognosis:** Stable fractures have excellent outcomes with conservative management.
- **Unstable fractures carry a high mortality rate, particularly with associated hemorrhage and organ injuries.**
- **Patient Education:** Patients and caregivers must be educated about the

severity of the injury, potential complications, and the importance of adherence to rehabilitation protocols for optimal recovery.

An open book fracture represents a critical injury requiring comprehensive, timely care to minimize complications and optimize functional recovery. Its management highlights the importance of advanced trauma care systems and interprofessional collaboration.

References

"Pelvic Fractures". OrthoInfo - AAOS. February 2016. Retrieved 17 May 2018.

ATLS - Advanced Trauma Life Support - Student Course Manual (10 ed.). American College of Surgeons. 2018. pp. 89, 96–97. ISBN 9780996826235.

Peitzman, Andrew B.; Rhodes, Michael; Schwab, C. William (2008). The Trauma Manual: Trauma and Acute Care Surgery. Lippincott Williams & Wilkins. p. 322. ISBN 9780781762755.

Walls, Ron; Hockberger, Robert; Gausche-Hill, Marianne (2017). Rosen's Emergency Medicine - Concepts and Clinical Practice E-Book. Elsevier Health Sciences. pp. 577, 588. ISBN 9780323390163.

Walker, J (Nov 9–15, 2011). "Pelvic fractures: classification and nursing management". Nursing Standard. 26 (10): 49–57, quiz 58. doi:10.7748/ns2011.11.26.10.49.c8816. PMID 22206172.

"Fracture of the Pelvis". OrthoInfo. American Academy of Orthopaedic Surgeons.

Dimon, Theodore Jr. (2010). The body in motion : its evolution and design. Berkeley, Calif.: North Atlantic Books. pp. 49–56. ISBN 978-1556439704.

Young, JW; Resnik, CS (December 1990). "Fracture of the Pelvis: Current Concepts of Classification". AJR. American Journal of Roentgenology. 155 (6): 1169–75. doi:10.2214/ajr.155.6.2122661. PMID 2122661.

Lee, C; Porter, K (February 2007). "The prehospital management of pelvic fractures". Emergency Medicine Journal. 24 (2): 130–3. doi:10.1136/emj.2006.041384. PMC 2658194. PMID 17251627.

"Pelvic Fractures". The Lecturio Medical Concept Library. Retrieved 3 October 2021.

"Anteroposterior Compression Fracture of Pelvis (Open Book Fracture)". Elsevier: Netter's Images.

Rothenberger, D; Velasco, R; Strate, R; Fischer, RP; Perry JF, Jr. (March 1978). "Open pelvic fracture: a lethal injury". The Journal of Trauma. 18 (3): 184–7. doi:10.1097/00005373-197803000-00006. PMID 642044.

"High Energy Fractures". International Society for Fracture Repair. Archived from the original on 2013-01-27.

Davis DD, Foris LA, Kane SM, et al. (January 2021). "Pelvic Fracture". National Center for Biotechnology Information, U.S. National Library of Medicine. PMID 28613485. Retrieved 2 October 2021.

Osgood-Schlatter disease

Overview

Osgood-Schlatter disease, more accurately termed Osgood-Schlatter condition, is an osteochondrosis of the tibial tuberosity. It is a common cause of knee pain in adolescents, affecting the area just below the kneecap where the patellar tendon inserts into the tibial tubercle. Clinical signs include localized pain, swelling, and tenderness, often aggravated by physical activity, especially those involving knee flexion and extension.

Historical Background

- **1891:** Sir James Paget first described a clinical syndrome resembling this condition.- 1903: Independently, Robert Bayley Osgood, an American orthopedic surgeon, and Carl B. Schlatter, a Swiss surgeon, detailed the condition as an inflammation of the tibial tuberosity due to overuse and repetitive strain.
- Over time, the condition came to bear their names, though some attribute earlier recognition to other clinicians such as Odilon Marc Lannelongue.

Purpose

- **Diagnosis and Management:**
- To identify and alleviate knee pain caused by tibial tubercle inflammation in adolescents.
- To prevent complications such as persistent pain or deformity of the tibial tuberosity.
- **Education and Prevention:** To guide

active adolescents and their families on activity modification during the growth phase.

Procedure Overview

Clinical Examination:

- Pain localized to the tibial tuberosity, often exacerbated by activities like jumping or kneeling.
- Swelling and tenderness at the site.

Imaging:

- X-rays may show fragmentation or irregularity of the tibial tuberosity in severe cases.
- MRI is rarely needed but can reveal soft tissue inflammation and tendon thickening.

Treatment:

- **Non-surgical Management:**
- Rest, ice, and anti-inflammatory medications.
- Physical therapy focusing on stretching the quadriceps and hamstring muscles.
- **Surgical Intervention:** Rarely needed but may be indicated for persistent symptoms or large ossicles causing pain.

Results and Interpretation

- **Short-Term Outcomes:** Pain and swelling improve with rest and activity modification.
- **Long-Term Prognosis:** Most adolescents outgrow the condition as the growth plates fuse.
- Rare complications include a persistent prominence at the tibial tuberosity or chronic pain.

Physiological Basis

- **Growth Phase Vulnerability:** The tibial tuberosity is a secondary ossification center, susceptible to stress during rapid growth spurts.
- **Repetitive Microtrauma:** Overuse or strain from sports causes microtrauma and inflammation at the patellar tendon's insertion.
- **Healing and Adaptation:** With reduced strain, the tibial tuberosity remodels, and symptoms typically resolve.

Clinical Applications

- **Orthopedic Assessment:** Diagnosis and management of adolescent knee pain.
- **Physical Therapy:** Rehabilitation programs emphasizing stretching and strengthening exercises.
- **Sports Medicine:** Guidance for athletes on modifying training regimens to prevent recurrence.

Limitations and Technical Considerations

- **Self-Limiting Nature:** The condition often resolves spontaneously, making aggressive treatments unnecessary.
- **Activity Modification:** Adolescents may struggle with restrictions on physical activity during treatment.
- **Diagnostic Challenges:** Differentiating Osgood-Schlatter disease from other causes of anterior knee pain, such as patellar tendinitis or Sinding-Larsen-Johansson syndrome.

Modern Relevance

- **Widespread Recognition:** Common among adolescent athletes, particularly in sports requiring jumping or running.
- **Preventive Strategies:** Emphasis on proper warm-up, stretching, and conditioning to minimize risk.
- **Multidisciplinary Approach:** Collaboration between orthopedists, physical therapists, and sports coaches ensures optimal outcomes.

Associated Conditions

- **Sinding-Larsen-Johansson Syndrome:** A similar condition affecting the lower pole of the patella.
- **Patellar Tendinitis:** Overlap in symptoms with Osgood-Schlatter disease.
- **Growth Plate Injuries:** Other apophyseal injuries in active adolescents.

Clinical Importance

- **Early Recognition:** Detecting the condition early prevents unnecessary pain and functional limitations.
- **Non-Invasive Management:** Highlights the importance of conservative treatments, avoiding unnecessary interventions.
- **Athletic Guidance:** Ensures active adolescents can return to sports safely and without long-term sequelae.
- **Prognostic Value:** Understanding the self-limiting nature reassures patients and families, emphasizing the importance of patience and adherence to treatment plans.

Osgood-Schlatter disease remains a classic condition in pediatric and sports orthopedics, emphasizing the interplay between growth and activity in adolescent health.

References

R. B. Osgood: Lesions of the tibia tubercle occurring during adolescence. Boston Medical and Surgical Journal, 1903, 148: 114-117.

C. Schlatter: Verletzungen des schnabelförmigen Forsatzes der oberen Tibiaepiphyse. [Bruns] Beiträge zur klinischen Chirurgie, 1903, 38: 874-887.

Pellegrini-Stieda disease

Overview

Pellegrini-Stieda disease refers to the ossification at the medial collateral ligament (MCL) of the knee or the insertion of the medial head of the gastrocnemius muscle, typically resulting from trauma. The term Pellegrini-Stieda syndrome is used when this ossification is associated with pain and restricted knee movement. Ossification represents a late-stage finding of past injury, and while asymptomatic cases are benign, symptomatic lesions may require intervention.

Historical Background

- **1903:** Alfred Stieda discovered the ossification on radiographs, attributing its origin to trauma at the insertion of the medial gastrocnemius muscle.
- **1905:** Augusto Pellegrini, in contrast, identified the ossification arising from the medial collateral ligament. His findings were supported by surgical removal of the lesion, which confirmed its MCL location.
- Later studies clarified that true *Pellegrini-Stieda lesions* might involve both structures, but the term is more commonly associated with MCL ossification.

Purpose

- **Diagnosis of Previous Injury:** Identifying Pellegrini-Stieda lesions helps recognize past trauma to the medial knee structures, often due to sports or high-impact activities.
- **Symptom Management:** Differentiating symptomatic Pellegrini-Stieda syndrome from incidental findings aids in guiding appropriate treatment.

Procedure Overview

- **Clinical Evaluation:** History of knee trauma, with or without current symptoms such as pain or restricted motion.
- Physical examination focuses on MCL stability and knee joint range of motion.
- **Imaging:**
- **X-rays:** Identify ossification near the medial femoral condyle.
- **MRI:** Evaluates associated soft tissue injuries, such as MCL disruption or gastrocnemius damage.

Treatment:

- **Conservative Management:** Rest, ice, compression, and elevation (RICE), along with physical therapy and anti-inflammatory medications.
- **Invasive Options:** Persistent symptoms may require local corticosteroid injections or surgical removal of ossified fragments.

Results and Interpretation

- **Radiographic Findings:** Ossification near the medial condyle, often described as elongated or irregular.
- Calcifications are typically dense and localized to the MCL or gastrocnemius insertion.
- **Symptom Resolution:** Asymptomatic lesions require no treatment.

- Symptoms associated with Pellegrini-Stieda syndrome generally improve with conservative therapy, though surgery may be necessary in resistant cases.

Physiological Basis

- **Trauma-Induced Ossification:** Repeated stress or acute trauma to the MCL or gastrocnemius muscle causes inflammation and subsequent calcification.
- **Healing Response:** The ossified lesion represents a late stage in the healing process, often without clinical significance unless symptomatic.

Clinical Applications

- **Diagnosis of Post-Traumatic Changes:** Aids in evaluating the long-term sequelae of knee injuries.
- **Symptom Relief in Pellegrini-Stieda Syndrome:** Directs appropriate interventions for pain and restricted motion.
- **Prevention of Recurrent Injury:** Highlights the need for MCL rehabilitation to ensure stability and prevent future damage.

Limitations and Technical Considerations

- **Asymptomatic Cases:** Many lesions are incidental findings with no clinical relevance.
- **Diagnostic Challenges:** Differentiating Pellegrini-Stieda lesions from other causes of knee pain, such as osteophytes or enthesopathy, requires careful imaging interpretation.
- **Surgical Risks:** Surgical removal carries risks, including potential instability if the MCL is disrupted.

Modern Relevance

- **Sports Medicine:** Frequently encountered in athletes with knee injuries, underscoring the importance of early diagnosis and management.
- **Advances in Imaging:** Modern MRI provides detailed evaluation of soft tissue injuries, enhancing diagnostic accuracy.
- **Conservative Treatment Strategies:** Emphasis on non-invasive interventions aligns with current trends in musculoskeletal injury management.

Associated Conditions

- **MCL Injuries:** Often coexists with acute or chronic MCL tears.
- **Post-Traumatic Ossification:** Commonly seen in other ligamentous or tendinous injuries.
- **Knee Osteoarthritis:** Chronic instability from unresolved injuries can predispose to degenerative changes.

Clinical Importance

- **Recognition of Injury Sequelae:** Identifying Pellegrini-Stieda lesions confirms past trauma and guides future management.
- **Differentiating Asymptomatic vs. Symptomatic Cases:** Distinguishes incidental findings from true Pellegrini-Stieda syndrome requiring intervention.
- **Focus on Knee Stability:** Emphasizes the importance of rehabilitating the MCL to ensure long-term joint stability and function.

- **Prognostic Insights:** Provides information on the potential for persistent symptoms and guides treatment decisions, balancing conservative and surgical options.

Pellegrini-Stieda disease and syndrome highlight the complexity of trauma-induced ossification and underscore the need for tailored approaches in diagnosing and managing post-traumatic knee injuries.

References

Pellegrini A (1905) Ossificazione traumatica del ligamento collaterale tibiale dell'articolazione del ginocchio sinistro. Clin Mod Firenze 11:433–439.

Houston AN, Roy WA, Faust RA, Ewin DM, Espenan PA (1968) Pellegrini–Stieda syndrome: report of 44 cases followed from original injury. South Med J 61:113–117.

Theivendran K, Lever CJ, Hart WJ (2009) Good result after surgical treatment of Pellegrini–Stieda syndrome. Knee Surg Sports Traumatol Arthrosc 17:1231–1233.

A. Pellegrini: Ossificazione traumatica del ligamento collaterale tibiale dell'articolazione del ginocchio sinistro. Clin Moderne Firenze, 1905, 11: 433-439.

A. Stieda: Über eine typische Verletzung am unteren Femurende. Archiv für klinische Chirurgie, Berlin, 1908, 85: 815-826.

A. Köhler: Die normale und pathologische Anatomie des Hüftgelenkes und Oberschenkels in röntgenographische Darstellung. Hamburg, 1905, page 140.

Pennal View

Overview

The Pennal View is a specialized radiographic projection used to assess pelvic injuries, particularly superior or inferior displacement in the anterior or posterior halves of the pelvis. The patient is positioned supine, and the X-ray beam is angled cranially at 40 degrees to capture detailed images. This view is commonly utilized in trauma cases to evaluate pelvic ring disruptions, such as those caused by anterior compression injuries (e.g., "open book" fractures).

Historical Background

- **1961:** Dr. George Pennal, in collaboration with Dr. Gordon Sutherland, a radiologist, described a comprehensive set of X-ray views, including the Pennal view (also called outlet view). These radiographs aimed to define patterns of pelvic ring disruptions, enhancing diagnostic precision in trauma cases.
- **Mid-20th Century:** Their contributions revolutionized pelvic imaging by introducing a systematic approach for identifying complex injury patterns in the pelvis.

Purpose

- **Evaluation of Pelvic Stability:** The Pennal view is critical for assessing vertical and rotational stability in pelvic fractures.
- Helps identify superior or inferior displacements in both anterior and posterior pelvic structures.

- **Trauma Management:** Used in the acute setting to evaluate pelvic ring disruptions caused by high-energy trauma, such as motor vehicle accidents or falls.

Procedure Overview

- **Patient Positioning:**
- The patient is placed in a supine position.
- The central ray is angled 40 degrees cranially and centered midline approximately 4 cm below the upper border of the symphysis pubis.
- **Imaging Technique:** X-rays are taken with precise angulation to ensure clear visualization of the pelvic ring and associated structures.
- **Complementary Views:** Anteroposterior View: For general assessment of pelvic fractures.
- **Inlet View:** Evaluates posterior displacement.
- **Outlet View (Pennal View):** Identifies superior or inferior displacement.

Results and Interpretation

- **Superior Displacement:** Reveals upward movement of the posterior half of the pelvis, often associated with vertical shear fractures.
- **Inferior Displacement:** Indicates downward displacement of the anterior portion of the pelvis, common in anterior compression injuries.
- **Fracture Patterns:** Demonstrates classic "open book" fractures with symphysis pubis separation and sacroiliac joint disruptions.

Physiological Basis

- **Pelvic Stability:**
- The pelvis is a ring structure supported by bony and ligamentous elements.
- Disruption of this ring, such as in vertical shear or anterior compression mechanisms, leads to instability, which is clearly visualized using the Pennal view.
- **Load Distribution:** The X-ray angle provides a tangential view of load-bearing regions, aiding in precise fracture alignment evaluation.

Clinical Applications

- **Trauma Assessment:** Crucial for evaluating pelvic injuries caused by high-energy trauma.
- **Pre-Surgical Planning:** Used to guide surgical intervention, such as reduction and fixation in unstable pelvic fractures.
- **Follow-Up:** Assesses healing progress and alignment following surgical or conservative treatment of pelvic injuries.

Limitations and Technical Considerations

- **Complexity of Positioning:** Requires precise angulation and positioning, which may be challenging in polytrauma patients.
- **Radiation Exposure:** Involves additional radiation compared to routine views, necessitating judicious use.
- **Limited Visualization:** The Pennal view may not adequately capture posterior pelvic injuries; complementary imaging (e.g., CT scan) is often necessary.

Modern Relevance

- **Role in Advanced Imaging:** While CT has become the gold standard for pelvic imaging, the Pennal view remains valuable in initial trauma assessment.
- **Integration in Trauma Protocols:** Commonly included in standardized imaging protocols for pelvic injuries.
- **Guidance for Minimally Invasive Surgery:** Helps determine fracture alignment and stability before minimally invasive procedures.

Associated Conditions

- **Open Book Fractures:** Caused by anterior compression, resulting in symphysis pubis separation and sacroiliac joint disruption.
- **Vertical Shear Injuries:** Upward displacement of the posterior pelvic ring, often associated with severe instability.
- **Combined Mechanism Injuries:** Complex fractures involving multiple planes of displacement.

Clinical Importance

- **Accurate Diagnosis:** Enables early and accurate identification of pelvic ring disruptions, critical for preventing complications such as hemorrhage or instability.
- **Guidance for Treatment:** Differentiates between stable and unstable fractures, directing appropriate surgical or conservative management.
- **Trauma Protocol Integration:** Plays a key role in multidisciplinary trauma care by providing rapid, detailed assessment of pelvic injuries.
- **Prognostic Significance:** Superior and inferior displacements seen on the Pennal view provide insight into the severity of injury and likelihood of long-term complications.

The Pennal View, with its focused visualization of pelvic displacement, remains a cornerstone in the evaluation and management of pelvic trauma, bridging the gap between traditional X-ray imaging and advanced modalities like CT.

References

Musculoskeletal Radiographic Views and Eponyms; 10.1594/essr2013/P-0158.

Piedmont Fracture

Overview

The Piedmont fracture refers to an isolated fracture of the radius at the junction of its middle and distal thirds, without disruption of the distal radioulnar joint (DRUJ). It is a specific type of radial shaft fracture that differs from a Galeazzi fracture, which involves DRUJ instability. This type of fracture is rare and is commonly caused by direct trauma to the dorsoradial aspect of the forearm.

Historical Background

- The *Piedmont fracture* was first described by the Piedmont Orthopedic Society, though their initial definition lacked clarity regarding associated ulnar dislocation.
- *Adam Greenspan* later clarified the distinction, emphasizing the lack of DRUJ disruption in a Piedmont fracture compared to a Galeazzi fracture.
- The term and its differentiation gained prominence in orthopedic literature in the mid-to-late 20th century.

Purpose

- **Primary Objective:** To restore forearm anatomy and function, including pronation and supination, by preventing complications such as malunion or interosseous space compromise.
- **Secondary Objective:** To differentiate Piedmont fractures from other radial fractures, particularly Galeazzi fractures, for appropriate management and surgical planning.

Procedure Overview

Diagnosis:

- **Clinical Examination:** Focus on forearm deformity, pain, swelling, and range of motion.
- **Imaging:** Radiographs (anteroposterior and lateral views) to confirm the fracture and assess alignment.
- **Differentiation:** Ensuring no DRUJ instability through clinical and radiographic evaluation.

Treatment Options:

- **Non-Surgical Management:** Reserved for non-displaced fractures with intact alignment.
- Immobilization in a long-arm cast for 4–6 weeks.
- **Surgical Intervention:** Open Reduction and Internal Fixation (ORIF) is the standard of care for displaced fractures.
- Ensures alignment of the radius and preserves interosseous space, crucial for forearm rotation.
- **Post-Treatment:**
- Rehabilitation through physical therapy to restore strength and motion.
- Monitoring for signs of complications such as malunion or loss of motion.

Results and Interpretation

- **Immediate Outcome:** Proper alignment of the radius is achieved, and interosseous space is preserved.
- **Long-Term Outcome:** Patients regain full pronation and supination, and the risk of chronic pain or functional

limitations is minimized when treated effectively.

Physiological Basis

- The radius plays a critical role in *forearm rotation*, with the interosseous membrane acting as a stabilizer and load distributor.
- A fracture at the middle to distal third disrupts this structural integrity. Improper treatment can compromise the interosseous space, leading to loss of pronation and supination.

Clinical Applications

- **Orthopedic Trauma Management:** Understanding the distinction between Piedmont and Galeazzi fractures is critical for appropriate treatment planning.
- **Surgical Techniques:** ORIF is preferred for displaced fractures to ensure optimal outcomes.

Limitations and Technical Considerations

- **Challenges in Diagnosis:** Differentiating a Piedmont fracture from a Galeazzi fracture requires thorough evaluation of the DRUJ.
- **Missed DRUJ instability may lead to chronic instability and poor outcomes.**
- **Surgical Considerations:** Inadequate fixation can result in malunion, nonunion, or compromised interosseous space.
- Care must be taken to avoid soft tissue injury during ORIF.

Modern Relevance

- Improved imaging and surgical techniques have made the management of Piedmont fractures more effective, minimizing complications.
- Continued education on distinguishing Piedmont fractures from Galeazzi fractures ensures better outcomes in orthopedic trauma settings.

Associated Conditions

- **Galeazzi Fracture:** Includes DRUJ instability, differentiating it from a Piedmont fracture.
- **Interosseous Membrane Injuries:** Though rare in Piedmont fractures, they may occur with severe trauma.
- **Forearm Compartment Syndrome:** A potential complication if the trauma causes severe soft tissue injury.

Clinical Importance

- **Early Diagnosis and Treatment:** Prompt recognition and differentiation from other radial fractures are essential for effective management.
- **ORIF ensures anatomical alignment and functional recovery in displaced fractures.**
- **Rehabilitation:** Physical therapy post-treatment is critical for regaining full range of motion and strength.
- **Prognosis:** Favorable outcomes are common when fractures are managed appropriately.
- Delay in treatment or misdiagnosis can lead to chronic pain, stiffness, and reduced forearm function.

The Piedmont fracture, though rare, highlights the importance of accurate diagnosis, differentiation, and surgical expertise in managing forearm injuries to optimize patient outcomes.

References

Greenspan A. Orthopedic Imaging. LWW. ISBN:1608312879.

HUGHSTON JC. Fracture of the distal radial shaft; mistakes in management. J Bone Joint Surg Am. 2002;39-A (2): 249-64.

Pilon Fracture

Overview

A pilon fracture refers to a fracture of the distal tibial plafond caused by high-energy axial compression forces, often involving the articular surface of the ankle joint. These fractures are frequently associated with severe bone comminution, metaphyseal extension, and significant soft tissue compromise. They account for 1% to 10% of tibial fractures and require meticulous assessment and management to achieve optimal outcomes.

Historical Background

- The term *"pilon,"* derived from the French word for "pestle," was first used by *Etienne Destot* in *1911* to describe the mechanical function of the distal tibia as it impacts the talus during high-energy axial loading.
- Early descriptions and classifications of pilon fractures were primarily based on surgical observations and outcomes, notably the *Ruedi-Allgower classification* introduced in the mid-20th century.

Purpose

- **The primary goals of managing pilon fractures are:** Restoring the congruence of the ankle joint to enable functional mobility.
- Preventing long-term complications such as post-traumatic arthritis and deformity.
- Minimizing soft tissue damage and maintaining vascular integrity to ensure proper healing.

Procedure Overview

Diagnosis:

- **Clinical Examination:** Assess neurovascular status, checking pulses and sensory function in the affected limb.
- Evaluate for compartment syndrome, a common complication in these fractures.
- **Imaging:** Radiographs in anteroposterior, lateral, and oblique views to assess fracture pattern.
- CT scans to evaluate articular involvement and guide surgical planning.
- **Classification:**
- **Ruedi-Allgower Classification:** Type I: Nondisplaced fractures.
- **Type II:** Displaced fractures without comminution.
- **Type III:** Comminuted fractures with metaphyseal impaction.
- **AO/OTA Classification:** 43A: Extra-articular fractures.
- **43B:** Partial articular fractures.
- **43C:** Intra-articular fractures.
- **Soft Tissue Damage:** Classified using Gustilo-Anderson (open fractures) or Tscherne (closed fractures) systems.

Treatment:

- **Non-Surgical:** Reserved for stable, nondisplaced fractures.
- **Immobilization with a cast or splint, followed by progressive weight-bearing as tolerated.**
- **Surgical:** Most cases require open reduction and internal fixation (ORIF).
- **Staged approaches are often used:**
- **Initial stage:** External fixation to stabilize the fracture and manage soft tissue swelling.
- **Definitive surgery:** ORIF to restore joint alignment and fix the fracture.
- Bone grafting may be required for metaphyseal voids.
- **Rehabilitation:**
- Physical therapy to restore range of motion and strength postoperatively.
- Weight-bearing is gradually reintroduced, typically 6–8 weeks after surgery, depending on fracture stability.

Results and Interpretation

- **Short-Term Outcomes:** Successful surgical reduction leads to restored joint congruence and alignment, enabling early mobilization.
- **Long-Term Outcomes:** Prognosis varies with the severity of the fracture and quality of reduction.
- Post-traumatic arthritis is a frequent complication, especially in cases with poor articular alignment or comminution.

Physiological Basis

- The distal tibial plafond serves as a key load-bearing surface in the ankle joint.
- Pilon fractures disrupt the normal articulation between the tibia and talus, leading to joint instability and altered biomechanics.
- High-energy trauma often compromises the soft tissue envelope, which is critical for vascular supply and healing.

Clinical Applications

- Pilon fractures represent a *critical challenge in orthopedic trauma management*, requiring a multidisciplinary approach involving surgeons, radiologists, and physical therapists.
- **Advances in** imaging and surgical techniques have improved outcomes for these complex injuries.

Limitations and Technical Considerations

- **Challenges in Management:** Severe comminution and soft tissue damage complicate surgical fixation.
- **Staged surgical approaches are often necessary to address swelling and prevent infection.**
- **Surgical Risks:** Infections, wound dehiscence, and implant failure are common complications.
- Postoperative stiffness and malunion can impact long-term functional outcomes.

Modern Relevance

- Improved imaging (CT scans) and surgical techniques, including minimally invasive fixation, have enhanced the precision of pilon fracture management.
- Research continues to refine treatment protocols and reduce complications, particularly post-traumatic arthritis.

Associated Conditions

- **Fibular Fractures:** Often accompany pilon fractures, requiring concurrent management for optimal stability.
- **Compartment Syndrome:** Common in high-energy trauma, necessitating urgent fasciotomy.
- **Soft Tissue Injuries:** Including degloving or vascular damage, significantly impacting treatment and prognosis.

Clinical Importance

- **Early Diagnosis:** Prompt imaging and assessment are critical to prevent delayed treatment and complications.
- **Surgical Expertise:** ORIF is technically demanding, requiring meticulous attention to soft tissue handling and joint alignment.
- **Patient Counseling:** Patients should be informed about the prolonged recovery period and potential for long-term complications.
- **Rehabilitation:** Aggressive physical therapy is essential to regain mobility and prevent joint stiffness.

The pilon fracture exemplifies the complexity of high-energy orthopedic trauma. Multidisciplinary care and advancements in surgical techniques continue to improve outcomes for these challenging injuries.

References

Michelson J, Moskovitz P, Labropoulos P. The nomenclature for intra-articular vertical impact fractures of the tibial plafond: pilon versus pylon. Foot Ankle Int. 2004 Mar;25(3):149-50. [PubMed]

Jacob N, Amin A, Giotakis N, Narayan D, Nayagam S, Trompeter AJ. Management of high-energy tibial pilon fractures. Strategies Trauma Limb Reconstr. 2015 Nov;10(3):137-47. [PMC free article] [PubMed]

Rüedi T. Fractures of the lower end of the tibia into the ankle joint: results 9 years after open reduction and internal fixation. Injury. 1973 Nov;5(2):130-4. [PubMed]

Rüedi TP, Allgöwer M. The operative treatment of intra-articular fractures of the lower end of the tibia. Clin Orthop Relat Res. 1979 Jan-Feb;(138):105-10. [PubMed]

Mauffrey C, Vasario G, Battiston B, Lewis C, Beazley J, Seligson D. Tibial pilon fractures: a review of incidence, diagnosis, treatment, and complications. Acta Orthop Belg. 2011 Aug;77(4):432-40. [PubMed]

Cole PA, Mehrle RK, Bhandari M, Zlowodzki M. The pilon map: fracture lines and comminution zones in OTA/AO type 43C3 pilon fractures. J Orthop Trauma. 2013 Jul;27(7):e152-6. [PubMed]

Ballal A, Rai HR, Shetty SM, Mathias LJ, Shetty V, Shetty A. A Prospective Study on Functional Outcome of Internal Fixation of Tibial Pilon Fractures with Locking Plate using Minimally Invasive Plate Osteosynthesis Technique. J Clin Diagn Res. 2016 Jan;10(1):RC01-4. [PMC free article] [PubMed]

Wyrsch B, McFerran MA, McAndrew M, Limbird TJ, Harper MC, Johnson KD, Schwartz HS. Operative treatment of fractures of the tibial plafond. A randomized, prospective study. J Bone Joint Surg Am. 1996 Nov;78(11):1646-57. [PubMed]

Anglen JO. Early outcome of hybrid external fixation for fracture of the distal tibia. J Orthop Trauma. 1999 Feb;13(2):92-7. [PubMed]

Chen SH, Wu PH, Lee YS. Long-term results of pilon fractures. Arch Orthop Trauma Surg. 2007 Jan;127(1):55-60. [PubMed]

Korkmaz A, Ciftdemir M, Ozcan M, Copuroğlu C, Sarıdoğan K. The analysis of the variables, affecting outcome in surgically treated tibia pilon fractured patients. Injury. 2013 Oct;44(10):1270-4. [PubMed]

Teeny SM, Wiss DA. Open reduction and internal fixation of tibial plafond fractures. Variables contributing to poor results and complications. Clin Orthop Relat Res. 1993 Jul;(292):108-17. [PubMed]

Topliss CJ, Jackson M, Atkins RM. Anatomy of pilon fractures of the distal tibia. J Bone Joint Surg Br. 2005 May;87(5):692-7. [PubMed]

Schulz AP, Fuchs S, Simon L, Seide K, Paech A, Queitsch C. Severe Fracture of the Tibial Pilon: Results with a Multidirectional Self-locking Osteosynthesis Plate Utilizing a Two-stage Procedure. Eur J Trauma Emerg Surg. 2008 Aug;34(4):391-6.

Pipkin classification of femoral head Fracture

Overview

The *Pipkin classification of femoral head fractures* is a system used to categorize fractures of the femoral head, usually occurring in association with hip dislocations. These injuries are often the result of high-impact trauma, such as motor vehicle accidents. The classification aids in determining the severity of the injury, the involvement of weight-bearing surfaces, and associated fractures, such as those of the femoral neck or acetabulum. Prompt management is critical to prevent complications like osteonecrosis and post-traumatic arthritis.

Historical Background

- **1957:** Dr. Garrett Pipkin introduced the classification system to differentiate femoral head fractures based on their location and associated injuries.- Pipkin's work highlighted the clinical importance of accurately identifying these fractures to guide treatment and reduce complications.

- The classification remains widely used in orthopedics, serving as a foundation for understanding and managing hip dislocations with associated femoral head fractures.

Purpose

- **Guidance for Treatment:** Provides a structured approach to determine the severity of the fracture and associated injuries, guiding surgical or conservative treatment.

- **Risk Stratification:** Identifies fractures with a higher risk of complications, such as avascular necrosis and post-traumatic arthritis.

- **Surgical Decision-Making:**Assists surgeons in selecting appropriate fixation techniques and managing associated injuries.

Procedure Overview

- **Imaging Evaluation:**
- **Radiographs:** Anteroposterior (AP) and lateral views of the hip are standard.
- **CT scans:** Provide detailed visualization of the fracture and associated dislocations or acetabular involvement.
- **Classification:**
- **Type I:** Femoral head fracture distal (inferior) to the fovea.
- **Type II:** Femoral head fracture proximal (superior) to the fovea, involving the weight-bearing surface.
- **Type III:** Type I or II fracture combined with a femoral neck fracture.
- **Type IV:** Type I or II fracture combined with an acetabular fracture, commonly of the posterior wall.
- **Reduction and Stabilization:**
- Emergency reduction of hip dislocation is crucial to restore vascular supply to the femoral head.
- Definitive management involves surgical fixation, total hip arthroplasty (THA), or conservative care based on the classification and patient factors.

Results and Interpretation

- **Type I Fractures:** Small fractures not involving the weight-bearing surface, generally associated with a favorable prognosis.
- **Type II Fractures:** Larger fractures involving the weight-bearing surface, increasing the risk of post-traumatic arthritis.
- **Type III Fractures:** High risk of avascular necrosis due to the femoral neck involvement disrupting blood supply.
- **Type IV Fractures:** Complex injuries with acetabular involvement, often necessitating extensive surgical intervention.

Physiological Basis

- **Blood Supply Disruption:** The femoral head is primarily supplied by the medial femoral circumflex artery. Fractures and dislocations can compromise this supply, leading to avascular necrosis.
- **Weight-Bearing Considerations:** Fractures involving the weight-bearing surface (Type II) are more likely to result in mechanical complications, such as cartilage loss and joint instability.

Clinical Applications

- **Emergency Management:** Immediate reduction of hip dislocations to minimize ischemic injury to the femoral head.
- **Pre-Surgical Planning:** Classification informs the selection of surgical approaches, such as internal fixation or hip replacement.
- **Rehabilitation Guidance:** Post-surgical rehabilitation protocols can be tailored based on the Pipkin classification.

Limitations and Technical Considerations

- **Overlapping Features:** Differentiation between Types I and II fractures may be challenging on imaging without detailed CT scans.
- **Complexity in Type IV:** The presence of acetabular fractures complicates treatment, requiring advanced surgical expertise.
- **Long-Term Complications:** Even with optimal treatment, there is a high risk of avascular necrosis, particularly in Type III fractures.

Modern Relevance

- **Role in Trauma Care:** Pipkin classification remains integral in trauma protocols for assessing hip dislocations and associated fractures.
- **Imaging Advances:** Modern imaging techniques, such as 3D CT reconstructions, have improved the precision of classification and surgical planning.
- **Guidance for Minimally Invasive Surgery:** Enables orthopedic surgeons to adopt less invasive approaches when managing Type I or II fractures.

Associated Conditions

- **Hip Dislocations:** Nearly all Pipkin fractures are associated with traumatic hip dislocations, requiring immediate attention.
- **Avascular Necrosis:** Common in Type III fractures due to disrupted blood supply to the femoral head.
- **Post-Traumatic Arthritis:** Risk increases in fractures involving the weight-bearing surface (Type II) or acetabular fractures (Type IV).

Clinical Importance

- **Emergency Response:** Early identification and reduction of hip dislocations are critical to preventing ischemic damage to the femoral head.
- **Prognostic Value:** The classification system predicts outcomes and guides discussions with patients about long-term risks.
- **Surgical Planning:** Facilitates decision-making for orthopedic surgeons, particularly in complex cases with multiple fracture components.
- **Rehabilitation Focus:** Ensures tailored rehabilitation programs to restore mobility and reduce the risk of complications.

The Pipkin classification remains a cornerstone in the evaluation and management of femoral head fractures, ensuring comprehensive care from diagnosis through rehabilitation.

References

Pipkin G. Treatment of grade IV fracture-dislocation of the hip. J Bone Joint Surg Am. 1957 Oct;39-A(5):1027-42 [PMID 13475403]

Brumback RJ, Kenzora JE, Levitt LE, Burgess AR, Poka A. Fractures of the femoral head. Hip. 1987:181-206. [PMID 3546215]

Pott's Fracture

Overview

Pott's fracture refers to a common ankle fracture involving one or both bones of the leg just above the ankle. It typically includes a fracture of the distal fibula and medial malleolus of the tibia, often accompanied by rupture of the internal lateral ligament of the ankle. The injury occurs due to outward and backward displacement of the leg while the foot is fixed. The fracture is historically significant, as it was first described in detail by Sir John Percivall Pott after experiencing the injury himself.

Historical Background

- **1756:** Sir John Percivall Pott sustained a compound fracture of the ankle, which was managed by Mr. Nourse in London.
- **1768:** Pott published his seminal work, *Some Few General Remarks on Fractures and Dislocations*, offering the first detailed description and classification of ankle fractures.
- **1769:** Pott's comprehensive classification included unimalleolar, bimalleolar, and trimalleolar fractures, emphasizing the fibula's critical role in ankle stability.
- Pott also highlighted the importance of proper limb positioning and management to prevent long-term complications like lameness or deformity.

Purpose

- **Classification and Diagnosis:** Provide a systematic approach to classifying ankle fractures, ensuring appropriate treatment and prognosis.
- **Emphasis on Fibula:** Demonstrate the fibula's structural and functional significance in maintaining ankle stability despite its slender anatomy.
- **Guide Treatment:** Advocate for precise limb positioning to promote proper healing and minimize complications.

Procedure Overview

- **Initial Assessment:** Detailed physical examination and history to assess displacement, ligament rupture, and potential deformity.
- **Imaging Studies:** X-rays to identify fractures and assess the involvement of malleoli. AP, lateral, and mortise views are standard.
- **Reduction:** Closed or open reduction to restore alignment, especially in cases involving dislocation or ligament damage.
- **Stabilization:** Methods may include casting, internal fixation with plates and screws, or external fixation in severe cases.

Results and Interpretation

- **Unimalleolar Fractures:** Involve a single malleolus, typically stable unless ligamentous injury is significant.
- **Bimalleolar Fractures:** Involve both the lateral malleolus (fibula) and medial malleolus (tibia), often resulting in ankle instability.
- **Trimalleolar Fractures:** Include the posterior malleolus, frequently associated with posterior displacement of the talus.

- **Ligamentous Involvement:** Rupture of the internal lateral ligament often accompanies the fracture, complicating treatment.

Physiological Basis

- **Structural Importance of Fibula:** Provides critical lateral support to the ankle joint. Its fracture compromises stability and predisposes to dislocation.
- **Ligamentous Integrity:** The medial collateral ligament and other structures maintain joint stability. Their rupture can lead to significant displacement and instability.
- **Healing Considerations:** Proper alignment is necessary to prevent malunion, which can result in chronic pain and deformity.

Clinical Applications

- **Immediate Management:** Early reduction and stabilization are critical to restore alignment and prevent long-term complications.
- **Surgical Techniques:** Internal fixation is often required for bimalleolar and trimalleolar fractures or cases with severe displacement.
- **Rehabilitation:** Focuses on restoring range of motion, strengthening, and preventing stiffness after immobilization or surgery.

Limitations and Technical Considerations

- **Complexity in Trimalleolar Fractures:** Involvement of the posterior malleolus complicates reduction and stabilization.
- **Risk of Chronic Complications:** Malunion, arthritis, and persistent instability can occur if reduction is incomplete.
- **Dependence on Proper Positioning:** Accurate positioning during treatment is critical to ensure alignment and healing.

Modern Relevance

- **Standardized Classification:** Pott's fracture serves as a foundational concept for understanding ankle fractures and their management.
- **Advances in Imaging:** CT and MRI provide detailed insights into fracture patterns and associated ligamentous injuries.
- **Minimally Invasive Techniques:** Modern surgical approaches focus on reducing tissue trauma while achieving stable fixation.

Associated Conditions

- **Open Book Injuries:** Severe ankle dislocations associated with ligamentous rupture.
- **Chronic Pain and Arthritis:** Long-term sequelae of improper alignment or healing.
- **Post-Traumatic Deformities:** Result from malunion or incomplete reduction.

Clinical Importance

- **Early Diagnosis:** Prompt identification of fracture patterns and ligamentous involvement is essential for effective treatment.
- **Restoration of Stability:** Accurate reduction and stabilization prevent chronic instability and deformity.

- **Historical Influence:** Pott's contributions laid the groundwork for the modern understanding and classification of ankle fractures.
- **Guidance for Rehabilitation:** Early mobilization and strengthening reduce the risk of stiffness and promote functional recovery.

The Pott's fracture remains a cornerstone in orthopedic education, offering insights into the mechanics, diagnosis, and management of ankle fractures. Its historical significance underscores the evolution of fracture care, from rudimentary treatments to modern surgical techniques.

References

Dobson J. Percivall Pott. Ann R Coll Surg Engl 1972; 50: 54–65.

BROWN JR, THORNTON JL. Percivall Pott (1714-1788) and chimney sweepers' cancer of the scrotum. Br J Ind Med 1957; 14: 68–70.

Peltier LF. Percivall Pott and Pott's fracture. Surgery 1962; 51: 280–6.

P. Pott: Some Few General Remarks on Fractures and Dislocations. London, Howes, 1769.

G. Dupuytren: Mémoire sur la fracture de l'extremité inferieure du peroné, les luxations et les accidents qui en sont la suite. Ann med.-chir Hôp Paris, 1819; 1: 2-212.

Of special interest in this treatise is his **Description** of experimental fractures produced in cadavers to elucidate the mechanism of injury.

Recklinghausen's disease

Overview

Recklinghausen's disease, also known as neurofibromatosis type 1 (NF1), is an inheritable disorder marked by café au lait spots (skin pigmentation) and multiple peripheral nerve tumors, including schwannomas and neurofibromas. It is also associated with dysplastic abnormalities affecting various organ systems, including the nervous system, skin, bones, endocrine organs, and blood vessels. Onset typically occurs in childhood and may intensify at life stages involving hormonal changes such as puberty, pregnancy, or menopause. The disease can present as asymptomatic or with pain from tumors pressing on adjacent structures. It affects 1 in 3,000 births.

Historical Background

- **1768:** The condition was first described by Mark Akenside.- 1793: Wilhelm Gottlieb Tilesius von Tilenau offered additional insights.
- **1849:** Robert William Smith of the University of Dublin provided detailed observations.
- **1863:** Rudolf Virchow documented further cases, particularly emphasizing the pathological features.
- **1882:** Friedrich Daniel von Recklinghausen conducted a thorough investigation of the disease. His findings, based on autopsies, linked the condition to nerve tissue and gave it its eponym.
- Recklinghausen's detailed account

included observations of peripheral nerve tumors, pigmentation abnormalities, and the systemic effects of the disorder.

Purpose

- **Diagnosis and Classification:** To provide a framework for identifying, diagnosing, and categorizing the clinical manifestations of NF1.
- **Understanding Tumor Biology:** To highlight the mechanisms underlying peripheral nerve tumors and their malignant potential.
- **Genetic Inheritance:** To clarify its autosomal dominant inheritance pattern and sporadic mutation cases.

Procedure Overview

- **Clinical Evaluation:** Observation of café au lait spots, axillary freckles, and peripheral nerve tumors.
- **Imaging Studies:** MRI and CT scans to detect tumors along cranial, spinal, or peripheral nerve roots.
- **Genetic Testing:** Identification of mutations in the NF1 gene for definitive diagnosis.
- **Ophthalmologic Examination:** Assessment for optic gliomas, glaucoma, or other ocular complications.
- **Histopathological Analysis:** Evaluation of excised tumors to distinguish between benign and malignant types.

Results and Interpretation

- **Skin Lesions:** Characterized by café au lait spots, which are diagnostic when six or more spots larger than 5 mm are observed in children (or >15 mm in adults).
- **Peripheral Nerve Tumors:** Schwannomas and neurofibromas vary in size, number, and location, and may cause localized pain or neurological deficits.
- **Skeletal Abnormalities:** Include scoliosis, bone dysplasia, and thinning of the cortex, which may lead to fractures or deformities.
- **Neurological Manifestations:** Include seizures, hydrocephalus, or mental retardation, depending on the extent of central nervous system involvement.

Physiological Basis

- **Tumor Pathophysiology:** Schwannomas and neurofibromas arise from Schwann cells or fibroblasts along nerves.
- **Genetic Mutation:** Caused by mutations in the NF1 gene on chromosome 17, which codes for neurofibromin, a tumor suppressor protein.
- **Systemic Effects:** Dysregulation of cell growth and differentiation leads to tumor formation and organ dysfunction.

Clinical Applications

- **Diagnosis and Monitoring:** Clinical evaluation and imaging are essential for early detection and follow-up of tumors.
- **Surgical Interventions:** Indicated for

symptomatic neurofibromas, particularly those causing pain or compressing vital structures.

- **Multidisciplinary Management:** Involves neurologists, geneticists, dermatologists, and orthopedic surgeons to address systemic manifestations.

Limitations and Technical Considerations

- **Variability in Presentation:** The disease exhibits wide phenotypic variability, complicating diagnosis and prognosis.
- **Malignancy Risk:** Neurofibromas can undergo malignant transformation, necessitating regular monitoring.
- **Incomplete Penetrance:** Not all cases exhibit the full spectrum of symptoms, posing challenges in early detection.

Modern Relevance

- **Genetic Research:** Advances in understanding the NF1 gene have facilitated targeted therapies for tumor management.
- **Precision Medicine:** Emerging treatments, such as MEK inhibitors, show promise in reducing tumor growth.
- **Awareness and Advocacy:** Greater awareness of the disease has led to earlier diagnosis and improved outcomes for affected individuals.

Associated Conditions

- **Optic Gliomas:** Common in children with NF1 and may cause visual impairment.
- **Scoliosis:** A frequent skeletal complication requiring orthopedic intervention.
- **Malignant Peripheral Nerve Sheath Tumors (MPNSTs):** A severe complication with poor prognosis if untreated.

Clinical Importance

- **Early Diagnosis:** Enables timely intervention, reducing complications and improving quality of life.
- **Genetic Counseling:** Essential for families with a history of NF1, as there is a 50% chance of inheritance.
- **Prognostic Value:** Regular monitoring can identify complications such as malignancy or progressive neurological deficits.
- **Comprehensive Care:** Requires a coordinated approach involving multiple specialties for optimal patient outcomes.

Recklinghausen's disease remains a cornerstone in the study of genetic disorders, illustrating the interplay between genetics, tumor biology, and systemic manifestations. Its historical and modern relevance highlights the evolution of understanding and managing complex hereditary conditions.

References

M. Akenside: Observations on cancers. Medical Transactions. Royal College of Physicians of London, 1768, 1: 64-92.

W. G. Tilesius von Tilenau: Historia pathologica singularis entis turpitudinus. Jo Godofredi Rheinhardi viri 50 Annorum. SL Crusins, Leipzig, 1793.

Robert W. Smith: Pathology, Diagnosis and Treatment of Neuroma. 1849.

R. Virchow: Die krankhaften Geschwülste. 3 volumes, Berlin, 1863-1867.

(On Multiple Fibromas in the Skin and their Relationship to Multiple Neuromas.)

Title page, translated from German: Festschrift in commemoration of the 25th anniversary of the founding of the Pathological

Institute of Berlin, presented to Professor Rudolf Virchow by F. von Recklinghausen, professor in Strasbourg". Berlin, A. Hirschwald, 1882.

Ribbing's Syndrome or disease

Overview

Ribbing's syndrome, or Ribbing's disease, is a hereditary condition characterized by progressive multiple diaphyseal sclerosis, a rare disorder involving osteosclerosis and hyperostosis predominantly affecting the shafts of long bones, such as the tibia and femur. It typically manifests as increased bone density that is symmetrical and confined to the diaphysis. The condition usually appears after puberty and has an autosomal dominant inheritance pattern.

Historical Background

- **1949:** Seved Ribbing, a Swedish physician, first described the syndrome. His work highlighted the familial nature of the disease, emphasizing the symmetrical involvement of long bones and its autosomal dominant inheritance.

- Ribbing's detailed observations established this as a distinct entity, differentiating it from other sclerosing bone disorders.

Purpose

- **Clarifying Pathophysiology:** To distinguish Ribbing's syndrome from other forms of osteosclerosis and diaphyseal conditions.

- **Improving Diagnosis:** Establishing radiological and clinical criteria for early and accurate identification of the condition.

- **Defining Management Approaches:** Developing treatment plans to alleviate symptoms and prevent complications.

Procedure Overview

- **Clinical Examination:** Assessment for symmetrical bone pain or tenderness, particularly in the lower limbs.
- **Radiological Imaging:** X-rays and CT scans reveal symmetrical osteosclerosis and hyperostosis localized to the diaphysis of long bones.
- **Histopathological Analysis:** Bone biopsy confirms increased bone density and cortical thickening without evidence of malignancy.
- **Genetic Testing:** Identification of autosomal dominant inheritance patterns through family history or genetic analysis.

Results and Interpretation

- **Radiological Findings:** Increased cortical thickness and dense bone lesions along the diaphysis of long bones, typically sparing the metaphysis and epiphysis.
- **Clinical Symptoms:** Onset of bone pain, limited joint movement, and occasional fractures. Symptoms are symmetrical and progressively worsen.
- **Histological Results:** Marked sclerosis and thickening of the bone, with no signs of inflammation or malignancy.

Physiological Basis

- **Bone Remodeling Dysregulation:** Imbalance between osteoblastic (bone-forming) and osteoclastic (bone-resorbing) activity leads to excessive bone deposition and sclerosis.
- **Genetic Influence:** The autosomal dominant inheritance suggests a mutation affecting bone metabolism pathways, though the exact gene remains unknown.

Clinical Applications

- **Diagnostic Tool:** Radiological imaging is the primary tool for diagnosing and monitoring disease progression.
- **Pain Management:** Use of nonsteroidal anti-inflammatory drugs (NSAIDs) and physical therapy to alleviate discomfort and maintain mobility.
- **Surgical Interventions:** In cases of significant deformity or functional impairment, corrective surgery may be indicated.

Limitations and Technical Considerations

- **Delayed Diagnosis:** Onset after puberty and nonspecific symptoms can delay recognition of the condition.
- **Overlap with Other Disorders:** Ribbing's syndrome can be confused with other osteosclerotic conditions, necessitating thorough differential diagnosis.
- **Genetic Variability:** Variability in the degree of expression complicates clinical and genetic assessment.

Modern Relevance

- **Advances in Imaging:** Modern imaging modalities like MRI and CT offer detailed evaluation of bone abnormalities, aiding early diagnosis.
- **Genetic Research:** Ongoing research aims to identify the genetic mutations responsible, which could lead to targeted therapies.

- **Awareness:** Increased understanding among clinicians ensures more timely and accurate diagnoses.

Associated Conditions

- **Osteopetrosis:** Shares features of increased bone density but differs in etiology and systemic manifestations.
- **Paget's Disease of Bone:** Characterized by abnormal bone remodeling, but typically involves multiple bone regions and older populations.
- **Melorheostosis:** Localized "dripping candle wax" appearance on imaging, differing from the symmetrical pattern of Ribbing's disease.

Clinical Importance

- **Early Diagnosis:** Radiological findings in early stages can prevent misdiagnosis and guide appropriate management.
- **Symptom Management:** Early intervention with NSAIDs or physical therapy improves patient quality of life by addressing pain and mobility issues.
- **Family Screening:** Identification of autosomal dominant inheritance underscores the importance of genetic counseling and screening of family members.
- **Research Value:** Ribbing's syndrome serves as a model for studying hereditary osteosclerotic disorders, enhancing understanding of bone metabolism.

Ribbing's syndrome remains a rare but clinically significant disorder, illustrating the interplay of genetics, bone physiology, and progressive skeletal abnormalities. Its recognition and management continue to benefit from **Advances in** *imaging and genetic research.*

References

S. Ribbing: Hereditary multiple diaphyseal sclerosis. Acta Radiologica, Stockholm, 1949; 31: 522-536.

Rookwood View

Overview

The Rockwood view is a specialized radiographic technique primarily used for assessing shoulder structures, specifically the anterior inferior acromion in cases of impingement syndrome. It involves an anteroposterior (AP) view with adjustments to accommodate the glenoid cavity's anatomy and beam angulation, providing a detailed visualization of relevant bony structures.

Historical Background

- **1970s:** Dr. Rockwood, a prominent figure in orthopedic radiology, developed this specialized view to enhance the evaluation of the acromion and its relationship to the supraspinatus tendon in impingement syndromes. This technique has since become a critical diagnostic tool in shoulder imaging.

Purpose

- **Assessment of Acromial Anatomy:** To evaluate the spur formation and morphology of the anterior inferior acromion, which can contribute to impingement syndromes.
- **Diagnosis of Impingement Syndrome:** Identifies mechanical impingement of the supraspinatus tendon caused by anatomical changes or bony overgrowths.
- **Pre-Surgical Planning:** Provides critical information for surgical interventions, such as acromioplasty.

Procedure Overview

- **Patient Positioning:** The patient is positioned in an anteroposterior view without correcting the anteversion of the glenoid cavity.
- **Beam Angulation:** The radiographic beam is angled 30 degrees caudally to optimize visualization of the anterior inferior acromion.
- **Radiographic Technique:** Low-penetration settings are used to ensure fine detail in the radiographic image, particularly of the bony structures.
- **Imaging Focus:** The view centers on the acromion, specifically to evaluate spur formation or other abnormalities.

Results and Interpretation

- **Normal Findings:** Smooth contour of the anterior inferior acromion without spur formation or narrowing of the subacromial space.
- **Abnormal Findings:** Presence of a bony spur or irregularity in the anterior inferior acromion.
- Narrowing of the subacromial space, suggesting mechanical impingement.
- **Implications for Impingement Syndrome:** Shortened acromion or prominent spur correlates with increased likelihood of supraspinatus tendon impingement.

Physiological Basis

- **Shoulder Impingement Mechanism:** In impingement syndrome, the supraspinatus tendon is compressed by the anterior acromion during abduction or forward flexion, leading to pain and inflammation.

- **Role of Acromion Anatomy:** Variations in acromial morphology, such as spur formation, exacerbate the impingement by reducing the subacromial space.

Clinical Applications

- **Diagnosis of Shoulder Disorders:** Useful in identifying anatomical factors contributing to rotator cuff impingement.
- **Guiding Surgical Decisions:** Provides preoperative insights for procedures like subacromial decompression or acromioplasty.
- **Monitoring Post-Surgical Outcomes:** Can be used postoperatively to assess the acromion and subacromial space.

Limitations and Technical Considerations

- **Limited Soft Tissue Visualization:** Primarily assesses bony structures; additional imaging modalities like MRI are required for evaluating soft tissues.
- **Patient Positioning Challenges:** Requires precise positioning for accurate results, which may be difficult in patients with severe pain or restricted mobility.
- **Radiographic Variability:** Image quality and interpretation can vary depending on technique and equipment.

Modern Relevance

- **Improved Imaging Technology:** Advances in digital radiography have enhanced the resolution and accuracy of the Rockwood view.
- **Integration with MRI and CT:** Often used in conjunction with advanced imaging modalities for comprehensive shoulder evaluation.
- **Broader Diagnostic Applications:** Continues to be a valuable tool for diagnosing impingement syndrome and related shoulder conditions.

Associated Conditions

- **Rotator Cuff Tendinopathy:** Often accompanies impingement syndromes, with degenerative changes visible on imaging.
- **Subacromial Bursitis:** Inflammation of the subacromial bursa commonly coexists with acromial spurs.
- **Acromioclavicular Joint Arthritis:** May contribute to altered acromion morphology and impingement.

Clinical Importance

- **Early Diagnosis:** Detecting acromial abnormalities early prevents progression of impingement syndrome to rotator cuff tears.
- **Preoperative Planning:** Assists surgeons in tailoring interventions like acromioplasty to individual patient anatomy.
- **Improved Patient Outcomes:** Accurate imaging guides effective treatment, reducing pain and improving shoulder function.
- **Educational Value:** Remains a standard imaging technique for training radiologists and orthopedic specialists in shoulder pathology assessment.

The Rockwood view is an essential diagnostic tool in orthopedic radiology, facilitating the evaluation and management of shoulder impingement and related conditions through detailed visualization of acromial anatomy.

References

Pavlov H, Warren RF, Weiss CB Jr, et al. The roentgenographic evaluation of anterior shoulder instability. Clin Orthop Relat Res. 1985; (194):153-8.

K.L. Bontrager, JP Lanpiglano. Tratado de posicionamento radiográfico e anatomia associada, 6th edition, Mosby, Elsevier, 2011: 195.

Rolando Fracture

Overview

The Rolando fracture is a comminuted, T- or Y-shaped intra-articular fracture of the base of the first metacarpal, involving three or more segments. This fracture is unstable and typically requires surgical intervention, as conservative management often leads to poor outcomes. It is considered a more severe variant of the Bennett fracture, distinguished by its comminuted nature and multi-fragmented configuration.

Historical Background

- **1910:** The fracture was first described by Silvio Rolando, who noted its distinct pattern in three of ten cases involving the base of the first metacarpal. Rolando's original publication, titled *Fracture de la base du premier metacarpien*, emphasized the need for specialized treatment distinct from the simpler Bennett fracture.
- *Edward Hallaran Bennett* (1837–1907) previously described the related *Bennett fracture*, but Rolando identified and characterized a more complex, comminuted variant.

Purpose

- **Detailed Classification:** To differentiate the Rolando fracture from the simpler Bennett fracture based on its comminuted, multi-fragmented nature.
- **Guidance for Management:** Provides a framework for surgical intervention and fixation techniques tailored to its instability.

Procedure Overview

- **Clinical Examination:**
- The fracture often follows trauma directed along the longitudinal axis of the thumb, typically resulting from high-energy impacts like falls or motor vehicle accidents.
- Patients present with localized pain, swelling, and deformity at the base of the thumb.
- **Imaging:**
- **Radiographs:** Anteroposterior, lateral, and oblique views confirm the comminuted fracture pattern.
- **CT scans:** May be used for detailed visualization of fragment alignment and intra-articular extension.
- **Management:** Initial Stabilization: Immobilization with a thumb spica splint for temporary support.
- **Definitive Treatment:** Surgical intervention, often involving external fixation, percutaneous pinning, or internal fixation using tension band wiring.

Results and Interpretation

- **Radiographic Findings:** A Y- or T-shaped fracture at the base of the first metacarpal with comminution.
- Displacement and instability of fragments may be evident.
- **Surgical Outcomes:** Proper alignment and fixation result in improved stability and preservation of thumb function.
- Delayed treatment or inadequate reduction may lead to arthritis or reduced grip strength.

Physiological Basis

- **Mechanism of Injury:** Typically caused by an axial load applied to the first metacarpal during a high-energy trauma, compressing the bone and causing comminution.
- The thumb's pivotal role in grip and opposition places additional stress on the joint, exacerbating instability.
- **Intra-Articular Nature:** The fracture extends into the carpometacarpal (CMC) joint, compromising the joint's integrity and mobility.

Clinical Applications

- **Orthopedic Surgery:** Commonly treated by hand surgeons to restore thumb function.
- **Rehabilitation:** Following surgical stabilization, patients often require physiotherapy to regain strength, mobility, and dexterity.

Limitations and Technical Considerations

- **Challenges in Reduction:** Fragmentation and comminution make anatomical reduction complex.
- **Surgical Risks:** Risk of complications such as infection, nonunion, or stiffness.
- **Post-Treatment Arthritis:** High likelihood of developing post-traumatic osteoarthritis due to the intra-articular nature of the fracture.

Modern Relevance

- **Enhanced Fixation Techniques:** Advances in surgical methods, such as locking plates and improved external fixators, have increased success rates.

- **Use of 3D Imaging:** Modern imaging modalities enable better preoperative planning and intraoperative precision.

Associated Conditions

- **Bennett Fracture:** Shares a similar mechanism but involves only two segments and less comminution.
- **Carpometacarpal Joint Arthritis:** A common sequela of inadequately treated Rolando fractures.
- **Collateral Ligament Injuries:** May coexist due to the force of injury.

Clinical Importance

- **Early Diagnosis:** Identifying a Rolando fracture promptly is critical to preserving thumb function and avoiding long-term complications.
- **Surgical Necessity:** Due to the unstable nature of this fracture, surgical intervention is often required for optimal outcomes.
- **Functional Restoration:** Accurate reduction and fixation are essential for maintaining the thumb's role in grip and precision tasks.
- **Post-Treatment Monitoring:** Long-term follow-up is necessary to monitor for arthritis, malunion, or functional deficits.

The Rolando fracture represents a severe injury to the base of the thumb, requiring a multidisciplinary approach involving radiologists, surgeons, and physiotherapists to achieve favorable outcomes. Its management remains a cornerstone of orthopedic hand surgery.

References

Rolando S. Fracture de la base du premier metacarpien et principalement sur une variété non encore décrite. Presse Med 1910; 33: 303–304. [Translated Meals RA. Fracture of the base of the first metacarpal and a variation that has not yet been described. Clin Orthop Relat Res. 2006 Apr;445:15-8. PMID8641081]

Proubasta IR. Rolando's fracture of the first metacarpal. Treatment by external fixation. J Bone Joint Surg Br. 1992 May;74(3):416-7. [PMID 1587892]

Howard FM. Fractures of the basal joint of the thumb. Clin Orthop Relat Res. 1987 Jul;(220):46-51. [PMID 3595009]

Edmunds JO. Traumatic dislocations and instability of the trapeziometacarpal joint of the thumb. Hand Clin. 2006 Aug;22(3):365-92. [PMID 16843802]

Rouvière ligament

Overview

The Rouvière ligament, also known as the "fibulotalocalcaneal ligament," is an extrinsic ligament located in the posterolateral corner of the ankle and the posterior aspect of the subtalar joint. It originates from the lateral malleolus and plays a role in stabilizing the ankle and subtalar joints. Although its exact biomechanical function remains unclear, it is notable for influencing posterior ankle arthroscopy.

Historical Background

- **1932:** The ligament was first described by Henri Rouvière and Miguel Canela Lázaro. They detailed its anatomical structure and its continuity with other ligaments in the posterolateral ankle region.
- **2000s:** The ligament gained renewed attention when van Dijk highlighted its relevance in posterior ankle arthroscopy, recommending its division to improve access without adverse biomechanical effects.

Purpose

- **Anatomical Definition:** To delineate the fibulotalocalcaneal ligament's structure and relationship to adjacent ligaments.
- **Arthroscopic Access:** To understand its role in obstructing the posterior portals during arthroscopy and justify its division during surgical procedures.

Procedure Overview

- **Anatomical Examination:** The ligament is identified as a sheath-like structure originating from the medial border of the peroneal groove of the lateral malleolus and extending toward the calcaneus and talus.
- **Surgical Context:** During posterior ankle arthroscopy (e.g., van Dijk hindfoot approach), the ligament obstructs direct access to the ankle joint through posterior portals.
- **Arthroscopic Technique:** The ligament is typically divided to facilitate joint entry, a step that has not been shown to compromise stability or function.

Results and Interpretation

- **Anatomical Observations:** The ligament often originates alongside the posterior tibiofibular ligament and may reach the calcaneofibular ligament, indicating its role in posterolateral stability.
- **Arthroscopic Outcomes:** Dividing the ligament during posterior arthroscopy provides improved access and visualization without biomechanical repercussions.

Physiological Basis

- **Structural Role:** The ligament is part of the posterolateral ankle stabilizers, working alongside the calcaneofibular and posterior tibiofibular ligaments.
- Its involvement with both the subtalar and ankle joints suggests a sheath-like function that supports joint congruency.
- **Biomechanical Ambiguity:** The

exact biomechanical significance remains unclear, as its division during arthroscopy does not appear to affect ankle or subtalar joint function significantly.

Clinical Applications

- **Posterior Ankle Arthroscopy:** Key consideration in procedures using the two-portal posterior approach, where division of the ligament is often required.
- **Ankle Stabilization:** Although its biomechanical role is uncertain, it is part of the broader network of ligaments stabilizing the posterolateral ankle and subtalar joints.

Limitations and Technical Considerations

- **Surgical Challenges:** Careful identification is necessary during arthroscopy to ensure precise division without damaging adjacent structures.
- **Lack of Biomechanical Evidence:** Despite its anatomical prominence, the exact functional role of the ligament remains undetermined, limiting its standalone significance in stability assessments.

Modern Relevance

- **Arthroscopic Techniques:** Awareness of the Rouvière ligament's anatomical position improves procedural efficacy in posterior ankle arthroscopy.
- Division of the ligament is a routine step in the van Dijk hindfoot approach, facilitating better visualization and access.
- **Surgical Anatomy:** The ligament's relationship with other stabilizers makes it a relevant feature in understanding complex ankle injuries and interventions.

Associated Conditions

- **Posterolateral Ankle Instability:** While not directly implicated, damage to this ligament may coexist with injuries to other posterolateral stabilizers.
- **Subtalar Joint Dysfunction:** The ligament's involvement in the subtalar joint suggests a potential, though minor, role in subtalar pathologies.

Clinical Importance

- **Arthroscopic Navigation:** Cutting the ligament during posterior ankle arthroscopy is a routine yet essential step to improve joint access and visualization.
- **Surgical Anatomy Awareness:** Understanding the ligament's anatomy prevents inadvertent damage to adjacent structures during surgical interventions.
- **Unresolved Biomechanics:** Further studies are needed to determine the ligament's specific role in ankle and subtalar stability.

The Rouvière ligament remains a focal point in ankle arthroscopy, offering both anatomical and clinical significance. While its biomechanical function is still under study, its routine division during posterior procedures highlights its surgical importance.

References

Pastore D, Cerri GG, Haghighi P, Trudell DJ, Resnick DL. Ligaments of the posterior and lateral talar processes: MRI and MR arthrography of the ankle and posterior subtalar joint with anatomic and histologic correlation. AJR Am J Roentgenol 2009; 192: 967–73.

van Dijk CN. Hindfoot Endoscopy. Foot Ankle Clin 2006; 11:

391–414.

van Dijk C, de Leeuw P, Scholten P. Hindfoot Endoscopy for Posterior Ankle Impingement. J Bone Jt Surgery-American Vol 2009; 91: 287–98.

van Dijk CN, Scholten PE, Krips R. A 2-portal endoscopic approach for diagnosis and treatment of posterior ankle pathology. Arthrosc J Arthrosc Relat Surg 2000; 16: 871–6.

Rotter-Erb Syndrome

Overview

Rotter-Erb syndrome is a rare skeletal dysplasia marked by deformities in bones, joints, and tendons. The syndrome presents with characteristic features such as dwarfism, brachycephaly, brachymetapody, multiple metaphyseal lesions, congenital dislocations, joint laxity, bilateral clubfoot, pterygium colli, vertebral deformities, hypertelorism, cleft palate, and nasal bridge depression. This familial disorder has been observed primarily in males, and while mental development is typically normal, respiratory difficulties may occur at a young age. Both autosomal dominant and recessive inheritance patterns have been recognized.

Historical Background

- **1947:** Werner Erb first described the condition in his doctoral dissertation, focusing on skeletal deformities and familial patterns.
- **1948:** Wolfgang Rotter, alongside Erb, expanded on the syndrome's clinical features and pathophysiological basis, providing a more comprehensive overview.
- **1950:** Loren Joseph Larsen further analyzed the condition, adding observations related to associated joint laxity and metaphyseal lesions.
- Subsequent contributions by B. L. McFarland and others questioned the distinctiveness of the syndrome, suggesting overlapping features with other skeletal dysplasias.

Purpose

- **Clinical Characterization:** To document and delineate the constellation of skeletal and connective tissue anomalies associated with this syndrome.
- **Inheritance Patterns:** To clarify the genetic basis of the condition and its transmission mechanisms.
- **Diagnostic Framework:** To aid in the early diagnosis and differentiation from other skeletal dysplasias.

Procedure Overview

- **Clinical Assessment:** Physical examination reveals short stature, brachycephaly, and joint laxity, alongside prominent skeletal abnormalities such as brachymetapody, clubfoot, and vertebral deformities.
- **Radiographic Imaging:** Imaging studies confirm multiple metaphyseal lesions, vertebral anomalies, and other skeletal deformities, essential for diagnosis.
- **Genetic Testing:** Conducted to determine inheritance patterns and identify any familial prevalence.
- **Differential Diagnosis:** Differentiation from other skeletal dysplasias such as Larsen syndrome and other connective tissue disorders is vital.

Results and Interpretation

- **Skeletal Findings:** Radiographic studies reveal metaphyseal lesions, brachymetapody, and vertebral anomalies.
- **Physical Characteristics:** Typical features include clubfoot, joint laxity, cleft palate, and hypertelorism.
- **Inheritance Patterns:** Both autosomal dominant and recessive forms are noted, with variable penetrance and expressivity.

Physiological Basis

- **Connective Tissue Dysplasia:** The syndrome affects bone and connective tissue development, leading to dwarfism, joint laxity, and metaphyseal lesions.
- **Skeletal Malformation:** Abnormal ossification and growth plate development result in deformities such as brachymetapody and clubfoot.

Clinical Applications

- **Early Diagnosis:** Early identification allows for orthopedic interventions to manage joint laxity, clubfoot, and other deformities.
- **Genetic Counseling:** Families with a history of the syndrome can benefit from genetic counseling to understand inheritance patterns and recurrence risks.
- **Multidisciplinary Management:** A combination of orthopedic, pediatric, and genetic specialists is essential for optimal care.

Limitations and Technical Considerations

- **Diagnostic Challenges:** The condition shares features with other skeletal dysplasias, making differential diagnosis complex.
- **Variable Expression:** Differences in severity and manifestations across individuals complicate standardized treatment approaches.

- **Lack of Specific Genetic Markers:** The absence of well-defined genetic markers limits precise molecular diagnosis.

Modern Relevance

- **Advances in Imaging:** Improved imaging modalities aid in earlier and more accurate diagnosis of skeletal anomalies.
- **Genetic Insights:** Ongoing research into the genetic basis of skeletal dysplasias may offer deeper understanding and novel treatment avenues.
- **Surgical Innovations:** Modern surgical techniques enhance outcomes for deformities such as clubfoot and joint laxity.

Associated Conditions

- **Larsen Syndrome:** Shares features like joint laxity and skeletal deformities, necessitating careful differentiation.
- **Other Skeletal Dysplasias:** Includes conditions with overlapping features such as achondroplasia and multiple epiphyseal dysplasia.

Clinical Importance

- **Early Diagnosis:** Prompt recognition prevents complications and enables targeted interventions.
- **Orthopedic Management:** Addressing deformities such as clubfoot and joint laxity improves mobility and quality of life.
- **Genetic Counseling:** Understanding inheritance patterns informs family planning and recurrence risk evaluation.
- **Long-term Monitoring:** Regular follow-ups are crucial for managing progressive skeletal deformities and potential complications.

Rotter-Erb syndrome represents a complex skeletal dysplasia with significant clinical and genetic implications. Advances in imaging and genetics continue to enhance our understanding and management of this rare disorder.

References

B. L. McFarland: Congenital dislocation of the knee. Journal of Bone and Joint Surgery, 1929, II: 281-285. BR or US?

W. Erb: Über eine seltene Systemerkrankung der Stützgewebe. Zugleich ein Beitrag zur Pathogenese der Wirbelbogenspalten. Diss med Kiel, 1947.

W. Rotter, W. Erb: Über eine Systemerkrankung des Mesenchyms mit multiplen Luxationen, angeborener Gelenkschlaffheit und über Wirbelbogenspalten. Virchows Archiv für pathologische Anatomie und Physiologie und für klinische Medizin, 1948, 316: 233-263.

Salter-Harris Classification

Overview

Salter-Harris Classification is a widely used system for categorizing fractures that involve the epiphyseal plate (growth plate) in growing patients. Recognizing these injuries is critical to avoiding complications such as growth disturbances, limb length discrepancies, and angular deformities. The classification system originally described five types of fractures, which have since been expanded by subsequent researchers.

Historical Background

- **1963:** Robert Bruce Salter and W. Robert Harris published their classification system, intending to improve the recognition and management of growth plate injuries. Harris insisted his name follow Salter's as he felt Salter's clinical research was more substantial than his basic science contributions.
- **1969:** Mercer Rang added Type VI fractures, which described peripheral epiphyseal injuries causing bridging bone formation and early closure of the growth plate.
- **1982:** J.A. Ogden expanded the classification further, detailing Types VII, VIII, and IX, which involve different anatomical structures surrounding the growth plate.

Purpose

- **Clinical Management:** To guide treatment strategies for epiphyseal injuries and mitigate long-term complications.
- **Understanding Prognosis:** To predict the likelihood of growth disturbances based on the type of fracture.
- **Standardized Communication:** To provide a universal framework for describing these injuries among healthcare professionals.

Procedure Overview

- **Radiographic Examination:** Initial imaging, typically plain X-rays, is used to identify the type of fracture and assess involvement of the epiphyseal plate.
- **Classification:** Fractures are classified into Types I-V based on the Salter-Harris system:
- **Type I:** Slipped; fracture through the growth plate.
- **Type II:** Above; fracture through the metaphysis and growth plate.
- **Type III:** Lower; fracture through the epiphysis and growth plate.
- **Type IV:** Through; fracture involving metaphysis, growth plate, and epiphysis.
- **Type V:** Rammed; compression injury to the growth plate.
- **Additional Types (Rang and Ogden):** Types VI-IX include periosteal and peripheral injuries, as well as injuries localized to the metaphysis or epiphysis.

Results and Interpretation

- **Type-Specific Outcomes:** Type I and II: Generally favorable outcomes with low risk of growth disturbance.
- **Type III and IV:** Higher risk due to involvement of the joint surface, often requiring surgical intervention.
- **Type V:** High likelihood of growth disturbance due to physeal compression.
- **Advanced Classification:** Types VI-IX describe rare or peripheral injuries and are often associated with significant deformity or growth plate dysfunction.

Physiological Basis

- **Growth Plate Vulnerability:** The epiphyseal plate is a zone of rapid cell division and matrix production, making it susceptible to disruption by trauma.
- **Healing Potential:** Younger patients have a higher capacity for bone remodeling, which is a critical factor in recovery and outcome.

Clinical Applications

- **Treatment Planning:** Differentiating types helps determine whether conservative management (casting) or surgical intervention (open reduction and fixation) is required.
- **Prognostic Evaluation:** The classification informs the risk of growth arrest, angular deformities, or joint dysfunction.
- **Follow-Up:** Regular imaging is needed to monitor healing and detect complications, particularly for higher-grade injuries.

Limitations and Technical Considerations

- **Overlap in Classification:** Some fractures may exhibit features of multiple types, complicating diagnosis.
- **Imaging Challenges:** Radiographs may fail to detect subtle injuries; advanced imaging like MRI may be required.
- **Rare Types:** Types VI-IX are less common and not always recognized, potentially delaying appropriate treatment.

Modern Relevance

- **Advanced Imaging Techniques:** MRI and CT provide better visualization of complex growth plate injuries, aiding in accurate classification and treatment planning.
- **Improved Surgical Interventions:** Advances in minimally invasive techniques improve outcomes for complex fractures.
- **Genetic Research:** Studies on bone growth and regeneration may offer insights into enhancing recovery after growth plate injuries.

Associated Conditions

- **Growth Arrest:** Common with Types IV and V fractures, leading to deformities or limb length discrepancies.
- **Joint Dysfunction:** Types III and IV may cause arthritis due to disruption of the articular surface.
- **Physeal Bar Formation:** Bone bridging across the growth plate may lead to asymmetric growth.

Clinical Importance

- **Early Diagnosis:** Prompt identification of epiphyseal injuries prevents long-term complications.
- **Standardized Approach:** The Salter-Harris classification provides a consistent framework for describing injuries and guiding treatment.
- **Preventing Growth Disturbances:** Accurate treatment minimizes risks of limb deformities and joint dysfunction.
- **Education and Research:** The classification remains a cornerstone in orthopedic education, promoting research into improving outcomes for pediatric fractures.

The Salter-Harris Classification revolutionized the understanding and management of growth plate injuries, providing a systematic and prognostically valuable tool that remains integral to pediatric orthopedics.

References

Salter RB, Harris WR. Injuries involving the epiphyseal plate. J Bone Joint Surg Am. 1963;45:587–622.

Rang M. The Growth Plate and Its Disorders. Livingstone, 1969

Peterson CA, Peterson HA. Analysis of the incidence of injuries to the epiphyseal growth plate. J Trauma. 1972 Apr;12(4):275-81. [PMID 5018408]

Ogden JA. Skeletal growth mechanism injury patterns. J Pediatr Orthop. 1982 Oct;2(4):371-7. [PMID 7142386]

Cepela DJ, Tartaglione JP, Dooley TP, Patel PN. Classifications In Brief: Salter-Harris Classification of Pediatric Physeal Fractures. Clin Orthop Relat Res. 2016 Nov; 474(11): 2531–2537. [PMC5052189]

Weissleder R, Wittenberg J, Harisinghani MGH, Chen JW. Primer of Diagnostic Imaging. Mosby

Schatzker classification of tibial plateau Fractures

Overview

The Schatzker Classification of tibial plateau fractures is one of the most widely used systems in orthopedic surgery. It categorizes fractures of the tibial plateau into six distinct types based on radiographic findings. These classifications aid in understanding fracture severity, predicting prognosis, and guiding treatment decisions.

Historical Background

- **1951:** Initial attempts at classifying tibial plateau fractures were introduced by Palmer.
- **1956:** Hohl and Luck further refined classifications, identifying key features such as condylar involvement and subchondral depression.
- **1967:** Hohl refined the classification further, introducing considerations for both fracture patterns and soft tissue involvement.
- **1979:** Joseph Schatzker formally published his six-type classification based on the radiographic analysis of 94 patients. The system emphasized the relationship between fracture patterns and treatment strategies.
- Subsequent classifications, such as those from Khan (2000), expanded on these systems, but the Schatzker and AO/OTA classifications remain the most commonly used today.

Purpose

- **Clinical Categorization:** Provides a standardized method to describe tibial plateau fractures.
- **Treatment Planning:** Guides surgical and non-surgical interventions based on the type and severity of the fracture.
- **Prognostic Insight:** Identifies factors such as depression, displacement, and bicondylar involvement that predict outcomes.

Procedure Overview

- **Imaging:**
- **Plain Radiographs (AP View):** Used as the basis for initial classification.
- Advanced imaging such as **CT or** MRI may be used for better visualization of complex fractures.
- **Classification:**
- **Type I:** Lateral tibial plateau fracture with minimal displacement (<4 mm).
- **Type II:** Lateral tibial plateau fracture with a depressed fragment.
- **Type III:** Compression fracture of the lateral or central plateau:
- **IIIA:** Lateral.
- **IIIB:** Central.
- **Type IV:** Medial tibial plateau fracture with split or depression.
- **Type V:** Bicondylar fracture involving both lateral and medial condyles.
- **Type VI:** Transverse tibial plateau fracture with metaphyseal-diaphyseal discontinuity.

Results and Interpretation

- **Type I and II:** Generally less severe and may be treated non-operatively in some cases.
- **Type III-IV:** More complex with involvement of weight-bearing articular surfaces, often requiring surgical intervention.
- **Type V and VI:** High-energy injuries with significant displacement and joint instability, often necessitating advanced surgical techniques.

Physiological Basis

- **Articular Surface Vulnerability:** The tibial plateau bears significant weight and is prone to fractures during high-energy trauma or falls.
- **Bone Quality:** Osteoporotic bones are more susceptible to complex fractures and have poorer outcomes when surgically managed.
- **Soft Tissue Considerations:** Associated injuries, such as meniscal tears and ligamentous damage, can complicate treatment and recovery.

Clinical Applications

- **Orthopedic Surgery:** Surgical fixation techniques are chosen based on the Schatzker classification type.
- **Rehabilitation:** The classification predicts the extent of recovery and the need for physical therapy.
- **Research and Training:** Provides a framework for studying outcomes and advancing treatment protocols.

Limitations and Technical Considerations

- **Imaging Limitations:** Plain radiographs may not capture complex fracture patterns, particularly in the coronal plane.
- **CT or** MRI enhances visualization but is not included in the original classification system.
- **Interobserver Reliability:** Interpretation varies among practitioners, especially for complex fractures.
- **Soft Tissue Injury:** Schatzker classification does not account for soft tissue injuries, which significantly impact treatment and outcomes.

Modern Relevance

- **Advanced Imaging:** Modern imaging modalities, such as CT and MRI, complement the Schatzker system for improved diagnostic accuracy and surgical planning.
- **Surgical Techniques:** Minimally invasive and robotic-assisted procedures have improved outcomes for complex fracture types.
- **Personalized Medicine:** The system informs tailored treatment plans based on fracture type, patient age, and bone health.

Associated Conditions

- **Osteoarthritis:** Long-term complication due to joint surface involvement.
- **Ligamentous Injuries:** Often associated with high-energy tibial plateau fractures.
- **Delayed Union or Nonunion:** Particularly in osteoporotic patients or those with complex fractures.

Clinical Importance

- **Early Diagnosis:** Prompt classification ensures appropriate management and reduces the risk of long-term complications.
- **Treatment Guidance:** Helps determine whether to pursue conservative or surgical treatment based on fracture complexity and patient factors.
- **Surgical Precision:** Aids in planning open reduction, internal fixation, or external fixation techniques.
- **Prognostic Value:** Identifies cases at high risk for complications, such as post-traumatic arthritis or joint instability.
- **Educational Framework:** Remains a cornerstone of orthopedic education for understanding tibial plateau fractures.

References

Schatzker J, McBroom R, Bruce D. The tibial plateau fracture. The Toronto experience 1968 – 1975. Clin Orthop Relat Res. 1979 Jan-Feb;(138):94-104. [PMID 445923]

Müller ME, Nazarian S, Koch P, Schatzker J. The Comprehensive Classification of Fractures of Long Bones. Springer 1990

Markhardt B, Gross J, Monu J. Schatzker Classification of Tibial Plateau Fractures: Use of CT and MR Imaging Improves Assessment. Radiographics. 2009;29 (2): 585-597.

Zeltser D, Leopold S. Classifications in Brief: Schatzker Classification of Tibial Plateau Fractures. Clin Orthop Relat Res. 2013 Feb; 471(2):371-374. [PMC3549155]

Palmer I. Fractures of the upper end of the tibia. J Bone Joint Surg Br. 1951;33:160-166 [PMID:14832314]

Hohl M, Luck JV. Fractures of the tibial condyle; a clinical and experimental study. J Bone Joint Surg Am. 1956 Oct;38-A(5):1001-18. [PMID: 13367078]

Hohl M. Tibial condylar fractures. J Bone Joint Surg Am. 1967;49:1455–1467 [PMID: 6053707]

Khan RM, Khan SH, Ahmad AJ, Umar M. Tibial plateau fractures: a new classification scheme. Clin Orthop Relat Res. 2000;375:231–242. [PMID: 10853174]

Walton NP, Harish S, Roberts C, Blundell C. AO or Schatzker? How reliable is classification of tibial plateau fractures? Arch Orthop Trauma Surg. 2003;123:396–398 [PMID: 14574596]

Schwartz-Jampel Syndrome

Overview

Schwartz-Jampel syndrome (SJS) is a rare genetic disorder characterized by growth retardation, distinctive facial features, skeletal abnormalities, and myotonia. The syndrome affects multiple systems, with hallmark features including muscle stiffness, joint limitations, and unique facial characteristics that evolve over time.

Historical Background

- **1962:** The condition was first described by Oscar Schwartz and Robert Steven Jampel, who identified the association between growth abnormalities, skeletal dysplasia, and myotonia in affected individuals.
- Subsequent studies expanded on their findings, recognizing the genetic nature of the syndrome and its autosomal recessive inheritance pattern.
- Additional insights into myotonia and its underlying pathophysiology were contributed by *Donald C. Aberfeld* and others.

Purpose

- **Diagnostic Recognition:** To identify a multisystem disorder that presents with myotonia, skeletal abnormalities, and characteristic facial dysmorphisms.
- **Treatment Guidance:** Provides a basis for managing symptoms such as muscle stiffness, joint limitations, and orthopedic complications.

Procedure Overview

- **Clinical Assessment:**
- Detailed physical examination focusing on facial features, muscle stiffness, and joint mobility.
- Evaluation of growth patterns and skeletal anomalies.
- **Diagnostic Imaging:** X-rays to evaluate short vertebrae, coxa vara, acetabular dysplasia, and femoral epiphysis abnormalities.
- **Electromyography (EMG):** Confirms the presence of myotonia by detecting electrical activity in muscles during relaxation.
- **Genetic Testing:** Identification of mutations in the HSPG2 gene, which encodes perlecan, a heparan sulfate proteoglycan.

Results and Interpretation

- **Facial Features:** Mask-like facies with puckered lips, upward-slanting eyes, blepharophimosis, and ptosis.
- **Musculoskeletal Findings:** Limited joint mobility, short stature, pectus carinatum, acetabular dysplasia, and fragmented femoral epiphyses.
- **Neuromuscular Symptoms:** Myotonia leading to muscle stiffness and hypertrophy.
- **Functional Impact:** Waddling gait, progressive difficulty with movement, and potential hip dislocation at birth.

Physiological Basis

- **Myotonia:** Caused by a defect in the relaxation of muscle fibers due to altered ion channel function.
- **Skeletal Abnormalities:** Result from disrupted cartilage and bone development due to the genetic mutation affecting extracellular matrix proteins.
- **Facial Dysmorphism:** Persistent muscle contractions contribute to the mask-like facial appearance and other distinctive features.

Clinical Applications

- **Orthopedic Management:** Addresses joint limitations and skeletal deformities through physical therapy, bracing, and surgical interventions.
- **Neurological Treatment:** Myotonia can be managed with muscle relaxants like carbamazepine or phenytoin.
- **Supportive Care:** Speech and occupational therapy for associated functional impairments.

Limitations and Technical Considerations

- **Heterogeneity:** Variable presentation of symptoms, ranging from mild to severe.
- **Genetic Testing Availability:** Limited access to confirmatory genetic testing in some settings.
- **Surgical Risks:** Orthopedic surgeries may pose challenges due to fragile skeletal structures and poor muscle relaxation.

Modern Relevance

- **Advances in** *genetic research* have improved the diagnostic accuracy of Schwartz-Jampel syndrome.
- Emerging therapies, such as *gene editing*, hold promise for addressing the underlying genetic mutation.
- Increased awareness among clinicians facilitates early diagnosis and intervention.

Associated Conditions

- **Congenital Hip Dislocation:** Common at birth due to acetabular dysplasia.
- **Scoliosis and Kyphosis:** Progressive spinal deformities may develop over time.
- **Respiratory Issues:** May arise from chest wall deformities and muscle stiffness.

Clinical Importance

- **Early Diagnosis:** Recognizing signs like facial dysmorphism and myotonia in infancy enables prompt intervention.
- **Comprehensive Management:** Involves a multidisciplinary approach, including neurologists, orthopedists, and geneticists.
- **Prognostic Insight:** Understanding the progressive nature of the condition helps in planning long-term care.
- **Quality of Life:** Treatment of symptoms improves mobility, reduces pain, and enhances overall functionality.

Schwartz-Jampel syndrome remains a significant focus in medical genetics and neurology due to its complex presentation and multidisciplinary management needs.

References

L. M. Pinto, J. S. De Spuza: Un caso de "doenca muscular" de difficil classificacao. Revista portuguesa de pediatria e puericultura, 1961, 6: 1.

O. Schwartz, R. S. Jampel: Congenital blepharophimosis associated with a unique generalized myopathy. Archives of Ophthalmology, Chicago, 1962, 68: 52.

D. C. Aberfeld, L. V. Hinterbuchner, M. Schneider: Myotonia, dwarfism, diffuse bone disease and unusual ocular and facial abnormalities (a new syndrome). Brain, Oxford, 1965, 88: 313-322.

D. C. Aberfeld et al: Chondrodystrophic myotonia: Report of two cases. Myotonia, dwarfism, diffuse bone disease and unusual ocular and facial abnormalities. Annals of Neurology. Boston, 1970, 22: 455-62.

Schanz' disease

Overview

Schanz' disease, also known as tendinitis achillea traumatica, is a condition characterized by traumatic inflammation of the Achilles tendon. It results from overuse, repetitive microtrauma, or acute injury to the tendon, leading to localized pain, swelling, and functional limitations in the ankle and lower leg.

Historical Background

- **1890s:** The condition was first described by Alfred Schanz, a German surgeon known for his work in orthopedics and traumatology.
- His focus on the Achilles tendon highlighted its vulnerability to trauma and repetitive strain, particularly in physically active individuals.

Purpose

- **Diagnostic Recognition:** To identify inflammation and injury to the Achilles tendon resulting from trauma or overuse.
- **Management and Prevention:** To guide treatment strategies that promote healing and prevent recurrence or chronic complications.

Procedure Overview

- **Clinical Examination:**
- Observation for swelling, redness, and tenderness along the Achilles tendon.
- Assessment of pain during palpation and movement of the ankle joint.
- **Imaging:** Ultrasound or MRI to

confirm tendon inflammation, assess severity, and rule out partial or complete rupture.

- **Functional Assessment:** Evaluation of range of motion and strength in the affected ankle.

Results and Interpretation

- **Clinical Findings:** Pain and tenderness localized to the Achilles tendon.
- Swelling and potential thickening of the tendon sheath.
- Pain exacerbated by activities such as walking, running, or climbing stairs.
- **Imaging:** Evidence of localized fluid accumulation or inflammation around the tendon.
- No signs of rupture in isolated Schanz' disease.

Physiological Basis

- **Inflammation Process:** Microtears in the Achilles tendon fibers lead to an inflammatory response, characterized by swelling and pain.
- **Trauma Contribution:** Direct trauma or repetitive stress disrupts the tendon's structural integrity, increasing vulnerability to inflammation.

Clinical Applications

- **Conservative Management:** Rest, ice, compression, and elevation (RICE) protocol for acute inflammation.
- Physical therapy to improve strength and flexibility of the tendon and surrounding muscles.
- **Pharmacological Intervention:** Non-steroidal anti-inflammatory drugs (NSAIDs) for pain and inflammation control.
- **Surgical Options:** Rarely required unless there is significant structural damage or chronic tendon degeneration.

Limitations and Technical Considerations

- **Chronicity Risk:** If untreated, Schanz' disease can progress to tendinosis or chronic pain.
- **Imaging Challenges:** Early-stage inflammation may not always be evident on imaging.
- **Activity Modification:** Patients must be cautious about returning to physical activities prematurely, which can exacerbate the condition.

Modern Relevance

- **Sports Medicine:** Increasing recognition of Schanz' disease in athletes highlights the need for preventive strategies and early intervention.
- **Rehabilitation Advances:** Improved physical therapy techniques and regenerative medicine (e.g., platelet-rich plasma) offer promising outcomes.

Associated Conditions

- **Achilles Tendinopathy:** Chronic degeneration of the Achilles tendon.
- **Plantar Fasciitis:** Inflammation of the plantar fascia, often coexisting with Achilles tendon injuries.
- **Heel Spur Syndrome:** Calcaneal bone spurs that may exacerbate Achilles tendon strain.

Clinical Importance

- **Early Detection:** Prompt diagnosis and treatment reduce the risk of progression to chronic conditions.
- **Functional Restoration:** Ensuring proper healing allows patients to regain full mobility and return to physical activities.
- **Prevention:** Educating patients on proper footwear, stretching, and warm-up techniques reduces recurrence risk.
- **Interdisciplinary Approach:** Collaboration between orthopedic specialists, physical therapists, and sports medicine practitioners ensures optimal care.

Schanz' disease remains a critical focus in orthopedic and sports medicine due to its implications for mobility and quality of life. Early intervention and comprehensive care are key to managing this condition effectively.

References

A. Schanz: Eine typische Erkrankung der Achillessehne. Zentralblatt für Chirurgie, Leipzig, 1905, 32: 1289-1291.

Schanz' Syndrome II

Overview

Schanz' syndrome II is a condition characterized by combined neurological features of lateral sclerosis and anterior cornual syndromes. The primary symptoms include fatigue and lumbar pain, especially when transitioning from an erect to a prone position. It reflects both motor and sensory dysfunctions associated with spinal cord pathology.

Historical Background

- **1907:** Alfred Schanz, a German surgeon, described this syndrome in his observations of combined lateral sclerosis and anterior cornual involvement, highlighting the interplay of motor and sensory components in spinal cord syndromes.

Purpose

- **Diagnostic Clarification:** To identify and differentiate combined motor and sensory spinal cord syndromes.
- **Therapeutic Planning:** To design management strategies that address the overlapping features of lateral sclerosis and anterior cornual syndromes.

Procedure Overview

- **Clinical Examination:**
- Observation for muscle weakness, spasticity, and sensory abnormalities.
- Assessment of pain and fatigue levels during positional changes.
- **Imaging Studies:** MRI to detect structural changes in the spinal cord.

- **Electrophysiological Testing:** Nerve conduction studies and electromyography (EMG) to assess motor and sensory nerve function.

Results and Interpretation

- **Clinical Findings:** Symptoms include lumbar pain, fatigue, and progressive difficulty with posture transitions.
- Evidence of spasticity and weakness from lateral sclerosis, combined with anterior horn cell dysfunction.
- **Imaging and Testing:** MRI shows abnormalities in the lateral columns and anterior horn cells of the spinal cord.
- EMG findings suggest lower motor neuron involvement.

Physiological Basis

- **Neurological Pathophysiology:** Lateral sclerosis affects the corticospinal tracts, leading to spasticity and hyperreflexia.
- Anterior cornual syndrome involves the anterior horn cells, causing flaccid weakness and muscle atrophy.
- **Biomechanical Factors:** Lumbar pain and fatigue result from impaired posture regulation and muscle weakness.

Clinical Applications

- **Rehabilitation:** Physical therapy focusing on strengthening and mobility restoration.
- **Pain Management:** Pharmacological interventions like NSAIDs or muscle relaxants.
- **Assistive Devices:** Braces or supports to aid posture and movement.

Limitations and Technical Considerations

- **Diagnostic Complexity:** Differentiating Schanz' syndrome II from similar neurological disorders is challenging.
- **Progressive Nature:** Symptoms may worsen over time, requiring ongoing monitoring.
- **Treatment Constraints:** Limited specific treatments for the combined motor and sensory pathology.

Modern Relevance

- **Neurology and Rehabilitation:** Advances in imaging and therapy provide better diagnostic precision and symptom management.
- **Patient-Centered Care:** Focus on improving quality of life despite chronic symptoms.

Associated Conditions

- **Lateral Sclerosis:** Progressive motor neuron disease affecting the corticospinal tracts.
- **Anterior Cornual Syndrome:** Conditions like poliomyelitis affecting the anterior horn cells.

Clinical Importance

- **Symptom Recognition:** Early identification of combined motor and sensory symptoms aids in timely intervention.
- **Functional Restoration:** Rehabilitation efforts aim to preserve mobility and reduce pain.
- **Chronic Care:** Long-term management

strategies enhance the quality of life for affected individuals.

- **Interdisciplinary Approach:** Neurologists, physiatrists, and physical therapists collaborate for optimal care delivery.

Schanz' syndrome II highlights the challenges of managing combined spinal cord syndromes and underscores the importance of an integrated clinical approach for effective treatment.

References

A. Schanz: Eine typische Erkrankung der Wirbelsäule (Insufficienta vertebrae). Berliner klinische Wochenschrift, 1907, 44: 989-992. 17: 986 ff.

Schauthauer-Marie-Sainton Syndrome

Overview

Schauthauer-Marie-Sainton syndrome, also known as cleidocranial dysostosis, is a hereditary skeletal disorder characterized by defective development of membranous bones, especially the clavicles and skull. The condition is marked by the absence or underdevelopment of clavicles, leading to hypermobility of the shoulders, and defective ossification of the skull, which results in persistent fontanels and abnormal skull shapes. Other features may include hypoplasia of facial bones, dental anomalies, and hip or pelvic deformities.

Historical Background

- **1897:** Pierre Marie and Paul Sainton provided the first comprehensive description of the condition in their study, naming it "cleidocranial dysostosis."
- **1913:** Gustav Scheuthauer described further associated osseous anomalies, contributing to the understanding of the syndrome.
- **1930s:** Johan Vilhelm Hultkrantz added clinical insights, including racial and ethnic variations in its presentation. Purpose
- **Diagnostic Clarity:** To identify skeletal dysplasias affecting the clavicles and skull, ensuring accurate diagnosis and differentiation from similar syndromes.
- **Treatment Guidance:** To inform appropriate interventions, including

surgical correction and dental management.

Procedure Overview

- **Clinical Examination:** Assessment of shoulder mobility, cranial shape, and dental anomalies.
- **Radiographic Studies:** X-rays to evaluate clavicular aplasia and cranial ossification.
- Imaging of the pelvis and other skeletal regions to identify additional anomalies.
- **Genetic Testing:** Identification of mutations in the RUNX2 gene, associated with autosomal dominant inheritance.

Results and Interpretation

- **Radiographic Findings:** Partial or complete absence of one or both clavicles.
- Persistent fontanels and wormian bones within the sutures.
- Hypoplasia or dysplasia of the pelvic bones and hip joints.
- **Clinical Presentation:** Hypermobile shoulders and an abnormal cranial shape.
- High-arched palate and dental abnormalities, including delayed eruption of teeth.

Physiological Basis

- **Genetic Mutation:** Mutation in the RUNX2 gene, critical for osteoblast differentiation and skeletal development.
- **Membranous Ossification Defect:** Affects clavicular and cranial bones, leading to delayed or incomplete ossification.

Clinical Applications

- **Orthopedic Management:** Surgical correction of clavicular defects and hip dislocations.
- **Dental Treatment:** Orthodontic interventions for delayed or abnormal tooth eruption.
- **Physical Therapy:** Strengthening exercises to improve shoulder function and mobility.

Limitations and Technical Considerations

- **Diagnostic Challenges:** Overlapping features with other skeletal dysplasias may complicate diagnosis.
- **Surgical Risks:** Procedures involving the clavicles or pelvis may carry significant risks due to structural abnormalities.

Modern Relevance

- **Genetic Insights:** Advances in molecular genetics have improved the ability to diagnose and understand the syndrome's inheritance patterns.
- **Multidisciplinary Care:** Collaboration among orthopedic surgeons, dentists, and geneticists enhances treatment outcomes.

Associated Conditions

- **Hereditary Cleidal Dysostosis:** A milder variant of the condition with less severe cranial involvement.
- **Hip Dysplasia:** Often associated with underdeveloped pelvic structures.

Clinical Importance

- **Early Diagnosis:** Identifying the syndrome in infancy allows for timely interventions to address skeletal and dental issues.
- **Functional Restoration:** Management of hypermobile shoulders and dental anomalies significantly improves quality of life.
- **Genetic Counseling:** Essential for families with a history of the syndrome to understand inheritance risks and recurrence.
- **Interdisciplinary Approach:** Orthopedic, dental, and genetic care is essential for comprehensive management.

Schauthauer-Marie-Sainton syndrome underscores the complexity of skeletal dysplasias and the importance of a tailored, multidisciplinary approach to diagnosis and treatment.

References

G. Scheutauer: Kombination rudimentärer Schlüsselbeine mit Anomalien des Schädels beim erwachsenen Menschen. Allgemeine Wiener medizinische Zeitung,1871,16:293-295.

P. Marie, P. Sainton: Observation d'hydrocéphalie héréditaire (père et fils), par vice de dévelopment du crâne et du cerveau. Bulletins et memoires de la Société medicale des hôpitaux de Paris, 1897, 14: 706-712.

P. Marie, P. Sainton: Sur la dysostose cléido-crânienne héréditaire. Bulletins et memoires de la Société medicale des hôpitaux de Paris, 1898, 15: 436.

Segond Fracture

Overview

Segond fracture is an avulsion fracture involving the lateral tibial condyle, often associated with anterior cruciate ligament (ACL) injuries, meniscal tears, and damage to other supporting structures of the knee. It is considered a pathognomonic radiographic finding indicative of rotational and varus stress injuries to the knee joint. The injury occurs due to tension on the lateral capsular ligament (LCL) caused by internal tibial rotation with varus stress.

Historical Background

- **1845:** Amédée Bonnet conducted the first cadaveric studies to explore the mechanism of knee ligament injuries, laying the groundwork for understanding related fractures.
- **1879:** Paul Ferdinand Segond expanded Bonnet's work, demonstrating that internal tibial rotation with knee flexion results in lateral capsular ligament tension, leading to avulsion of the lateral tibial plateau. Segond described this fracture and its clinical association with ACL ruptures.
- **1936:** Henry Milch reported the first radiographic observations of Segond fractures in patients with acute knee injuries, establishing its clinical and diagnostic significance.

Purpose

- **Diagnostic Indicator:** The Segond fracture serves as a key radiographic marker for ACL injuries and associated knee ligament pathologies.

- **Treatment Planning:** Identifying this fracture aids in assessing the extent of associated ligamentous and meniscal injuries, informing surgical or conservative management.

Procedure Overview

- **Radiographic Evaluation:** Standard anterior-posterior and lateral knee X-rays often reveal the small avulsion fragment on the lateral tibial condyle.
- Advanced imaging, such as MRI, is used to evaluate soft tissue injuries (e.g., ACL rupture, meniscal tears) associated with the Segond fracture.
- **Physical Examination:** Clinical signs, such as joint effusion, anterior-posterior instability, and pain during movement, complement imaging findings.
- **Intraoperative Assessment:** During surgical intervention for ACL reconstruction, the extent of associated injuries is often further clarified.

Results and Interpretation

- **Radiographic Findings:** A small bony fragment avulsed from the lateral tibial plateau is the hallmark radiographic sign.
- Associated findings include widening of the lateral joint space, indicative of ligamentous laxity.
- **MRI Insights:** Reveals concomitant soft tissue injuries, including ACL tears (present in over 75% of cases) and meniscal damage.

Physiological Basis

- **Mechanism of Injury:** Excessive internal tibial rotation combined with varus stress increases tension on the lateral capsular ligament, leading to its avulsion.
- **Capsular Involvement:** The avulsion typically occurs at the insertion of the lateral capsular ligament into the lateral tibial plateau.

Clinical Applications

- **Diagnostic Value:** Early detection of Segond fractures provides critical insight into the likelihood of associated ACL and meniscal injuries.
- **Surgical Planning:** Knowledge of this fracture informs the surgeon about the extent of soft tissue involvement, guiding comprehensive reconstruction procedures.

Limitations and Technical Considerations

- **Diagnostic Challenges:** Subtle fractures may be missed on plain radiographs without proper positioning or high-quality imaging.
- **MRI Dependency:** While X-rays confirm the fracture, MRI is essential to assess associated ligamentous and meniscal injuries.

Modern Relevance

- **Enhanced Imaging Techniques:** The use of high-resolution MRI and CT scans improves detection of Segond fractures and their associated injuries.
- **Orthopedic Advances:** Modern surgical techniques, including arthroscopic ACL reconstruction, have

been refined using insights gained from Segond fractures.

Associated Conditions

- **Anterior Cruciate Ligament (ACL) Tears:** Commonly associated with Segond fractures and often require surgical intervention.
- **Meniscal Injuries:** Medial and lateral meniscal tears frequently accompany this type of fracture.
- **Posterolateral Corner Injuries:** Additional ligamentous damage in severe cases.

Clinical Importance

- **Early Diagnosis:** Prompt recognition of a Segond fracture aids in the early detection of ACL injuries, improving outcomes.
- **Predictive Marker:** The presence of this fracture strongly indicates associated soft tissue damage, guiding further diagnostic evaluation.
- **Interdisciplinary Approach:** Collaboration between radiologists, orthopedic surgeons, and physical therapists is essential for effective management.

Segond fractures remain a crucial diagnostic finding in knee trauma, providing insight into the biomechanics of injury and aiding in the management of complex knee ligament reconstructions.

References

Segond P. Recherches cliniques et expérimentales sur les épanchements sanguins du genou par entorse. Prog Med 1879; 16: 297–299, 319–321, 340–341

Milch H. Cortical avulsion fracture of the lateral tibial condyle. J Bone Joint Surg 1936;18:159e64.

Gottsegen CJ, Eyer BA, White EA, Learch TJ, Forrester D. Avulsion fractures of the knee: imaging findings and clinical significance. Radiographics. 2008 Oct;28(6):1755-70. [PMID 18936034]

Dietz GW, Wilcox DM, Montgomery JB. Segond tibial condyle fracture: lateral capsular ligament avulsion. Radiology. 1986 May;159(2):467-9. [PMID 3961179]

Campos JC et al. Pathogenesis of the Segond fracture: anatomic and MR imaging evidence of an iliotibial tra**CT or** anterior oblique band avulsion. Radiology. 2001 May;219(2):381-6. [PMID 11323461]

Schindler OS. Surgery for anterior cruciate ligament deficiency: a historical perspective. Knee Surg Sports Traumatol Arthrosc. 2012 Jan;20(1):5-47. [PMID 22105976]

Goldman AB, Pavlov H, Rubenstein D. The Segond fracture of the proximal tibia: a small avulsion that reflects major ligamentous damage. AJR Am J Roentgenol. 1988 Dec;151(6):1163-7. [PMID 3263770]

Sever Disease

Overview

Sever disease, or calcaneal apophysitis, is a common cause of heel pain in growing children. It is an overuse syndrome involving inflammation of the growth plate (apophysis) at the posterior calcaneus where the Achilles tendon inserts. The condition typically affects active children, often between the ages of 7 and 15 in boys and 8 and 13 in girls, and is more prevalent in overweight children and boys. Symptoms include localized heel pain, often bilateral, and discomfort exacerbated by physical activity.

Historical Background

- **1912:** James Warren Sever first described the condition, identifying it as a traction apophysitis at the insertion of the Achilles tendon on the calcaneus in growing children.
- Since then, it has been recognized as a common musculoskeletal injury in pediatric populations, particularly in those engaged in sports or physical activities involving running and jumping.

Purpose

- **Diagnosis:** To identify the cause of heel pain in pediatric patients and differentiate it from other conditions such as plantar fasciitis or Achilles tendonitis.
- **Management Guidance:** Understanding the underlying cause aids in determining appropriate interventions to reduce pain and prevent recurrence.

Procedure Overview

- **Clinical Examination:**
- Observation of heel pain localized to the posterior calcaneus, often elicited by palpation or squeezing the heel.
- Evaluation of gait and assessment of tightness in the Achilles tendon or calf muscles.
- **Radiographic Evaluation:**
- X-rays may be performed to rule out fractures or other bony abnormalities, although they are not typically required for diagnosis.
- Findings of sclerosis or fragmentation at the calcaneal apophysis may be noted but are nonspecific.
- **Symptom Assessment:** Pain severity and impact on daily activities or sports participation are evaluated.

Results and Interpretation

- **Clinical Findings:** Pain localized to the calcaneal apophysis that worsens with physical activity and improves with rest.
- Tenderness when the heel is compressed medially and laterally (positive "squeeze test").
- **Radiographic Findings:** Fragmentation or sclerosis of the calcaneal apophysis may be seen but is not definitive.

Physiological Basis

- **Traction Stress:** The Achilles tendon exerts repetitive tension on the calcaneal apophysis during activities involving running, jumping, or rapid changes in direction.

- **Growth Plate Vulnerability:** The apophysis is a cartilaginous area weaker than surrounding bone, making it susceptible to overuse and inflammation.

Clinical Applications

- **Symptom Relief:** Provides a framework for managing heel pain in active children.
- **Activity Modification:** Advising reduced participation in high-impact sports or activities can help alleviate symptoms.
- **Rehabilitation:** Incorporation of stretching and strengthening exercises to address tightness in the Achilles tendon and calf muscles.

Limitations and Technical Considerations

- **Non-Specific Radiographic Features:** Imaging findings are not always definitive, and diagnosis is primarily clinical.
- **Self-Limiting Nature:** The condition resolves with skeletal maturity, making aggressive interventions unnecessary.

Modern Relevance

- **Increasing Incidence:** With the rise in sports participation among children, Sever disease remains a common concern for pediatric and sports medicine clinicians.
- **Focus on Conservative Management:** Emphasis on non-invasive treatments like rest, ice, and activity modification reflects modern approaches to managing the condition.

Associated Conditions

- **Plantar Fasciitis:** Differential diagnosis, especially in cases with heel pain.
- **Achilles Tendonitis:** May co-exist with or mimic Sever disease in some children.
- **Obesity-Related Stress:** Overweight children are more prone to developing Sever disease due to increased stress on the heel.

Clinical Importance

- **Early Diagnosis:** Identifying Sever disease early can prevent prolonged pain and disruptions to physical activity.
- **Management Guidance:** Offers clinicians strategies to reduce pain and inflammation through conservative measures.
- **Pediatric Awareness:** Educating parents and coaches about Sever disease helps in early recognition and appropriate activity modification for affected children.

Sever disease remains a critical consideration in evaluating heel pain in pediatric populations, with its resolution closely tied to skeletal maturity and effective management of activity levels.

References

Orava S, Puranen J. Exertion injuries in adolescent athletes. Br J Sports Med 1978; 12: 4–10.

Kaeding CC, Whitehead R. Musculoskeletal injuries in adolescents. Prim Care 1998; 25: 211–23.

Brantigan CO. Calcaneal apophysitis. One of the growing pains of adolescence. Rocky Mt Med J 1972; 69: 59–60.

Listed N. Obituary. N Engl J Med 1964; 271: 475.

Mehlman CT, Koepplinger ME. Hyphenated history: the Sever-L'Episcopo procedure. J Pediatr Orthop 2007; 27: 533–6

Sherpherd Fracture

Overview

Shepherd Fracture refers to a fracture of the lateral tubercle of the posterior process of the talus. This injury typically results from inversion or extreme equinus stress on the ankle. It is often observed on lateral radiographs but may require advanced imaging techniques for definitive diagnosis. Complications include chronic pain, arthrosis, and occasionally avascular necrosis.

Historical Background

- **1882:** First described by Francis John Shepherd through a dissection of a single fracture case, later expanded into a series of three cases.
- Over time, the fracture was differentiated from the *os trigonum*, a secondary ossification center accessory ossicle that can mimic the fracture radiographically.
- *Cedell's Fracture*, involving the medial tubercle of the posterior process of the talus, was later described as a related injury with distinct mechanisms of forced dorsiflexion and pronation.

Purpose

- **Diagnostic Clarity:** To distinguish between a Shepherd fracture and an os trigonum using radiological and clinical findings.
- **Preventive Measures:** Understanding the injury mechanism to guide prevention strategies for high-risk activities.
- **Treatment Guidance:** To establish appropriate treatment protocols, including conservative management or surgical intervention for symptomatic cases.

Procedure Overview

- **Imaging:**
- Lateral radiographs of the ankle to visualize the posterior talar process.
- If radiographic findings are inconclusive or significant trauma is suspected, CT imaging is recommended for enhanced sensitivity and specificity.
- **Clinical Examination:** Evaluation of posterior ankle pain, particularly in patients with a history of inversion injury or extreme equinus movements.
- **Differentiation:** Distinguishing the fracture from an os trigonum by examining the sharp, irregular, non-corticated outline of a fracture versus the smooth, corticated appearance of an os trigonum.

Results and Interpretation

- **Radiographic Findings:** A fracture line across the lateral tubercle of the posterior talar process. Sensitivity of lateral X-rays is approximately 78%.
- **CT Imaging:** Offers higher accuracy in confirming the fracture and identifying fragment displacement.

Physiological Basis

- **Stress Mechanism:** Inversion or extreme plantar flexion places significant stress on the lateral tubercle, leading to fracture.
- **Comparative Anatomy:** The posterior process of the talus comprises lateral and medial tubercles, both of which

can sustain fractures under distinct biomechanical forces (e.g., Cedell's fracture for the medial tubercle).

Clinical Applications

- **Conservative Management:** Immobilization of the ankle with a cast or boot to allow healing.
- **Surgical Intervention:** Rarely required; delayed excision of fragments may be necessary in cases of persistent pain or significant displacement.

Limitations and Technical Considerations

- **Radiographic Sensitivity:** Lateral X-rays have a limited sensitivity of 78%, leading to potential misdiagnosis.
- **Differentiation Challenges:** Misidentification of an os trigonum as a fracture can result in unnecessary interventions.

Modern Relevance

- **Improved Imaging Techniques:** The use of CT scans ensures accurate diagnosis and differentiation from accessory ossicles like the os trigonum.
- **Sports Medicine Applications:** The injury is particularly relevant in athletes, such as soccer players and ballet dancers, due to the frequent stress placed on the posterior talus.

Associated Conditions

- **Cedell's Fracture:** A related injury involving the medial tubercle of the posterior talus caused by forced dorsiflexion and pronation.
- **Os Trigonum Syndrome:** May mimic Shepherd fracture symptoms but involves a developmental accessory ossicle.
- **Ankle Instability:** Chronic instability may predispose individuals to repeated talar fractures.

Clinical Importance

- **Accurate Diagnosis:** Differentiating between a Shepherd fracture and os trigonum is critical to avoid mismanagement.
- **Prevention of Chronic Pain:** Early intervention can prevent complications like arthrosis and avascular necrosis.
- **Rehabilitation Guidance:** Emphasis on gradual return to activity and strengthening of ankle stabilizers.

The Shepherd fracture remains a clinically significant injury, particularly in active individuals and athletes, requiring precise diagnosis and appropriate management to ensure optimal recovery and functional outcomes.

References

Shepherd FJ. A Hitherto Undescribed Fracture of the Astragalus (talus). J Anat Physiol. 1882 Oct; 17(Pt 1): 79–81. [PMC1310130]

Hodge JC. Clinics in diagnostic imaging (42). Shepherd's fracture. Singapore Med J. 1999 Oct;40(10):666-8.[PMID 10741198]

Haddad FS, Bartlett M, Singh D. The sequelae of posterior talar fractures. Injury. 2000 Mar;31(2):107-11. [PMID 10748813]

Ahmad R, Ahmed AMY. Fracture of the posterior process of the talus: an unusual injury. Emerg Med J. 2007 Dec; 24(12): 867. [PMC2658382]

Early JS. Talus fracture management. [PMID 19013400]

Summers NJ, Murdoch MM. Fractures of the talus: a comprehensive review. Clin Podiatr Med Surg. 2012 Apr;29(2):187-203, vii [PMID 22424484]

Dale JD, Ha AS, Chew FS. Update on talar fracture patterns: a large level I trauma center study. AJR Am J Roentgenol. 2013 Nov;201(5):1087-92. [PMID 24147480]

Skier's Thumb

Overview

Skier's thumb, also referred to as gamekeeper's thumb, is a ligamentous injury to the ulnar collateral ligament (UCL) of the thumb's metacarpophalangeal joint (MCPJ). This injury results from trauma, typically hyperabduction of the thumb, and can present acutely or as a chronic condition. Acute cases are termed skier's thumb, while chronic repetitive stress-related injuries are called gamekeeper's thumb. Left untreated, these injuries may lead to significant joint instability and functional impairment.

Historical Background

- The term *gamekeeper's thumb* originated from the chronic thumb injuries observed in Scottish gamekeepers who repetitively killed small animals by twisting their necks, leading to repetitive stress on the UCL.
- *Skier's thumb* emerged as a modern descriptor, reflecting the acute nature of UCL injuries common among skiers who experience sudden hyperabduction trauma when falling with a ski pole in hand.

Purpose

- **The primary goal of diagnosing and managing skier's thumb is to:** Restore the stability of the MCPJ.
- Preserve pinch strength and pain-free motion.
- Prevent long-term complications like instability, weakened grip, and chronic pain.

Procedure Overview

- **Clinical Evaluation:**
- Patients typically report pain and weakness in the thumb, particularly during pinch or grip activities.
- Acute cases present with swelling, tenderness, and bruising along the ulnar aspect of the MCPJ.
- A palpable mass (indicating a Stener lesion) may be felt proximal to the MCPJ.
- **Diagnostic Imaging:**
- **Ultrasound:** The preferred imaging modality to confirm UCL rupture or displacement.
- **X-rays:** Used to identify associated fractures or avulsion injuries.
- **MRI:** Occasionally employed to evaluate ligament integrity and diagnose a Stener lesion.
- **Management:**
- **Non-Surgical:** Partial UCL tears and strains are managed with immobilization using a thumb splint or cast for 4–6 weeks.
- **Rehabilitation with physical therapy follows to restore motion and strength.**
- **Surgical:** Required for complete ruptures, Stener lesions, or significant instability.
- Techniques include direct ligament repair, augmentation with grafts, or treatment of associated fractures.

Results and Interpretation

- **Short-Term Results:** Successful non-surgical or surgical management restores thumb function and prevents chronic instability.
- **Long-Term Results:** Patients with timely treatment generally regain full strength and range of motion.
- Delayed treatment or misdiagnosis may lead to chronic pain, joint instability, or weak pinch grip.

Physiological Basis

- The UCL of the MCPJ provides critical *valgus stability* to the thumb during pinch and grip activities.
- A rupture or attenuation of the UCL disrupts this stability, leading to thumb *hyperextension* and *functional weakness.*
- Chronic injury can result in *ligament elongation*, causing progressive instability and pain.

Clinical Applications

- Skier's thumb is commonly encountered in *sports medicine, orthopedics,* and *emergency settings.*
- Prompt diagnosis and management prevent long-term disability and ensure optimal functional recovery.

Limitations and Technical Considerations

- **Diagnostic Challenges:** Differentiating partial from complete UCL tears can be difficult without imaging.
- **Missed or delayed diagnosis of a Stener lesion complicates treatment and worsens outcomes.**
- **Surgical Risks:** Infection, stiffness, and incomplete ligament healing may occur postoperatively.

Modern Relevance

- With the increasing popularity of skiing and other high-velocity sports, *skier's thumb* remains a prevalent injury.
- **Advances in** imaging, minimally invasive surgical techniques, and tailored rehabilitation protocols have improved the management of these injuries.

Associated Conditions

- **Stener Lesion:** A complication where the ruptured UCL's distal end is displaced and interposed by the adductor aponeurosis, preventing spontaneous healing.
- **Avulsion Fractures:** Often associated with UCL tears, requiring concurrent management.

Clinical Importance

- **Timely Diagnosis:** Early identification and treatment prevent complications like chronic instability and recurrent pain.
- **Comprehensive Management:** An interdisciplinary approach involving orthopedic surgeons, radiologists, and physiotherapists ensures optimal recovery.
- **Patient Education:** Patients should be counseled on preventing re-injury by avoiding activities that place excessive stress on the thumb.

Skier's thumb exemplifies the importance

of a systematic approach to diagnosis and treatment to restore function and prevent long-term morbidity.

References

Ritting AW, Baldwin PC, Rodner CM. Ulnar collateral ligament injury of the thumb metacarpophalangeal joint. Clinical Journal of Sports Medicine. 2010 Mar 1;20(2):106-12.

Mahajan M, Rhemrev SJ. Rupture of the ulnar collateral ligament of the thumb–a review. International journal of emergency medicine. 2013 Dec;6(1):1-6.

Tsiouri C, Hayton MJ, Baratz M. Injury to the ulnar collateral ligament of the thumb. Hand. 2009 Mar;4(1):12-8.

Mahajan M, Rhemrev SJ. Rupture of the ulnar collateral ligament of the thumb–a review. International journal of emergency medicine. 2013 Dec;6(1):1-6.

Ritting AW, Baldwin PC, Rodner CM. Ulnar collateral ligament injury of the thumb metacarpophalangeal joint. Clinical Journal of Sport Medicine. 2010 Mar 1;20(2):106-12.

Anna Pickens . Game keepers thumb. EM in 5. Available from: https://www.youtube.com/watch?v=0ZUtTT9v3r0 (last accessed 15.4.2019)

Ebrahim FS et al. US diagnosis of UCL tears of the thumb and Stener lesions: technique, pattern-based approach, and differential diagnosis. Radiographics. 2006; 26(4): 1007-20

ORTHOfilms . Stener Lesion. EM in 5. Available from: https://www.youtube.com/watch?v=RLskrc7qifY(last accessed 15.4.2019)

Patel S, Potty A, Taylor EJ, Sorene ED. Collateral ligament injuries of the metacarpophalangeal joint of the thumb: a treatment algorithm. Strategies in trauma and limb reconstruction. 2010 Apr;5(1):1-0.

Sebastin S, et al. Overview of a finger, hand, and wrist fractures. http://www.uptodate.Foye PM et al, Skler's Thumb. Medscape. 2010

American Society for Surgery of the Hand. Thumb sprains. www.assh.org/Public/HandConditions/Pages/ThumbSprains.aspx (accessed 18 March 2011)

Pediatric Trauma Care II: A clinical reference for physicians and nurses caring for the acutely injured child. AHC Media. LLC. 2014;6:52-53.

Leggit JC, Meko CJ. Acute finger injuries: part II. Fractures, dislocations, and thumb injuries. American Family Physician. 2006 Mar 1;73(5):827-34.

Nakayama M, Sakuma Y, Tobimatsu H. Recurrent volar dislocation of the metacarpophalangeal joint of the thumb with radial collateral ligament injury: a case report. International Journal of Surgery Case Reports. 2020 Jan 1;68:96-9.

C. Fusetti. The ECRL bone-tendon ligamentoplasty for chronic ulnar instability of the metacarpophalangeal joint of the thumb. Hand Surgery Unit, Chirurgie de la Main. 2005; Vol 24:5:217–221

Başar H. Comparison of results after surgical repair of acute and chronic ulnar collateral ligament injury of the thumb. Chirurgie de la Main. 2014;vol 33:6:384–389

Smith Fracture

Overview

The *Smith fracture*, also referred to as the *reverse Colles fracture*, is a transverse fracture of the distal radius with volar displacement and/or angulation of the distal fracture fragment. This injury typically results from a fall onto a flexed wrist. It is also known as the *Goyrand fracture* in French literature or the *reverse Barton's fracture* when involving the articular surface. The fracture is commonly diagnosed with AP and lateral X-rays, and treatment ranges from closed reduction and immobilization to surgical fixation in more complex cases.

Historical Background

- **1832:** Jean-Gaspard-Blaise Goyrand described fractures of the distal forearm that could be displaced palmarly as well as dorsally.
- **1847:** Robert William Smith provided a detailed account of this fracture in his book *A Treatise on Fractures in the Vicinity of Joints and on Certain Forms of Accidents and Congenital Dislocations*.
- He expanded on the characteristics of Colles' fracture and highlighted the volar displacement pattern, which he attributed to specific mechanisms of injury.

Purpose

- **Accurate Classification:** To differentiate Smith fractures from Colles fractures and other distal radius injuries based on displacement direction.
- **Guided Treatment:** To determine appropriate management strategies, including reduction techniques and the need for surgical intervention.

Procedure Overview

- **Imaging:**
- **X-rays:** AP and lateral views of the wrist are essential to confirm the diagnosis and assess displacement.
- **CT scans:** May be necessary in complex cases to evaluate articular involvement and fracture comminution.
- **Closed Reduction:**
- Performed in cases without severe comminution or instability. The wrist is manipulated to restore alignment and immobilized with a cast or splint.
- **Surgical Intervention:**
- Indicated in cases of significant comminution, articular involvement, or failure of closed reduction. Open reduction and internal fixation (ORIF) are commonly used techniques.

Results and Interpretation

- **X-Ray Findings:** Transverse fracture line through the distal radius with volar displacement or angulation of the distal fragment.
- Associated injuries may include fractures of the ulnar styloid or dislocation of the distal radioulnar joint (DRUJ).
- **CT Results:** Detailed assessment of comminution and articular surface involvement, critical for surgical planning.

Physiological Basis

- **Mechanism of Injury:** A fall onto a flexed wrist transmits force through the distal radius, resulting in a volar displacement pattern.
- **Anatomical Considerations:** The distal radius is the primary load-bearing structure in the wrist, making it prone to fractures under compressive and shear forces.

Clinical Applications

- **Non-Surgical Management:** Closed reduction and immobilization are effective for simple, stable fractures without articular involvement.
- **Surgical Management:** ORIF is preferred in unstable fractures, comminution, or those involving the articular surface.
- **Rehabilitation:** Gradual mobilization and physiotherapy are essential for restoring function and preventing stiffness.

Limitations and Technical Considerations

- **Imaging Limitations:** Plain radiographs may not provide sufficient detail in complex fractures, necessitating advanced imaging modalities like CT scans.
- **Reduction Challenges:** Achieving and maintaining reduction can be difficult in severely comminuted or unstable fractures.
- **Surgical Risks:** Potential complications include infection, nonunion, and stiffness.

Modern Relevance

- **Widespread Recognition:** Smith fractures remain an important consideration in wrist injuries, especially in falls involving flexed wrists.
- **Improved Techniques:** Advances

in imaging and surgical methods have significantly enhanced diagnostic accuracy and treatment outcomes.

Associated Conditions

- **Reverse Barton's Fracture:** An intra-articular variant of the Smith fracture involving volar displacement of the articular surface.
- **Ulnar Styloid Fractures:** Commonly associated with distal radius fractures and may complicate management.
- **DRUJ Dislocation:** Disruption of the distal radioulnar joint may occur in conjunction with Smith fractures.

Clinical Importance

- **Accurate Diagnosis:** Early identification and differentiation from Colles fractures are crucial to appropriate management.
- **Functional Preservation:** Proper reduction and stabilization are essential for preserving wrist function and preventing long-term complications.
- **Patient Education:** Educating patients on injury mechanisms and preventive measures, particularly in at-risk populations like the elderly.

References

Smith RW. On Fractures of the Bones of the Fore-arm in the Vicinity of the Wrist Joint. In: A Treatise on Fractures in the Vicinity of Joint and on Certain Forms of Accidental and Congenital Dislocations. Dublin: Hodges Smith. 1847:129-175.

Thurston AJ. 'Ao' or eponyms: the classification of wrist fractures. ANZ J Surg. 2005 May;75(5):347-55. [PMID 15932450]

Zhang Y. Clinical Epidemiology of Orthopedic Trauma. Thieme. 2012

Sprengel's deformity

Overview

Sprengel's deformity is a congenital anomaly characterized by elevation of the scapula, often accompanied by medial rotation of its inferior angle toward the spine. It typically presents with restricted shoulder abduction above 90 degrees and may occur unilaterally or bilaterally. Frequently associated with scoliosis and occasionally torticollis, Sprengel's deformity results from the failure of the scapula to descend from its embryonic position in the neck to its normal location in the posterior thorax. This condition is more common in girls and may have a genetic basis, with familial forms known as Corno's disease. It is often seen in conjunction with Klippel-Feil syndrome.

Historical Background

- **1863:** Moritz Michael Eulenburg (1811–1877) is believed to have first described the condition.
- **1891:** Otto Gerhard Karl Sprengel provided a detailed account of the deformity and its spectrum.
- **1908:** Vittorio Putti expanded upon the understanding of Sprengel's deformity, offering further insights into its morphology and associations.

Purpose

- **Diagnostic Clarity:** To identify and classify the deformity, distinguishing it from other shoulder or thoracic abnormalities.
- **Treatment Planning:** To provide a framework for surgical or non-surgical

interventions aimed at improving shoulder function and aesthetics.

Procedure Overview

- **Clinical Examination:**
- Visible elevation of the scapula with the medial rotation of its lower angle.
- Restricted shoulder abduction above 90 degrees.
- Assessment for scoliosis, torticollis, or other associated syndromic features.
- **Imaging Studies:**
- **X-rays:** To evaluate the scapular position, thoracic abnormalities, and associated scoliosis.
- **CT Scans or MRI:** To assess bone and soft tissue structures in complex cases or before surgical intervention.
- **Surgical Intervention (for severe cases):** Techniques such as the Woodward procedure or scapular relocation surgeries aim to improve shoulder function and cosmetic outcomes.

Results and Interpretation

- **Radiographic Findings:** High-riding scapula with medial rotation of its lower angle.
- Associated anomalies such as fused cervical vertebrae (in Klippel-Feil syndrome) or spinal curvature.
- **Post-Surgical Outcomes:** Improved shoulder mobility and appearance, though complete normalization is often not achievable.

Physiological Basis

- **Embryonic Development:** During fetal development, the scapula migrates from the neck to its normal position in the thorax. Failure of this descent leads to Sprengel's deformity.
- **Muscle and Ligament Involvement:** Soft tissue anomalies, including tight or shortened muscles and ligaments, further contribute to the deformity and restricted movement.

Clinical Applications

- **Non-Surgical Management:** Physical therapy to improve range of motion and strengthen surrounding muscles.
- **Surgical Management:** Reserved for severe cases where function and aesthetics are significantly impaired.

Limitations and Technical Considerations

- **Residual Deformity:** Even with surgical intervention, some degree of scapular elevation or asymmetry often persists.
- **Risk of Complications:** Surgery may carry risks such as nerve damage or impaired shoulder function.
- **Diagnostic Complexity:** Associated conditions such as Klippel-Feil syndrome may complicate diagnosis and management.

Modern Relevance

- **Advances in Surgery:** Modern surgical techniques offer better outcomes with reduced complication rates.
- **Multidisciplinary Approach:** Collaboration between orthopedists,

physiotherapists, and geneticists has improved patient care.

Associated Conditions

- **Klippel-Feil Syndrome:** A common association, characterized by fused cervical vertebrae.
- **Corno's Disease:** The familial form of Sprengel's deformity.
- **Scoliosis and Torticollis:** Frequently present as co-morbidities.

Clinical Importance

- **Early Detection:** Essential for planning interventions that optimize functional outcomes.
- **Functional and Cosmetic Impact:** Severe deformities can impair shoulder mobility and cause psychosocial distress due to appearance.
- **Patient Education:** Families benefit from genetic counseling and understanding the condition's progression and management options.

Sprengel's deformity highlights the intricate interplay between embryonic development, musculoskeletal anomalies, and clinical interventions, emphasizing the importance of tailored approaches for each patient.

References

Goldfarb CA, Yin Y, Gilula LA, Fisher AJ, Boyer MI. Wrist fractures: what the clinician wants to know. Radiology. 2001;219(1):11–28.

Ellis J. Smith's and Barton's fractures. A method of treatment. J Bone Joint Surg (Br). 1965;47(4):724–7.

M. M. Eulenburg: Hochgradige Dislocation der Scapula, bedingt durch Retraction des M. levator anguli und des oberen Teiles des M. cucullaris. Heilung mittels subcutaner Durchschneidung beider Muskeln und entsprechender Nachbehandlung. Archiv für klinische Chirurgie, Berlin, 1863, 4: 304.

O. K. Sprengel: Die angeborene Verschiebung des Schulterblattes nach oben. Archiv für klinische Chirurgie, Berlin, 1891, 42: 545-549.

V. Putti: Beitrag zur Aetiologie, Pathogenese und Behandlung des angeborenen Hochstandes des Schulterblattes. Fortschritte auf dem Gebiete der Röntgenstrahlen, 1908, 12: 328.

R. Corno: Scapolo alta congenita a carattere familiare. Clinca Pediatrica, Bologna, 1956, 38: 948-952.

Stieda Process

Overview

The Stieda process refers to the lateral tubercle of the posterior talar process, a bony structure on the talus that plays a critical role in the anatomy and biomechanics of the ankle. It consists of two tubercles, medial and lateral, separated by a groove through which the flexor hallucis longus (FHL) tendon passes. The Stieda process is associated with critical ligamentous attachments and, when prominent or ossified, is implicated in conditions such as posterior ankle impingement syndrome.

Historical Background

- **1908:** Christian Hermann Ludwig Stieda described this anatomical structure, linking it to posterior ankle pathologies.
- Subsequent studies clarified the functional anatomy and its implications in clinical conditions such as impingement syndromes.

Purpose

- **Anatomical Understanding:** To delineate the structure and role of the Stieda process in ankle biomechanics and its relationship to surrounding tendons and ligaments.
- **Diagnostic Relevance:** To aid in identifying posterior ankle impingement and differentiate it from related entities such as the os trigonum.
- **Surgical Planning:** Provides a framework for addressing conditions involving the Stieda process, such as chronic pain or impingement.

Procedure Overview

- **Clinical Examination:**
- Assessment of posterior ankle pain exacerbated by plantarflexion.
- Identification of swelling or tenderness in the posterior ankle region.
- **Imaging Studies:**
- **X-ray:** Identification of the prominent Stieda process or os trigonum.
- **MRI or CT Scan:** Detailed imaging to evaluate soft tissue involvement, including FHL tendon impingement or ligamentous injuries.
- **Surgical Intervention (if needed):**
- **Open Surgery:** Removal of the os trigonum or prominent Stieda process.
- **Arthroscopic Surgery:** A minimally invasive alternative for excising impinging structures.

Results and Interpretation

- **Radiographic Findings:** Ossified lateral tubercle visible on lateral ankle radiographs.
- Signs of posterior impingement, including soft tissue inflammation or FHL tendonopathy.
- **Post-Surgical Outcomes:** Relief from posterior ankle pain and improved range of motion, though recovery varies by severity.

Physiological Basis

- The *Stieda process* plays a key role in ankle stability, serving as an attachment site for the posterior talofibular ligament.
- The groove between the medial and lateral tubercles guides the FHL tendon, facilitating its smooth function.
- A prominent or ossified Stieda process may compress adjacent soft tissues during plantarflexion, leading to impingement syndromes.

Clinical Applications

- **Diagnostic Utility:** Imaging and clinical evaluation of the Stieda process help diagnose posterior ankle impingement and associated pathologies.
- **Surgical Intervention:** For persistent pain or functional limitations, surgical excision of the Stieda process or os trigonum is performed.

Limitations and Technical Considerations

- **Complex Anatomy:** The close proximity of ligaments, tendons, and the posterior ankle joint requires precise imaging and surgical technique.
- **Recovery Challenges:** Post-surgical recovery may be prolonged due to the intricate nature of posterior ankle structures.
- **Variable Symptomatology:** The Stieda process may be asymptomatic, complicating the decision for intervention.

Modern Relevance

- **Arthroscopic Advances:** Arthroscopic procedures have significantly reduced recovery times and complications associated with surgical treatment of posterior ankle impingement.
- **Wider Recognition:** Increasing awareness of posterior ankle pathologies has led to earlier diagnosis and management of conditions involving the Stieda process.

Associated Conditions

- **Posterior Ankle Impingement Syndrome:** Caused by compression of the Stieda process or os trigonum against posterior ankle structures during plantarflexion.
- **Flexor Hallucis Longus Tendinopathy:** Due to repetitive irritation within the groove between the tubercles.
- **Os Trigonum Syndrome:** An unossified Stieda process may present as an os trigonum with similar clinical manifestations.

Clinical Importance

- **Early Diagnosis:** Identification of the Stieda process in symptomatic patients prevents chronic impingement and tendon damage.
- **Surgical Relevance:** Surgical excision significantly improves outcomes in patients with persistent pain or limited ankle function.
- **Functional Restoration:** Enhances athletic performance and everyday mobility, especially in active individuals prone to repetitive ankle stress.

The Stieda process underscores the intricate interplay between bone, ligament, and tendon in the posterior ankle, emphasizing the need for precise diagnosis and tailored management approaches.

References

van Dijk C, de Leeuw P, Scholten P. Hindfoot Endoscopy for Posterior Ankle Impingement. J Bone Jt Surgery-American Vol 2009; 91: 287–98.

van Dijk CN, Scholten PE, Krips R. A 2-portal endoscopic approach for diagnosis and treatment of posterior ankle pathology. Arthrosc J Arthrosc Relat Surg 2000; 16: 871–6.

Stieda CHL. Über secundare Fusswurzelknochen. Arch Physiol Wissensch Med 1869; : 108–11.

Abramowitz Y, Wollstein R, Barzilay Y, et al. Outcome of resection of a symptomatic os trigonum. J Bone Joint Surg Am 2003; 85–A: 1051–7.

Straddle Fractures

Overview

Straddle fractures are a severe and distinct type of pelvic injury involving bilateral fractures of the pubic rami with potential disruption of the pelvic ring. These injuries often result from high-energy trauma, such as motor vehicle accidents, falls from heights, or crush injuries. Straddle fractures are associated with significant complications, including urogenital injuries, hemorrhage, and pelvic instability, requiring a multidisciplinary treatment approach.

Historical Background

- The term "straddle fracture" is descriptive, derived from the bilateral nature of the fractures resembling the positioning of the pelvis over an object. While the concept of pelvic ring fractures dates back to early anatomical studies, modern characterization and management strategies have evolved over the last few decades, particularly with advancements in radiological imaging and trauma surgery.

Purpose

- **The management of straddle fractures aims to:**
- Stabilize the *pelvic ring*.
- Control *hemorrhage.*
- Address *associated injuries*, especially urogenital trauma.
- Prevent long-term complications such as *pelvic instability* and *malunion.*
- Optimize recovery through *rehabilitation*

and *multidisciplinary care.*

Procedure Overview

- **Initial Assessment:** Patients often present after high-energy trauma with severe pelvic pain and visible deformity.
- Advanced Trauma Life Support (ATLS) principles guide initial evaluation to stabilize the patient and identify life-threatening conditions.
- **Imaging:**
- **X-rays:** Anteroposterior views are essential for identifying fractures.
- **CT scans:** Provide detailed information on fracture patterns, pelvic ring stability, and associated injuries.
- **MRI:** Occasionally used to evaluate soft tissue injuries or vascular complications.
- **Management:**
- **Hemorrhage Control:** Application of a pelvic binder or external fixation to control bleeding.
- **Angiographic embolization for vascular injuries.**
- **Surgical Intervention:** Open reduction and internal fixation (ORIF) for unstable fractures.
- **Percutaneous screw fixation for minimally displaced fractures.**
- **External fixation for temporary stabilization in hemodynamically unstable patients.**
- **Rehabilitation:** Early mobilization and physical therapy begin post-stabilization to restore function.

Results and Interpretation

- **Short-Term Outcomes:** Hemorrhage control and stabilization reduce early morbidity and mortality.
- **Surgical repair of pelvic instability improves pain and mobility.**
- **Long-Term Outcomes:** Successful management results in restored pelvic stability and function.
- Poor outcomes may include chronic pain, leg-length discrepancies, and urogenital dysfunction.

Physiological Basis

- The pelvic ring serves as the structural base for the spine and lower extremities, protecting vital organs within the pelvic cavity.
- High-energy trauma disrupts the bony and ligamentous integrity of the pelvic ring, leading to instability and associated injuries to vascular, urogenital, and neural structures.

Clinical Applications

- Straddle fractures are most commonly encountered in *trauma centers* and require *interdisciplinary care* involving trauma surgeons, orthopedic specialists, urologists, and rehabilitation therapists.
- Understanding the biomechanics of pelvic injuries is crucial for developing individualized treatment plans.

Limitations and Technical Considerations

- **Diagnostic Challenges:** Subtle fractures or incomplete disruptions may be missed on initial imaging.

- **Associated injuries to the urogenital system, bladder, or rectum require a high index of suspicion.**
- **Surgical Risks:** Infection, nonunion, and hardware failure are potential complications of surgical fixation.
- Managing soft tissue injuries alongside skeletal stabilization can be complex.

Modern Relevance

- With increasing incidences of high-speed vehicular trauma, *straddle fractures* remain a critical area of focus in modern trauma care.
- **Advances in** *angiographic embolization*, *minimally invasive surgery*, and *postoperative rehabilitation* have improved patient outcomes significantly.

Associated Conditions

- **Urogenital Injuries:** Bladder and urethral tears are common and require surgical repair.
- **Vascular Injuries:** Hemorrhage from pelvic vessels is life-threatening and necessitates prompt intervention.
- **Neurological Injuries:** Nerve damage in the pelvic region can lead to chronic pain and motor dysfunction.

Clinical Importance

- **Early Diagnosis:** Prompt identification of straddle fractures ensures timely intervention, reducing morbidity and mortality.
- **Comprehensive Management:** Multidisciplinary care is essential for addressing associated injuries and optimizing recovery.
- **Patient Counseling:** Patients should be informed about the risks of long-term complications, including pain, instability, and functional impairments, and the importance of adherence to rehabilitation protocols.

Straddle fractures underscore the complexity of managing high-energy pelvic injuries and the critical role of coordinated trauma care in improving patient outcomes.

References

"Pelvic Fractures". OrthoInfo - AAOS. February 2016. Retrieved 17 May 2018.

ATLS - Advanced Trauma Life Support - Student Course Manual (10 ed.). American College of Surgeons. 2018. pp. 89, 96–97. ISBN 9780996826235.

Peitzman, Andrew B.; Rhodes, Michael; Schwab, C. William (2008). The Trauma Manual: Trauma and Acute Care Surgery. Lippincott Williams & Wilkins. p. 322. ISBN 9780781762755.

Walls, Ron; Hockberger, Robert; Gausche-Hill, Marianne (2017). Rosen's Emergency Medicine - Concepts and Clinical Practice E-Book. Elsevier Health Sciences. pp. 577, 588. ISBN 9780323390163.

Walker, J (Nov 9–15, 2011). "Pelvic fractures: classification and nursing management". Nursing Standard. 26 (10): 49–57, quiz 58. doi:10.7748/ns2011.11.26.10.49.c8816. PMID 22206172.

"Fracture of the Pelvis". OrthoInfo. American Academy of Orthopaedic Surgeons.

Dimon, Theodore Jr. (2010). The body in motion : its evolution and design. Berkeley, Calif.: North Atlantic Books. pp. 49–56. ISBN 978-1556439704.

Young, JW; Resnik, CS (December 1990). "Fracture of the Pelvis: Current Concepts of Classification". AJR. American Journal of Roentgenology. 155 (6): 1169–75. doi:10.2214/ajr.155.6.2122661. PMID 2122661.

Lee, C; Porter, K (February 2007). "The prehospital management of pelvic fractures". Emergency Medicine Journal. 24 (2): 130–3. doi:10.1136/emj.2006.041384. PMC 2658194. PMID 17251627.

"Pelvic Fractures". The Lecturio Medical Concept Library. Retrieved 3 October 2021.

Silber J. & Flynn J. Changing Patterns of Pediatric Pelvic Fractures with Skeletal Maturation: Implications for Classification and Management. J Pediatr Orthop 2002;22:22-26

Torode I & Zieg D. Pelvic Fractures in Children J Pediatr Orthop 1985;5(1)76-84

Amorosa, L. High Energy Pediatric Pelvic and Acetabular Fractures Orthop Clin N Am 2014;45(4);483-500

Syme's amputation

Overview

Syme's amputation is a surgical procedure performed at the ankle joint, involving the removal of the foot while preserving the heel pad to create a weight-bearing residual limb. This technique revolutionized the approach to lower limb amputations by allowing patients to retain a functional, sensate stump capable of supporting prostheses and providing proprioception. The procedure remains an important option for lower limb salvage in severe trauma or disease.

Historical Background

- **1843:** James Syme, a Scottish surgeon, introduced this technique as a method to improve outcomes for patients requiring amputation due to severe trauma, gangrene, or infection.
- Prior to Syme's innovation, amputations for compound fractures of the tibia and fibula were typically performed at the thigh, leading to reduced mobility and functionality.
- Syme first demonstrated his procedure on a young woman with severe foot infection, emphasizing the preservation of the heel pad for weight-bearing.

Purpose

- **Functional Restoration:** To create a weight-bearing residual limb that retains proprioception and sensation.
- **Improved Mobility:** To provide patients with a stable base for prosthetic attachment, enabling ambulation.
- **Preservation of Limb Length:** To avoid the loss of the entire lower leg, improving patient quality of life and mobility.

Procedure Overview

- **Preoperative Preparation:**
- Evaluation of vascular supply, infection control, and patient-specific factors.
- Imaging studies to assess bone and soft tissue involvement.
- **Surgical Steps:**
- **Incision and Flap Creation:** A circular or elliptical incision around the ankle joint is made, extending to create a heel flap from the plantar surface.
- **Bone Resection:** Removal of the malleoli and talus while preserving the tibia and fibula.
- **Flap Positioning:** The heel flap is carefully placed over the distal tibia and fibula to form a cushion for weight-bearing.
- **Closure:** Secure suturing of the heel flap to ensure vascularity and stability.
- **Postoperative Care:**
- Monitoring for infection, vascular compromise, and proper wound healing.
- Gradual introduction of weight-bearing and prosthetic fitting.

Results and Interpretation

- **Functional Outcomes:** High patient satisfaction with the ability to bear weight directly on the residual limb.
- Enhanced mobility with prosthetic devices compared to higher-level amputations.

- **Complications:** Risks of wound dehiscence, infection, or necrosis of the heel flap.
- Occasional need for revision surgery due to poor healing or stump discomfort.

Physiological Basis

- The preservation of the heel pad provides a natural, sensate cushion for weight-bearing.
- Retention of tibial and fibular length allows for a biomechanically advantageous alignment for prostheses.
- Maintenance of proprioception aids in balance and coordination during ambulation.

Clinical Applications

- **Indications:** Severe trauma to the foot with preserved vascular supply to the heel pad.
- Chronic infections or non-reconstructable deformities.
- Malignant or benign tumors localized to the foot.
- **Rehabilitation:** Early prosthetic fitting enhances functional recovery and reduces dependency on assistive devices.

Limitations and Technical Considerations

- **Heel Pad Viability:** Success depends on ensuring adequate vascular supply to the heel flap.
- **Stump Management:** Improper alignment or flap tension can lead to complications like ulceration or delayed healing.
- **Prosthetic Design:** Requires specialized prostheses to account for the unique shape and load distribution of the Syme stump.

Modern Relevance

- **Prosthetic Advances:** Modern prostheses provide enhanced functionality and cosmetic outcomes for Syme amputees.
- **Global Accessibility:** The technique remains vital in regions where advanced reconstructive options are unavailable.
- **Surgical Refinements:** Improvements in surgical techniques and postoperative care have reduced complications and improved long-term outcomes.

Associated Conditions

- **Trauma:** Severe crush injuries or non-viable lower extremity conditions.
- **Infections:** Chronic osteomyelitis or soft tissue infections resistant to other treatments.
- **Vascular Disorders:** Critical limb ischemia with preserved heel pad perfusion.

Clinical Importance

- **Preservation of Function:** Retains proprioception and weight-bearing ability, enhancing patient mobility.
- **Improved Quality of Life:** Provides a stable and functional limb that enables walking and independence.
- **Versatility:** Offers a reliable alternative to higher-level amputations, especially in resource-limited settings.

Syme's amputation exemplifies how a surgical innovation can drastically improve patient outcomes, offering a balance between limb salvage and prosthetic adaptation.

References

J. Syme: Amputation at the ankle-joint. London and Edinburgh Monthly Journal of Medical Science, 1843, 3: 93-94.

The operation was first successfully performed by Syme on September 8, 1842.

A modification of Syme's amputation, known as Mackenzie's operation, was introduced by the Scottish surgeon Richard James Mackenzie (1821-1854) six years later:

R. J. Mackenzie: On amputation at the ankle-joint by internal lateral flap. Monthly Journal of Medical Science, Edinburgh, 1849, 9: 951-954.

Thomas View

Overview

Thomas View is a specialized radiographic projection used to assess the shoulder girdle, particularly in cases of acute trauma and shoulder pathologies. It involves positioning the patient to optimize visualization of the shoulder structures, including the glenohumeral joint, clavicle, and scapula. This view is crucial for diagnosing injuries and conditions affecting the shoulder girdle.

Historical Background

- **19th Century:** Hugh Owen Thomas, widely regarded as the "father of British Orthopaedics," pioneered various orthopedic practices, including diagnostic and therapeutic advancements.

- Thomas's influence extended to standardized approaches in imaging and treatment, setting the groundwork for radiographic techniques such as the *Thomas View.*

- The Thomas family had a long lineage of bone-setters, dating back to the mid-18th century, which heavily influenced Hugh Thomas's orthopedic innovations.

Purpose

- **Diagnostic Clarity:** To provide a detailed radiographic view of the shoulder girdle, particularly in trauma cases.

- **Fracture Identification:** Essential for detecting fractures of the clavicle, scapula, or proximal humerus.

- **Joint Assessment:** Aids in evaluating

dislocations and other abnormalities of the glenohumeral joint.

Procedure Overview

- **Patient Positioning:**
- The patient is either sitting or lying down, with the cassette placed on the shoulder region.
- The arm may need to be positioned according to the specific injury or suspected pathology.
- **Beam Orientation:** The radiographic beam is directed toward the armpit, ensuring proper alignment with the shoulder structures.
- **Monitoring:** In cases of acute trauma, the physician should personally monitor and assist in positioning to avoid exacerbating the injury.
- **Image Capture:** High-quality radiographs are obtained with precise beam angulation to capture the shoulder anatomy comprehensively.

Results and Interpretation

- **Fracture Visualization:** Clear imaging of fractures in the scapula, clavicle, or humerus.
- **Joint Evaluation:** Identifies dislocations or malalignment in the glenohumeral or acromioclavicular joints.
- **Soft Tissue Assessment:** Although limited, can provide indirect signs of soft tissue injury or swelling.

Physiological Basis

- The shoulder girdle is a complex anatomical structure composed of bones, joints, ligaments, and muscles. The *Thomas View* leverages the axillary perspective to minimize overlap of surrounding structures, offering an unobstructed view of the shoulder anatomy.

Clinical Applications

- **Trauma Cases:** Critical for assessing fractures or dislocations in the shoulder region.
- **Chronic Conditions:** Useful in diagnosing degenerative changes or deformities in the shoulder girdle.
- **Pre-Surgical Planning:** Provides detailed imaging for orthopedic surgical interventions.

Limitations and Technical Considerations

- **Positioning Challenges:** Acute pain or trauma may make positioning difficult without causing patient discomfort.
- **Radiation Exposure:** Care must be taken to minimize unnecessary exposure, especially in younger patients.
- **Soft Tissue Limitations:** Limited capability to assess soft tissue injuries, which may require complementary imaging modalities like MRI.

Modern Relevance

- **Advances in Imaging:** While modern imaging methods like CT and MRI are increasingly used, the Thomas View remains a vital, cost-effective tool for initial assessments.

- **Trauma Care:** Still widely utilized in emergency settings to rapidly evaluate shoulder injuries.
- **Standardization:** Continues to serve as a benchmark for shoulder radiography in orthopedic diagnostics.

Associated Conditions

- **Fractures:** Scapula, clavicle, or proximal humerus fractures.
- **Dislocations:** Glenohumeral or acromioclavicular joint dislocations.
- **Arthritic Changes:** Degenerative joint disease or osteoarthritis.

Clinical Importance

- **Trauma Diagnosis:** Provides critical information for immediate management of shoulder injuries.
- **Surgical Planning:** Essential for orthopedic surgeons to determine the extent of injury and guide surgical interventions.
- **Accessibility:** An important tool in settings where advanced imaging modalities may not be readily available.

The Thomas View exemplifies the enduring relevance of foundational radiographic techniques in orthopedic diagnostics and trauma care, highlighting Hugh Thomas's lasting legacy in the field.

References

Pavlov H, Warren RF, Weiss CB Jr, et al. The roentgenographic evaluation of anterior shoulder instability. Clin Orthop Relat Res. 1985; (194):153-8.

Tillaux Fracture

Overview

Tillaux Fracture is a Salter-Harris Type III fracture of the anterolateral tibial epiphysis, typically occurring in adolescents due to a rotational injury. It is often associated with avulsion of the anterior tibiofibular ligament. This injury is frequently underdiagnosed as a sprain, but accurate detection is crucial for proper management to prevent long-term complications.

Historical Background

- **1822:** Sir Astley Paston Cooper described fractures of the lateral tibia in adults, setting the foundation for understanding tibial injuries.
- **1876:** Paul Jules Tillaux conducted cadaveric studies demonstrating that rotational stress on the anterior inferior tibiofibular ligament could result in avulsion fractures of the anterolateral tibial epiphysis.
- **1899:** Henri Chaput expanded on Tillaux's findings by utilizing roentgenograms to identify fractures in the dorsal lip of the tibia. His observations were later linked to Tillaux's descriptions, leading to the term Tillaux-Chaput fracture.

Purpose

- **Accurate Diagnosis:** To differentiate Tillaux fractures from simple ankle sprains, which they are often mistaken for in adolescents.
- **Treatment Guidance:** To assess fracture displacement, which determines

whether conservative or surgical intervention is required.

Procedure Overview

- **Imaging Modalities:**
- Conventional X-rays (AP, lateral, and mortise views) are the initial diagnostic tools.
- CT scans provide superior sensitivity, especially for detecting displacements >2 mm, which are indications for surgical intervention.
- **Clinical Examination:** The injury may present as swelling and localized tenderness at the anterior ankle with a history of twisting trauma.
- **Surgical Indications:** Open reduction is considered if there is significant displacement or joint incongruity.

Results and Interpretation

- **X-ray Findings:** Visible fracture line through the anterolateral tibial epiphysis on conventional radiographs.
- **CT Findings:** Accurate measurement of fracture displacement and identification of associated injuries.
- **Clinical Features:** Pain exacerbated by movement, swelling, and tenderness localized to the lateral ankle.

Physiological Basis

- The tibial epiphysis ossifies in a sequence, beginning medially and progressing laterally. During late adolescence, the medial portion of the growth plate is fused, while the lateral portion remains open, making the anterolateral epiphysis vulnerable to avulsion injuries caused by rotational forces.

Clinical Applications

- **Orthopedic Trauma:** Used to diagnose and manage adolescent ankle injuries.
- **Surgical Planning:** Guides surgeons in deciding whether open reduction is necessary based on fracture displacement.
- **Rehabilitation:** Informs physiotherapists about appropriate weight-bearing protocols and exercises for recovery.

Limitations and Technical Considerations

- **Diagnostic Challenges:** May be misdiagnosed as an ankle sprain, especially in cases without significant fracture displacement.
- **Imaging Limitations:** Conventional X-rays may not detect minor displacements, necessitating CT scans for accurate diagnosis.
- **Surgical Risks:** Open reduction can lead to complications such as infection or delayed healing.

Modern Relevance

- **Advancements in Imaging:** The availability of CT scans has significantly improved diagnostic accuracy and treatment planning for Tillaux fractures.
- **Increased Awareness:** Greater understanding among clinicians has reduced the misdiagnosis rate of these injuries as simple sprains.

Associated Conditions

- **Chaput Fracture:** A similar injury involving the posterolateral tibial epiphysis.
- **Anterior Tibiofibular Ligament Injury:** Commonly associated with Tillaux fractures.
- **Ankle Sprains:** Often misdiagnosed as sprains due to overlapping clinical features.

Clinical Importance

- **Early Detection:** Identifying the injury early prevents long-term complications like growth disturbances and joint incongruity.
- **Surgical Indications:** Displacement >2 mm requires surgical intervention for proper realignment.
- **Prognostic Value:** Proper management ensures favorable outcomes, including restored joint function and alignment.

The Tillaux Fracture represents a critical orthopedic condition that underscores the importance of combining clinical vigilance with advanced imaging for accurate diagnosis and effective management.

References

Cooper AP. On dislocation of the ankle joints. In: A treatise on dislocations and on fractures of the joints. London, 1822

Tillaux PJ. Recherches expérimentales et cliniques sur le mécanisme de la production des luxations coxo-fémorales en arrière. 1876

Tillaux PJ. Traité de chirurgie clinique. Volume II p856-868. 1891

Chaput H. Les fractures malléolaires du cou-de-pied et les accidents du travail. [Malleolar instep fractures and occupational injuries] Paris, Masson 1908.

von Laer L. Classification, diagnosis, and treatment of transitional fractures of the distal part of the tibia. J Bone Joint Surg Am. 1985 Jun;67(5):687-98. [PMID 3997921]

Lebrun A. L'appareil de Tillaux dans les fractures de la diaphyse du fémur. Bruxelles: 1880

Dias LS, Giegerich CR. Fractures of the distal tibial epiphysis in adolescence. J Bone Joint Surg Am. 1983 Apr;65(4):438-44. [PMID 6833316]

Kumar N, Prasad M. Tillaux fracture of the ankle in an adult: a rare injury. J Foot Ankle Surg. 2014 Nov-Dec;53(6):757-8. [PMID 25128312]

Sharma B, Reddy IS, Meanock C. The adult Tillaux fracture: one not to miss. BMJ Case Rep. 2013; 2013: bcr2013200105. [PMC3736651]

Koury SI, Stone CK, Harrell G, La Charité DD. Recognition and management of Tillaux fractures in adolescents. Pediatr Emerg Care. 1999 Feb;15(1):37-9. [PMID 10069311]

Duchesneau S, Fallat LM. The Tillaux fracture. J Foot Ankle Surg. 1996 Mar-Apr;35(2):127-33; discussion 189. [PMID 8722880]

Horn BD, Crisci K, Krug M, Pizzutillo PD, MacEwen GD. Radiologic evaluation of juvenile tillaux fractures of the distal tibia. J Pediatr Orthop. 2001 Mar-Apr;21(2):162-4. [PMID 11242242]

Toddler's Fracture

Overview

Toddler's fracture, also referred to as childhood accidental spiral tibial (CAST) fracture, is a type of nondisplaced spiral or oblique fracture of the distal tibia that commonly affects ambulatory children aged 9 months to 3 years. This injury typically occurs due to rotational forces applied to the tibia while the foot remains fixed, such as during tripping or falling. These fractures are challenging to diagnose because they often present without a clear history of trauma and with nonspecific symptoms like limping or refusal to bear weight.

Historical Background

The term toddler's fracture was introduced in 1964 by Dunbar et al. to describe the characteristic fracture of the distal tibia in young children. The injury was reclassified in the 1990s to CAST fracture to account for a broader age range of up to 8 years. Since its initial description, the understanding and management of toddler's fractures have evolved, particularly with advancements in diagnostic imaging and treatment protocols.

Purpose

- **The goals of managing toddler's fractures are:**
- *Early diagnosis* to minimize unnecessary pain and immobilization.
- *Appropriate immobilization* to allow healing while avoiding complications.
- *Exclusion of differential diagnoses*, including nonaccidental trauma, malignancy, or infections.

Procedure Overview

- **Clinical Presentation:**
- Symptoms include refusal to bear weight, limping, or localized tenderness on the tibia.
- Often no overt history of trauma; parents may report mild falls or tripping episodes.
- **Diagnostic Workup:**
- **Radiographs:** Initial imaging includes anteroposterior and lateral views. Fracture lines may be difficult to detect early but become apparent on follow-up radiographs within 10–14 days.
- **Internal Oblique Views:** Help improve fracture detection rates in some cases.
- **Ultrasound:** Can be utilized to detect fracture-associated hematoma in ambiguous cases.

Treatment:

- **Conservative Management:** Immobilization with a controlled ankle motion (CAM) boot or a short leg back slab for 3–4 weeks.
- **Rehabilitation:** Gradual return to weight-bearing and normal activity following immobilization.

Results and Interpretation

- **Short-Term Outcomes:** Most fractures heal uneventfully with conservative treatment, and children regain full function within weeks.
- **Follow-Up:** Repeat imaging may show evidence of healing, confirming the diag-

nosis in cases initially suspected but not visualized.

Physiological Basis

- Toddler's fractures occur due to the biomechanical vulnerability of the pediatric tibia to rotational forces. The tibia in young children has a more pliable cortical structure than in adults, allowing for spiral fractures under stress without significant displacement.

Clinical Applications

- **Pediatric Orthopedics:** Routine cases of limping or refusal to walk in toddlers often necessitate consideration of toddler's fractures in the differential diagnosis.
- **Emergency Medicine:** Early recognition in emergency settings prevents unnecessary delays in immobilization and reduces parental anxiety.

Limitations and Technical Considerations

- **Challenges in Diagnosis:** Absence of a clear trauma history and nonspecific symptoms can lead to delayed recognition.
- **Initial radiographs may fail to identify fractures; repeated imaging is often necessary.**
- **Differential Diagnosis:** Conditions such as malignancy, infections (osteomyelitis), or nonaccidental injuries must be ruled out, especially in ambiguous cases.

Modern Relevance

- Toddler's fractures remain a common pediatric injury in ambulatory children. **Advances in** imaging, such as the use of ultrasound, have improved diagnostic accuracy. The focus on noninvasive and family-friendly treatment strategies, like CAM boots, highlights modern trends in pediatric orthopedic care.

Associated Conditions

- **Nonaccidental Trauma:** Spiral fractures in young children can sometimes indicate abuse; careful documentation and evaluation of the history are essential.
- **Infections or Malignancy:** Differential diagnoses must include osteomyelitis and neoplasms, particularly when clinical findings are atypical.

Clinical Importance

- **Timely Diagnosis:** Early recognition and management ensure rapid recovery and prevent unnecessary complications.
- **Conservative Treatment:** CAM boots and short leg splints reduce the need for more restrictive casting, offering a child- and family-friendly option.
- **Educational Counseling:** Parents should be reassured about the benign nature of the injury and educated on avoiding further trauma during recovery.

Toddler's fractures illustrate the importance of a careful clinical assessment and family-centered management approach in pediatric care. Despite their challenging diagnosis, these injuries generally have excellent outcomes when properly managed.

References

Tenenbein M, Reed MH, Black GB. The toddler's fracture revisited. Am J Emerg Med. 1990;8(3):208–11. [PubMed]

Sarmah A. 'Toddler's fracture'? A recognised entity. Arch Dis Child. 1995;72(4):376. [PMC free article] [PubMed]

Dunbar JS, Owen HF, Nogrady MB, Mcleese R. Obscure tibial fracture of infants: the toddler's fracture. J Can Assoc Radiol. 1964;15:136–44. [PubMed] [Google Scholar]

Mellick LB, Milker L, Egsieker E. Childhood accidental spiral tibial (CAST) fractures. Pediatr Emerg Care. 1999;15(5):307–9. [PubMed] [Google Scholar]

Clancy J, Pieterse J, Robertson P, McGrath D, Beattie TF. Toddler's fracture. J Accid Emerg Med. 1996;13(5):366–7. [PMC free article] [PubMed] [Google Scholar]

Sapru K, Cooper JG. Management of the toddler's fracture with and without initial radiological evidence. Eur J Emerg Med. 2014;21(6):451–4. [PubMed] [Google Scholar]

Lewis D, Logan P. Sonographic diagnosis of toddler's fracture in the emergency department. J Clin Ultrasound. 2006;34(4):190–4. [PubMed] [Google Scholar]

Seguin J, Brody D, Li P. Nationwide survey on current management strategies of toddler's fractures. CJEM. 2017 Jul;:26. Epub ahead of print. [Google Scholar]

Halsey MF, Finzel KC, Carrion WV, Haralabatos SS, Gruber MA, Meinhard BP. Toddler's fracture: presumptive diagnosis and treatment. J Pediatr Orthop. 2001;21(2):152–6. [PubMed] [Google Scholar]

Schuh AM, Whitlock KB, Klein EJ. Management of toddler's fractures in the pediatric emergency department. Pediatr Emerg Care. 2016;32(7):452–4. [PMC free article] [PubMed] [Google Scholar]

Bauer JM, Lovejoy SA. Toddler's fractures: time to weight-bear with regard to immobilization type and radiographic monitoring. J Pediatr Orthop. 2017 Jan;:30. Epub ahead of print. [PubMed] [Google Scholar]

Adamich JS, Camp M. Do all toddler's fractures need to be managed by orthopaedic surgeons? CJEM. 2017;19(Suppl 1):S77–8. [Google Scholar]

Shravat BP, Harrop SN, Kane TP. Toddler's fracture. J Accid Emerg Med. 1996;13(1):59–61. [PMC free article] [PubMed] [Google Scholar]

Mellick LB, Reesor K. Spiral tibial fractures of children: a commonly accidental spiral long bone fracture. Am J Emerg Med. 1990;8(3):234–7. [PubMed] [Google Scholar]

Roche A, Brown P, Rani S, Landes C, Sampath J. "Toddlers" fracture: the importance of a complete clinical assessment. Emerg Med J. 2009;26(Suppl 1):11.

Torus Fracture

Overview

Torus fracture, also known as a buckle fracture, is a common injury in children caused by compressive forces applied to a long bone, usually following a fall. It occurs when the bony cortex on one side compresses and bulges without breaking completely. Torus fractures are stable, low-risk injuries that typically heal without complications. These fractures are most commonly seen in the distal radius and result from falls, particularly onto an outstretched hand (FOOSH).

Historical Background

The term torus derives from the Latin word meaning "protuberance" or "swelling," reflecting the bulging deformation seen in this type of fracture. While the exact historical documentation of torus fractures is unclear, their recognition became prominent as pediatric orthopedic care evolved, highlighting the unique biomechanical properties of children's bones.

Purpose

- **The management of torus fractures aims to:**
- *Alleviate pain* and ensure comfort.
- *Facilitate natural healing* with minimal intervention.
- *Prevent unnecessary treatment* and follow-up, as highlighted by recent research like the FORCE study.

Procedure Overview

- **Clinical Presentation:**
- Pain and tenderness localized to the fracture site, commonly the distal radius.
- Swelling and discomfort, often exacerbated by movement or palpation.
- No significant deformity due to the stability of the fracture.

Diagnosis:

- **Radiographic Imaging:** Torus fractures are best visualized on X-rays, with anterior/posterior and lateral projections revealing the characteristic bulging of the cortex.
- Differentiation from other fractures is crucial to prevent overtreatment.

Treatment:

- **Immobilization Options:** Splinting for comfort and stabilization.
- Bandaging without follow-up, as shown to be effective in the FORCE study.
- Routine follow-ups and interventions are typically unnecessary.

Results and Interpretation

- **Healing Process:** Most torus fractures heal within 2–4 weeks without complications.
- **Pain and swelling subside quickly with conservative treatment.**
- **Outcomes:** Comparable pain relief, function, and complication rates between splinting and simple bandaging, as demonstrated by the FORCE study.

Physiological Basis

- Children's bones have a higher collagen-to-bone ratio, making them more pliable and less prone to complete fractures. The trabecular structure of the bone absorbs compressive forces, leading to buckling rather than fracturing. This unique biomechanical property explains why torus fractures are common in the pediatric population and rarely occur in adults.

Clinical Applications

- **Pediatric Orthopedics:** Torus fractures serve as a classic example of the need for age-specific approaches in managing orthopedic injuries.
- **Emergency Medicine:** Efficient and accurate diagnosis in emergency settings prevents overtreatment and unnecessary follow-ups.

Limitations and Technical Considerations

- **Overtreatment:** Historically, torus fractures were immobilized in casts, leading to unnecessary medical visits and discomfort.
- **Diagnosis Challenges:** Differentiating between torus fractures and more severe injuries (e.g., greenstick fractures) requires careful evaluation of radiographs.
- **Parent Education:** Clear communication is essential to reassure parents about the benign nature of this injury.

Modern Relevance

- The *FORCE study (2022)* demonstrated that immobilization in a splint or cast is not always necessary for torus fractures. The study revolutionized treatment protocols, emphasizing the efficacy of simple bandaging and no routine follow-up. This approach reduces healthcare costs, minimizes patient inconvenience, and aligns with evidence-based practices.

Associated Conditions

- **Greenstick Fractures:** While both involve incomplete fractures, greenstick fractures result in bending with cortical disruption on one side, distinguishing them from torus fractures.
- **Soft Tissue Injuries:** Occasionally, minor swelling or bruising accompanies torus fractures but resolves with rest and immobilization.

Clinical Importance

- **Rapid Recovery:** Torus fractures typically heal quickly and uneventfully, ensuring a swift return to normal activities.
- **Avoidance of Complications:** The stability of these fractures reduces the risk of long-term sequelae.
- **Evidence-Based Practice:** Recent studies provide robust data supporting non-invasive management, reshaping the standard of care for pediatric fractures.
- **Reassurance for Parents:** Clear guidance and simple management strategies improve patient and caregiver satisfaction.

Torus fractures exemplify the resilience of pediatric bones and highlight the importance of tailoring treatment approaches to the unique needs of children. By embracing modern evidence-based protocols, healthcare providers can deliver effective, efficient, and patient-centered care.

References

Naranje, SM; Erali, RA; Warner WC, Jr; Sawyer, JR; Kelly, DM (June 2016). "Epidemiology of Pediatric Fractures Presenting to Emergency Departments in the United States". Journal of Pediatric Orthopedics. 36 (4): e45-8. doi:10.1097/BPO.0000000000000595. PMID 26177059. S2CID 36351361.

Della-Giustina, K; Della-Giustina, DA (November 1999). "Emergency department evaluation and treatment of pediatric orthopedic injuries". Emergency Medicine Clinics of North America. 17 (4): 895–922, vii. doi:10.1016/s0733-8627(05)70103-6. PMID 10584108.

Sharp, JW; Edwards, RM (August 2019). "Core curriculum illustration: pediatric buckle fracture of the distal radius". Emergency Radiology. 26 (4): 483–484. doi:10.1007/s10140-017-1524-4. PMID 28593329. S2CID 3984890.

Wheeless, Clifford R.; Nunley, James A.; Urbaniak, James R. Wheeless' Textbook of Orthopaedics. Data Trace Internet Publishing, LLC.

Randsborg, PH; Sivertsen, EA (October 2009). "Distal radius fractures in children: substantial difference in stability between buckle and greenstick fractures". Acta Orthopaedica. 80 (5): 585–9. doi:10.3109/17453670903316850. PMC 2823323. PMID 19916694.

van Bosse, HJ; Patel, RJ; Thacker, M; Sala, DA (July 2005). "Minimalistic approach to treating wrist torus fractures". Journal of Pediatric Orthopedics. 25 (4): 495–500. doi:10.1097/01.bpo.0000161098.38716.9b. PMID 15958903. S2CID 33574847.

Firmin, F; Crouch, R (July 2009). "Splinting versus casting of "torus" fractures to the distal radius in the paediatric patient presenting at the emergency department (ED): a literature review". International Emergency Nursing. 17 (3): 173–8. doi:10.1016/j.ienj.2009.03.006. PMID 19577205.

Patrice Eiff, M.; L. Hatch, Robert (2003). "Boning up on common pediatric fractures". Contemporary Pediatrics.

Perry, Daniel C.; Achten, Juul; Knight, Ruth; Appelbe, Duncan; Dutton, Susan J.; Dritsaki, Melina; Mason, James M.; Roland, Damian T.; Messahel, Shrouk; Widnall, James; Costa, Matthew L.; Ahmad, Rahail; Alcock, Anastasia; Appelboam, Andrew; Armour, Lisa (2022-07-02). "Immobilisation of torus fractures of the wrist in children (FORCE): a randomised controlled equivalence trial in the UK". The Lancet. 400 (10345): 39–47. doi:10.1016/S0140-6736(22)01015-7. ISSN 0140-6736. PMID 35780790.

Nice.org.uk. 2020. Overview | Fractures (Non-Complex): Assessment And Management | Guidance | NICE. [online] Available at: <https://www.nice.org.uk/guidance/ng38> [Accessed 21 December 2020].

Trendelenburg's symptom

Overview

Trendelenburg's Symptom is a clinical sign indicative of static insufficiency in the gluteal muscles, most notably seen in cases of congenital hip dislocation and other hip joint pathologies. It is characterized by the tilting of the pelvis towards the unaffected side when weight-bearing on the affected leg, often accompanied by a compensatory shift in the upper body. This symptom can occur unilaterally or bilaterally and is associated with a waddling gait in bilateral cases.

Historical Background

- **1860s:** Friedrich Trendelenburg, a German surgeon, formally described this clinical observation in relation to hip joint pathologies, giving it his name.
- **1867:** Guillaume Benjamin Amand Duchenne de Boulogne, a French neurologist, correlated the symptom with gluteal muscle paralysis, extending its clinical understanding to neurological causes. Purpose
- **Diagnostic Tool:** To identify conditions involving hip joint dysfunction or gluteal muscle weakness.
- **Assessment of Gait Abnormalities:** Evaluates the extent of pelvic instability during ambulation.

Procedure Overview

- **Clinical Examination:**
- The patient is asked to stand on one leg (the affected side).
- Observations are made for pelvic tilt and compensatory body movements.
- **Trendelenburg Test:** Positive if the pelvis tilts downward on the side opposite to the weight-bearing leg.

Results and Interpretation

- **Positive Sign:** Indicates weakness or paralysis of the gluteus medius and minimus muscles.
- Suggestive of conditions such as hip dislocation, gluteal muscle paralysis, or advanced hip osteoarthritis.
- **Negative Sign:** Suggests intact gluteal muscle function and stable hip joint mechanics.

Physiological Basis

- The *gluteus medius* and *gluteus minimus* muscles stabilize the pelvis during single-leg stance by counteracting the pull of gravity on the unsupported side.
- In cases of weakness or dysfunction of these muscles, the pelvis tilts downward on the contralateral side, causing the characteristic Trendelenburg gait.

Clinical Applications

- **Orthopedics:** Diagnosis of hip dislocation, Perthes disease, and femoral neck fractures.
- **Neurology:** Identifies gluteal muscle paralysis due to conditions such as poliomyelitis or nerve injuries.
- **Rehabilitation:** Guides physical therapists in designing strengthening programs for the hip abductors.

Limitations and Technical Considerations

- **Non-Specificity:** The sign can be caused by various conditions, necessitating further diagnostic tests for accurate identification.
- **Observer Dependence:** Clinical skill and experience are required to accurately interpret the sign.
- **Bilateral Cases:** In bilateral hip dislocations or gluteal muscle weakness, the swaying gait may complicate the interpretation of individual leg involvement.

Modern Relevance

- **Refined Diagnostics:** Advances in imaging, such as MRI and gait analysis, complement Trendelenburg's symptom in confirming the underlying pathology.
- **Continued Use:** Despite technological advancements, it remains a valuable bedside test due to its simplicity and effectiveness in clinical settings.

Associated Conditions

- **Congenital Hip Dislocation:** Most commonly associated with Trendelenburg's symptom.
- **Perthes Disease:** Late stages of osteochondropathia deformans coxae juvenilis.
- **Gluteal Muscle Paralysis:** Due to poliomyelitis or nerve injury.
- **Advanced Osteoarthritis:** Leading to functional weakness of the hip abductors.
- **Femoral Neck Fractures:** Impacting hip joint stability and muscle attachment.

Clinical Importance

- **Early Detection:** Identifying congenital hip dislocation or muscle weakness early can prevent long-term complications like gait abnormalities.
- **Monitoring Progression:** Used in rehabilitation settings to assess improvement in muscle strength and hip stability.
- **Prognostic Value:** Indicates the severity of pelvic instability and aids in planning surgical or therapeutic interventions.

Trendelenburg's Symptom remains a cornerstone in clinical orthopedics and neurology, bridging historical insights with modern diagnostic precision to address a range of hip joint and muscular pathologies.

References

F. Trendelenburg: Über den Gang bei angeborener Hüftgelenksluxation. Deutsche medicinische Wochenschrift, Berlin, 1895, 21: 21-24.

Trevor's disease

Overview

Trevor's Disease, also known as dysplasia epiphysealis hemimelica, is a rare congenital bone developmental disorder characterized by localized overgrowth of cartilage, primarily affecting one limb. The condition typically involves the lower extremities, most commonly in the ankle region, although the upper limbs can be affected in rarer cases. The overgrowth resembles osteochondromas histologically, but the disorder is distinct and isolated to a single limb, often favoring one side (medial or lateral). The exact cause of Trevor's disease remains unknown, with an uncertain genetic basis.

Historical Background

- **1926:** The condition was first described by French surgeons Albert Mouchet and Joseph Belot, who documented localized cartilage overgrowth causing limb deformities.- 1956: Thomas John Fairbank proposed the term "dysplasia epiphysealis hemimelica" to describe the disease's unique presentation and predilection for one side of a limb.- 1959: David Trevor further refined the description and boundaries of the disorder, lending his name to the condition. Purpose
- **Diagnostic Understanding:** To recognize and classify an uncommon skeletal disorder causing asymmetrical limb deformity.
- **Guidance for Management:** To determine appropriate treatment approaches to alleviate symptoms and restore limb function.

Procedure Overview

- **Clinical Presentation:**
- Patients often present with an asymmetrical limb deformity, noticeable by uneven limb growth or swelling, typically around the ankle.
- Symptoms may include pain, joint stiffness, and limited range of motion.
- **Diagnostic Imaging:**
- **X-rays:** Reveal irregular cartilaginous overgrowth and bone deformity.
- **MRI/CT scans:** Provide detailed views of cartilage involvement and the extent of deformity, aiding surgical planning.
- **Histological Examination:** Confirms the cartilaginous growth's resemblance to osteochondroma.

Results and Interpretation

- **Typical Findings:**
- Localized cartilaginous overgrowth confined to a single limb, often centered around epiphyses or joints.
- Asymmetry and predilection for either the medial or lateral side of the affected limb.
- **Prognosis:** While not life-threatening, untreated cases may result in functional impairment and chronic pain.

Physiological Basis

- The condition arises from an abnormal proliferation of cartilage in the epiphyses, leading to asymmetric limb growth and deformity.
- The cartilage overgrowth mimics the histological characteristics of

osteochondroma but differs in its localized and unilateral presentation.

Clinical Applications

- **Orthopedic Surgery:** Used to correct deformities, relieve joint pain, and restore function.
- **Physical Therapy:** Helps in managing stiffness and improving the range of motion post-surgery.
- **Pediatric Monitoring:** Vital for early detection and management, especially during growth spurts.

Limitations and Technical Considerations

- **Misdiagnosis Risk:** Can be mistaken for osteochondroma or other bone growth disorders.
- **Complexity of Surgery:** Requires precise imaging to ensure complete excision of cartilaginous overgrowth without damaging surrounding structures.
- **Recurrence Potential:** Incomplete surgical removal may lead to recurrence.

Modern Relevance

- **Advancements in Imaging:** MRI and CT provide improved diagnostic accuracy, enabling detailed mapping of affected areas for surgical intervention.
- **Refined Surgical Techniques:** Arthroscopic and minimally invasive approaches have reduced morbidity associated with traditional surgeries.
- **Genetic Studies:** Ongoing research aims to uncover potential genetic links to enhance early detection and preventive measures.

Associated Conditions

- **Osteochondroma:** Histological resemblance but distinct in its systemic, rather than localized, presentation.
- **Developmental Limb Deformities:** Trevor's disease is often considered in differential diagnosis alongside conditions such as Ollier's disease or multiple epiphyseal dysplasia.

Clinical Importance

- **Early Diagnosis:** Critical to prevent long-term functional impairment and deformity.
- **Surgical Correction:** Essential for alleviating symptoms and improving quality of life, especially in severe cases.
- **Prognostic Value:** Early intervention typically results in good functional outcomes, with minimal recurrence.
- **Pediatric Relevance:** Focused monitoring during growth periods is essential to manage progression effectively.

Trevor's disease remains a significant, albeit rare, condition in pediatric orthopedics, with modern diagnostic and surgical advancements improving outcomes and offering a better quality of life to affected individuals.

References

A. Mouchet, J. Belot:La tarsomégalie. Journal de radiologie et d'electrologie, Paris, 1926, 10: 289-293.

D. Trevor: Tarso-epiphyseal aclasis: A congenital error of epiphyseal development. Journal of Bone and Joint Surgery, London, 1950; 32B: 204-213.

T. J. Fairbank: Dysplasia epiphysealis hemimelica (tarso-epiphyseal aclasis). Journal of Bone and Joint Surgery, London, 1956, 38B: 237-257.

H.-R. Wiedemann, M. Mann, P. Spreter von Kreudenstein: Dysplasia epiphysealis hemimelia. Trevor disease: Severe manifesstation in a child. European Journal of Pediatrics, Berlin, 1982, 136: 311-316.

Unsolved Fracture

Overview

Unsolved fracture refers to the intracapsular fracture of the neck of the femur, a condition historically and contemporarily marked by challenges in treatment and outcomes. This type of fracture continues to elude definitive solutions due to high failure rates in union, frequent complications, and the debate between surgical and conservative management. Such fractures are increasingly common in aging populations, particularly in individuals with osteoporosis, and are accompanied by significant disability and morbidity.

Historical Background

- The term "unsolved fracture" was coined by *Kellogg Speed in 1934* during a presentation to the American College of Surgeons. He highlighted the longstanding controversies and suboptimal outcomes associated with femoral neck fractures, a challenge persisting for over a century.
- In *1824*, Sir Astley Cooper described the fragility of elderly bones due to aging and identified osteoporosis as a significant contributor to femoral neck fractures.
- By the mid-20th century, advancements in surgical techniques and implants began to shift treatment trends. However, the persistent high failure rates and complications continued to deem the fracture "unsolved."

Purpose

- To identify and improve upon treatment methods for femoral neck fractures.
- To minimize complications and maximize the likelihood of union.
- To develop strategies and implants that provide better outcomes, especially in elderly and osteoporotic populations.
- To bridge the gap between clinical observations and experimental evidence for more efficient fracture healing.

Procedure Overview

Diagnosis:

- Clinical presentation includes pain in the hip or groin, inability to bear weight, and reduced mobility.
- Imaging techniques such as X-rays, CT scans, or MRI are used to classify the fracture and evaluate displacement or vascular compromise.

Treatment Modalities:

- **Conservative Management:** Plaster immobilization (e.g., Whitman method) involves traction, gentle reduction, and immobilization in specific postures.
- **Surgical Options:** Internal fixation using screws or nails for stabilization.
- Arthroplasty (joint replacement), particularly in elderly patients with significant displacement or vascular compromise.
- **Challenges:**
- Rupture of vessels supplying the femoral head during injury complicates healing.
- Achieving and maintaining alignment and immobilization for sufficient union remains difficult.

Results and Interpretation

- **Conservative Treatment:** Lower surgical risk but associated with prolonged immobilization, delayed rehabilitation, and higher rates of nonunion.
- **Surgical Intervention:** Initially better results with primary arthroplasty or fixation, though long-term outcomes often deteriorate.
- Reports suggest a failure rate of 30-50% for displaced fractures, with high rates of nonunion and avascular necrosis.

Physiological Basis

- Intracapsular fractures disrupt the blood supply to the femoral head, primarily via the medial circumflex femoral artery. This vascular disruption contributes to nonunion and avascular necrosis.
- Osteoporosis in elderly patients further compromises bone density and healing capacity, increasing fracture susceptibility and complicating treatment outcomes.

Clinical Applications

- Management of femoral neck fractures forms a cornerstone of geriatric orthopedics, with implications for improving mobility, reducing disability, and ensuring independence in aging populations.
- **Advances in** surgical techniques and implants aim to provide better fixation and long-term functionality.

Limitations and Technical Considerations

- **Conservative Management:** Prolonged recovery and immobility increase the risk of complications like bedsores, deep vein thrombosis, and muscle atrophy.
- **Surgical Management:** Risks include infection, implant failure, and the need for revision surgeries.
- Challenges in elderly or comorbid patients include balancing surgical risks with the benefits of earlier mobilization.

Modern Relevance

- The global aging population has resulted in an increased incidence of femoral neck fractures. It is estimated that cases will rise from *1.6 million currently to 6.5 million by 2050.*
- Innovations in implants, minimally invasive techniques, and **Advances in** materials science continue to refine treatment approaches.
- Evidence-based guidelines now emphasize early mobilization, patient-specific treatment plans, and interdisciplinary approaches to optimize outcomes.

Associated Conditions

- **Osteoporosis:** Primary risk factor due to reduced bone density and strength.
- **Avascular Necrosis:** Common complication due to disrupted blood supply.
- **Postoperative Complications:** Include infection, malunion, nonunion, and implant failure.
- **Arthritis:** Degeneration of the hip joint is a frequent long-term sequela.

Clinical Importance

- **Improving Patient Outcomes:** Early intervention and tailored treatment plans can reduce mortality and enhance quality of life.
- **Geriatric Implications:** Reducing the disability burden and healthcare costs associated with long-term immobility.
- **Focus on Innovation:** Research into biomechanical factors, healing mechanisms, and novel materials for implants may address the current challenges.
- **Comprehensive Care:** Multidisciplinary teams, including orthopedic surgeons, physical therapists, and geriatric specialists, play a critical role in managing these fractures effectively.

The unsolved fracture remains a challenge in orthopedic care. However, advancements in technology and a deeper understanding of fracture biomechanics offer hope for better outcomes in the future.

References

Clin Orthop Relat Res. 1975 Jan-Feb;(106):279-84.

The Journrtl of the Royal Medico-Cl~irurgical Society of Qlssgow, the Medico-Chimgical biety 0, ,in,, the Edinbu~gh obstetrim, society ME D I C AIL and the Scottish Society for Experimental Medicine ~oi,,me 9 WEBEUAXY 1964 Number 2.

JAMA. 1953;153(6):536-540. doi:10.1001/jama.1953.02940230008004.

Dilip Shah. "Intertrochanteric Fractures - Unsolved Enigma". Acta Scientific Orthopaedics 5.6 (2022): 39-42.

Van Bogaert-Hozay Syndrome

Overview

Van Bogaert-Hozay Syndrome is a rare familial form of acro-osteolysis, characterized by mild mental retardation, facial dysmorphism, skin atrophy, and ocular defects. It manifests with distinctive facial features, short extremities, underdeveloped ulna, and aplastic fingers and toes, which retain an infantile appearance. The syndrome typically has an onset around the age of three years and affects both sexes. The etiology is unknown, and inheritance is suspected to be autosomal recessive.

Historical Background

- **1952:** Ludo Van Bogaert, a prominent neurologist, first described this condition in siblings with unique craniofacial, ocular, and skeletal anomalies.
- **1953:** Jean Hozay, collaborating with Van Bogaert, further expanded on the clinical presentation and familial occurrence of the syndrome.
- These early descriptions established the foundational understanding of this disorder and led to its eponymous naming.

Purpose

- **Diagnostic Clarity:** To identify a rare, hereditary skeletal and craniofacial disorder with systemic implications.
- **Genetic Study:** To explore patterns of inheritance and potential genetic mutations underlying the syndrome.

Procedure Overview

- **Clinical Evaluation:** Initial diagnosis is based on observable craniofacial, ocular, and skeletal deformities, along with developmental delays.
- **Imaging Studies:** Radiographs: Reveal acro-osteolysis, underdeveloped ulnas, and skeletal abnormalities.
- **CT/MRI:** Provide detailed views of craniofacial and skeletal structures.
- **Genetic Testing:** Investigates possible autosomal recessive mutations, though no definitive genetic markers have been identified.

Results and Interpretation

- **Characteristic Findings:**
- **Facial anomalies:** Flat nose with a broad bridge, thickened cheeks, malformed ears, hypertelorism, and micrognathia.
- **Ocular defects:** Ptosis, alternating squint, astigmatism, and myopia.
- **Skeletal abnormalities:** Acro-osteolysis of fingers and toes, short extremities, and underdeveloped distal ulna.
- **Developmental Impact:** Normal to mild mental retardation with no significant systemic organ involvement.

Physiological Basis

- The syndrome affects bone growth and integrity, particularly in the distal phalanges and ulna, leading to acro-osteolysis.
- Abnormal craniofacial and ocular development suggests disruption in early embryological patterning and tissue differentiation.
- The mild mental retardation points to potential but limited neurodevelopmental involvement.

Clinical Applications

- **Early Diagnosis:** Enables timely intervention to manage complications like malocclusion or severe visual impairment.
- **Orthopedic Interventions:** Corrective procedures for limb deformities and associated mobility challenges.
- **Multidisciplinary Care:** Collaboration among geneticists, ophthalmologists, neurologists, and orthopedic surgeons for comprehensive management.

Limitations and Technical Considerations

- **Lack of Genetic Clarity:** No definitive genetic mutation has been identified, making prenatal diagnosis difficult.
- **Variability in Presentation:** Symptoms can vary widely between affected individuals, complicating diagnosis and management.
- **Limited Treatment Options:** Current management focuses on symptomatic relief rather than addressing underlying causes.

Modern Relevance

- **Advances in Genetic Research:** Ongoing studies may uncover the genetic basis of the syndrome, leading to better diagnostic and therapeutic approaches.
- **Imaging Innovations:** High-resolution imaging helps in accurately

identifying skeletal and craniofacial anomalies.

- **Improved Support Systems:** Availability of multidisciplinary care ensures better quality of life for affected individuals.

Associated Conditions

- **Acro-Osteolysis Syndromes:** Shares features with other forms of acro-osteolysis, requiring differential diagnosis.
- **Craniofacial Syndromes:** Overlaps with conditions like Treacher Collins and Noonan syndrome.

Clinical Importance

- **Early Identification:** Recognition of craniofacial and skeletal anomalies is critical for managing associated complications.
- **Functional Restoration:** Timely orthopedic and dental interventions improve mobility and quality of life.
- **Multisystem Surveillance:** Regular monitoring prevents progression of ocular or skeletal impairments.
- **Research Implications:** Understanding this syndrome may provide insights into the genetic and developmental pathways influencing bone growth and craniofacial development.

References

J. Hozay: Sur une dystrophie familiale particulière. Inhibition précoce de la croissance et ostéolyse non mutilante acrale avec dysmorphie faciale. Revue neurologique, Paris, 1953, 89: 245-258.

L. van Bogaert: Essai de classement et d'interprétation de quelques acro-ostéolyses mutilantes et non mutilantes actuellement connues. Acta neurologica et psychiatrica Belgica, Brussels, 1953, 53: 90-115.

van der Hoeve's Syndrome

Overview

Van der Hoeve's Syndrome is a hereditary disorder characterized by brittle bones, blue sclerae, and the absence of deafness, distinguishing it from other types of osteogenesis imperfecta. Patients present with multiple fractures from minimal trauma, opalescent teeth, translucent skin, joint instability, and a small, triangular facial appearance. Most cases follow an autosomal dominant inheritance pattern, with some rare autosomal recessive forms. Variants include Ekman-Lobstein (adult form) and Vrolik's disease (infantile, recessive, and lethal form).

Historical Background

- **1,000 BC:** The earliest evidence of this condition is a skeleton of an Egyptian mummy preserved in the British Museum.
- **7th Century:** An Anglo-Saxon burial revealed an abnormal femur possibly indicative of the condition.
- **1788:** Olof Jakob Ekman described osteogenesis imperfecta in his doctoral thesis, coining the term "osteomalacia congenita."
- **1833:** Jean Fréderic Lobstein described the adult form, calling it "osteopsathyrosis idiopathica."
- **1849–1854:** Willem Vrolik made significant observations and distinctions regarding the disorder.
- **1905:** Charles Porak and Gustave Durante in Paris identified additional

cases and broadened the understanding of the condition.

- Other contributors included *Heinrich Stilling* (histopathological features, 1889) and *Martin Benno Schmidt* (linking newborn and adult forms, 1897).

Purpose

- **Clinical Identification:** To diagnose a hereditary bone fragility disorder distinct from other forms of osteogenesis imperfecta.
- **Family Counseling:** To understand inheritance patterns and manage familial cases.

Procedure Overview

- **Clinical Examination:** Focus on skeletal fragility, blue sclerae, and dental abnormalities.
- **Imaging:** X-rays reveal fractures, skeletal deformities, and reduced bone density.
- **Genetic Testing:** Identifies mutations associated with autosomal dominant or recessive inheritance.
- **Histopathology:** Histological examination shows structural abnormalities in collagen and bone matrix.

Results and Interpretation

- **Key Findings:**
- Fragile bones with a propensity for fractures.
- Blue sclerae, translucent skin, and opalescent teeth.
- Absence of deafness differentiates it from other forms of osteogenesis imperfecta.
- **Inheritance Patterns:** Predominantly autosomal dominant; some recessive cases have been observed.

Physiological Basis

- **Bone Fragility:** Caused by defects in collagen synthesis and structural integrity, leading to brittle bones.
- **Scleral Coloration:** Blue sclerae result from thinning of the sclera, exposing the underlying choroid.
- **Skin and Ligaments:** Abnormal connective tissue contributes to translucency and joint laxity.

Clinical Applications

- **Early Diagnosis:** Identifies affected individuals to implement fracture prevention strategies.
- **Supportive Therapy:** Includes physical therapy, bracing, and surgical interventions for severe deformities.
- **Genetic Counseling:** Helps families understand inheritance risks and recurrence in future generations.

Limitations and Technical Considerations

- **Variable Presentation:** Clinical manifestations can range from mild to severe, complicating diagnosis.
- **Overlap with Other Conditions:** Differentiating from other types of osteogenesis imperfecta may require advanced genetic testing.
- **Treatment Limitations:** Current therapies focus on symptom management rather than addressing the

underlying defect.

Modern Relevance

- **Genetic Advances:** Research into collagen and connective tissue disorders continues to improve diagnostic accuracy.
- **Therapeutic Innovations:** Development of bisphosphonates and other drugs to improve bone density.
- **Global Awareness:** Increased understanding and documentation of the disorder enhance patient outcomes.

Associated Conditions

- **Ekman-Lobstein Syndrome:** A milder, adult-onset variant.
- **Vrolik's Disease:** An infantile, recessive, and lethal form.

Clinical Importance

- **Early Recognition:** Enables timely interventions to prevent fractures and manage skeletal deformities.
- **Quality of Life:** Improves mobility, reduces pain, and enhances overall well-being.
- **Research Implications:** Understanding the genetic basis may lead to targeted therapies for connective tissue disorders.

Van der Hoeve's Syndrome remains a critical area of interest for its unique presentation and challenges, with ongoing research offering hope for improved management and patient care.

References

Olaus Jacob Ekman: Dissertatio medica **Description**em et casus aliquot osteomalaciæ sistens. Upsaliæ, J. Edman, 1788. In his doctoral thesis Ekman gave an account of osteogenesis imperfecta in three generations. English translation in Knud Stakemann Seedorff, Osteogenesis imperfecta. A study of clinical features and heredity based on 55 Danish families comprising 180 affected members. Århus, Universitetsforlaget, 1949. Also gives a case reported in 1678.

D. F. Sartorius: Medical dissertation, Leipzig. 1826.

E. Axmann: Merkwürdige fragilität der Knochen ohne dyskrastische Ursache als krankhafte Eigenthümlichkeit dreier Geschwister. Annalen für die gesammte Heilkunde, Karlsruhe, 1831, 4: 58-68.

Axmann of Wertheim described osteogenesis imperfecta occurring in himself and his two brothers. He referred to the occurrence of articular dislocations and blue sclerotics.

J. F. Lobstein: De la fragilité des os, ou l'ostéopsathyrose. In his: Traité de l'anatomie pathologique. Paris, 1833, 2: 204-212.

Lehrbuch der pathologischen Anatomie. Stuttgart, 1835. 179 pages.

W. Vrolik: Tabulae ad illustrandam embryogenesin hominis et mammalium, tam naturalem quam abnormem. G. M. P., Londinck, 1849. Lipsiae, Weigel, 1854 (German and Latin).

H. Stilling: Osteogenesis imperfecta. [Virchows] Archiv für pathologische Anatomie und Physiologie und für klinische Medicin, Berlin, 1889, 115: 357.

Velpeau View

Overview

Velpeau View is a radiographic technique used in patients with immobilized upper limbs, often following reduction or surgery, to obtain an axillary profile view of the shoulder. It is particularly helpful when standard axillary radiographs cannot be performed due to patient immobilization. The view involves positioning the patient with a shoulder sling (Velpeau bandage) while leaning backward, allowing the X-ray beam to pass vertically through the shoulder joint.

Historical Background

- **1795:** Alfred Armand Marie Velpeau was born. He was a celebrated French surgeon, anatomist, and obstetrician known for his prolific contributions to medical science.
- **1827:** Velpeau provided the first accurate description of leukemia and contributed significantly to the fields of anatomy and surgery.
- The Velpeau bandage, used to immobilize the arm against the chest wall, is one of the many medical innovations associated with his name.
- Other terms associated with Velpeau include "Velpeau hernia" (femoral hernia), "Velpeau's canal" (inguinal canal), and "Velpeau's fossa" (ischiorectal fossa).

Purpose

- **Primary Use:** To provide an axillary profile view of the shoulder in patients who cannot tolerate standard positioning due to immobilization.
- **Secondary Use:** Assessment of shoulder joint alignment and postoperative or post-reduction imaging.

Procedure Overview

- **Patient Positioning:**
- The patient, with a Velpeau bandage or shoulder sling in place, sits or stands at the edge of the X-ray table.
- The patient leans backward 20 to 30 degrees over the table.
- **X-ray Setup:**
- The X-ray cassette is placed directly beneath the shoulder on the table.
- The X-ray beam is positioned vertically, passing superior to inferior through the shoulder joint.
- **Radiographic View:**
- A modified axillary profile of the shoulder joint is captured.

Results and Interpretation

- **Expected Outcomes:** Visualization of the shoulder joint in profile to assess alignment and potential pathology.
- **Key Findings:**
- Useful for identifying shoulder joint dislocations, post-reduction positioning, or surgical outcomes.
- Not recommended for diagnostic purposes as a replacement for standard axillary radiographs.

Physiological Basis

- **Shoulder Joint Assessment:** The view allows visualization of the glenohumeral joint, ensuring proper alignment and positioning without the need for extensive arm movement.

Clinical Applications

- **Post-Surgical Imaging:** Used to evaluate surgical outcomes or reduction procedures in immobilized patients.

- **Alternative to Axillary Radiographs:** Provides a suitable alternative when patients cannot tolerate standard axillary views.

Limitations and Technical Considerations

- **Limitations:**

- Not intended for primary diagnostic purposes, particularly in non-immobilized patients.

- Limited sensitivity compared to standard axillary radiographs for detecting subtle abnormalities.

- **Technical Challenges:**

- Requires precise positioning to avoid suboptimal imaging.

- Relies on patient cooperation to maintain the leaning-backward posture.

Modern Relevance

- **Continued Utility:** Remains relevant for patients with shoulder immobilization, particularly in orthopedic and trauma settings.

- **Historical Significance:** While other imaging techniques have largely replaced the Velpeau View, it continues to be an important tool in specific clinical contexts.

Associated Conditions

- **Post-Reduction Shoulder Imaging:** Ensures proper alignment following shoulder dislocations.

- **Postoperative Shoulder Assessment:** Evaluates the outcomes of shoulder surgeries while minimizing patient discomfort.

Clinical Importance

- **Alternative for Immobilized Patients:** Enables imaging without disrupting immobilization devices such as the Velpeau bandage.

- **Reduced Discomfort:** Provides a less painful alternative for patients with acute trauma or restricted shoulder mobility.

- **Support for Diagnosis:** Offers a secondary view when standard radiographic techniques are not feasible.

The Velpeau View continues to be a valuable radiographic tool for managing complex shoulder conditions in immobilized patients, underscoring the enduring legacy of Alfred Velpeau's contributions to medicine.

References

Pavlov H, Warren RF, Weiss CB Jr, et al. The roentgenographic evaluation of anterior shoulder instability. Clin Orthop Relat Res. 1985; (194):153-8.

Jacobson JA, Lin J, Jamadar DA et al.Aids to Successful Shoulder Arthrography Performed with a Fluoroscopically Guided Anterior Approach.Radiographics 2003; 23(2):373-378.

Sanders TG, Jersey SL. Conventional Radiography of the Shoulder. Seminars in Roentgenology 2005; 40:207-222

Volkmann's canals

Overview

Volkmann's canals are vascular channels in compact bone that serve as conduits for blood vessels from the periosteum. These canals connect to the Haversian canals, forming a network for the transport of nutrients and waste products within the bone. Unlike Haversian canals, Volkmann's canals are not surrounded by concentric lamellae, distinguishing their structure and function within the bone matrix.

Historical Background

- **1800–1877:** Alfred Wilhelm Volkmann, a prominent German physiologist, anatomist, and philosopher, described these canals. His research significantly contributed to the understanding of bone vascularity and the microscopic anatomy of skeletal structures.
- Volkmann's contributions extended beyond anatomy, including studies on the nervous system and philosophical discourses on human nature and free will.

Purpose

- **Primary Function:** To carry blood vessels from the periosteum into the bone and link them with the Haversian system, ensuring efficient vascular supply to compact bone.
- **Secondary Role:** To facilitate the transport of nutrients, oxygen, and waste products between the periosteum, compact bone, and deeper structures.

Procedure Overview

- **Structural Description:**
- Volkmann's canals are oriented perpendicular or oblique to the Haversian canals, connecting them to the periosteal surface.
- They carry blood vessels and nerves, forming an essential component of the bone's microvascular system.
- **Histological Features:** Unlike Haversian canals, Volkmann's canals are not surrounded by concentric lamellae, providing a clear histological distinction.

Results and Interpretation

- **Observational Findings:**
- Histological sections reveal transverse or oblique canals connecting the periosteal vessels to the Haversian system.
- The structure ensures bone vitality and structural integrity through continuous vascular communication.
- **Implications:** Damage or obstruction to Volkmann's canals can impair bone health, leading to conditions like ischemia or delayed healing.

Physiological Basis

- **Vascular Integration:**
- Volkmann's canals are integral to the hierarchical vascular system in bones, maintaining a steady supply of nutrients and oxygen to osteocytes within compact bone.
- They also provide an essential pathway for metabolic waste removal, ensuring bone tissue remains healthy and functional.

Clinical Applications

- **Bone Healing and Surgery:** Understanding the vascular architecture, including Volkmann's canals, is critical in surgical interventions and bone repair processes.
- **Pathological Analysis:** Histological examination of these canals aids in diagnosing bone disorders, including osteoporosis and osteonecrosis.

Limitations and Technical Considerations

- **Histological Challenges:** Identifying Volkmann's canals requires precise histological preparation and staining techniques to distinguish them from other bone structures.
- **Functional Vulnerability:** As conduits for blood vessels, these canals can become pathways for infection or metastatic spread in pathological conditions.

Modern Relevance

- **Ongoing Research:** Current studies continue to explore the role of Volkmann's canals in bone remodeling and response to injury.
- **Orthopedic Significance:** Knowledge of these canals enhances surgical precision and postoperative outcomes, particularly in procedures involving compact bone.

Associated Conditions

- **Osteoporosis:** Impairment in the vascular supply through Volkmann's canals contributes to reduced bone density and fragility.
- **Osteonecrosis:** Obstruction in the vascular channels, including Volkmann's canals, may lead to ischemia and necrosis of bone tissue.

Clinical Importance

- **Bone Health and Healing:** The integrity of Volkmann's canals is critical for maintaining bone vitality, particularly during growth, repair, and remodeling.
- **Diagnostic Relevance:** Pathological alterations in these canals provide insights into systemic conditions affecting bone, such as metabolic disorders and cancer metastasis.
- **Surgical Planning:** An understanding of the vascular architecture aids in the development of surgical techniques that minimize disruption to the bone's vascular network.

Volkmann's canals play a foundational role in bone physiology, ensuring vascular integration and systemic communication within the skeletal system. Their relevance extends from basic anatomy to advanced clinical applications, reflecting Alfred Wilhelm Volkmann's enduring legacy in the field of medical science.

References

A. W. Volkmann: Ueber die naheren Bestandtheile der menschlichen Knochen. Berichte über die Verhandlungen der königlichen sächsischen Gesellschaft der Wissenschaften zu Leipzig, Mathematisch Physikalische Klasse. 1873. volume 25, page 275. 5: 1863.

Volkmann's contracture

Overview

Volkmann's contracture refers to an ischemic muscle contracture resulting from impaired circulation, leading to necrosis of muscle tissue. This condition is characterized by flexion contractures, particularly of the hand and fingers, resulting in a "claw hand" deformity. It is commonly seen in children and is often a complication of untreated or improperly treated injuries to the elbow or forearm, or from prolonged external pressure such as a tight bandage or tourniquet.

Historical Background

- **1875:** Richard von Volkmann, a German surgeon, first described this condition in his studies on the effects of ischemia in muscle tissue. He identified the role of vascular compromise in causing muscle necrosis and subsequent contracture.
- Volkmann's research marked a paradigm shift in understanding contractures, emphasizing ischemia rather than nerve compression as the primary cause.

Purpose

- **Clinical Recognition:** To identify early signs of ischemia in muscles, preventing irreversible damage.
- **Treatment Guidance:** To establish treatment protocols that restore circulation and minimize functional impairments.

Procedure Overview

- **Diagnosis:**
- **Based on Clinical Presentation:** claw-like deformities, burning pain, weakness, or paralysis in the hand and forearm.
- Imaging and vascular studies may help assess the extent of damage.
- **Treatment:**
- Immediate interventions to restore blood flow, such as removing constrictive dressings or performing fasciotomy.
- Long-term management may include physical therapy or reconstructive surgery for severe contractures.

Results and Interpretation

- **Clinical Findings:**
- Irreversible muscle necrosis if ischemia persists beyond a critical threshold, leading to fibrosis and contractures.
- Successful early intervention often results in full recovery of function.
- **Prognostic Factors:** The duration and severity of ischemia largely determine outcomes. Delayed treatment significantly increases the risk of permanent disability.

Physiological Basis

- **Pathophysiology:**
- Prolonged ischemia results in necrosis of muscle fibers, followed by fibrosis and shortening of the involved muscles.
- The flexor group of forearm muscles is most commonly affected due to their anatomical vulnerability to compartment syndrome.
- **Vascular and Muscular Compromise:** Tight bandages, fractures, or external compression

reduce arterial flow and venous return, causing hypoxia and eventual necrosis.

Clinical Applications

- **Preventative Measures:**
- Early detection of compromised circulation in orthopedic injuries.
- Proper application of casts, bandages, and tourniquets to avoid excessive pressure.
- **Therapeutic Interventions:**
- Surgical release via fasciotomy for compartment syndrome.
- Tendon transfers or reconstructive procedures for chronic contractures.

Limitations and Technical Considerations

- **Diagnostic Challenges:** Early symptoms may be mistaken for nerve compression, delaying intervention.
- **Surgical Risks:** Fasciotomy and reconstructive surgeries carry risks of infection, scarring, and incomplete functional restoration.

Modern Relevance

- **Awareness and Education:** Emphasis on recognizing early signs of ischemic damage among healthcare providers to prevent Volkmann's contracture.
- **Advances in Surgical Techniques:** Minimally invasive procedures and improved reconstructive options have enhanced outcomes.

Associated Conditions

- **Compartment Syndrome:** A common precursor to Volkmann's contracture, involving increased pressure within the muscle compartments.
- **Elbow Fractures:** Particularly supracondylar fractures, which may impair vascular supply to the forearm.

Clinical Importance

- **Early Intervention:** Recognizing and promptly treating ischemic injuries prevent irreversible muscle damage and disability.
- **Functional Restoration:** Advanced surgical and rehabilitative techniques aim to restore hand function in affected individuals.
- **Patient Education:** Awareness of the risks associated with tight bandages or prolonged external pressure can reduce the incidence of Volkmann's contracture.

Volkmann's contracture remains a significant concern in orthopedic and trauma care. Richard von Volkmann's insights laid the foundation for understanding ischemic muscle damage, emphasizing prevention, early recognition, and timely intervention to preserve limb function and quality of life.

References

R. Volkmann: Krankheiten der Bewegungsorgane. In: Pitha-Billroth, publishers: Handbuch der allgemeinen und speciellen Chirurgie, volume 2: 845-920. Erlangen, 1869.

Die ischämischen Muskellähmungen und Kontracturen. Centralblatt für Chirurgie, Leipzig, 1881, 8: 801-803.

Volkmann's triangle

Overview

Volkmann's triangle refers to an avulsion fracture of the posterior lateral edge of the distal tibia, also known as a posterior malleolus fracture. This injury is typically associated with fracture-dislocations of the ankle. While historically attributed to Richard von Volkmann, the eponym is debated due to earlier descriptions by Henry Earle. This fracture is of clinical importance due to its involvement in ankle stability and potential complications.

Historical Background

- **1828:** Henry Earle first described an avulsion fracture of the posterior part of the tibia.
- **1881:** Richard von Volkmann provided detailed descriptions of injuries, including the contraction of fingers (now known as Volkmann's contracture) and lateral tibial avulsion fractures.
- **Debate:** Volkmann's original article focused primarily on lateral avulsions in the sagittal plane, raising questions about the accuracy of the eponym "Volkmann's triangle."

Purpose

- **Understanding Ankle Stability:** To identify and manage fractures affecting the posterior tibial edge, which plays a crucial role in ankle stability.
- **Guiding Surgical Interventions:** To determine when surgical fixation is required based on the size and displacement of the fracture fragment.

Procedure Overview

- **Diagnosis:**
- **Imaging:** Diagnosis is made through X-rays, often supplemented by CT scans for detailed visualization of the posterior malleolus and its involvement in joint congruency.
- **Treatment:**
- **Non-Surgical:** Immobilization is considered for small, stable fractures without significant displacement.
- **Surgical:** Larger, displaced fractures or those involving >25–30% of the tibial articular surface require open reduction and internal fixation (ORIF).

Results and Interpretation

- **Clinical Findings:** Patients with posterior malleolus fractures often present with pain, swelling, and limited range of motion in the ankle.
- **Prognosis:** Early intervention results in better outcomes, with reduced risks of post-traumatic arthritis or chronic instability.

Physiological Basis

- **Anatomical Role:** The posterior tibial edge contributes to the stability of the ankle mortise and prevents posterior subluxation of the talus.
- **Injury Mechanism:** Typically caused by rotational forces during high-energy trauma, such as motor vehicle accidents or sports injuries.

Clinical Applications

- **Orthopedic Surgery:** Essential in surgical planning and execution for managing posterior malleolus fractures.
- **Rehabilitation:** Post-treatment physical therapy focuses on restoring ankle stability and mobility.

Limitations and Technical Considerations

- **Imaging Challenges:** Plain radiographs may miss subtle fractures; CT is often needed for accurate assessment.
- **Surgical Risks:** Risks include infection, delayed union, or hardware complications in cases requiring ORIF.

Modern Relevance

- **Advanced Imaging:** The use of 3D imaging techniques has improved the diagnosis and classification of posterior malleolus fractures.
- **Evolving Fixation Techniques:** Newer implants and fixation strategies enhance outcomes, particularly in complex fracture-dislocations.

Associated Conditions

- **Fracture-Dislocations:** Commonly associated with lateral and medial malleolus fractures, forming part of trimalleolar fracture patterns.
- **Post-Traumatic Arthritis:** A long-term complication due to articular surface involvement.

Clinical Importance

- **Preservation of Joint Function:** Accurate reduction and stabilization of the posterior malleolus are critical for maintaining ankle biomechanics.
- **Timely Diagnosis:** Early identification of posterior malleolus involvement ensures appropriate treatment and minimizes complications.
- **Interdisciplinary Management:** Collaboration between radiologists, orthopedic surgeons, and physical therapists enhances patient outcomes.

Volkmann's triangle remains a significant concept in orthopedic trauma, emphasizing the importance of understanding posterior tibial avulsions in ankle fractures for optimal patient care.

References

Earle H. Simple, succeeded by compound dislocation forwards, of the inferior extremity of the tibia, with fracture of its posterior edge comminuted fracture of the fibula, amputation of the leg and death. Lancet 1929; II: 346–8.

Volkmann R. Beiträge zur Chirurgie anschliessend an einen Bericht über die Thätigkeit der chirurgischen Universitatsklinik zu Halle um Jahre 1873. Leipzig: Breitkopf und Härtelm, 1875.

Bartonícek J. Avulsed posterior edge of the tibia. Earle's or Volkmann's triangle? J Bone Joint Surg Br 2004; 86: 746–50. R. Volkmann, in Centralblatt für Chirurgie, Leipzig, 1875: 358.

Kai Witzel, Christoph Raschka: Ist die Fraktur des Volkmannschen Dreiecks eine typische Snowboard-Verletzung? Sport-Orthopädie - Sport-Traumatologie, 2001, 17

E. Neumaier Probst, R. Maas, N. M. Meenen: Isolated fracture of the posterolateral tibial lip (Volkmann's triangle). Acta radiologica, 1997, 38 (3) 359-362.

Volkmann's deformity

Overview

Volkmann's deformity refers to a congenital luxation of the talus, often described as a tibiotarsal dislocation resulting in a deformity of the foot. It is a rare condition involving structural abnormalities in the ankle joint and surrounding structures, affecting both function and appearance.

Historical Background

- **1881:** Richard von Volkmann, a German surgeon, provided detailed insights into musculoskeletal injuries and deformities, including those involving the ankle joint. His extensive work on contractures and deformities of the lower limbs brought recognition to the condition bearing his name.

Purpose

- **Defining Congenital Deformities:** To categorize and understand congenital luxations and dislocations, particularly of the talus, for better diagnosis and management.
- **Optimizing Treatment:** To develop effective surgical and non-surgical interventions aimed at improving foot function and correcting deformity.

Procedure Overview

- **Diagnosis:** Clinical Examination: Observation of the foot's appearance, range of motion, and alignment.
- **Imaging:** X-rays and MRI scans are used to assess the talus position, joint involvement, and any associated structural abnormalities.
- **Treatment Options:**
- **Non-Surgical:** Orthotic devices or casting in mild cases to improve alignment.
- **Surgical:** Corrective osteotomies or talar realignment for severe deformities or cases resistant to conservative management.

Results and Interpretation

- **Clinical Findings:** Affected individuals typically present with limited range of motion, visible foot deformity, and potential functional impairment.
- **Prognosis:** Early intervention leads to better outcomes, including improved joint mobility and reduced risk of secondary complications like arthritis.

Physiological Basis

- **Anatomical Abnormalities:** Congenital displacement of the talus disrupts normal biomechanics of the tibiotarsal joint, leading to deformities and altered gait.
- **Biomechanical Impact:** The luxation affects the stability of the ankle joint and the distribution of weight during movement, contributing to functional limitations.

Clinical Applications

- **Orthopedic Management:** Insight into the deformity guides both corrective procedures and post-operative rehabilitation.
- **Rehabilitation:** Focused physical therapy programs aim to restore mobility and improve gait mechanics.

Limitations and Technical

Considerations

- **Challenges in Early Diagnosis:** Subtle cases may be missed in infancy, delaying treatment until more pronounced deformities or functional impairments develop.
- **Surgical Risks:** Procedures may involve complications such as infection, non-union of osteotomy sites, or overcorrection.

Modern Relevance

- **Advancements in Imaging:** High-resolution imaging, including 3D CT scans, enhances the diagnostic accuracy for congenital foot deformities.
- **Innovations in Orthopedic Surgery:** Improved surgical techniques and implant designs facilitate more precise correction of deformities.

Associated Conditions

- **Other Congenital Foot Deformities:** Clubfoot (talipes equinovarus) and other tarsal dislocations may co-exist with Volkmann's deformity.
- **Arthritis:** Long-term misalignment or untreated cases can lead to early-onset osteoarthritis in the ankle joint.

Clinical Importance

- **Improved Functional Outcomes:** Correct diagnosis and timely treatment can significantly enhance the quality of life for affected individuals.
- **Preventing Secondary Complications:** Early intervention minimizes the risk of associated conditions such as joint instability or arthritis.
- **Holistic Management:** Collaboration among orthopedic surgeons, radiologists, and physical therapists ensures comprehensive care and optimal results.

Volkmann's deformity underscores the importance of recognizing and treating congenital foot abnormalities early, leveraging modern diagnostic and surgical advancements to improve outcomes.

References

R. Volkmann: Ein Fall von hereditärer kongenitaler Luxation beider Sprunggelenke. Deutsche Zeitschrift für Chirurgie, Leipzig, 1873, 2: 538-542.

Voorhoeve's disease

Overview

Voorhoeve's disease, also referred to as osteopathia striata with cranial sclerosis, is a rare genetic condition characterized by radiographic evidence of parallel linear striations in long bones and fan-shaped sclerotic patterns in the iliac bones. These findings are often accompanied by varying degrees of cranial sclerosis and minimal clinical symptoms. Both sexes are affected, and inheritance is typically autosomal dominant.

Historical Background

- **1924:** Nicolaas Voorhoeve, a Dutch radiologist, initially described the condition in terms of its peculiar striated radiological appearance in the bones.
- **1953:** R.L. Hunt recognized the association between osteopathia striata and cranial sclerosis, consolidating it into a single syndrome and introducing the eponym Voorhoeve's disease.
- Harold Arthur Thomas Fairbank further elaborated on the radiographic characteristics of osteopathia striata, contributing to the understanding of the disease.

Purpose

- **Identification of Skeletal Abnormalities:** To distinguish Voorhoeve's disease from other forms of osteosclerosis or dysplasias through its unique radiological patterns.
- **Understanding Genetic Inheritance:** To study the autosomal dominant transmission and its implications for genetic counseling.

Procedure Overview

- **Diagnostic Imaging:** Radiographs: Linear striations in the metaphyseal regions of long bones and fan-shaped sclerotic patterns in the pelvis are hallmark findings.
- **CT or MRI:** Utilized for detailed imaging of cranial sclerosis and associated skeletal changes.
- **Clinical Assessment:** Evaluation of craniofacial features, skeletal deformities, and any associated hearing or spinal abnormalities.

Results and Interpretation

- **Key Findings:**
- Parallel sclerotic striations in long bones.
- Fan-like sclerotic patterns in iliac bones interspersed with areas of rarefaction.
- Cranial thickening or sclerosis may vary from mild to severe.
- **Prognosis:** Typically benign with minimal clinical symptoms. Rare complications such as hearing loss or spinal deformities may arise.

Physiological Basis

- **Osteosclerotic Changes:** Result from abnormal bone remodeling processes leading to areas of increased density (sclerosis) and striation patterns.
- Cranial sclerosis is likely due to excessive periosteal and endosteal bone formation.
- **Genetic Basis:** Autosomal dominant inheritance with variable expressivity. The exact genetic mutation remains unidentified but is suspected to involve

pathways regulating bone density and remodeling.

Clinical Applications

- **Differential Diagnosis:** Helps differentiate Voorhoeve's disease from other conditions like osteopoikilosis, melorheostosis, and pyknodysostosis.
- **Monitoring:** Regular follow-up imaging is essential to monitor cranial changes or potential complications such as scoliosis or spondylolisthesis.

Limitations and Technical Considerations

- **Diagnostic Challenges:** Mild cases may be misdiagnosed due to subtle radiographic findings, especially in asymptomatic individuals.
- **Treatment Limitations:** There is no specific treatment for the condition itself; management focuses on addressing associated complications.

Modern Relevance

- **Advances in Imaging:** High-resolution imaging techniques like CT and MRI have improved diagnostic accuracy, enabling earlier identification of skeletal and cranial abnormalities.
- **Genetic Insights:** Ongoing genetic research aims to uncover the mutations responsible for this rare disorder, potentially offering targeted therapies in the future.

Associated Conditions

- **Craniofacial Abnormalities:** Pierre Robin sequence, characterized by a small jaw, cleft palate, and airway obstruction, has been occasionally linked to Voorhoeve's disease.
- **Hearing Defects:** Sensorineural or conductive hearing loss may occur due to cranial sclerosis affecting auditory structures.
- **Spinal Deformities:** Scoliosis and spondylolisthesis are potential complications requiring orthopedic evaluation.

Clinical Importance

- **Accurate Diagnosis:** Recognizing the characteristic radiographic features aids in early diagnosis and prevents unnecessary interventions for misdiagnosed conditions.
- **Genetic Counseling:** Essential for affected families due to the autosomal dominant inheritance pattern, providing guidance on recurrence risk in offspring.
- **Management of Complications:** Proactive management of hearing defects, craniofacial abnormalities, and spinal deformities improves quality of life for affected individuals.

Voorhoeve's disease exemplifies the interplay between clinical radiology and genetic inheritance in diagnosing and managing rare skeletal dysplasias. **Advances in** *imaging and genetics continue to refine our understanding of this unique condition.*

References

N. Voorhoeve: L'image radiologique non encore décrite d'une anomalie du squélette. Ses rapports avec la dyschondroplasie et l'osteopathia condensans disseminata. Acta Radiologica, Stockholm, 1924, 3: 407-427.

H. A. T. Fairbank:A case of unilateral affection of the skeleton of unknown origin. The British Journal of Surgery, London, 1925, 12: 594-597. Osteopathia striata.

Proceedings of the Royal Society of Medicine, 1935, 28: 1616.

The Journal of Bone and Joint Surgery, London, 1950, 32: 117-

125. An Atlas of General Affections of the Skeleton. Edinburgh, Livingstone, 1951.

Baltimore, Williams & Wilkins, 1951. Pages 181-183.

R. L. Hurt: Osteopathia striata – Voorhoeve's disease. The Journal of Bone and Joint Surgery, London, 35: 89-96.

F. Horan, P. Beighton: Osteopathia striata with cranial sclerosis. An autosomal dominant entity. Clinical Genetics, Copenhagen, 1978, 13: 201-206.

Vrolik's Syndrome

Overview

Vrolik's syndrome, also known as congenital bone fragility, is a rare genetic disorder characterized by generalized hypostosis, leading to abnormally brittle and thick bones that are prone to fractures. This condition often results in severe skeletal deformities, short-limb dwarfism, and a variety of associated abnormalities such as blue sclerae, wide fontanels, and muscle hypotonia. Affected infants typically do not survive beyond the neonatal period. The condition follows an autosomal recessive inheritance pattern.

Historical Background

- **1849:** Willem Vrolik, a Dutch anatomist and embryologist, published a detailed treatise on embryogenesis. He documented the skeletal abnormalities of an infant with multiple fractures and characteristic Wormian bones in the skull, offering one of the earliest accounts of this syndrome.

- **1905:** Charles Porak and Gustave Durante further described the condition, referring to it as a form of "achondroplasia" in French medical literature. However, this terminology has since been abandoned due to its inaccuracy.

Purpose

- **Clinical Characterization:** To identify the unique skeletal and systemic manifestations of Vrolik's syndrome for differential diagnosis.

- **Genetic Insights:** To study its autosomal recessive inheritance pattern, aiding in genetic counseling for affected families.

Procedure Overview

- **Diagnostic Imaging:**
- **Radiographs:** Show multiple fractures, generalized hypostosis, and Wormian bones in the skull.
- **CT or MRI:** Provide detailed visualization of skeletal abnormalities and cranial deformities.
- **Histopathological Examination:** Confirms structural defects in bone remodeling and mineralization.
- **Genetic Testing:** Identifies mutations associated with the autosomal recessive inheritance pattern.

Results and Interpretation

- **Radiological Findings:** Thickened but brittle bones with multiple fractures.
- Wormian bones in the skull and large caput membranaceum (caoutchouc head).
- **Clinical Observations:** Infants are often stillborn or die shortly after birth due to respiratory failure or other complications.
- Severe short-limb dwarfism and deformed extremities are hallmark features.

Physiological Basis

- **Bone Fragility:** Results from defective bone remodeling, leading to thickened yet brittle bones that lack structural integrity.
- **Skeletal Dysplasia:** Affects endochondral ossification, leading to short-limb dwarfism and other skeletal deformities.
- **Associated Features:** Blue sclerae due to thinning of collagen fibers in the sclera and other connective tissue abnormalities.

Clinical Applications

- **Differential Diagnosis:** Differentiates Vrolik's syndrome from other skeletal dysplasias, such as osteogenesis imperfecta and achondroplasia.
- **Prenatal Diagnosis:** High-resolution ultrasound can identify severe skeletal abnormalities in utero.
- **Genetic Counseling:** Assists families in understanding recurrence risks in subsequent pregnancies.

Limitations and Technical Considerations

- **Diagnostic Challenges:** Severe cases may be misdiagnosed as other forms of skeletal dysplasia due to overlapping features.
- **Management Difficulties:** There is no curative treatment, and management is limited to supportive care, which is often insufficient due to the severity of the condition.

Modern Relevance

- **Advances in Genetic Testing:** Next-generation sequencing aids in the identification of causative mutations, enabling more precise diagnosis and counseling.
- **Prenatal Screening:** Improvements in fetal imaging provide earlier detection and diagnosis of severe skeletal dysplasias like Vrolik's syndrome.

Associated Conditions

- **Blue Sclerae:** Thinning of collagen layers in the sclera, a common feature in connective tissue disorders.
- **Respiratory Distress:** Results from underdeveloped ribcage and associated skeletal deformities.
- **Wormian Bones:** Additional small bones within the cranial sutures, a characteristic finding in Vrolik's syndrome.

Clinical Importance

- **Early Detection:** Crucial for anticipating complications and providing appropriate palliative care for affected neonates.
- **Genetic Counseling:** Assists families in understanding the autosomal recessive inheritance and potential outcomes in future pregnancies.
- **Research Implications:** Insights into bone fragility syndromes contribute to understanding other genetic skeletal disorders.

Vrolik's syndrome, though rare, underscores the importance of integrating radiological, genetic, and clinical assessments for accurate diagnosis and management of congenital skeletal disorders. Advances in prenatal and genetic diagnostics continue to enhance our understanding and approach to this condition.

References

W. Vrolik: Tabulae ad illustrandam embryogenesin hominis et mammalium, tam naturalem quam abnormem. Amsterdam, G. M. P., Londinck, 1849; Lipsiae, Weigel, 1854 (German and Latin).

Won a Monthyon prize in Paris. The 100 plates of this volume contain some of the most accurate and beautiful depictions of human and animal malformations ever published.

B. Porak, G. Durante: Les micromélies congénitales. Achondroplasie vraie et dystrophie périostale. Nouvelle iconographie de la Salpêtrière, Paris, 1905, 18: 181-538.

Emil Looser (1877-1936): Zur Kenntnis der osteogenesis imperfecta congenita et tarda. Mittheilungen aus dem Grenzgebieten der Medizin und Chirurgie, 1906, 15: 161-207.

Waldenström's disease

Overview

Waldenström's disease is a chronic inflammatory condition affecting the head of the femur in children. The disease is characterized by progressive atrophy and shortening of the femoral neck and shaft, often accompanied by a wide and flattened femoral head. It is considered a form of osteochondritis deformans juvenilis, though its relationship to other conditions like Scheuermann's disease remains debated.

Historical Background

- **1934:** Johann Henning Waldenström, a Swedish internist, described the clinical and pathological features of the disease, focusing on the chronic inflammation and deformities of the femoral head.
- Waldenström is also known for his contributions to hematology, particularly describing Waldenström's macroglobulinemia.

Purpose

- **Understanding Juvenile Osteochondritis:** To clarify the pathophysiological mechanisms behind chronic inflammation and deformity in the juvenile femoral head.
- **Differentiating Related Conditions:** To distinguish Waldenström's disease from other juvenile osteochondritic conditions, such as Scheuermann's disease.

Procedure Overview

- **Diagnostic Imaging:**
- **X-rays:** Show a widened, flattened femoral head with atrophy of the femoral neck.
- **MRI or CT scans:** Provide detailed imaging of inflammation and structural deformities.
- **Histopathology:** Examination of affected bone tissue reveals chronic inflammatory changes and osteonecrosis.
- **Clinical Assessment:** Includes evaluation of joint pain, mobility, and limb-length discrepancies.

Results and Interpretation

- **Radiological Findings:** Flattened femoral head with a widened appearance and shortened femoral neck.
- **Clinical Presentation:** Children often present with limping, restricted hip motion, and occasional pain in the groin or thigh region.
- **Differential Diagnosis:** Requires exclusion of conditions such as Legg-Calvé-Perthes disease or Scheuermann's disease.

Physiological Basis

- **Chronic Inflammation:** Persistent inflammatory processes affect the growth and development of the femoral head.
- **Osteonecrosis and Remodeling:** Decreased blood supply to the femoral epiphysis results in necrosis, followed by inadequate remodeling and deformity.

Clinical Applications

- **Early Intervention:** Early recognition of Waldenström's disease can prevent severe deformities and improve long-term outcomes.
- **Guided Rehabilitation:** Physical therapy helps improve mobility and strengthen supporting musculature around the hip.
- **Surgical Management:** In severe cases, surgical interventions like femoral osteotomy may be required.

Limitations and Technical Considerations

- **Diagnostic Challenges:** Waldenström's disease is often misdiagnosed or conflated with other conditions such as Legg-Calvé-Perthes disease, leading to delays in treatment.
- **Management Complexity:** Treatment is largely symptomatic and aimed at preventing deformity progression, with no definitive cure available.

Modern Relevance

- **Advancements in Imaging:** Modern imaging techniques, including MRI, provide earlier and more accurate diagnosis.
- **Genetic Insights:** Research into genetic predispositions and inflammatory pathways may offer new treatment avenues in the future.

Associated Conditions

- **Legg-Calvé-Perthes Disease:** Shares clinical and radiographic similarities but differs in etiology and progression.
- **Scheuermann's Disease:** Though debated, Scheuermann's disease has been considered a broader term encompassing similar juvenile osteochondritic processes.

Clinical Importance

- **Early Detection and Monitoring:** Regular imaging and clinical follow-up are crucial for minimizing deformities and maintaining hip function.
- **Differential Diagnosis:** Accurate diagnosis ensures appropriate management and distinguishes it from similar conditions like Perthes disease.
- **Multidisciplinary Approach:** Collaboration between pediatricians, orthopedic surgeons, and physiotherapists is essential for optimal care.

Waldenström's disease remains a significant pediatric orthopedic condition requiring early recognition and proactive management to prevent long-term disability. **Advances in** *imaging and therapeutic strategies continue to improve outcomes for affected children.*

References

H. Waldenström: Die Tuberkulose des Collum femoris im Kindesalter und ihre Beziehungen zur Hüftgelenkentzündung. Stockholm, 1910.

Weber Ankle Fracture Classification

Overview

The Weber Ankle Fracture Classification is a radiographic system used to categorize fractures of the lateral malleolus based on their relationship to the syndesmosis, the fibrous connection between the distal tibia and fibula. First introduced in 1949 by Robert Danis and refined by Bernhard Georg Weber in 1972, it remains an essential tool in assessing the stability of ankle fractures and guiding treatment decisions. The classification identifies three main fracture types: A, B, and C, corresponding to the distal, syndesmotic, and proximal locations of the fracture.

Historical Background

- **1949:** Robert Danis, a Belgian surgeon, described the initial classification system for lateral malleolar fractures.
- **1972:** Bernhard Georg Weber, a Swiss orthopedic surgeon, refined and popularized the system. The Weber classification has since become a cornerstone in orthopedic practice for assessing ankle fractures.

Purpose

- To classify lateral malleolar fractures based on their anatomical position relative to the syndesmosis.
- To predict the stability of the fracture and determine the need for surgical intervention.
- To provide a standardized system for communication among healthcare providers and for research purposes.

Procedure Overview

- **Imaging:**
- X-rays in multiple views (anteroposterior, lateral, and oblique) are obtained to visualize the fracture.
- The relationship of the fracture line to the syndesmosis and the integrity of surrounding structures, such as the deltoid ligament, are assessed.
- **Classification:**
- **Type A:** Fracture below the syndesmosis. Typically stable and managed conservatively.
- **Type B:** Fracture at the level of the syndesmosis. Stability is variable, often requiring further assessment of ligamentous injury.
- **Type C:** Fracture above the syndesmosis, usually involving syndesmotic injury and requiring surgical fixation.
- **Management:**
- Type A fractures are usually treated with immobilization using a cast or orthosis.
- Types B and C, due to their association with instability, frequently require surgical intervention, such as open reduction and internal fixation (ORIF).

Results and Interpretation

- **Type A:** Stable fractures with intact syndesmosis.
- **Good prognosis with conservative treatment.**
- **Type B:** Variable stability depending on associated ligamentous injuries.

- **Prognosis depends on proper reduction and stabilization.**
- **Type C:** High instability with syndesmotic disruption.
- Poorer prognosis without surgical intervention.

Physiological Basis

- The ankle joint is stabilized by the syndesmosis, ligaments, and bony architecture.
- Fractures disrupting these stabilizing structures result in varying degrees of instability, affecting joint function and healing.
- Syndesmotic injury, particularly in Type C fractures, compromises the joint's biomechanical integrity, necessitating surgical repair.

Clinical Applications

- **Treatment Planning:** Guides the decision between conservative and surgical management.
- **Helps identify the need for syndesmotic stabilization in Types B and C.**
- **Prognostic Assessment:** Predicts the likelihood of complications such as post-traumatic arthritis.

Limitations and Technical Considerations

- **Type B Ambiguity:** Stability assessment is variable and often requires additional imaging, such as stress X-rays or MRI.
- **Accessory Ossicles:** Misinterpretation of anatomical variants as fractures can lead to unnecessary interventions.
- **Syndesmotic Injury:** Hidden ligamentous damage in Type B and C fractures may not be evident on standard radiographs, requiring advanced imaging.

Modern Relevance

- With the increase in sports and occupational injuries, the Weber classification provides a reliable framework for evaluating ankle fractures.
- **Advances in** imaging, such as CT and MRI, have enhanced the precision of fracture assessment and detection of associated injuries.
- The system continues to evolve with research into biomechanical stability and fixation techniques.

Associated Conditions

- **Deltoid Ligament Injury:** Common in Type B and C fractures.
- **Syndesmotic Disruption:** Integral to Type C fractures.
- **Post-Traumatic Arthritis:** Long-term complication of improperly treated unstable fractures.

Clinical Importance

- **Early Diagnosis and Treatment:** Prevents complications such as malunion, chronic pain, and joint instability.
- **Standardization:** Facilitates uniform communication in clinical practice and research.
- **Comprehensive Management:** Encourages interdisciplinary collaboration

among orthopedic surgeons, radiologists, and physical therapists to optimize outcomes.

Enhancing Healthcare Outcomes

- **Emergency Management:** Application of Advanced Trauma Life Support (ATLS) principles for associated injuries.
- **Imaging Expertise:** Radiologists play a critical role in accurately identifying fracture types and associated injuries.
- **Multidisciplinary Approach:** Physical therapists aid in postoperative recovery to restore range of motion and strength.
- **Patient Education:** Counseling on rehabilitation, weight-bearing protocols, and lifestyle modifications to prevent recurrence.

The Weber Ankle Fracture Classification remains a fundamental tool in orthopedic care, guiding effective management of lateral malleolar fractures and contributing to improved patient outcomes.

References

Barker HB, Beynnon BD, Renstrom PA. Ankle injury risk factors in sports. Sports Med. 1997;23:69–74.

Boszczyk A, et al. X-ray features to predict ankle fracture mechanism. Forensic Sci Int. 2018;291:185–192.

Boyce SH, Quigley MA. Review of sports injuries presenting to an accident and emergency department. Emerg Med J. 2004;21:704–706.

Eastgate P, Davidson R, McPhail SM. Radiographic imaging for traumatic ankle injuries: a demand profile and investigation of radiological reporting timeframes from an Australian tertiary facility. J Foot Ankle Res. 2014;7:25.

Browner BD. Skeletal trauma, basic science, management, and reconstruction. W B Saunders Co. (2003) ISBN:0721691757.

Hunter TB, Peltier LF, Lund PJ. Radiologic history exhibit. Musculoskeletal eponyms: who are those guys? Radiographics. 20 (3): 819-36. Radiographics (full text) - Pubmed citation

Skinner HB. Current diagnosis & treatment in orthopedics. McGraw-Hill Medical. (2006).

Scheer RC, Newman JM, Zhou JJ, Oommen AJ, Naziri Q, Shah NV, Pascal SC, Penny GS, McKean JM, Tsai J, Uribe JA. Ankle Fracture Epidemiology in the United States: Patient-Related Trends and Mechanisms of Injury. J Foot Ankle Surg. 2020 May-Jun;59(3):479-483. [PubMed]

Delco ML, Kennedy JG, Bonassar LJ, Fortier LA. Post-traumatic osteoarthritis of the ankle: A distinct clinical entity requiring new research approaches. J Orthop Res. 2017 Mar;35(3):440-453. [PMC free article] [PubMed]

Brockett CL, Chapman GJ. Biomechanics of the ankle. Orthop Trauma. 2016 Jun;30(3):232-238.

Kašper Š, Bartoníček J, Kostlivý K, Malík J, Tuček M. Maisonneuve fracture. Rozhl Chir. 2020 Winter;99(2):77-85. [PubMed]

Möllenhoff G, Walz M. [Tibial pilon fracture]. Unfallchirurg. 1998 May;101(5):395-401. [PubMed]

Martin-Somoza FJ, Picazo DR, Cabezuelo JAM, González AV. Bosworth fracture. An atypical case of irreducible ankle fracture-dislocation. Trauma Case Rep. 2020 Aug;28:100322. [PMC free article] [PubMed]

Planas JH, Waseem M, Sigmon DF. StatPearls [Internet]. StatPearls Publishing; Treasure Island (FL): Aug 7, 2022. Trauma Primary Survey. [PubMed]

Stiell I. Ottawa ankle rules. Can Fam Physician. 1996 Mar;42:478-80.

Wegner's disease

Overview

Wegner's disease is a condition characterized by pseudoparalysis in infants due to the separation of orthochondritic epiphyses. It is associated with congenital syphilis and typically manifests as disabling pain on movement. The condition most often affects the upper extremities and typically occurs within the first three weeks of life, rarely presenting after three months.

Historical Background

- **1747:** Swedish physician Niels Rosén von Rosenstein (1706–1773) provided the earliest description of the disease.
- **1870:** Friedrich Rudolf Georg Wegner further elaborated on the clinical and pathological aspects of the condition.
- **1871:** Joseph Marie Jules Parrot contributed additional insights, describing epiphyseal separation in infants with congenital syphilis.
- Alois Bednar also investigated related phenomena in congenital syphilis, broadening understanding of skeletal involvement.

Purpose

- **Recognizing Congenital Syphilis:** To identify early skeletal manifestations in infants with congenital syphilis.
- **Preventing Long-term Disability:** To address early signs of pseudoparalysis and prevent irreversible skeletal deformities.

Procedure Overview

- **Clinical Examination:** Infants present with reduced limb movement (pseudoparalysis) and pain during passive motion.
- **Imaging Studies:**
- **X-rays:** Show characteristic separation of the epiphyses, often with periosteal reactions.
- **Ultrasound:** May be used to confirm joint involvement and effusions.
- **Serological Tests:** Specific tests for syphilis (e.g., VDRL, RPR) confirm the underlying congenital infection.

Results and Interpretation

- **Radiological Findings:** Separation of the epiphyses and widening of the metaphysis in affected bones.
- **Clinical Features:** Pseudoparalysis with localized tenderness and swelling, most commonly affecting the humerus or femur.
- **Laboratory Confirmation:** Positive serological markers for syphilis confirm the diagnosis in the context of clinical and radiological findings.

Physiological Basis

- **Pathophysiology:** Congenital syphilis induces inflammatory changes at the epiphyseal junctions, disrupting normal ossification.
- Vascular compromise and inflammatory cytokines contribute to pain and separation of epiphyses.
- **Skeletal Vulnerability:** The immature skeleton in infants is particularly

susceptible to disruptions in blood supply and structural integrity.

Clinical Applications

- **Early Diagnosis:** Identification of Wegner's disease enables timely treatment of congenital syphilis, preventing further systemic complications.
- **Targeted Therapy:** Specific treatment with penicillin addresses the underlying syphilitic infection, halting disease progression.
- **Rehabilitation:** Physical therapy aids in restoring movement and preventing muscle atrophy after resolution of the infection.

Limitations and Technical Considerations

- **Challenges in Diagnosis:**
- The subtle and nonspecific nature of early symptoms can delay diagnosis.
- Radiographic changes may not be apparent in very early stages, requiring high clinical suspicion.
- **Residual Effects:** Despite treatment, some infants may experience persistent deformities or impaired joint function.

Modern Relevance

- **Syphilis Resurgence:** Increasing cases of congenital syphilis worldwide underscore the importance of recognizing conditions like Wegner's disease.
- **Enhanced Diagnostic Tools:** Advanced imaging techniques improve early detection and accurate assessment of skeletal involvement.
- **Public Health Interventions:** Improved maternal screening and treatment during pregnancy reduce the incidence of congenital syphilis.

Associated Conditions

- **Congenital Syphilis:** Wegner's disease is a direct manifestation of untreated syphilis in neonates.
- **Skeletal Dysplasia:** Differential diagnosis includes other conditions affecting epiphyseal and metaphyseal regions.

Clinical Importance

- **Prompt Recognition:** Early diagnosis and treatment prevent severe skeletal deformities and systemic complications.
- **Public Health Screening:** Maternal screening programs for syphilis play a critical role in preventing conditions like Wegner's disease.
- **Interdisciplinary Management:** Collaboration between pediatricians, radiologists, and infectious disease specialists ensures comprehensive care.

Wegner's disease remains a critical condition to recognize in neonates, reflecting the systemic impact of congenital syphilis. Advances in diagnosis and treatment, coupled with preventive measures, continue to improve outcomes for affected infants.

References

F. R. G. Wegner: Über hereditäre Knochensyphilis bei jungen Kindern. [Virchows] Archiv für pathologische Anatomie und Physiologie und für klinische Medicin,1870,50:305-322.

J. M. Parrot: Sur une pseudo-paralysie causée par une altération du système osseux chez les nouveau-nés atteints de syphilis héréditaire. Archives de physiologie normale et pathologique Paris, 1871-1872, 4: 319-333, 470-490, 612-623.

Wegner's sign

Overview

Wegner's sign is a radiological finding indicative of osteochondritis syphilitica, typically observed in congenital syphilis. It refers to a wavy or jagged line at the boundary between the epiphysis and diaphysis of the femur, which normally follows a straight course. This sign is significant for diagnosing syphilitic involvement in the skeletal system of infants and young children.

Historical Background

- **1870:** Friedrich Rudolf Georg Wegner described this diagnostic radiological feature in the context of congenital syphilis.
- His observations built on earlier work regarding syphilis-related skeletal deformities, providing a specific radiological marker for osteochondritis syphilitica.

Purpose

- **Diagnostic Indicator:** To detect syphilitic involvement in the long bones of infants and young children, particularly when other clinical signs may be subtle.
- **Early Identification:** Facilitates the diagnosis of congenital syphilis, allowing for prompt treatment to prevent systemic complications.

Procedure Overview

- **Radiographic Examination:** X-rays of the femur, particularly focusing on the metaphyseal region, are used to identify the characteristic wavy or jagged line.
- **Differential Diagnosis:** Other conditions affecting bone formation, such as rickets or metabolic disorders, must be ruled out through clinical correlation and additional testing.

Results and Interpretation

- **Normal Appearance:** A straight boundary line between the epiphysis and diaphysis.
- **Wegner's Sign:** A jagged or wavy line indicative of syphilitic osteochondritis, often accompanied by other radiological signs like periosteal reaction or metaphyseal irregularities.
- **Correlative Diagnosis:** Positive syphilis serological tests confirm the infectious etiology in the presence of Wegner's sign.

Physiological Basis

- **Bone Development:** Syphilitic osteochondritis disrupts normal endochondral ossification at the growth plate, leading to irregularities in bone architecture.
- **Inflammatory Mechanism:** Chronic inflammation induced by syphilitic spirochetes contributes to the irregular appearance of the metaphyseal-diaphyseal junction.

Clinical Applications

- **Screening for Congenital Syphilis:** A helpful tool in diagnosing skeletal manifestations of congenital syphilis, especially in neonates and infants.
- **Monitoring Disease Progression:** Radiographic follow-ups assess the

response to treatment and resolution of bone abnormalities.

- **Guiding Therapy:** Identification of skeletal involvement aids in determining the severity of syphilis and tailoring treatment regimens.

Limitations and Technical Considerations

- **Specificity:** While characteristic, the sign is not exclusive to syphilis and may be confused with other bone disorders.
- **Radiographic Expertise:** Accurate interpretation requires skilled radiologists familiar with congenital syphilis presentations.
- **Early Detection Challenges:** Changes may not be apparent in the earliest stages of the disease, necessitating high clinical suspicion.

Modern Relevance

- **Resurgence of Congenital Syphilis:** Increasing global cases make recognition of Wegner's sign critical for early intervention.
- **Improved Imaging Modalities:** Advances in radiographic and cross-sectional imaging enhance the detection and evaluation of bone involvement.
- **Public Health Impact:** Routine maternal screening and neonatal assessments reduce the prevalence and complications of congenital syphilis.

Associated Conditions

- **Congenital Syphilis:** Wegner's sign is a hallmark finding in syphilitic osteochondritis.
- **Other Bone Disorders:** Differential considerations include rickets, scurvy, and metabolic bone diseases.

Clinical Importance

- **Diagnostic Value:** Wegner's sign provides a radiological clue for diagnosing congenital syphilis in symptomatic or at-risk infants.
- **Guidance for Treatment:** Identifying syphilitic involvement allows for targeted penicillin therapy to prevent further skeletal and systemic complications.
- **Historical and Modern Relevance:** As a foundational radiological finding, Wegner's sign bridges historical medical discoveries with current diagnostic practices, emphasizing the enduring importance of early recognition in managing congenital infections.

Wegner's sign remains an essential diagnostic feature in pediatric radiology, particularly in the context of congenital syphilis, and highlights the intersection of clinical observation and radiological expertise.

Whiplash Associated Disorders

Overview

Whiplash Associated Disorders (WAD) refers to the range of injuries and symptoms caused by a sudden acceleration-deceleration mechanism, commonly seen in motor vehicle accidents. The term encompasses the clinical manifestations such as neck pain, stiffness, headaches, and psychological distress following trauma, particularly in the absence of identifiable structural damage. Whiplash is a mechanical term, while WAD emphasizes the resultant symptoms and injuries.

Historical Background

- **1919:** The term "railway spine" was used to describe severe neck pain observed in train collisions. This concept evolved into whiplash with the rise of automobile accidents.
- **1995:** The Quebec Task Force on Whiplash-Associated Disorders coined the term "WAD" to classify and describe the range of symptoms following a whiplash mechanism.
- Whiplash-related insurance claims increased sharply with the advent of motor vehicles, significantly impacting healthcare and economic systems in countries like the United Kingdom and the United States.

Purpose

- To provide a standardized classification system for diagnosing and managing injuries caused by the whiplash mechanism.
- To improve understanding of the complex interplay between biomechanical forces and the resulting clinical symptoms.
- To identify and manage the physical, sensory, motor, and psychological effects of WAD effectively.

Procedure Overview

- **1. Mechanism of Injury:**
- Sudden hyperextension followed by hyperflexion of the cervical spine, often caused by rear-end motor vehicle collisions or high-impact sports.
- Results in ligament sprains, muscle strains, and potential cervical spine alignment issues.
- **2. Clinical Presentation:**
- Suboccipital headache and neck pain (constant or motion-induced).
- Sensory symptoms such as tingling or numbness in the arms.
- Delayed symptom onset, sometimes up to 48 hours post-trauma.
- **3. Diagnostic Measures:**
- **Physical Examination:** Identifying tenderness, reduced range of motion, and neurological deficits.
- **Imaging:** X-rays, CT scans, or MRI may be used to rule out fractures or severe structural damage.
- **4. Treatment:**
- Conservative management with physical therapy, pain management, and education.
- For severe cases, multidisciplinary inter-

ventions addressing both physical and psychological components.

Results and Interpretation

- WAD recovery rates vary widely. While most acute cases resolve within weeks, a subset of patients may develop chronic symptoms lasting months or years.
- Symptom severity does not always correlate with the mechanism of injury, making individualized care essential.
- Early identification and appropriate management significantly reduce the risk of chronicity.

Physiological Basis

- **Biomechanical Injury:** Sudden forces lead to deformation of the cervical spine, placing stress on ligaments such as the anterior longitudinal ligament and nuchal ligament.
- Muscle spasms and inflammation may further contribute to symptoms.
- **Neurovascular Impact:**
- Stretching of cervical nerve roots may lead to radiculopathy.
- Potential disruption of blood flow in cervical arteries can exacerbate symptoms.
- **Psychological and Sensory Factors:**
- Chronic pain may result from central sensitization, where the nervous system amplifies pain signals.
- Anxiety and depression can aggravate symptoms.

Clinical Applications

- **Acute Care:** Effective for managing soft tissue injuries and preventing progression to chronic pain.
- **Chronic Cases:** Cognitive behavioral therapy (CBT) combined with physiotherapy can improve outcomes.
- **Workplace and Insurance Claims:** Accurate diagnosis and documentation of WAD are critical in legal and insurance cases.

Limitations and Technical Considerations

- **Subjective Symptoms:** Pain and psychological distress are difficult to quantify, complicating diagnosis and treatment planning.
- **Variable Outcomes:** Recovery is highly individualized, with some patients progressing to chronic WAD despite appropriate management.
- **Imaging Limitations:** Often fails to reveal structural abnormalities in mild to moderate cases, leading to underdiagnosis.

Modern Relevance

- **Advances in** imaging and biomechanical modeling have improved understanding of the injury mechanism.
- Multidisciplinary approaches, including physical therapy, pharmacotherapy, and psychological interventions, have enhanced patient outcomes.
- Increased awareness has led to improved prevention strategies, such as headrest positioning in vehicles to minimize cervical spine hyperextension.

Associated Conditions

- **Cervical Radiculopathy:** Resulting from nerve root irritation or compression.
- **Post-Traumatic Stress Disorder (PTSD):** Common in severe cases with psychological trauma.
- **Chronic Pain Syndrome:** Persistent symptoms due to central sensitization.
- **Cervical Spondylosis:** Accelerated degenerative changes secondary to trauma.

Clinical Importance

- **Early Intervention:** Prompt management reduces the risk of chronic WAD.
- Identifying risk factors for delayed recovery (e.g., high initial pain intensity, psychological distress) allows targeted interventions.
- **Economic Impact:** WAD represents a significant burden on healthcare and insurance systems due to frequent claims and prolonged treatment.
- **Multidisciplinary Care:** Coordinated care involving physicians, physical therapists, psychologists, and case managers ensures optimal recovery and minimizes long-term disability.

Enhancing Healthcare Outcomes

- **Education and Prevention:** Public awareness campaigns on safe driving practices and proper headrest positioning.
- **Personalized Management:** Tailored rehabilitation plans addressing both physical and psychological needs.
- **Research and Innovation:** Ongoing studies into biomechanical mechanisms and central sensitization are paving the way for novel therapeutic approaches.

Whiplash-associated disorders remain a common yet complex clinical challenge. Effective management requires a combination of early diagnosis, multidisciplinary care, and preventive strategies to optimize outcomes and mitigate the socioeconomic impact.

References

Insurance Institute for Highway Safety. "Q&A: Neck Injury". Retrieved 2007-09-18.

"whiplash" at Dorland's Medical Dictionary

Krafft, M; Kullgren A; Lie A; Tingval C (2005-04-01). "Assessment of Whiplash Protection in Rear Impacts" (PDF). Swedish National Road Administration & Folksam. Retrieved 2016-01-10.

"Whiplash". 2017-10-23.

(2010). Retrieved January 16, 2013 from http://www.njpcc.com/conditions-of-the-spine/neck-paininjury.html

"Warning over whiplash 'epidemic'". BBC News. 2008-11-15. Retrieved 2010-04-06.

"Whiplash Statistics • Whiplash Prevention". 2022-09-30. Retrieved 2022-11-25.

Desapriya, Ediriweera (2010). Head restraints and whiplash : the past, present, and future. New York: Nova Science Publishers. ISBN 978-1-61668-150-0.

NY Times - In one country chronic whiplash is uncompensated - and unknown

Bismil QM, Bismil MS (2012). "Myofascial-entheseal dysfunction in chronic whiplash injury". J R Soc Med Sh Rep. 3 (8): 57. doi:10.1258/shorts.2012.012052. PMC 3434435. PMID 23301145.

Gorski JM and Schwartz LH, Shoulder Impingement Presenting as Neck Pain. The Journal of Bone and Joint Surgery Vol 85-A · Number 4 · April 2003 p635-638

Chauhan SK, Peckham T, Turner R (2003). "Impingement Syndrome Associated with Whiplash Injury". J Bone Joint Surg. 85-B (3): 408–410. doi:10.1302/0301-620X.85B3.13503. PMID 12729119.

Umaar W. Yew KIM; Zenios M.; Brett I.; Sharma Y. (2005). "Whiplash Injury of the Shoulder: Is it a Distinct Clinical Entity?". Acta Orthop. Belg. 71 (4): 385–387. PMID 16184990.

Abbassian A.; Giddins G. (2008). "Subacromial Impingement in Patients with Whiplash Injury to the Cervical Spine". Journal of Orthopaedic Surgery and Research. 3 (25): 1749. doi:10.1186/1749-799X-3-25. PMC 2443117. PMID 18582391.

Yersinia-arthritis

Overview

Yersinia arthritis refers to acute joint inflammation (monoarthritis or oligoarthritis) caused by bacterial infection with Yersinia enterocolitica or Yersinia pseudotuberculosis. This condition typically develops as a reactive arthritis following a gastrointestinal or systemic infection caused by these bacteria. Symptoms include joint pain, swelling, and stiffness, commonly affecting larger joints such as the knees and ankles.

Historical Background

- **1894:** Alexandre-Émile-John Yersin discovered Yersinia pestis, the bacterial genus associated with the bubonic plague. Subsequent research identified related species, Yersinia enterocolitica and Yersinia pseudotuberculosis, as causative agents of gastrointestinal and systemic infections.
- The association between *Yersinia* infections and post-infectious arthritis was first documented in the mid-20th century, coinciding with Advances in microbiology and epidemiology.

Purpose

- **Disease Identification:** To recognize arthritis resulting from Yersinia infection as part of a post-infectious syndrome.
- **Treatment Planning:** To determine appropriate antibiotic therapy and manage symptoms of joint inflammation.

Procedure Overview

- **Clinical Assessment:** Joint pain, swelling, and stiffness, often following gastrointestinal symptoms such as diarrhea or abdominal pain.
- **Laboratory Diagnosis:**
- Stool cultures to identify *Yersinia* species.
- Serological testing for antibodies against *Yersinia enterocolitica* or *Yersinia pseudotuberculosis*.
- **Imaging Studies:** Radiographs or ultrasound may be performed to rule out other joint pathologies.
- **Arthrocentesis:** Joint fluid aspiration may be conducted to exclude septic arthritis and confirm reactive arthritis.

Results and Interpretation

- **Positive Stool or Serological Tests:** Confirmation of Yersinia infection.
- **Synovial Fluid Analysis:** Typically sterile with inflammatory markers such as elevated white blood cells.
- **Imaging Findings:** May show nonspecific signs of joint inflammation, such as effusion or synovitis, without structural damage.

Physiological Basis

- **Infectious Trigger:** Yersinia species initiate gastrointestinal or systemic infections.
- **Immune Response:** Cross-reactivity of bacterial antigens with host tissues leads to joint inflammation through molecular mimicry.

- **HLA-B27 Association:** Individuals with HLA-B27 genotype are at higher risk of developing reactive arthritis following *Yersinia* infection.

Clinical Applications

- **Diagnosis and Treatment of Reactive Arthritis:** Identification of *Yersinia*-associated arthritis is essential for targeted therapy and symptom management.
- **Antibiotic Therapy:** Effective treatment of the underlying infection with antibiotics such as doxycycline or ciprofloxacin.
- **Management of Joint Symptoms:** Anti-inflammatory medications, including NSAIDs or corticosteroids, are used to reduce joint inflammation.

Limitations and Technical Considerations

- **Diagnostic Challenges:** Symptoms of reactive arthritis may overlap with other arthritic or autoimmune conditions.
- Stool cultures may yield negative results if the initial infection has resolved.
- **Variable Severity:** Disease presentation ranges from mild and self-limited to chronic and debilitating arthritis.

Modern Relevance

- **Emerging Infections:** Increased global travel and foodborne outbreaks have heightened the relevance of *Yersinia* infections.
- **Advances in Diagnostics:** Improved molecular techniques have enhanced the ability to detect *Yersinia* infections and associated complications.
- **Immunogenetic Insights:** Understanding the role of HLA-B27 in reactive arthritis has implications for personalized treatment strategies.

Associated Conditions

- **Reactive Arthritis Spectrum:** *Yersinia*-induced arthritis is part of a broader category of post-infectious or reactive arthritis conditions.
- **Other Reactive Arthritides:** Infections with *Salmonella*, *Shigella*, or *Chlamydia* can produce similar joint symptoms.
- **HLA-B27-Associated Diseases:** Ankylosing spondylitis and other spondyloarthropathies.

Clinical Importance

- **Recognition of Reactive Arthritis:** Identifying *Yersinia*-associated arthritis ensures prompt and appropriate treatment, reducing complications.
- **Public Health Implications:** Outbreaks of *Yersinia* infections highlight the need for robust food safety measures and early infection control.
- **Research and Therapeutics:** Ongoing studies into the pathogenesis of reactive arthritis offer the potential for novel therapeutic approaches.

Yersinia arthritis represents a distinct form of reactive arthritis, with significant clinical and public health implications. Early diagnosis and treatment are critical to managing symptoms and preventing long-term sequelae.

Zanca View

Overview

The Zanca view is a specialized radiographic technique designed to evaluate the acromioclavicular (AC) joint. It involves an anteroposterior (AP) projection with a cranial tilt of 20 degrees. This angulation reduces the overlapping of the acromion and clavicle, allowing clearer visualization of the AC joint. The technique is particularly useful for diagnosing AC joint injuries or degenerative changes.

Historical Background

- Peter Zanca, a prolific researcher and radiologist, introduced this imaging view during his career as a means to improve the evaluation of the AC joint. Zanca contributed extensively to the field of radiology, publishing over 75 articles and exhibits.
- The technique was formalized in the mid-20th century as a valuable diagnostic tool for shoulder injuries, gaining widespread adoption due to its simplicity and effectiveness.

Purpose

- **Diagnostic Objective:** To provide a clear and unobstructed view of the acromioclavicular joint.
- **Clinical Utility:** Useful in diagnosing AC joint injuries, osteoarthritis, or other degenerative conditions affecting the joint.

Procedure Overview

- **Patient Positioning:**
- The patient is positioned standing or sitting upright.
- The radiographic cassette is placed posterior to the shoulder, centered over the AC joint.
- **Beam Angulation:** The X-ray beam is angled cranially at 20 degrees to reduce overlapping structures, particularly the acromion.
- **Radiographic Settings:** A low-penetration radiographic technique is used to enhance contrast in the AC joint region.

Results and Interpretation

- **Normal Findings:** Well-defined AC joint with no widening, narrowing, or displacement.
- **Pathological Findings:**
- Joint space widening indicative of ligamentous injury.
- Bone irregularities or osteophytes suggestive of degenerative changes.
- Clavicular displacement, which may indicate a grade of AC joint separation.

Physiological Basis

- **Imaging Clarity:** The cranial tilt of the beam prevents superimposition of the acromion on the clavicle, providing a detailed view of the AC joint.
- **Structural Focus:** Allows visualization of subtle injuries to the joint capsule and surrounding ligaments.

Clinical Applications

- **Trauma Assessment:** Identification of AC joint injuries, including sprains, dislocations, or fractures.

- **Degenerative Disease:** Evaluation of osteoarthritis or calcific changes within the joint.
- **Postoperative Monitoring:** Assessment of surgical outcomes, such as after AC joint reconstruction or fixation.

Limitations and Technical Considerations

- **Imaging Limitations:**
- May not capture injuries involving surrounding soft tissues or subtle fractures.
- Overlying anatomical structures could still obscure findings if improperly positioned.
- **Patient Comfort:** Standing or upright positioning may be difficult for patients with severe shoulder pain or restricted mobility.
- **Supplementary Imaging:** CT or MRI may be required for detailed evaluation of soft tissue structures or complex injuries.

Modern Relevance

- **Enhanced Diagnostics:** The Zanca view remains a cornerstone in diagnosing AC joint pathology due to its reliability and ease of use.
- **Standardized Protocols:** It is frequently included in imaging protocols for shoulder injuries, particularly in sports medicine.

Associated Conditions

- **Acromioclavicular Joint Separation:** Commonly graded from I to III based on displacement visible on Zanca views.
- **Osteoarthritis of the AC Joint:** Presents as joint space narrowing, osteophytes, and subchondral sclerosis.
- **Clavicular Fractures:** Fractures near the AC joint are often evaluated using this view.

Clinical Importance

- **Accurate Diagnosis:** Early and precise identification of AC joint injuries ensures timely treatment, preventing chronic instability or arthritis.
- **Guidance for Management:** The Zanca view helps determine the severity of injuries, guiding nonoperative versus surgical management.
- **Sports Medicine Applications:** Widely used in athletes to evaluate AC joint trauma, aiding in return-to-play decisions.

The Zanca view has become an indispensable tool in shoulder imaging, offering a clear perspective of the AC joint while maintaining simplicity and effectiveness. Its clinical utility is demonstrated in both acute and chronic conditions, making it a gold standard in orthopedic radiology.

References

Pavlov H, Warren RF, Weiss CB Jr, et al. The roentgenographic evaluation of anterior shoulder instability. Clin Orthop Relat Res. 1985; (194):153-8.

Jacobson JA, Lin J, Jamadar DA et al.Aids to Successful Shoulder Arthrography Performed with a Fluoroscopically Guided Anterior Approach.Radiographics 2003; 23(2):373-378.

Sanders TG, Jersey SL. Conventional Radiography of the Shoulder. Seminars in Roentgenology 2005; 40:207-222.